EveryWoman's® Guide to Prescription and Nonprescription Drugs

EveryWoman's® GUIDE TO PRESCRIPTION AND NONPRESCRIPTION DRUGS

BY **Kathleen Cahill Allison**

Lynne M. Sylvia, Pharm.D., MEDICAL EDITOR

WITH DRUG PROFILES BY U.S. Pharmacopeia

PRODUCED BY ALISON BROWN CERIER
BOOK DEVELOPMENT, INC.

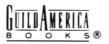

DOUBLEDAY DIRECT, INC.
GARDEN CITY, NEW YORK

Printed in the United States of America
Published by GuildAmerica® Books,
an imprint of Doubleday Direct, Inc., Dept. GB,
401 Franklin Avenue, Garden City, New York 11530

EveryWoman's®, EveryWoman's Library®, and GuildAmerica® Books
are registered trademarks of Doubleday Direct, Inc.

ISBN: 1-56865-248-8

Although the information and guidance in this book are appropriate in most cases, and may supplement your physician's advice, it is recommended that you consult your own physician concerning your personal medical condition.

Book design by Vertigo Design
Art direction by Nanna Tanier for Doubleday Direct, Inc.

The USP has provided the drug profiles and color photographs contained herein. All other information provided is the sole responsibility of Alison Brown Cerier Book Development, Inc.

The information about drugs contained herein is general in nature and is intended to be used in consultation with your health care providers. It is not intended to replace specific instructions or directions or warnings given to you by your physician or other prescriber or accompanying a particular product. The information is selective and it is not claimed that it includes all known precautions, contraindications, effects, or interactions possibly related to the use of a drug. The information may differ from that contained in the product labeling which is required by law. The information is not sufficient to make an evaluation as to the risks and benefits of taking a particular drug in a particular case and is not medical advice for individual problems and should not alone be relied upon for these purposes. Since the inclusion or exclusion of particular information about a drug is judgmental in nature and since opinion as to drug usage may differ, you may wish to consult additional sources. Should you desire additional information or if you have any questions as to how this information may relate to you in particular, ask your doctor, nurse, pharmacist, or other health care provider.

The listing of selected brand names is intended only for ease of reference. The inclusion of a brand name does not mean the USP, Broadway Books, or Doubleday Direct has any particular knowledge that the brand listed has properties different from other brands of the same drug, nor should it be interpreted as an endorsement by the USP, Broadway Books, or Doubleday Direct. Similarly, the fact that a particular brand has not been included does not indicate that the product has been judged to be unsatisfactory or unacceptable.

The inclusion in this book of a monograph on any drug in respect to which patent or trademark rights may exist shall not be deemed, and is not intended as, a grant of, or authority to exercise, any right or privilege protected by such patent or trademark. All such rights and privileges are vested in the patent or trademark owner, and no other person may exercise the same without express permission, authority, or license secured form such patent or trademark owner.

The following profiles have been developed by the USP based primarily on labeling provided by the manufacturer at the time of its approval. This information is intended for use as a temporary educational aid until the drug has been assessed by USP advisory panels. The information does not cover all possible uses, actions, precautions, side effects, or interactions of this medicine. It is not intended as medical advice for individual problems.
- Alendronate (Oral)
- Butalbital, Acetaminophen, and Codeine (Oral)
- Fentanyl (Transdermal)

Requests for permission to reprint drug profiles contained in this book should be made to:
Secretary
United States Phamacopeial Convention
12601 Twinbrook Parkway
Rockville, Maryland 20852

All material contained herein has been compiled specifically with the United States reader in mind. Readers outside of the United States should be aware that the laws and regulations regarding prescription and nonprescription drugs may differ from country to country.

CONTENTS

HOW TO USE
THIS BOOK

EveryWoman's Guide to Prescription and Nonprescription Drugs will help you use medications more effectively, more comfortably, and more safely. It answers questions that many women have when purchasing a medicine over the counter (nonprescription) or with a doctor's prescription. It will make you an informed consumer of the drugs that play important roles in the health and well-being of yourself, your daughter, your mother, and other women among your family and friends.

The first three parts of the book contain general, easy-to-understand information about drugs and about drug treatments for specific health problems. Then the Drug Profiles provide specific information about the most common drugs. To get the complete picture, you should read all of Part 1, the sections in Parts 2 or 3 that cover your specific health concern, and the profile of the drug that you want to learn about.

You can use this book two different ways. If you have a health problem, you can look up your condition or disease in the General Index or the table of contents and find a description of the symptoms and treatments as well as self-help information where appropriate. Information specific to women can be found here as well. If, instead, you want to find out more about a specific drug you are taking or considering taking, you can look it up in the Drug Profiles in the second half of the book. Then, in the front half of the book, you can read about the condition the drug is being used to treat. You may find other possible treatments here.

Understanding medications and drug treatments

In Part 1, "Understanding Medications," you will learn about drug testing, side effects and adverse reactions, drug interactions, avoiding drug dependence, storing and taking drugs, and other topics of great importance to every drug consumer. This section answers such questions as: What should I do if I forget to take a dose? Which drugs will make birth-control pills less effective? What are the signs of an allergic reaction? Also in this section is a chapter with straight talk on diet aids, the nicotine patch, sunscreens, and other drugs that have helped some people live more healthfully.

Part 2, "For Women Only," covers reproductive health and pregnancy. It will help you make choices about contraceptives, hormone replacement therapy, treatments of common reproductive-system disorders, infertility treatments, and more. There are separate chapters about special concerns during pregnancy and breast-feeding.

Part 3, "Drugs to Treat Disease," describes the treatments you and your doctor will consider if you develop heart disease, osteoporosis, cancer, diabetes, infection, or pain. There is also a chapter about drugs that can help with depression, anxiety, and insomnia.

The drug profiles

The second half of the book contains profiles of 200 commonly used drugs and drug groups, encompassing over 1,000 of the brand and generic drugs taken most often by women. Each profile includes:

- About Your Medicine—the drug's purpose
- Before Using This Medicine—information you must tell your doctor or pharmacist
- Proper Use of This Medicine—administering the drug, correcting skipped doses, and so on
- Precautions While Using This Medicine—activities to avoid, food interactions, and other warnings
- Possible Side Effects of This Medicine—common and rare side effects

Each profile describes either an individual drug or a family of similar drugs. The profiles are listed under the generic names that all manufacturers must use. Some manufacturers also market drugs under brand names. To find the profile of a drug, look up either the generic or brand name in the Drug Index. A brand name that appears on your bottle or label will probably not appear in the profile itself, but will be listed in the drug index. Since the drug you're interested in may appear in a profile along with other closely related drugs and only under its generic or group name, the index is the only way to find what you're looking for. Let's say that your doctor has prescribed the drug widely known by the brand name Prozac. Looking up "Prozac" in the Drug Index, you will be referred to the profile "Fluoxetine (Oral)."

There are many brand names on the market. The index includes the most common generic and brand names for ease of reference only. The inclusion of a brand name is not an endorsement of that product, nor is the omission of a brand name a rejection of its quality.

Some drugs have separate profiles for different ways to take the drug. A drug taken in a lotion will have different information than the same drug taken in an oral tablet. There are also some separate entries for drugs taken for different purposes; for example, benzodiazepines are used differently for anxiety, insomnia, and epilepsy, and profiles are included for all three uses as well as for other oral uses.

Color photographs of most of the pills appear in the identification guide.

Because of space restraints, not all drugs could be included. Also, new drugs are constantly being marketed, and new side effects being reported. Ask your pharmacist whether there have been new developments affecting your drug treatment.

About the United States Pharmacopeia

The Drug Profiles have been culled from the vast database of the U.S. Pharmacopeial Convention, the organization that sets the official standards of strength, quality, purity, packaging, and labeling for medical products sold in the United States. In a unique private/public sector relationship, the USP standards are recognized as official by the Federal Food, Drug, and Cosmetic Act and are enforced by the Food and Drug Administration (FDA). USP also disseminates information about drugs to health-care professionals and consumers.

The USP is an independent, not-for-profit corporation composed of delegates from the accredited colleges of medicine and pharmacy in the United States; state medical and pharmaceutical associations; many national associations concerned with medicines, such as the American Medical Association, the American Nurses Association, the American Dental Association, the National Association of Retail Druggists, and the American Pharmaceutical Association; and various departments of the federal government, including the Food and Drug Administration. In addition, four members of the Convention are appointed by the Board of Trustees to represent the public. The USP was established in 1820.

The work of the USP is carried out by the Committee of Revision, which includes over one hundred outstanding physicians, pharmacists, dentists, nurses, chemists, microbiologists, and other individuals particularly qualified to judge the merits of drugs and the standards and information that should apply to them. Committee members serve without pay and are assisted by advisory panels, outside reviewers, and USP staff. The database is constantly updated with the current judgments of these experts. This intensive and objective review process makes the USP drug information the most reliable and unbiased available. (In contrast, other information sources and books rely on the package inserts and other information supplied directly by the drug manufacturers.)

You may have seen the initials "USP" on the label of a drug product. They assure that legal standards of strength, quality, purity, packaging, and labeling exist for the medicine inside the package.

The drug profiles in *EveryWoman's Guide to Prescription and Nonprescription Drugs* have been chosen from the USP database called Patient Education Leaflets. This authoritative drug information program is used by many pharmacies, managed care organizations, and hospitals.

Your doctor and pharmacist are there to help you

This book contains general answers to common questions as well as suggestions for correct use of medicines. It is important to remember, however, that the human body is very complex, and medicines may act differently on different people—and even on the same person at different times. If you want additional information about your medicine or its possible side effects, ask your doctor, nurse, or pharmacist.

If any of the information in this book causes you special concern, do not decide against taking any medicine prescribed for you without first checking with your doctor.

part one

UNDERSTANDING MEDICATIONS

chapter 1

UNDERSTANDING
DRUGS

$\mathcal{A}$ DRUG IS A CHEMICAL THAT CAN CHANGE THE course of a disease, alter the function of body organs, relieve symptoms, or ease pain. Although many substances can affect the body in these ways, the Food and Drug Administration (FDA) defines a drug more narrowly, as a substance, other than a food, intended to affect the structure or function of the body and intended for use in the diagnosis, cure, treatment, or prevention of a disease.

This book will focus on drugs with proven benefits that are sold either with a doctor's prescription or "over the counter" in a pharmacy without a prescription. Other kinds of drugs include recreational substances such as alcohol, caffeine, and nicotine, and illegal drugs such as cocaine and heroin. Vitamins, homeopathic remedies, and herbal medicines also contain chemicals, but they are recognized by the government as nutritional supplements, not drugs. This book will discuss the benefits and risks associated with the use of all of these chemicals and drugs in women.

Until the twentieth century, all drugs were derived from herbs, minerals, or plant extracts. Some common drugs are still derived from natural sources; for example, the pain relievers morphine and codeine are made from poppy plants. Some newer drugs are extracted from natural sources too; for example, paclitaxel (commonly known as Taxol), a treatment for ovarian cancer, is extracted from the Pacific yew tree. Many modern drugs are synthetic versions of substances found in nature. Penicillin, for example, is a synthetic version of a substance discovered on bread mold, and some synthetic estrogens are imitations of the body's natural estrogens.

Other drugs come not from nature but from the laboratory. For example, scientists combined chemicals to make cimetidine, which relieves heartburn by reducing the secretion of stomach acid.

Some drugs enhance the actions of hormones or other chemicals the body needs. The drug L-Dopa supplements the brain with the chemical messenger dopamine, helping people with Parkinson's disease, whose brains do not have enough dopamine. Other drugs work by blocking the effects of hormones or chemicals in the body, such as methimazole, which treats hyperthyroidism (overactive thyroid gland).

Scientists are also producing a limited but growing number of drugs through genetic engineering. They isolate a gene that instructs cells to create a specific hormone or body chemical, then insert copies of the gene into a microorganism such as a yeast or bacterium. They grow the microorganisms in vats, producing large amounts of the desired substance. This new technology has already produced drugs to treat diabetes, hemophilia, pituitary deficiency, cystic fibrosis, and chronic bronchitis. Hundreds more genetically engineered drugs are being tested.

Drug testing

In the United States, the Food and Drug Administration (FDA) governs the long and expensive process of testing and approving new drugs. This process, perhaps the most rigorous in the world, can be frustratingly slow, but it protects patients from most life-threatening and many potentially harmful drug effects. Even after rigorous tests over five to ten years, though, some questions usually remain, often concerning a drug's adverse effects or its interactions with other drugs.

Most research on drugs is performed by a research team comprising physicians practicing in teaching hospitals, clinical scientists in medical schools, and medicinal chemists and doctors working for drug companies. When researchers think a new chemical has potential for treating disease, they first test it on animals in the laboratory. Federal regulations do not allow testing of a new drug on humans until tests have clearly demonstrated that it is safe for animals.

Once a drug is approved for testing on humans, researchers follow three steps. In phase one, they test the drug on a small number (usually fewer than 100) of healthy people to establish the drug's safety and determine how it acts on the body and is removed by the body's organs. Phase two is a carefully controlled test of a few hundred people who have the condition that researchers hope the drug will help. The goal is to see if the drug is effective. In phase three, testing is expanded to a thousand or more patients. Altogether, premarketing studies of a new drug on humans may take 5 to 10 years and usually involve no more that 3,000 patients in total. Following premarketing study, a number of questions regarding the drug remain unanswered, such as the risk of drug interactions, long-term effects of the drug, and the use of the drug by patients with other conditions or diseases.

Next, the research team files an application for FDA approval. The FDA's review may take another two to three years. If the drug represents a major therapeutic advance, as with some therapies for AIDS, cancer, or rare diseases, the drug may be fast-tracked by the FDA and be reviewed in less than a year. If the drug is approved, the study process is not over. The company must continue to submit reports on quality control and on adverse drug effects, particularly during the first five years after drug approval. Because of the limitations of a premarketing study, if you are taking a newly introduced drug, tell your doctor if you experience any unusual effects.

Sometimes patients can take advantage of drugs still being tested by joining a clinical trial at a major medical center. If you are in treatment, ask your doctor about drug trials in your area. To join a clinical trial, you will have to sign a consent form and accept that you may receive not the active drug being tested but instead a placebo (inactive medication being compared to the active drug). If you do get the placebo, you can feel good that other people will be benefiting from your participation in the trial.

Frustrated by the long wait for testing and approval, some people have bought drugs outside the United States, usually through informally organized clubs. Generally the FDA does not interfere with these clubs but cautions that because unapproved drugs have not been subjected to the U.S. approval process, they may contain impurities, come in doses that have not been well studied, or cause dangerous side effects.

If a proposed drug would treat a condition that affects fewer than

200,000 people in the United States, or if the cost of developing and marketing the drug would not be profitable, the manufacturer can apply for a special "orphan drug" status. The government then provides tax incentives to encourage the development of the drug. Over 400 orphan drugs exist, including drugs for cystic fibrosis, multiple sclerosis, Gaucher's disease, Wilson's disease, and hereditary blood disorders. If you have an unusual condition, you may not be aware of these drug options. Talk to your physician or call the National Organization for Rare Disorders.

DRUG STUDIES AND WOMEN

Until recently, drug studies were conducted with the assumption that men's and women's bodies were the same except for their reproductive functions. Most studies included only men, but the results were applied to both men and women. Bernadine Healy, M.D., the first woman to direct the National Institutes of Health, explains, "Women's health still meant maternal health only. Studies of estrogen and heart attacks were conducted only in men, of aspirin and mortality only in men, of vitamins and cancer only in men, of cholesterol only in men and so forth. The results of these studies have been released to the media as if they applied to men and women."

Women were excluded from studies because should a woman become pregnant, the drug might harm the fetus. For this reason, the Food and Drug Administration used to prohibit all women capable of becoming pregnant from early studies of new drugs. Women who had passed through menopause were generally excluded too.

In recent years, women have stepped forward to question the assumption that research on men should be applied routinely to women. This groundswell of concern increased awareness among medical professionals and health officials. In 1991 the American Medical Association Council on Ethical and Judicial Affairs declared, "The results of medical research on men are generalized to women without sufficient evidence of applicability to women," citing as one example the widespread recommendation of prescribing aspirin to prevent heart disease, which was derived almost exclusively from research on men.

The year 1991 also saw the launch of the Women's Health Initiative, a $625 million, 15-year study involving more than 150,000 postmenopausal women. The study is intended to narrow the knowledge gap for women in crucial areas including heart disease, stroke, cancer, osteoporosis, and depression. This large, long-term study should yield a series of practical recommendations on diet, hormone replacement therapy, vitamin and mineral supplements, exercise, and other behaviors that affect women's health. It will also examine the interactions between different health issues (for example, hormone replacement therapy helps prevent heart disease and osteoporosis but might raise the risk of breast cancer).

In 1993 the FDA rescinded its 16-year-old guideline excluding women of childbearing age from the early stages of drug trials. Now it says that "reasonable numbers" of women of all age groups should be included. The new guidelines also require more careful study of the ways a person's gender may affect the way a drug works in the body. During the menstrual cycle, for example, the changing levels of female hormones may affect the speed at which the drug is absorbed by the intestine or leaves the body. The new guidelines call for study of the effects of estrogen medications such as birth control pills and hormone replacement therapy on the removal of other drugs taken by a woman.

New studies are including women in greater numbers than ever before, and there will gradually be answers to many pressing questions about women's health and drug use. Some drugs have already been shown to affect women differently than men because of women's lower body weight, higher percentage of body fat, different metabolic rate, and fluctuating hormone levels. (For more about these differences and their effects on dosing, see page 24.)

Until enough new studies include women, you must be your own health-care advocate. You can take a variety of steps, explained throughout this book, to make sure the medications you take are right for you.

Types of drugs

A typical pharmacy contains a vast and sometimes confusing variety of drugs. Pharmacists are often asked about the differences between prescription and over-the-counter drugs, about generics, and about the variety of brand names for the same drugs.

PRESCRIPTION VERSUS OVER THE COUNTER

Some drugs are sold only by prescription. This is not because they are always stronger or more effective than over-the-counter drugs, but because the FDA has ruled that they cannot be used safely without a doctor's guidance. Available only at licensed pharmacies, prescription drugs include most antibiotics, pain killers derived from opiates, anticancer medications, and many other drugs.

A wide array of medications is available without a prescription, including cold and allergy remedies, pain relief medication, laxatives, and diet aids. These drugs are considered relatively safe without the supervision of a physician. Of the 400,000 drugs currently marketed in the United States, more than 300,000 are sold without prescription. They contain, however, only about 700 active ingredients.

In 1972 the FDA began a comprehensive review of the active ingredients in nonprescription drugs. It appointed advisory panels to study the safety and effectiveness of the ingredients in each group of over-the-counter drugs (antacids, cough and cold remedies, laxatives, etc.). The panels designated each active ingredient as category I (generally recognized as safe and effective, or "GRASE"), category II (not recognized as safe and effective), or category III (having insufficient data to determine whether safe and effective). In 1984 the panels submitted their recommendations to the FDA for final evaluation. About one-third of the drugs were GRASE, one-third were found largely ineffective, and one-third needed additional information. The panels also recommended that a number of drugs or drug doses that had been restricted to prescription status be made available over the counter. At least 40 of these drugs have already been reclassified by the FDA.

Some drugs once available only by prescription now have FDA approval to be sold over the counter as well. Examples include remedies for vaginal infections, antihistamines (Benadryl), and topical hydrocortisone cream 0.5% to 1%.

Some drugs are available both by prescription and over the counter under different names. Often the only difference is the dose. For example, Motrin-IB and Advil (available as 200 mg tablets) are over-the-counter versions of the pain reliever ibuprofen, which is available by prescription as Motrin in doses of 300 to 800 mg per tablet. Tagamet HB is available over the counter in 100 mg tablets for treatment of heartburn. By prescription, Tagamet is available in various doses and by tablet, liquid, or injection in strengths of at least 300 mg per unit. Consumers can sometimes save money by buying the store-brand, over-the-counter version of a drug prescribed by their doctors. When you have a prescription filled, ask your pharmacist about over-the-counter options and alternatives.

Although over-the-counter drugs do not require a doctor's supervision, they are not harmless if used incorrectly. It is important to follow the directions on the package exactly. Do not exceed the recommended dose, and note any precautions or warnings. Many over-the-counter drugs should not be taken by women who are pregnant or breast-feeding (see page 132). Others are unsafe for children or older people, or in combination with alcohol or other drugs.

DECODING YOUR PRESCRIPTION

When doctors write prescriptions, they use the following abbreviations:

prn—as needed

a.c.—before meals

p.c.—after meals

b.i.d.—twice a day

t.i.d.—three times a day

q.i.d.—four times a day

h.s.—at bedtime

p.o.—by mouth

q.4h/q.8h—every 4 to 8 hours

ut dict—as directed by doctor

d.a.w.—dispense as written (no brand name or generic substitutions)

GENERIC VERSUS BRAND NAME

When a laboratory first develops a drug, a panel of drug experts gives it a unique generic name to distinguish it from all other drugs. The drug's developer can apply for a patent that prevents anyone else from selling the drug for a set time, usually 25 years. The company sells its drug under a brand name, which is usually shorter and easier to remember than the generic name. When the patent expires, other companies may decide to manufacture and sell the drug, usually for a lower price, in a generic version or under their own brand names.

Drug manufacturers must prove to the FDA that the generic drugs they sell by prescription or over the counter are "bioequivalent" to the brand-name drugs. When two drugs are bioequivalent, they have the same purity, strength, and chemical composition; disintegrate at the same rate; and are absorbed by the body at the same rate.

Because many newer drugs are protected by patent laws, not all drugs have generic counterparts. However, there are thousands of FDA-approved generic versions of brand-name drugs. In fact, many generic drugs are made by the same company that manufactures the brand-name versions. Generics usually cost less, so you can save money by asking your doctor to prescribe a generic version if it is available. Many health maintenance organizations, as well as Medicare and Medicaid, favor or require the use of generics to reduce costs.

Sometimes when your doctor prescribes a brand-name drug, you may find that the pharmacist fills it with the generic version. This usually happens because your state, hospital, or health plan requires generic substitution. Usually this is a good idea. But sometimes you and your doctor may decide that the brand-name drug is the one that works best for you (generics can vary about 10 percent in bioavailability). If this is the case, your doctor should write "No substitution, brand name medically necessary" on the prescription form.

WAYS TO TAKE DRUGS

From simple tablets to skin patches and implants, each method of getting drugs into the body has advantages and disadvantages. Many drugs can be taken several different ways depending on the health of the patient and the purpose of the drug. Following are the most common methods for delivering medications.

CUTTING THE COST OF YOUR MEDICATIONS

When you buy a drug, consider not only the price but the patient services that come with your purchase. There are costs if you use the drug improperly because you lack information about it. It is best to buy drugs where pharmacists are available to provide information, counseling, and answers to questions you may have about your medications. But because the cost of drugs can be imposing, consider the following cost-saving measures.

- Shop around. Many people don't realize that drug prices vary depending on where you shop. The most convenient place may not be the least expensive. Call several pharmacies in your area. Large chains often have low prices, but many small, independent pharmacies match prices to compete. Also, find out whether your health plan offers a pharmacy service with low prices.
- Ask your doctor if there is a cheaper medication that will do the same job.
- Ask your doctor or pharmacist if there is a generic drug, which will probably be cheaper.
- Look into buying drugs by mail. Mail order is not always cheaper, but it sometimes provides substantial savings, particularly if you will be taking the drug for a long time and buy a large quantity (but no more than a year's supply). If you have not taken a drug before and expect to have questions about its use, mail order may not be your best choice.

Oral

It is usually easiest and least expensive to take drugs by mouth as a tablet, capsule, or liquid. However, not all drugs can be taken by mouth. A drug taken orally must pass through the liver before entering the general blood circulation and before reaching the parts of the body where they will act. Some drugs are quickly broken down in this "first pass" through the liver and are inactivated before they reach the circulation. Others are quickly broken down during the first pass through the liver into substances that have minimal benefits and dangerous side effects. Depending on its chemistry, a drug may also be rapidly destroyed in the acid environment of the stomach and not be absorbed into the bloodstream. When taken orally as tablets, drugs generally act slowly because the tablet must be dissolved in the digestive system, then processed by the liver before the body can use it. Drugs in liquid forms, such as solutions, elixirs, syrups, or suspensions, act more quickly because they do not require disintegration and dissolution. Some oral drugs can be made available in extended-release, timed-release, or sustained-release forms, which slowly and steadily release the drug over a set number of hours. Whenever you are given an oral drug, ask your doctor or pharmacist whether its action will be affected by the presence of food or if it may irritate the stomach and should therefore be taken with food.

Sublingual drugs

Some drugs can be placed under the tongue and absorbed directly into the bloodstream. This method administers the drug much faster than the oral route because it bypasses the digestive system. One well-known example of sublingual delivery is the use of nitroglycerin during an acute angina attack to quickly alleviate symptoms. Only a few drugs are made in a sublingual dosage form. Buccal administration—in the side of the cheek near the gum line—also allows a rapid drug response, but is even rarer.

Injected drugs

Many drugs can be injected directly into the bloodstream (intravenous, or IV), into the subcutaneous tissue (just beneath the skin, or SC), or into the muscle (intramuscular, or IM). Compared to oral use, these methods provide more immediate effects, usually within minutes, so they are a good choice in an emergency such as during a heart attack or asthma attack. Injections are also used when a drug cannot survive the digestive process. For example, lidocaine is usually given by IV injection for life-threatening abnormal heart rhythms; it is not given orally because it is rapidly inactivated by the liver and converted into toxic by-products. Intravenous administration is the fastest method of drug delivery, followed by injection into the subcutaneous fat and muscle. Subcutaneous administration allows the drug to be slowly absorbed into the bloodstream over a number of hours. For example, insulin is usually given subcutaneously rather than intravenously to avoid a rapid fall in blood sugar and to allow for a more prolonged effect.

Topical drugs

Topical drugs are applied directly to the affected area, have a potent local effect, and are only minimally absorbed into the bloodstream. They include ointments; lotions; eye, ear, and nose drops; and vaginal creams or suppositories.

Rectal drugs

Some drugs can be administered by rectal enema or rectal suppository to treat systemic conditions such as ulcerative colitis and nausea and vomiting. Drugs administered high into the anal canal can be absorbed by the rectum or lower intestine and work throughout the body. For example, 5-aminosalicylic acid can be administered by rectal suppository or by enema for the treatment of ulcerative colitis. This treatment is usually reserved for those people with colitis at the far end of the colon, near the rectum. The rectal route of administration is used for a relatively small number of drugs under certain conditions. It may be used to treat nausea and vomiting when people cannot tolerate an oral medication, and it is particularly useful in children who have febrile seizures or require a preoperative medication.

Inhaled drugs

Some drugs work best when inhaled into the lungs in the form of metered dose inhalers (MDIs) or nasal spray solutions. Examples are bronchodilators (Ventolin, Serevent) and corticosteroids (Beclovent, Azmacort) to prevent asthma attacks, and ipratropium (Atrovent) to treat chronic lung conditions. Inhaled drugs of these types are absorbed quickly into the bronchioles (small airways in the lungs) and reach minimal levels in the bloodstream.

Transdermal skin patches

Skin patches adhere to the skin and slowly release a dose of medication from a reservoir into the body. Drugs that can now be delivered this way include estrogen replacement therapy, nicotine replacement therapy, nitrates to treat angina, and scopolamine for motion sickness.

Subdermal implants

Implants are capsules that are placed surgically under the skin, gradually releasing a drug from a reservoir over a long period of time. The hormonal contraceptive Norplant is administered through small implants under the skin of the arm. An implant is a convenient and reliable way of taking a drug for months or years, but insertion and removal of the implant require minor surgical procedures.

Alternative remedies

Many conventional drugstores and pharmacies are now selling herbal and homeopathic remedies over the counter. These alternative medicinal products are becoming more popular in the United States and abroad. The result is the widespread use of products that are legally available and in some cases have medicinal value but have not been proven therapeutically effective through the FDA approval process.

Although these substances are often lumped together under the label of "natural remedies," homeopathics and herbals are very different. Herbals come from plants and often (but not always) contain active ingredients that may have medicinal value. Homeopathics are highly diluted substances that often have no active ingredient.

One thing that herbals and homeopathics have in common is that they are regulated by the federal government as dietary supplements, not drugs, and are limited in the kinds of health claims they can make on their labels and package inserts. It is important to obtain information about how to use the products from reliable, knowledgeable sources, such as trained experts in naturopathic, homeopathic, or herbal medicines. Good information about these substances is hard to find, largely because sufficient scientific research has not been conducted.

Although many alternative medications may be helpful or at least do no harm, alternative medications can be harmful, in some cases, if they are used instead of conventional medicines to treat serious diseases. This can cost precious time that would be better spent tackling the disease with scientifically proven methods. With some diseases, the delay can make treatment more difficult or even impossible.

This book does not include a detailed discussion of individual herbal and homeopathic remedies, but such remedies will be discussed throughout if scientific evidence supports their use.

HERBAL REMEDIES

Herbal medicine is the use of parts of plants to treat symptoms and promote health. Herbs are not inert substances that can be taken in any amount. Many herbal remedies contain active ingredients that act on the body in the same way that some drugs do. In fact, most drugs originally came from plant sources. But most herbal remedies are prepared in low doses and act gently on the body. Herbs are typically not aggressive enough to treat acute or emergency situations. For example, bacterial infections are best treated with antibiotics (page 233). For information about using herbs to treat specific conditions, it is best to consult a health practitioner trained in using herbal preparations. Most medical doctors are not trained in the use of herbs.

Herbal remedies do not possess any magical, mystical, or spiritual healing properties. Herbs work because of their chemical properties and like other drugs must be administered in proper dosage to be effective. While some herbs are safe and effective, some are neither. Herbs can produce some undesirable effects as well as some benefits. Exercise the same caution in using herbal preparations that you would with any medication. They may cause unwanted side effects such as allergic reactions, change in blood sugar, and liver disease, and may interact adversely with other drugs or chemicals. If you experience any ill effects that you think might be caused by an herbal preparation you are using, report your symptoms to your doctor.

While some herbs contain active ingredients, other herbal remedies appear to work primarily as the result of what is known as the placebo effect. The placebo effect is a well-documented psychological effect in which a certain proportion of people, given a tablet containing no active ingredient, will report an improvement in their condition even though the tablet contains no medication.

Dosages have not been clearly established for most herbal products. As a result, it may take some experimentation with a product to find out the correct dosage and length of treatment. Work with a trained expert in herbal remedies to help make this determination. For example, you may want to start with a low dose and gradually increase it over time to the desired dose. The lack of information about correct dosages is one reason some medical experts raise cautions about the uses of herbal preparations. Also, herbal and natural preparations are not subject to standard testing for safety and effectiveness and not subject to the Good Manufacturing Practice Standards that govern pharmaceutical companies to ensure quality control. Manufacturers do not have to show purity of the product or even prove that the product contains what is listed on the label. Unsafe impurities and even prescription drugs have sometimes been found in products when tested—substances that have not appeared on the labels. Not all the products are sold in childproof containers.

However, advocates of herbal medicine rightly argue that countries that have embraced herbal medicines more widely than the United States have made important information about the use of these substances available. The FDA has allowed them to remain on the market as dietary supplements. Recent changes in regulation have made it possible for the manufacturers to include more information about the health effects of their products on the labels, an important step in increasing the flow of information to the consumer.

Herbal medicines come in many forms ranging from tablets and potions to teas and tinctures. Here is a basic rundown on each form:

- Herbal powders usually come in capsule form or compressed into tablets.
- Herbal teas may come loose or in tea bags. They can be prepared by steeping the herb in hot water (called an infusion) or by boiling the herbs in water for a more concentrated tea.
- Tinctures are prepared by soaking an herb in a solvent such as alcohol or water for several hours, days, or weeks, depending on the herb. A fluid extract is a more concentrated form of tincture.
- Solid extracts are the most concentrated form of herbal product and result when all of the liquid is evaporated off, leaving a solid residue.
- Standardized extracts are products that contain a guaranteed level of a certain herb or group of herbs, usually expressed as percentage of the total weight of the product. Standardization is becoming more common and allows for more accurate dosing.

DON'T MIX YOUR REMEDIES

If you choose to use herbal or natural remedies, it is best to avoid taking more than one remedy at a time so you can determine whether the product is effective and can watch for any side effects it might be causing. Some products contain more than one active ingredient, but it is better to choose a single-ingredient remedy. If you should experience any unpleasant side effects and you are taking more than one substance at a time, it will be more difficult to determine which substance may be causing the problem. Conversely, if you are experiencing benefits, it will be difficult to know which substance may be helping you. Also, one ingredient may cancel out the beneficial effects of another ingredient. Also avoid mixing alternative medicines with conventional prescription or over-the-counter medications.

HOMEOPATHIC REMEDIES

Homeopathy is a holistic system of medical diagnosis and treatment that is widespread in parts of Europe and growing in popularity in the United States. Most practitioners of conventional Western medicine do not accept the validity of homeopathic medicine.

Homeopathic remedies often contain no active ingredients. Instead, they are based on the idea that "like cures like"—that the substance causing a problem can cure that problem when administered in minute doses. With this in mind, the active ingredient is placed in solution and diluted so many times that it is likely that not even a single molecule of the active ingredient is left. The idea that a substance with essentially no active ingredient can have any chemical effect on the body defies the laws of conventional science. Practitioners of homeopathy argue that the diluted solution may contain a memory of the active substance that has effects on the body. They say the method is not based on any molecular or chemical mechanism and they do not claim to understand how homeopathic medicine works. They base their confidence on their clinical experience in which the treatments appear to work.

Homeopathic products can now be found in most stores. Products that could formerly be found only in health food or nutrition stores are now on the shelves in conventional pharmacies right next to the medications that have been subjected to lengthy scientific testing and approval. For example, several homeopathic remedies for vaginal yeast (fungal) infections are available in many stores along with conventional antifungal medicines for vaginal infections. If you look closely at the labels, some products indicate that they are homeopathically prepared. This means that they have been prepared by the homeopathic method of dilution—there may be no active ingredient at all in the preparation, although the ingredients list may mention *Candida albicanus*, a fungus that causes vaginal infections.

As with the apparently successful results of some herbal remedies, some of the success of homeopathic medicine may result from the placebo effect: a well-documented psychological effect in which some people report an improvement in their symptoms when given a "dummy" tablet containing no active ingredients. The power of the placebo effect cannot be dismissed, and people who perceive an improvement in their condition are probably gaining some benefit from their treatment even if the medication they are taking has no active ingredient.

chapter 2

DRUG SAFETY

$\mathcal{B}$ECAUSE DRUGS ARE AVAILABLE EVERYWHERE these days, not just in pharmacies but in supermarkets, convenience stores, and even vending machines, it may appear they are harmless. In fact, drugs, including those sold over the counter, are powerful substances that can be harmful or even life-threatening. To use drugs safely, you need to follow the instructions carefully, report side effects and adverse reactions to your doctor, avoid interactions with other drugs or foods, and recognize that certain drugs can cause psychological or physical dependence.

Communicating with your doctor and pharmacist

Drug safety begins with an exchange of information between you and the doctor or nurse practitioner prescribing the medication. Information about your health, other medications you are taking, and your lifestyle will help your doctor choose the right medication and dose. Bringing a list of questions and concerns to the doctor and writing down the answers will help make the exchange of information clear and complete.

TELL YOUR DOCTOR

Before a drug is prescribed and while you are taking it, talk with your doctor about:

- **Your health problems.** Make sure your doctor knows about all of your health conditions, particularly those being treated currently. If you're seeing a doctor for the first time, don't assume other doctors or clinics have passed along your records. Assume the doctor knows nothing about you except what you tell him or her.
- **Possible or current pregnancy.** Before a drug is prescribed, tell your doctor if you are pregnant, suspect you may be pregnant, are trying to become pregnant, or are planning a pregnancy soon. Also tell your doctor if you are breast-feeding. Don't assume that you can simply stop taking a medication if you later become pregnant. With some medications, it is detrimental to your health to abruptly stop taking the drug. Also, some medications can harm a fetus in its first weeks, before you even know you are pregnant, and others take weeks or even months to clear from the body.
- **Drug allergies.** Alert your doctor if you have allergies to drugs, foods, or other substances. An allergic reaction may occur not just to the drug's active ingredient, but to binders, coloring, or preservatives in the drug.
- **Other medications.** Bring to your appointment a list of all other drugs you are taking or are likely to take, including prescription and over-the-counter drugs and any natural, herbal, or homeopathic remedies. Note their doses as well. Even easier is to put all the medications in a bag and bring them with you, so the doctor can see exactly which drugs you are taking and their doses. This information is particularly important if you are going to have blood tests, as medications can affect the results of some tests. Some drugs, both OTC and prescription, interfere with the body's ability to absorb other drugs. For example, antacids interfere with the absorption of a number of drugs, specifically antibiotics and antifungal drugs, and need to be taken at least two hours later. Other drugs may interact by exaggerating or reducing each other's effects.
- **Alcohol and smoking.** Tell your doctor if you drink alcohol,

smoke cigarettes, or use any other legal or illegal substances that might interact with medications.

- **New symptoms.** While you are taking the medication, assume that any new symptom, discomfort, or mood change may be the result of the medication. If the new symptom interferes with your daily functioning, report it to your doctor as soon as possible. Many women tend to attribute such problems to other causes, particularly aging. But even if you are taking medications that you have taken in the past with no ill effects, a new combination with other drugs or new dosages can produce different effects. Also, as you get older, your body's ability to remove a drug by the kidneys or liver decreases, necessitating a reduction in your dose.

- **Changes you make.** While you are on the medication, it is best to follow the instructions exactly. But tell your doctor if you do make a change, such as reducing or increasing the dose, taking it less frequently, or stopping it. Don't be embarrassed to tell your doctor that you are not following instructions. There is probably a good reason you made these changes. But do tell your doctor.

ASK YOUR DOCTOR OR PHARMACIST

Studies show that the main reason drugs are not effective is that the patient does not have enough information. Some people walk out of their doctor's office not even knowing what the drug is supposed to do. Don't assume your doctor or pharmacist will remember to tell you everything you need to know to get the most from your medicine. Ask:

- **What am I taking?** Write down the drug's brand and generic names and find out what it is intended to do for you. When you pick up the prescription, check the label to make sure your name is on it and that the drug is the one the doctor prescribed.

- **How soon is the drug supposed to start working?** Some drugs, such as antidepressants, don't begin to work for two or more weeks, but their side effects often occur much sooner. If you think a drug isn't working fast enough, don't increase the dose yourself—talk to your doctor.

- **When do I take the drug?** How many times a day? What time of the day? If the prescription says every six hours, you may need

to take one every six hours while you are awake, including one before bed and one in the morning. Or you may need to wake up in
the middle of the night to take your medication. Ask your doctor
or pharmacist.

- **Do certain foods interact with the medication?** You may need
  to take the medication with meals or only on an empty stomach,
  or you may need to avoid certain foods or alcohol.
- **Are there any special ways to take the tablets?** Some drugs
  should be dissolved under the tongue and should not be swallowed. Some coated or slow-releasing oral dosage forms must be
  taken whole and should not be crushed, chewed, or split.
- **How long should I take the medication?** Until the symptoms
  stop, or until the prescription is finished? Are there any refills?
- **What are the possible side effects or adverse reactions?** See
  below.
- **Are there any habits or activities I should avoid?** For example, some drugs increase the effects of sun exposure, and some
  may initially impair your concentration and make it hazardous to
  drive or operate machinery.

SPECIAL QUESTIONS FOR WOMEN

When you receive a prescription, ask your doctor or pharmacist about
any of the following concerns that apply to you.

- **Will the medication interact with my birth-control pills?**
  Some drugs can make birth-control pills less effective, so you may
  need to use a backup form of contraception (see list of medications on page 38). Combined oral contraceptives containing estrogen and progestin decrease the removal of drugs from the liver,
  including some benzodiazepines (for anxiety or to induce sleep),
  antidepressants, and theophylline (for bronchial conditions). If
  you are on a combined oral contraceptive, you may need a lower
  dose of these medications, and you should watch for side effects
  and signs of an excessive dose.
- **Will hormone replacement therapy affect this medication?**
  Interactions between the estrogen in hormone replacement therapy and a number of antidepressants may occur. Some drugs for
  seizure disorders reduce the effectiveness of estrogen.

- **Can I take this if I am pregnant or thinking of becoming pregnant?** If you are pregnant, do not take any prescription or over-the-counter drug without consulting with your doctor. If you are contemplating pregnancy, consider that certain drugs take several weeks to clear from your system, so they should be discontinued before you try to become pregnant (see page 131). Other drugs may reduce the chance of conception.
- **Can I take this medication if I am breast-feeding my baby?** Find out if a medication will be passed through the breast milk to your baby and might cause unwanted effects in the baby such as diarrhea, change in sleep pattern, or change in heart rate. However, just because a drug passes into the breast milk, that does not mean you cannot take it. The baby may be able to eliminate it normally with no problem. Also, some medications will reduce your milk production. (For more on medications and breast-feeding, see chapter 8.)
- **Will this medication reduce the density of my bones?** If taken for a long time, some medications, including corticosteroids, de-

DO'S AND DON'TS OF TAKING YOUR MEDICATION

- Do take your medication at the time recommended.
- Do take all the medication unless your doctor tells you to stop when the symptoms subside.
- Do take your medication in a well-lighted place where you can read the label.
- Do make sure the expiration date on your medication hasn't passed.
- Don't take more or less than the recommended dose without calling your doctor first.
- Don't keep medications at your bedside, where you are more likely to take an overdose accidentally while half asleep.
- Don't take a medication that was prescribed for another person.
- Do use a standard measuring device available from a pharmacy when taking liquid drugs. Household measuring devices such as tablespoons, cups, and glasses may be inaccurate.

crease bone density and can contribute to the development of osteoporosis in later life. If taken for a short time, they do not cause this problem.

- **Will my monthly menstrual cycle affect how this medication works?** There is emerging evidence that the menstrual cycle affects the absorption of some medications in the body. (For more about hormone-drug interactions, see page 37.)

SWALLOWING TABLETS OR CAPSULES

- If you can, stand up when you swallow a tablet or capsule to help prevent it from lodging in your esophagus, where it may cause irritation and inflammation. If you cannot stand, sit as upright as possible.
- Before taking the tablet, sip some water.
- Put the tablet far back on your tongue.
- Wash it down with a 4-ounce glass of water.
- Continue standing or sitting upright for two to three minutes to allow the tablet to reach your stomach.
- If a tablet becomes stuck, eat a few bites of bread.

Wrong, missed, and extra doses

If you take an incorrect dose or you miss or add a dose, the drug may act differently on your body than it's supposed to. Much depends on your involvement. Carefully monitor the way the drug is acting, and carefully take all doses as prescribed.

GETTING THE DOSE RIGHT FOR WOMEN

Now that drug studies are including women, they are revealing differences between the ways women's and men's bodies handle some drugs. These important differences can make a dose that is right for a man (and probably has been studied only in men so far) not right for a woman.

The simplest and most likely reason that drugs affect women and men differently is body composition. Differences in sex hormones and body size also play a role. These factors can influence what is known as the drug's pharmacodynamics—your body's response to a certain concentration of a drug.

As a woman, it is especially important that you observe the ways a drug affects your body and report any unexpected observations or problems to your doctor. Your doctor may be able to reduce the dose without reducing the benefits of the drug. Depending on your medical problem, it may be more appropriate for you to start on a new medication or a similar drug at a lower dose. Find out the likely side effects and get information from your pharmacist on how they may be minimized or prevented. For some drugs, your doctor may recommend that you self-monitor your pulse or blood pressure to ensure that the drug is working effectively, or that you have levels of the drug in your blood measured periodically. With some drugs, it is best to have blood tested monthly or every three months to measure for markers of an impending adverse drug reaction, such as changes in liver function or kidney function. In any case, review your medications and treatment plan with your doctor every three to six months.

Body composition, metabolism, and hormones

To grasp the importance of self-monitoring, consider that a 120-pound, 52-year-old woman doesn't need as much medication as a 250-pound, 32-year-old man, and yet the same dosage is often prescribed. That's an extreme difference, but as a group women weigh less than men. Women also have a higher percentage of body fat, while men have more muscle tissue. Many drugs, including alcohol, are distributed in the water component of the body. There is more water in muscle than in fat. If you are smaller and also have more fat, there is less water in your body for the drug to be distributed in. The result: the drug may become concentrated in your body and cause an exaggerated effect, as well as more side effects or adverse reactions (see page 30).

Women also eliminate certain drugs from their bodies much more slowly than men do. For example, women's digestive tracts secrete less alcohol dehydrogenase, the enzyme that helps remove alcohol from the body. In addition to having less body water, this is the reason why women become intoxicated on less alcohol than men. In the liver, a number of the enzymes that are responsible for inactivating and removing drugs from the body are influenced by both estrogen and progesterone. Changes in these hormone levels during the normal menstrual cycle, and the loss of these hormones following menopause may influence the rate at which a woman's body removes common drugs throughout her life. Compared to men, women have been shown to remove more slowly acetaminophen (Tylenol), aspirin, several benzodiazepines (used for anxiety and as a sleep aid), lidocaine (an anesthetic), ondansetron (for nausea), and mephobarbital (a barbiturate). Women may need lower doses of some of these drugs during some stage of their life. Most important, you should closely monitor yourself for side effects or unusual reactions that may indicate your dose is too high.

For some drugs, the dose may need to be adjusted to reflect changing hormone levels during the menstrual cycle. The rise and fall of the female hormones estrogen and progesterone may affect your body's response to some drugs. For example, estrogen and progesterone influence insulin's ability to regulate blood sugar. For a woman with type 1 (insulin-dependent) diabetes, blood sugar may rise excessively at certain times during the menstrual cycle, particularly the luteal phase following ovulation. If she is taking insulin, she and her doctor must work together to adjust her dosages during the month.

Women's bodies take much longer to break down one of the most popular drugs, propranolol (Inderal), a beta-blocker used to treat high blood pressure and heart disease and to prevent migraines. The probable reason is that estrogen and progesterone regulate some of the enzymes that metabolize this drug. The higher concentrations of the drug in a woman's body may lead to bothersome side effects, such as profound tiredness and nausea. Also, you should monitor your heart rate and blood pressure closely when this drug is started.

The blood levels of some drugs for mental health conditions also rise and fall with a woman's hormones. The concentration of some antidepressants tends to fluctuate during women's hormonal cycles, with the result that a woman may be getting too large a dose at one part of her cycle and too small a dose during another part.

Hormones are complicated and intricate, and their interactions with drugs must be much more carefully studied before they can be truly understood.

MISSED DOSES

When you miss a dose of your medicine, there is temporarily less drug in your body. Whether or not this will affect your treatment depends on the drug and the condition being treated. Usually one missed dose is not a problem. In some cases, however, your symptoms might return.

If you miss more than one dose of any medication, call your doctor or pharmacist. For some drugs, you need to take immediate action if you miss even one dose. For example, if you miss a dose of a combination oral contraceptive, you need to take one missed pill as soon as you remember it. For specific guidance on missed doses, see the Drug Profiles in this book.

EXTRA DOSES

It's almost as easy to mistakenly take an extra dose of your medication as it is to miss a dose. An extra dose will raise the level of the drug in

TIPS FOR REMEMBERING YOUR MEDICATION

- Take your medication on an empty stomach at least one hour before meals unless specifically told to take with food.
- Carry birth-control pills in your purse so that if you miss a pill you will have it with you when you remember.
- If you are taking several medications, draw up a time chart telling you when to take each medication.
- Use a pill organizer, which can be purchased at most pharmacies, unless you are taking medication that must stay in its original container (ask your doctor or pharmacist).
- Use a digital watch with a beeper to remind you of your next medication time.

your body, and the result will vary depending on the type of medication. A single extra dose of most medications is usually nothing to worry about, but an extra dose of some medications is cause for concern. Check the Drug Profiles in this book for the symptoms to watch for if you have exceeded the recommended dosage.

Sometimes people take a higher dose hoping it will better relieve their symptoms. With most medications, more is not better. It is true, though, that people build up a tolerance for some drugs and need to take a higher dose to get the same effect. This happens with some sleeping pills, pain relievers, and sedatives. If the effects of your drug are waning, don't increase your dose on your own. Talk with your doctor. Depending on the situation, it may be best to switch to a different medication or temporarily discontinue the drug.

Sometimes people take extra doses because they are confused or forgetful—sometimes because the drug itself is making them drowsy or confused. In this case, a pill organizer that dispenses a single dose at a time can be useful.

If you have kidney, liver, or heart problems, which are common among older people, you need to be especially careful about extra doses. Most drugs are removed from the body by either the kidneys or liver or by both organs. The delivery of drugs to these organs is dependent on your blood flow, which is determined by the functioning of your heart. If you have any of these problems, the doses of your drugs have most likely been carefully determined by your doctor. Taking an extra dose may lead to a buildup of the drug in your blood and an excessive, potentially harmful response.

Signs of drug poisoning vary with each drug, and in some cases, there are no immediate signs to alert you. If you think you or someone you know may have taken an overdose, call your local poison control center or 911 immediately. Do not wait for symptoms to occur before calling. When you place the call, have the container of the drug with you. Keep in mind that the treatment of a poisoning differs depending on the drug. Follow the advice of the poison control experts. In many situations, you will be told to induce vomiting with syrup of ipecac, a nonprescription drug that should be a standard item in your medicine cabinet. Do not induce vomiting unless this is recommended by a poison specialist. If there is a seizure, unconsciousness, vomiting, or irregular breathing, call for an ambulance.

If the overdose was deliberate, tell a doctor, who can arrange for

SAFE STORING AND DISPOSING

- Shield your medications from excess light, heat, and humidity. Bathrooms are often too warm and humid, so a better place to store drugs is high in a kitchen or bedroom closet or cabinet.
- Close lids and caps tightly.
- To avoid confusion, store your drugs in the original containers or in a drug organizer. Keep in childproof containers.
- Dispose of medications by throwing them down the toilet so kids and pets can't get to them.
- Twice a year, go through your medicine closet and throw away any medications that have expired dates or are more than two years old. Get rid of any tablets that are cracked, chipped or crumbling; ointments, creams, or lotions that are discolored, hardened, or separated; any tube that is cracked or leaking; any liquid that is thickened or discolored; and any bottle of eye drops that has been open over a month.

the person to receive appropriate psychological treatment and support.

Drugs that you may consider as relatively harmless, such as vitamins, may cause toxic effects when taken in excess. Vitamins A, D, E, and K can be toxic. Extra amounts of these fat-soluble vitamins are not excreted in the urine, but are stored in fat and can build up to toxic levels. Don't exceed the recommended dietary allowance unless you and your doctor agree you need to take more.

Side effects and adverse reactions

Drugs often cause not only benefits but also unwanted but predictable side effects such as nausea, dry mouth, or drowsiness. Less often, they cause unexpected and serious effects called adverse reactions. Adverse drug reactions cause 3 to 5 percent of all hospital admissions per year. Some adverse reactions are caused by allergies.

Women report more adverse reactions, including drug allergies, than men do. For example, women of age 20 to 39 report twice as many adverse reactions as men the same age. The reason for this isn't fully studied, but it is probably because women take more drugs than men, are more likely to notice symptoms, and are more likely to report a health problem to their doctors.

SIDE EFFECTS

Many drugs cause not only benefits but also unwanted effects on other parts of the body. These "side effects" occur because the drug affects the whole body, not just the part you are trying to treat. For example, some antihistamines for sinus allergies can make you drowsy, and the tricyclic antidepressants can cause a dry mouth. Some side ef-

---

SIDE EFFECTS OF COMMON DRUGS

ACE INHIBITORS: headache, dizziness, cough, nausea, diarrhea, skin rash

ANTIBIOTICS: nausea, vaginal yeast (fungal) infection, diarrhea, skin rash

BENZODIAZEPINES: drowsiness, dizziness, change in concentration

CHEMOTHERAPY DRUGS: nausea, vomiting, diarrhea, fatigue, hair loss, mouth sores

CORTICOSTEROIDS: stomach upset, bone thinning, osteoporosis following long-term use

HORMONE REPLACEMENT THERAPY: vaginal bleeding, tender breasts, nausea, cramping, headaches, fluid retention, bloating, weight gain, irritability, depression

NITRATES: headache, dizziness, nausea

NONSTEROIDAL ANTI-INFLAMMATORY DRUGS (NSAIDS, MAINLY FOR PAIN RELIEF): heartburn, nausea, diarrhea, indigestion

ORAL CONTRACEPTIVES: mood changes, headaches, weight gain, acne, breakthrough bleeding, tender breasts

TRICYCLIC ANTIDEPRESSANTS: dry mouth, drowsiness, constipation, blurred vision

DEALING WITH DRY MOUTH

Dry mouth is one of the most common and annoying side effects of medications. Decreased saliva in the mouth not only is uncomfortable but can contribute to tooth decay and gum disease. It can also make eating, talking, and wearing dentures difficult. Besides medications, other causes are aging and breathing through your mouth because of allergies, cold, or flu. If you are experiencing dry mouth and suspect the cause is your medication, ask your doctor about it. It may be possible to change the dose or medication. If not, try these suggestions.

- Periodically sip small amounts of water throughout the day to keep your mouth moist.
- Keep a glass of water beside your bed at night.
- Don't drink alcohol, caffeinated coffee, caffeinated tea, or soft drinks. All will make your mouth dry.
- Don't smoke.
- Help prevent tooth decay by brushing frequently with a soft brush and using dental floss daily.
- Try artificial saliva products, such as Salivart or Salix, which are available without prescription.

fects, such as nausea, stomach upset, dizziness, and drowsiness, gradually disappear as your body becomes accustomed to the drug, but others persist. Surprisingly, not all side effects appear in the first few days of taking a new drug; some appear only after months or years of use, and they can even appear after you stop taking the drug.

Most side effects are well known. If your doctor or pharmacist does not tell you about potential side effects, ask if there are any. Some side effects are easier to live with than others. If side effects are causing you discomfort or are interfering with your normal activities, don't stop taking the drug, but do call your doctor. A change of dose or medication may be possible. It is especially important to report side effects if you are taking a drug that is relatively new on the market. Side effects are usually not fully understood until a drug has been widely used for several years.

One way to avoid side effects is to take medication only when necessary, especially if you are already taking medications for other problems. All drugs are chemicals that can be toxic. When you and your doctor decide medication is necessary, be sure to learn about the potential side effects. Ask your doctor and pharmacist about them, and read the labels and package inserts that come with your medication. Never take more of a medication than was prescribed. More medication will not improve your symptoms faster and may increase the risk of serious side effects.

ADVERSE REACTIONS

An adverse reaction is an unpleasant or harmful reaction to the normal dose of a drug. While side effects are predictable, an adverse reaction is often unexpected. It is also more serious. It can be caused by an allergy, a genetic predisposition, or an interaction with other drugs you are taking. Health conditions that interfere with your body's ability to absorb and eliminate drugs (such as kidney or liver disease) can increase your risk of adverse reactions. Some adverse reactions cause permanent damage to part of the body.

Possible adverse reactions include a skin rash such as hives, mouth sores, increased sensitivity to sun exposure, mood change, excessive drowsiness, unsteady gait, or confusion. If any of these adverse reactions occur, report them to your doctor as soon as possible. Your doctor may be able to solve the problem by reducing the dose, changing the timing of the medication, or changing the drug.

A fetus or breast-feeding infant may suffer adverse reactions to a drug you take. Many drugs cross the placenta and others pass into breast milk. See the chapters on drug use during pregnancy and breast-feeding.

Some adverse reactions are not obvious at first. For example, gold compounds and penicillamine used to treat rheumatoid arthritis may damage the kidneys over time. Blood counts and urine samples are taken regularly during treatment to test for this adverse reaction.

DRUGS AND SUN EXPOSURE

A number of common medications cause your skin to become more sensitive to sun exposure, a condition called photosensitivity. While taking the medication, you must carefully protect your skin from the sun. Otherwise, you could suffer a severe burn or increase your risk of skin cancer. If you have fair skin, you are particularly vulnerable. There are two kinds of photosensitivity reactions: phototoxic and photoallergic.

Phototoxic reactions are relatively common and usually result in exaggerated sunburns. Drugs that cause these reactions are deposited in the skin, where they absorb UVA or UVB light and destroy surrounding tissues. Common symptoms are a burning sensation in areas exposed to light (face, neck, chest, hands), pain, inflammation, and blistering. Phototoxic reactions can occur the first time you take a drug. With some drugs, the reaction can even occur from light exposure through a window. Drugs that cause these reactions are tetracyclines (specifically demeclocycline), fluoroquinolones (such as ciprofloxacin and lomefloxacin), topical preparations containing coal tar and psoralens, phenothiazines, antiarrhythmic amiodarone, piroxicam (Feldene), and estrogens in oral contraceptives and estrogen replacement products.

The second type of photosensitivity reaction to drugs is called photoallergic reaction. In this rarer reaction, exposure to light in the UVA band causes an allergic reaction to the drug, with an extremely itchy, inflamed, severe skin condition. This allergic reaction usually occurs on your second exposure to the drug. Areas of the body not directly exposed to light may be affected. Drugs that cause photoallergic reactions include quinidine, the sulfa drugs (thiazide diuretics, hypoglycemic drugs, sulfa antibiotics), and PABA-containing sunscreens. If you are taking any of these medications and plan to be in the sun, protect yourself by limiting time outside and using a sunscreen that blocks both UVA and UVB light.

DRUG ALLERGY

Less than 25 percent of adverse drug reactions are caused by allergic reactions to drugs. Although these reactions are relatively rare, they can be severe. In an allergic reaction, your body produces antibodies to the drug. The antibody binds to the drug to rid it from the body. In the process, the drug-antibody complex destroys body tissues or interferes with normal body functions. Although allergic reactions are often confined to the skin and cause hives and itching, they may also destroy cells in the kidney, liver, joints, and blood. In its most severe

DRUGS THAT INCREASE VULNERABILITY TO SUN

If you are taking any of the following medications, see chapter 3 for information on sun screens and other ways to protect your skin.

Type of Medication	Generic Name	Brand Name
ANTIARRHYTHMICS	amiodarone	Cordarone
	quinidine	Quinaglute, Quinora, Quinidex Extentabs
ANTIBIOTICS	tetracycline	Many generic, Sumycin, Achromycin
	demeclocycline	Declomycin
	doxycycline	Vibra-tabs, Vibramycin
	quinolones	Cipro, Maxaquin, Noroxin, Floxin
ANTINAUSEA	prochlorperazine	Compazine
COAL TAR	coal tar	Denorex, DHS Tar Gel, Medotar, Tegrin
NONSTEROIDAL ANTI-INFLAMMATORY DRUGS	naproxen piroxicam	Naprosyn Feldene
ORAL CONTRACEPTIVES	estrogen progestin	All combination estrogen-progestin
SULFA DRUGS (URINARY INFECTIONS)	sulfamethoxazole sulfasalazine sulfisoxazole trimethoprim-sulfamethoxazole	Gantanol Azulfidine Gantrisin Bactrim, Septra
THIAZIDE AND LOOP DIURETICS	furosemide chlorothiazide	Lasix Diuril
	hydrochlorothiazide	Esidrix, Hydro-D, HydroDIURIL, Oretic
RETINOIDS	isotretinoin	Accutane

form, an allergic drug reaction can lead to anaphylactic shock (see box).

While allergic reactions are unpredictable, several factors make them more likely. Drugs applied topically in a cream or lotion are more likely to cause allergic reactions than orally administered drugs. Certain drugs, particularly sulfa drugs and the penicillin class of antibiotics, are more likely than others to cause allergy. Allergic skin reactions to these drugs—the sulfas and penicillins—are more likely to occur on your second exposure to the drug rather than during the initial 10-day or 7-day course of therapy. Drug allergies are more common among people with certain conditions. For example, the risk of having an allergic reaction to a sulfa drug is much higher in people with AIDS than in the general population.

ANAPHYLACTIC SHOCK

Anaphylactic shock is a severe allergic reaction. Blood pressure drops, and the airways may become so narrow that the person can't breathe. Anaphylactic shock is extremely dangerous and requires emergency medical treatment. The warning signs include, in order from most to least significant:

* Loss of consciousness
* Difficulty breathing
* Difficulty swallowing
* Tightness in the chest
* Swollen face, lips, or tongue
* Hives or rash, specifically on the neck, face, or chest
* Nausea, vomiting
* Pale skin

If the person has stopped breathing, apply mouth-to-mouth resuscitation. Call an ambulance immediately. Do not give any food or drink.

Drug interactions

A drug interaction is an unpleasant or dangerous result of the combination of two or more drugs, or the combination of a drug with food.

DRUG-DRUG INTERACTIONS

Drugs can interact in many different ways. One drug can increase the effects of another. This can be useful—for example, your doctor may prescribe two different drugs for high blood pressure—but it may also be dangerous to combine two drugs that have similar effects. For example, sedatives and alcohol are a life-threatening combination. Sometimes two similar drugs can create a more profound effect, such as when combining alcohol with an antianxiety medication. Uncontrolled bleeding can occur if warfarin (Coumadin), a blood thinner (anticoagulant), is combined with certain nonsteroidal anti-inflammatory drugs (NSAIDS), which have the ability to inhibit platelets, a type of cell involved in blood clotting.

Sometimes one drug makes another less effective. For example, some antibiotics make birth-control pills less effective.

Sometimes a drug changes the body's ability to absorb, distribute, or eliminate another drug, causing a toxic buildup. For example, it is dangerous to combine the popular drugs ketoconazole (Nizoral), a prescription treatment for fungal and yeast infections, and the antihistamine terfenadine (Seldane). Ketoconazole interferes with the liver's ability to eliminate the antihistamine, which builds to levels that may adversely affect the rhythm of the heart.

Types of drugs that commonly interact with other drugs include antacids, antibiotics, anticonvulsants, antidepressants, oral antidiabetic drugs, blood thinners, decongestants, high blood pressure medications, and sedatives.

To reduce your risk of drug interactions, when a new drug is being prescribed always tell your doctor all the drugs you take currently or occasionally. Also, try to have your prescriptions filled at the same pharmacy, where your drug history can be maintained and monitored by your pharmacist. Also check the Drug Profiles in this book for warnings about interactions.

Alcohol

When you start a new medication, watch for side effects of fatigue, dizziness, or confusion. If you have these side effects, alcohol use may add to them. If you don't, you probably can drink alcohol in moderation with the drug. Also, consider that alcohol is frequently used in the formula of liquid drugs (for example, Nyquil). Check the package for the alcohol content.

If the drug you are taking is a central nervous system depressant, do not take alcohol at all. Alcohol is a central nervous system depressant; it decreases your reflexes and concentration, and it often makes you drowsy. Therefore it may have an additive, detrimental effect with similar depressants such as the benzodiazepines and barbiturates. It may also have an additive effect with any other drug that causes sedation as a side effect, such as the tricyclic antidepressants and some antihistamines.

Alcohol also irritates the stomach and so should not be combined with other drugs that can do this, including aspirin, ibuprofen, and corticosteroids such as prednisone. Also because of this irritation, alcohol increases your risk of bleeding from the gut, which can be dangerous if you are on a blood thinner such as warfarin (Coumadin).

Alcohol also reduces blood sugar and so should not be combined with oral antidiabetic drugs.

Alcohol and the popular pain reliever acetaminophen (Tylenol) may also be a poor mix, particularly for heavy drinkers. Heavy or chronic drinkers should take no more than 2 grams of acetaminophen per day.

Overall, avoid alcohol if you are on another central nervous system depressant, if you are on another drug that causes sedation, if you take a drug that can irritate your stomach and may cause ulceration, if you are on a blood thinner, or if you are on a drug for treatment of diabetes.

Interactions with hormonal contraceptives or hormone replacement therapy

Taking estrogen, in a combined birth-control pill or as part of hormone replacement therapy, can affect the concentrations of other drugs in your body. For example, prednisolone, a corticosteroid used to control inflammation, may accumulate in the body. If so, the dose may need to be lower. Cyclosporine, which suppresses the immune

COMMON DRUG INTERACTIONS

DRUG: WARFARIN ANTICOAGULANT

INTERACTING DRUGS: Aspirin, nonsteroidal anti-inflammatory drugs (including naproxen, Aleve, ibuprofen, Advil, Motrin), alcohol, trimethoprim-sulfamethoxazole (Bactrim Septra), cimetidine (Tagamet), amiodarone, and omeprazole (Prilosec)

RESULT: Even small doses of the interacting drug can increase the risk of uncontrolled bleeding.

DRUG: CYCLOSPORINE

INTERACTING DRUGS: Oral contraceptives, diltiazem, erythromycin, fluconazole, metoclopramide, nicardipine, verapamil

RESULT: Increased cyclosporine blood levels and increased risk of kidney damage

DRUG: MONOAMINE OXIDASE INHIBITOR ANTIDEPRESSANTS (Marplan, Nardil, Parnate)

INTERACTING DRUGS AND FOODS: Fluoxetine, levodopa, meperidine (Demerol); decongestants containing ephedrine, phenylephrine, or phenylpropanolamine; amphetamines, tricyclic antidepressants, aged cheeses, aged meats, concentrated yeast extracts, and some red wines and beers

RESULT: Shivering, nausea, confusion, dangerous rise in blood pressure, heart arrhythmia, seizures, brain hemorrhage, death

DRUG: BIRTH-CONTROL PILLS

INTERACTING DRUGS: Barbiturates, tetracycline, penicillin, sulfa antibiotics, griseofulvin, rifampin, anticonvulsants (carbamazepine, phenytoin)

RESULT: Reduced effectiveness of contraceptive

DRUG: QUINOLONE ANTIBIOTICS such as ciprofloxacin (Cipro) or ofloxacin (Floxin)

INTERACTING DRUG: Antacids containing aluminum, magnesium, or calcium; iron preparations

RESULT: Antibiotic loses 80 to 90 percent of its effectiveness if the antacid or iron was taken less than 4 hours earlier

(continued)

DRUG: SEDATIVES, SLEEPING PILLS, ANTIANXIETY
MEDICATION, NARCOTIC ANALGESICS,
ANTIHISTAMINES, ALCOHOL, and other drugs that
depress the central nervous system
INTERACTING DRUGS: Depressants of the central nervous system,
including alcohol, sedatives, sleeping pills, antianxiety
medications, narcotic analgesics, antihistamines
RESULT: Excessive sedation, lethargy, respiratory failure

DRUG: TETRACYCLINE ANTIBIOTICS
INTERACTING DRUGS AND FOODS: Antacids containing aluminum,
magnesium or calcium, dairy products, iron supplements,
bismuth subsalicylate (Pepto-Bismol)
RESULT: Antibiotic less effective if substance is taken less than 2
hours earlier

DRUG: THE ANTIHISTAMINES, TERFENADINE, (Seldane)
AND ASTEMIZOLE (Hismanal)
INTERACTING DRUGS: Cimetidine, clarithromycin, erythromycin,
fluconazole, itraconazole, fluconazole, nefazodone
RESULT: Increased blood level of the antihistamine, which
increases the risk of a life-threatening abnormal heart rhythm

system after a transplant operation, may reach high levels and damage
the kidneys. If you are taking oral contraceptives or estrogen replacement therapy, make sure you tell your doctor before you get a new
prescription.

Women who take oral contraceptives should also know that certain medications can make their birth-control pills less effective.
Among them are broad-spectrum antibiotics such as tetracycline,
some anticonvulsant medications such as carbamazepine and phenytoin, the anti-tubercular agent rifampin, and the antifungal medication griseofulvin.

DRUG-FOOD INTERACTIONS

Some drugs interact with food. Sometimes the drug becomes less potent; for example, the antibiotic tetracycline becomes less effective if taken with dairy products or iron supplements. In other cases, a drug becomes dangerous if taken with the wrong foods. A group of antidepressants called the monoamine oxidase inhibitors (MAOIs, Marplan, Nardil, Parnate) can cause a potentially fatal rise in blood pressure if taken with foods containing the chemical tyramine, found in aged cheeses, concentrated yeast extracts, aged meats (salami, sausages), broad bean pods, and sauerkraut. Tyramine in varying amounts is also present in alcoholic beverages, including beers and wines. Before taking an MAOI, speak to your doctor and pharmacist about both foods and drugs to avoid.

Most drugs can be taken safely with most foods in your normal diet, but always ask your doctor or pharmacist about possible drug-food interactions. The Drug Profiles in the back of this book list drug interactions to watch for when taking each medication. The most common offenders are dairy products, caffeine, salt, and grapefruit juice.

Drug dependence

Most people associate drug abuse with illegal drugs like cocaine, but it is far more common to be dependent on alcohol, caffeine, nicotine, or prescription drugs such as sleeping pills and tranquilizers.

Women are more likely than men to become dependent on prescription drugs. Again, they are more frequent users of these drugs, which affects the statistics.

Drug dependence is an uncontrollable desire to experience the pleasurable effects of a drug or to prevent the unpleasant effects of withdrawal. Drug dependence can be psychological, physical, or both. Physical dependence happens when the body has so adapted to the drug that stopping it causes severe withdrawal symptoms. Physical dependence also results when the body builds up a tolerance for the drug, so that the dose must be constantly increased to get the same results. This effect, called "drug tolerance," is a characteristic of most commonly abused drugs, including alcohol, nicotine, caffeine, and certain prescription drugs.

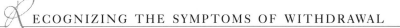 RECOGNIZING THE SYMPTOMS OF WITHDRAWAL

If you have been taking one of the following prescription medications, watch for these symptoms when you stop. You may need to reduce your use gradually, under the supervision of a doctor, to avoid these withdrawal symptoms associated with physical addiction.

AMPHETAMINES: Fatigue, need for long periods of sleep, dizziness, increased appetite, muscle pain, chills, abdominal pain

BENZODIAZEPINES: Anxiety, sleeplessness, sweating, shaking, increased heart rate, rapid breathing

BARBITURATES: Anxiety, sleeplessness, twitching, nightmares, convulsions, coma, dizziness, weakness

CORTICOSTEROIDS: Dizziness, fatigue, fainting, fever, loss of appetite, muscle or joint pain, nausea, reappearance of disease symptoms

People taking medications often worry that they will become dependent on the drug. In reality, only a few types of drugs are likely to cause physical dependence. Most are mood-altering drugs: narcotic pain relievers (morphine), sleeping pills, antianxiety drugs (benzodiazepines and barbiturates), nervous system depressants, and stimulants.

Some prescription drugs are prescribed less often than they once were because they tend to cause dependence. Examples are amphetamines as diet aids or barbiturates for anxiety or sleeplessness.

Psychological dependence occurs when the effects of the substance become necessary to maintain feelings of well-being. Psychological dependence is always part of substance abuse, but physical dependence may not always be present. Many people who abuse drugs are psychologically dependent but may not experience significant or severe physical withdrawal symptoms when they stop using the drug.

Steps you can take to avoid developing a dependence include:

- Take the drug as directed.
- Be aware of the signs of dependency for each drug.
- Use the drug for short-term treatment if possible and look for other, nondrug methods of treating the underlying problem.

chapter 3

DRUGS FOR A HEALTHIER LIFESTYLE

SOME OF THE MOST WIDELY USED MEDICATIONS help women quit smoking, lose weight, protect their skin from sun exposure, or relieve constipation. These drugs have helped some women increase their health and well-being, but they are also among the most misused and overused drugs. Some of the drugs in these categories can be addictive or can cause health problems rather than prevent them. This chapter will help you choose when and how to take these drugs.

Aids to quitting smoking

If you smoke, quitting is the most important thing you can do for your health; it will reduce your risk of lung cancer, emphysema, and heart disease. If you are pregnant, it will reduce health risks for both you and your baby.

Like most smokers, you may have tried to quit before and failed. The leading reason for such failures is physical and psychological addiction to the nicotine in tobacco smoke. Stopping suddenly can cause withdrawal symptoms including headache, hunger, cravings for sweet foods, anxiety, restlessness, inability to concentrate, irritability, anger, insomnia, and a depressed mood.

Some people overcome their addiction to nicotine through nicotine replacement therapy. A gum, skin patch, or nasal spray satisfies the body's craving for nicotine while you quit smoking. Nicotine replacement therapy can prevent withdrawal symptoms during the first weeks or months after quitting. However, the approach is successful only if you are motivated to stop smoking and have developed methods to cope without smoking. It is dangerous to use nicotine replacements and continue to smoke at the same time because of possible nicotine overdose. Though addictive, nicotine is not the part of tobacco smoke that causes lung cancer, so a short time of this therapy is less dangerous than continuing the habit of smoking.

If you are a smoker, talk to your doctor about whether these drugs might help you. Nicotine therapy is most helpful to people who have a high physical dependence on nicotine. A telling sign is a habit of smoking a cigarette within 30 minutes of waking up in the morning. You are more likely to be helped by nicotine replacement if several of these traits are true for you:

- You smoke more than 15 cigarettes a day.
- You prefer brands with more than 0.9 mg of nicotine.
- You usually inhale deeply and frequently.
- You smoke your first cigarette within 30 minutes of waking in the morning.
- You find your first cigarette of the day the hardest to give up.
- You smoke more frequently during the day than at night.
- You find it difficult to refrain from smoking where it is forbidden.
- You smoke even when you are so ill that you are confined to bed.
- You have made four unsuccessful attempts to quit.

If you choose to use nicotine replacement therapy, start by choosing a quit date within the next two weeks and prepare yourself mentally, physically, and environmentally by changing some of your behaviors. For example, if your quit date is a week from now, you can prepare yourself by removing ashtrays from your home or office and staying away from smoke-filled environments. You can start a low-energy exercise program and talk with your doctor about the availability of self-help manuals or support groups.

Immediately after quitting, you start on a dose of nicotine through the patch, gum, or nasal spray. Once you have kicked the cigarette habit, you will gradually reduce and finally eliminate the dose of nicotine. The process usually takes three to five months.

Nicotine aids cannot make you stop smoking. You have to be

motivated to quit. For the best chance of success, you should also seek help in changing behaviors linked to your smoking. Talk to your doctor about behavioral therapy, such as weekly counseling or local support groups such as Smokenders and Nicotine Anonymous.

If anxiety has been or is a major part of your withdrawal from smoking, ask your doctor about taking antianxiety medication—buspirone or alprazolam—starting two to four weeks before your quit date. These drugs are commonly used for this purpose.

PATCH, GUM, OR SPRAY?

Each method—gum, patch, or spray—has advantages and disadvantages. Talk with your doctor about which method may be best for you. With each method, women sometimes remain addicted to nicotine and feel the need to continue with the gum, patch, or spray for a long time. The best way to avoid this is to develop coping methods by seeking support from groups or a behavioral therapist.

Nicotine gum

Nicotine gum delivers a dose of nicotine each time you chew a piece. You chew one every 30 to 60 minutes. While a cigarette delivers nicotine to your body within 1 to 2 minutes after starting to smoke, the gum takes about 15 minutes to release nicotine, so don't wait until you have a craving for a cigarette before using the gum. Discuss with your doctor how many pieces of gum you can safely chew each day and which dose (2 or 4 mg) to use at first. If you smoke one pack a day, a good starting dose is 12 to 15 pieces a day of the 2-mg gum. The maximum number of pieces of gum per day is 30 pieces of the 2-mg-per-piece gum and 20 pieces per day of the 4-mg-per-piece gum.

Unlike the patch, gum replaces some of the oral gratification lost when you quit smoking. Another advantage is that, unlike the patch, which delivers a steady dose of nicotine, the gum may cause a rush similar to that of a cigarette. On the minus side, because the gum does not provide a consistent, uninterrupted level of nicotine, women sometimes feel cravings and begin smoking again. Also, the carefully prescribed chewing regimen can be a bother.

After two or three months, you will be ready to gradually reduce the number of pieces you chew each day. Do not reduce the amount

USING NICOTINE GUM

- Chew regularly—every 30 to 60 minutes (10 to 20 pieces a day for the first week).
- Do not take within 15 minutes of drinking an acidic beverage such as coffee, cola, wine, or orange juice—all can reduce the effectiveness of the gum. Overall, it is best to avoid eating or drinking 15 minutes before or after using the gum.
- Begin by chewing very slowly to release the nicotine. If you chew it too quickly, you may release too much nicotine from the gum and feel like someone smoking a cigarette for the first time. Symptoms can include a light head, nausea, vomiting, hiccups, and mouth or throat soreness.
- If you notice a peppery taste or tingling in your mouth, stop chewing and park the gum between your teeth and lower lip in front of the mouth. When the sensation is almost gone, start chewing again. If you do not get this tingling sensation from the 2-mg-per-piece gum, talk to your doctor. You may need the 4-mg dose.
- When the tingling returns, stop chewing and park the gum in a different place in your mouth. Chew each piece of gum for 30 minutes, then discard.

of nicotine too quickly. Every four to seven days, decrease the number of pieces chewed per day. Some people replace the nicotine gum with sugarless gum to keep the same oral gratification. You can also reduce the chewing time from 30 minutes per piece to 15 minutes to reduce the amount of nicotine released. If you started on the 4-mg dose, consider switching to the 2-mg dose after two months. Overall, do not use nicotine gum longer than six months.

Don't worry if you swallow the gum by accident. The nicotine can only be released from the gum by the vigorous chewing. Keep nicotine gum out of the reach of children and pets.

If you begin smoking again but continue the gum, you can get an overdose of nicotine (see box on page 48). Talk to your doctor about restarting your quit-smoking program.

Nicotine patch

A transdermal nicotine patch, worn on the skin, delivers a continuous dose of nicotine. One type of patch stays on your skin 24 hours a day (Habitrol, Nicoderm, ProStep), the other for only 16 hours when you are awake (Nicotrol). Both must be replaced every day. Talk with your doctor about which kind is best for you. The 24-hour patch may cause insomnia for some people. Your doctor will set your dose according to how much you used to smoke. Generally, if you weigh more than 100 pounds, do not have cardiovascular disease, and smoke at least a half pack per day, you will be started on the 21- or 22-mg-per-day 24-hour patch or the 15-mg-per-day 16-hour patch.

The patch is easier to use than gum and provides a steady amount of nicotine that prevents cravings; however, it takes about two days for this level of nicotine to stabilize in your system. Some people find the patch more socially acceptable because it is easily hidden and does not require chewing. Plus, you have to apply it only once a day. You are also less likely to receive an overdose of nicotine with a patch than with gum. Half of the people who use the patch get an irritating skin rash. Caused by the adhesive backing of the patch, this rash can be extremely bothersome and can last for weeks.

Apply your first patch the night before or on the morning of your quit day. Put it on a clean, dry, nonhairy area of your upper body or the outer side of your upper arm. Replace a 24-hour patch at the same time each day. Remove a 16-hour patch at bedtime and replace it in the morning. To avoid skin irritation, place the patch in a different place each day. Do not use the same spot on your skin more than once a week. Do not apply the patch on skin that is already irritated. Your doctor will gradually reduce your dose over 20 or fewer weeks.

If you are unable to stop smoking after four weeks, stop the replacement treatment and consult with your doctor. Smokers who do not use cigarettes for the first two weeks after starting the patch have the highest quit rates. If you resume smoking, your doctor may withhold the patch until you set a new quit date, then try it again, possibly at a higher dose. It is extremely important to stop smoking while you are on the patch. Symptoms of nicotine overdose (see box) have been reported in patients who continue to smoke while on the patch.

The used patch contains residual amounts of nicotine. To properly dispose of the patch, fold it over and place it into the protective

WARNING SIGNS OF NICOTINE OVERDOSE

Nicotine gum and the nicotine patch are not intended to be used by smokers. If you combine smoking and a nicotine aid, the nicotine in your body can reach a toxic level. You can also overdose on nicotine if you use the gum or patch incorrectly or if your dose is too high. A high level of nicotine causes uncomfortable symptoms and can be dangerous, particularly for people with heart disease. When using stop-smoking aids, watch for the following signs of nicotine overdose:

- Headache
- Dizziness
- Abdominal pain
- Drooling
- Nausea or vomiting
- Diarrhea
- Cold sweat
- Blurred vision
- Disturbed hearing
- Confusion
- Weakness
- Fainting

If you experience the following signs of severe overdose, seek emergency medical help:

- Difficulty breathing
- Low blood pressure, fainting, and profuse sweating
- Unconsciousness

If you suspect an overdose, remove the patch or gum immediately. Flush the skin or your mouth with water (soap increases the absorption of the nicotine delivered via the patch). Call your doctor immediately. If you use a patch, keep in mind that a depot (an accumulation of the drug) in the skin will continue to release nicotine for at least 6 to 10 hours.

pouch that contains the new system to be applied. Make sure it is out of the reach of children.

Nasal spray

The most recently developed form of nicotine replacement therapy is a nasal spray (Nicotrol NS). Available by prescription only, it is intended to be used along with a behavior modification program. It may be a good choice for heavily dependent smokers because the nasal spray delivers the nicotine more quickly to the system than nicotine gum, relieving cravings immediately. Like other nicotine replacement therapies, the nicotine spray may cause dependence. It is recommended that the spray be used for three months, and it should not be used for more than six. The spray causes nasal or throat irritation in most users and is not recommended for people with sinus conditions, allergies, or asthma.

You should not inhale, sniff, or swallow when using the spray. The spray is intended to be absorbed through the membranes of the nose, not breathed into the lungs or swallowed into the digestive tract.

To use the spray, tilt your head back slightly and place the tip of the bottle into the nostril as far as is comfortable. Squeeze the pump bottle once in each nostril. Wait two to three minutes before blowing your nose.

Your doctor will base your dose on your level of nicotine dependence. A typical regimen is 1 or 2 doses per hour (one dose is a spray in each nostril). The maximum dose is 40 per day. For best results, use at least 8 doses per day.

Weight-loss drugs

If, like many women, you have had trouble losing weight, you may have considered taking a weight-loss drug. These drugs, some sold by prescription and others over the counter, have helped some women, particularly those severely overweight. However, none of them can be taken for a long time, and women tend to gain the weight back after stopping the drug unless they have also made long-term changes in their diet and exercise habits.

Before taking a diet aid, first ask your doctor to determine your ideal weight for good health. There are charts on ideal body weight that are based on height and frame size, as well as a body-mass index chart and simple tests that can be used to measure subcutaneous fat thickness. If you do not need to lose weight, you can save yourself not only a lot of trouble, but also the risk of harming your health through unnecessary dieting. However, if you weigh 20 percent more than your ideal weight or have gained more than 20 pounds since reaching your adult height, you can improve your health by losing some weight. If you are overweight, losing even 10 to 15 pounds will reduce your risk of heart disease, high blood pressure, high cholesterol, diabetes, and cancer.

One of the best ways to assess your weight is by finding your waist-to-hip ratio. Waist-to-hip ratio is a comparison of your waist measurement to your hip measurement. You should strive for a waist-to-hip ratio of less than 85 percent, or 0.85. Calculate it by dividing your waist measurement by your hip measurement (For example, 28inches/38inches=0.73, or 73 percent).

Losing weight lowers blood pressure and sugar and improves your cholesterol ratio. For most women, though, losing weight and keeping it off is not easy. Can drugs help? Most of them offer only limited help to a limited number of women, and too often the weight comes back. The best way to lose weight and keep it off is to reduce the number of calories you take in and increase your aerobic exercise (walking, biking, swimming, aerobic dance). Weight lifting can help too, but not as much as aerobic exercise.

Nonprescription Diet Aids

Most diet aids are appetite suppressants. Some women who take them feel less hungry and so eat less, though others do not. Other types of diet aids offered over the counter, such as fat burners, are even less effective. Based on an FDA advisory panel review of nonprescription weight reduction products, only two ingredients are generally recognized as safe and effective: phenylpropanolamine and benzocaine. However, they provide only short-term benefits and they shouldn't be used unless a reducing diet has already been established. No diet aid should be taken by women who are pregnant or breast-feeding.

- **Phenylpropanolamine.** Phenylpropanolamine (Acutrim, Dexatrim) is an appetite suppressant approved by the FDA for over-the-counter sale. It is a mild stimulant that promotes weight loss when combined with diet and exercise. It becomes less effective after eight weeks and should not be taken longer than three months. Women tend to regain the weight once they stop taking the pills. Phenylpropanolamine is available in both immediate-release tablets and capsules and in timed-release capsules. Taking more than the recommended dose or taking the drug with caffeine can cause irritability, sleeplessness, anxiety, headache, or irregular heartbeat. There is evidence that the drug may also contribute to hemorrhagic stroke. It is not recommended for anyone under age 18 or for pregnant or breast-feeding women; it is known to cross the placenta and reach the fetus, and it may decrease blood flow and oxygen supply to the uterus. It also enters breast milk and may make a nursing infant hyperactive or constantly sleepy. It is not recommended if you have diabetes (it may increase blood sugar), heart disease, hyperthyroidism, or high blood pressure or are currently being treated with a monoamine oxidase inhibitor drug (Marplan, Parnate).

- **Benzocaine.** Benzocaine is an anesthetic found in diet candies, chewing gums, and capsules. When taken in candy or gum just before eating, it is intended to temporarily deaden the taste receptors on the tongue, so food isn't as appealing as usual. Benzocaine in these forms may reduce snacking, which may help because constant snacking is a common cause of excess calories. However, there are minimal data to support the effectiveness of benzocaine in this form as an appetite suppressant. The oral capsule is not believed to directly affect taste, so it is not clear how it works. Also, the oral capsules containing both phenylpropanolamine and benzocaine have not been shown to be more effective than the former alone. Do not take a benzocaine-containing product for longer than 10 weeks. If you exceed the recommended dose, you may experience blurred or double vision, confusion, convulsions, dizziness, drowsiness, feeling hot or cold, numbness, headache, increased sweating, ringing or buzzing in the ears, shivering, or trembling. Try a piece and determine how it makes your mouth feel. Does it numb it totally? Does it really curb your appetite?

- **Fat burners.** Some products claim to stimulate the body's metabolism so it burns more fat. The most common ingredient, chromium picolinate, has not been proven to burn fat. Other products contain caffeine, a stimulant that may boost your energy but does not burn fat. As a weak diuretic, caffeine may initially help you lose weight by losing body water. If taken in excess, it may cause gastritis and irregular heart rhythms. A dietary supplement, guarana or kola nuts, sold in health food stores for weight loss and energy contains high concentrations of caffeine and should be used with caution if you have high blood pressure, an irregular heart rhythm, or a history of ulcers. Ephedrine, a decongestant found in some fat burner products and available in herbs (*ma huang*), increases metabolism in some obese women, but there is no evidence that it has this effect in women who are not obese. Ephedrine can also cause irregular heart rhythms and hypertension and it should not be combined with caffeine. The FDA has received many reports regarding severe adverse effects from dietary supplements such as ma huang for weight loss. Adverse effects have ranged from mild symptoms (increased nervousness, headache) to chest pain, stroke, heart attack, psychoses, and death. These reactions have occurred in healthy young people and persons with underlying conditions like high blood pressure. The only real fat burner is exercise.

PRESCRIPTION APPETITE SUPPRESSANTS

Amphetamines, once the preferred prescription drug for weight control, are rarely prescribed now because they are addictive. They are often abused because they cause a euphoric state. Some relatively safer prescription drugs, known as the anorectics, are available by prescription as short-term weight reduction therapy. Although these drugs are effective, they are not recommended for long-term use, and the weight often comes back.

The anorectics include fenfluramine (Pondimin) and phentermine (Ionamin), which are often prescribed together to suppress appetite. The drugs in this class act on chemical pathways in the brain that influence your appetite center. With the exception of fenfluramine, these anorectics are stimulating and may cause nervousness, increased blood pressure, and heart palpitations. Fenfluramine, which affects the appetite center differently, is more likely to cause agitation, drowsiness, and confusion. All of these anorectics should not be used if you have high blood pressure, hyperthyroidism, or heart disease or are currently being treated with a monoamine oxidase inhibitor. All of these drugs, including fenfluramine, can cause dependence and should not be used longer than three months. Women tend to regain the weight once they stop taking the pills.

A newer, FDA-approved antiobesity drug is dexfenfluramine (Redux). It is the first new antiobesity drug to be approved in 22 years. Dexfenfluramine is chemically related to fenfluramine (Podimin), but it targets more directly serotonin, a chemical that decreases carbohydrate craving in the brain. Weight loss is usually seen within four weeks, peaks at four to six months, and is maintained for a year. Dexfenfluramine is available only by prescription and it is to be used with a low-calorie diet. It is specifically for people with a body mass index (see above) greater than 30. Side effects are dry mouth, tiredness, and diarrhea. Like the anorectics, it cannot be combined with an MAOI drug. There is no evidence yet that Dexfenfluramine causes physical or psychological dependence.

PRESCRIPTION APPETITE SUPPRESSANTS

Women respond in a wide variety of ways to the more than a dozen prescription appetite suppressants. Your doctor may suggest one of the following medications based on your medical history and your overall health.

amphetamines	dexfenfluramine (Redux)
dextroamphetamine	phendimetrazine (Plegine)
(Dexedrine)	diethylpropion (Tenuate)
methamphetamine (Desoxyn)	fenfluramine (Pondimin)
anorectics	mazindol (Mazanor, Sanorex)
benzphetamine (Didrex)	phentermine (Ionamin, Fastin)

Laxatives

Laxatives relieve constipation, which is difficulty or discomfort in passing stool. They can be useful occasionally, but should not be relied on all the time to achieve regularity. Laxatives that contain chemical stimulants are particularly dangerous; daily use can cause abdominal cramps, fluid loss, and colon damage.

Women who have eating disorders often abuse laxatives. If you often use laxatives to purge food from your body, particularly after eating, talk to your doctor. If you do not get help, you will permanently damage your health.

WHEN TO USE A LAXATIVE

You do not need to have a bowel movement every day. If you have bowel movements fairly regularly (and regular can range from three times a day to three times a week) and they are not uncomfortable, then you are probably not constipated. If you have fewer than two bowel movements a week, if you feel discomfort or pain during bowel movements, or if you experience a change in bowel movements, you may be constipated and treatment may help.

Constipation is usually caused by a lack of fiber and fluid in the diet. Before reaching for laxatives, your first step should be to eat more fiber and drink plenty of fluids (without caffeine or alcohol). A diet that includes fruits, vegetables, and whole grains will go a long way toward preventing constipation. An easy way to boost your fiber is to eat a bowl of bran cereal with skim milk each day.

Sometimes constipation has causes other than diet. It is common during pregnancy because high levels of progesterone relax the muscles of the colon, thereby decreasing the passage of stool. Also, the iron in prenatal vitamins is constipating, and as pregnancy progresses, the increased size of the uterus compresses the colon. Not all pregnant women complain of constipation, though—probably because they have made the necessary dietary changes to prevent the problem.

Constipation can also be caused by a wide range of diseases including metabolic and endocrine disorders such as diabetes and hypothyroidism, neurologic disorders such as multiple sclerosis and Parkinson's disease, and gastrointestinal disorders (diverticular disease, irritable bowel disease).

Constipation often becomes more common with age, not only because of increased illness and medications, but also because of changes in diet, insufficient fluid, and lack of exercise.

CHOOSING A LAXATIVE

Often you can alleviate constipation by getting more fiber and fluid in your diet, but if you need faster, short-term relief, there are a variety of nonprescription remedies. Fiber-based laxatives and stool softeners are the slowest but safest methods. Chemical stimulants act more quickly but are more easily misused and abused.

Bulk-forming agents

Bulk-forming agents like Metamucil and Citrocel usually come in granular or powdered form and are considered safe and effective for daily use. Unlike many other kinds of laxatives, they may be used daily over the long term because their action is mechanical, not chemical. They contain natural dietary fiber (methylcellulose, polysaccharides, psyllium) which absorbs water to form large, soft stools. As the fecal mass enlarges, it causes the intestinal muscles to move the bulk along, allowing it to pass comfortably from the body. Bulk-forming agents may not produce results for one to three days.

Bulk-forming agents are usually the best choice when constipation occurs. Also, they are safe to use even every day for those who are on a low-residue diet, have irritable bowel disease or diverticular disease, or are taking a medication that is known to be constipating. Pregnant and breast-feeding women can take these laxatives safely.

If you are diabetic, you should be aware that many psyllium products (such as regular Metamucil) contain high amounts of dextrose and should be avoided. Products without added sugar (Metamucil SF, Fiberall Natural Fiber) should be used instead.

Do not use bulk-forming agents if you have nausea, vomiting, intestinal ulceration, or intestinal stenosis.

These laxatives need to be take with an 8-ounce glass of fluid. To mask the taste of the powder, you can mix it into juice, a fruit drink, or soda rather than water. If you do not take the laxative with 8 ounces of fluid, not only will it not be as effective, but the fiber may form a blockage in the esophagus or intestines. If the drug forms an immov-

DRUGS THAT CAN CAUSE CONSTIPATION

Doctors know that some drugs can cause constipation, so they often prescribe a stool-softening agent or mild laxative at the same time. If you are taking a new medication and become constipated, ask your doctor or pharmacist whether the drug is the problem. The following medications are most likely to cause constipation:

antacids containing aluminum
 or calcium (not aluminum-
 magnesium antacids)
antiarrhythmic
 disopyramide (Norpace)
antihypertensives
 clonidine
 guanabenz
 guanfacine
antihistamines
 diphenhydramine
 orphenadrine
antiparkinson drugs
 amantadine

benztropine
trihexyphenidyl
calcium channel blockers
 diltiazem
 verapamil
iron preparations
opiate analgesics
 codeine
 morphine
phenothiazine antipsychotics
 chlorpromazine (Thorazine)
tricyclic antidepressants
 amitriptyline
 imipramine

able mass, you may experience chest pain and have the urge to vomit. To prevent intestinal blockage it is best to drink at least six 8-ounce glasses of water throughout the day.

Stool softeners

Stool softeners, also called emollients, contain docusate, which draws water into the stool to make it easier to pass. These are a safe form of laxative and can be taken daily. Like bulk-forming agents, they may need one to three days to work. These agents are often best for prevention of constipation rather than treatment and are good to use if you notice that the stool is hard and has been difficult to pass.

Stool softeners are a good choice for pregnant women, particularly when constipation is caused by iron supplements. They are also a good choice before labor to prevent constipation after delivery. They are safe while a woman is breast-feeding.

Stimulant laxatives

This category of laxatives consists of a number of stimulants with varying potencies.

Bisacodyl (Dulcolax), phenolphthalein (Ex-Lax, Correctol, Feen-a-Mint), and senna (Senokot) are the three most common stimulant laxatives. Available for oral use and as rectal suppositories, these laxatives directly irritate the intestine causing an increased passage of stool, and they also increase the amount of water and electrolytes in the intestine. They work quickly (ranging from 15 minutes with a rectal product to within 12 hours with an oral drug), but are the most commonly overused and abused laxatives. Daily use can cause severe abdominal cramps as well as a loss of fluid and potassium.

These laxatives should be used cautiously during pregnancy because they may interfere with water, sodium, and potassium balance and may thereby affect blood pressure and heart rate. Castor oil, a stimulant laxative, can cause premature labor and rupture of uterine tissues.

Stimulant laxatives are often abused by people with the eating disorder bulimia to purge their bodies of food after binge eating. This is a dangerous practice that can damage the colon. Large doses of stimulant laxatives can cause diarrhea and abnormal colon activity (similar to ulcerative colitis).

Phenophthalein can cause a pink or red discoloration of the urine or stool at almost any dose. This is a normal function of the chemical and is not a cause for concern. It can also cause a rash called a fixed drug eruption. This allergic reaction is not a sign of toxicity, but can permanently discolor the skin. A burning or itching on the skin is an early warning sign of this rash; if you notice this, stop the drug and notify your doctor as soon as possible.

Saline cathartics

Nicknamed "liquid dynamite" by medical professionals, saline cathartics are available over the counter as rectal enemas and oral liquids and produce quick and intense evacuation of the bowel. Saline cathartics are often used for rapid and complete evacuation of the bowel before you undergo a gastrointestinal procedure such as endoscopy or have gastrointestinal surgery. They deliver to the intestine a large amount of a charged particle (sulfate, citrate, or phosphate)

PREVENTING CONSTIPATION

Constipation is usually related to diet and other habits. Before reaching for chemical laxatives, try making these changes.

- Cut down on high-fat, highly processed foods.
- Choose high-fiber natural foods like fruits, vegetables, and whole grains.
- Eat dried fruit like raisins, prunes, and apricots.
- Drink six to eight large glasses of water per day.
- Avoid caffeine and alcohol, which draw water from your system.
- Do regular, moderate exercise like brisk walking to stimulate your digestive tract.

that quickly pulls water into the stool. A laxative effect occurs within 30 minutes to 6 hours after an oral preparation and within 2 to 15 minutes after a rectal product. These substances should not be used regularly to treat constipation but may be useful to relieve fecal impaction. They may cause a rapid loss of fluids and changes in electrolytes.

Saline cathartics, including magnesium citrate and Fleet's Phosphosoda enemas, can cause a high load of magnesium or sodium and cause dehydration. They should not be used during pregnancy or by people with kidney disease, high blood pressure, heart failure, or low-salt diet.

An alternative to chemicals is an enema of plain water. Administering ²/₃ cup of room temperature tap water into the rectum often leads to a bowel movement within a half hour.

Sunscreens

Over the years, sun exposure can cause wrinkles and skin cancer. The right sunscreen can help, but you also need to limit your hours in the sun (particularly at midday) and wear protective clothing and a hat. And you need to choose the right kind of sunscreen and use it correctly. The many products on the market are not equally effective.

Your skin is the largest organ of your body. It regulates body temperature and transforms light into vitamin D, which is essential for the regulation of calcium absorption. It protects the body from sunlight by acting as a physical barrier and also by producing the dark pigment melanin. The outer layer of the skin, the epidermis, consists of three sublayers; in order from the deepest, they are the basal cells, squamous cells, and stratum corneum. Underlying the epidermis is the thicker layer called the dermis, containing hair follicles, sweat glands, and nerve fibers.

TWO KINDS OF RAYS

Two kinds of ultraviolet rays from the sun pass through the atmosphere and damage skin. The UVB rays, which are shorter, are the primary burning rays. UVB radiation is most concentrated during the summer and at midday, which is why the best way to avoid a sunburn is to stay out of the sun between 10 and 2 o'clock. UVB rays do not pass through glass. When UVB rays reach your skin, they are absorbed in the outer layer, the epidermis, damaging the DNA, the genetic material in your cells. The rays also stimulate the cells to produce more melanin, the pigment that turns your skin brown, to try to protect themselves from the damaging rays. Melanin physically blocks and scatters the UV rays. UVB rays are thought to cause the two less dangerous forms of skin cancer, basal cell and squamous cell carcinomas.

Until recently, scientists thought UVA rays were relatively harmless. They were sometimes called the "tanning rays," as opposed to the UVB rays, which were called the "burning rays." We now know that UVA rays may be almost as harmful because they are more constant and plentiful. Also, they can penetrate glass, so you receive some indoors. UVA rays also penetrate the skin more deeply and may be responsible for most cases of malignant melanoma. Don't be misled by the claims of tanning salons that their equipment is safe because it uses only UVA rays. UVA rays can cause burning, wrinkles, and skin cancer.

Besides harming the skin, ultraviolet light can also damage the eyes and cause cataracts (a blurring of the lens). You can protect your eyes with sunglasses and a brimmed hat.

EVERYONE NEEDS PROTECTION

Every woman should limit her exposure to the sun, even if she lives in a cloudy region. Skin cancer is the leading cause of cancer in women between the ages of 24 and 29, and risk increases with age. You are particularly vulnerable if you have fair or freckled skin, but you can develop skin cancer even if you have dark skin or tan easily. Sunscreens are safe for women who are pregnant or breast-feeding. Older women particularly need protection because age thins the skin and makes it more vulnerable to the sun. Regardless of age, smokers also need more protection because of similar skin changes.

You must especially be careful about sun protection if you are taking a drug known to increase the skin's vulnerability to the sun. Some drugs absorb ultraviolet light and can cause either photoxicity or photosensitivity. (For more about these drugs, see page 32.)

INGREDIENTS TO LOOK FOR

Every sunscreen contains one or more active ingredients. There are more than 20 sunscreen agents, each protecting against a different range of rays.

Most products screen rays with chemicals that can absorb different wavelengths of light. Some absorb only UVB rays. The new broad-spectrum sunscreens are better because they absorb both UVB rays and at least some UVA rays. Even better are sunscreens that contain the right combination of chemicals to cover the whole spectrum: UVB rays from 290 to 320 wavelengths and UVA rays from 320 to 400. A good choice is a product that combines an ABA-containing sunscreen (Padimate O) for UVB rays with Avobenzone for UVA rays. Here are the most common active ingredients.

- **Aminobenzoic acid and derivatives (ABA or PABA).** These screen UVB rays. They bind well to proteins in the skin and provide lasting protection. Ironically, ABA-containing sunscreens make some people even more susceptible to the sun's rays and can cause photoallergic reactions (see page 32). Of the ABA products, Padimate O is least likely to cause a photoallergic reaction, and it is not washed off the skin as easily as PABA. ABA-containing sunscreens containing alcohol often cause stinging on application.

HOW MUCH PROTECTION DO YOU NEED?

Each sunscreen has a sun protection factor (SPF) rating of its degree of protection against UVB light. A sunscreen with a higher SPF protects you longer. To find out how long, multiply the SPF by the length of time you can normally spend in the sun without burning. For example, if you normally burn after 15 minutes and are using SPF 20, you should come out of the sun after 5 hours (15 times 20 is 300 minutes).

Ordinarily, a product with an SPF of 15 or higher is appropriate unless you have particularly dark skin, in which case you may choose a lower-SPF product. More than 30 SPF is usually not necessary.

Thus far, there is no method for rating the UVA protection of sunscreens. However, it is best to choose a product which offers both UVA and UVB protection.

Reaction to sun	SPF
Always burns, rarely tans	20 to 30
Burns easily, tans slightly	15 to 20
Burns moderately, tans gradually	15
Minimal burn, tans well	4 to 8
Rarely burns, tans deeply	2 to 4

- **Anthranilate.** Because it covers some of the UVA range and only part of the UVB rays. Anthranilate is often combined with other, more powerful sunscreens to provide broader coverage.
- **Benzophenones.** Benzophenones (dioxybenzone, oxybenzone, sulisobenzone) primarily block UVB rays but extend into the UVA range. Oxybenzone, the most common ingredient, blocks some UVA rays up to 350 wavelengths. As single agents, these sunscreens are weaker against UVB than the ABA agents. They can also cause photosensitivity reactions and are often combined with other ingredients (such as Padimate O) to provide broad coverage.
- **Cinnamates.** Cinnamates (cinoxate, octyl-methoxycinnamate) screen all of the UVB range and some of the UVA range. Because they do not bind well to the skin, cinnamates are combined with

other sunscreens (such as benzophenones) and with emulsifiers that help them cling to the skin.

- **Dibenzoylmethane derivatives.** A new group of sunscreens, dibenzoylmethane derivatives (avobenzone, Parsol 1789), effectively screen UVA rays. Look for the ingredient avobenzone or butyl-methoxydibenzoylmethane (Parsol 1789) in combination with other ingredients. A dibenzoylmethane derivative absorbs ultraviolet radiation through the UVA range, though its effectiveness drops off above 370. Studies have shown that a combination of Padimate O and avobenzone produces the most effective coverage.

- **Salicylates and salicylic acid derivatives.** These weak UVB sunscreens must be used in high concentrations. They do not adhere well to the skin and so must be combined with emulsifiers. However, they are extremely safe and are often used to raise the SPF of combination products.

- **Physical sunscreens.** Because they scatter all UVA, UVB, and visible light, physical sunscreens offer an even broader range of coverage than chemical sunscreens. Zinc oxide and titanium dioxide block the sun's UVB and UVA rays almost like clothing does. They are available in a variety of colors, and are generally used in small areas such as the nose or tops of ears. Though effective, they are not routinely used for all-body protection because application is messy and has to be thick. They should be used for sensitive areas that get repeated, heavy sun exposure. They also offer effective protection from drug-induced photosensitivity reactions. Titanium dioxide is more transparent than zinc oxide, and it is now included in some chemical sunscreen products to broaden the range.

HOW TO USE A SUNSCREEN

Sunscreens should not be your first line of defense against the sun. Stay inside between 10 and 2 o'clock, or at least stay in the shade as much as possible, even on cloudy or hazy days. Wear protective clothing and hats. Tightly knit or woven material provides full-spectrum protection. Dark clothing is better than light clothing. A white T-shirt, for example, has an SPF as low as 4—less if it gets wet. A general rule is that, if light can pass through dry clothing when held up to the light, then UV light will also pass through it. A hat will protect some of the areas most vulnerable to skin cancer: your nose, lips, ears, and scalp.

After limiting your exposure at midday and wearing protective clothing, your third line of defense is a sunscreen. You have to use the sunscreen properly to get the best protection:

- Apply the sunscreen 30 minutes before you go out in the sun so that it can bind to the proteins in the outermost layer of the skin.
- Apply it liberally (2 to 2.5 ounces) to all exposed skin surfaces.
- Reapply it if you perspire, swim, or wipe off with a towel or clothing. A good rule of thumb is to reapply sunscreen every 90 minutes. However, reapplying sunscreen does not extend the amount of time you can spend in the sun without burning. Water-resistant products protect for up to 40 minutes of continuous water exposure before they need to be reapplied. Waterproof products protect for up to 80 minutes.
- Limit your time in the sun to the number of hours your sunscreen can protect you (see box, How Much Protection Do You Need?").
- If itching, redness, or a rash develops, stop using the product and ask your doctor or pharmacist about alternatives. Face lotions and moisturizers that contain sunscreen agents can also cause itching and redness, particularly when they come in contact with the eyes.

If you get a sunburn, take oral analgesics (aspirin or ibuprofen are better than acetaminophen because they help reduce the inflammation of sunburn). Also use cool compresses and a cool bath. Topical anesthetics such as benzocaine or lidocaine sprays will relieve pain for 15 to 45 minutes, but they should not be used on damaged, peeling skin because they (particularly lidocaine) may be absorbed and cause toxicity (confusion, dizziness).

part two

FOR
WOMEN ONLY

chapter 4

CONTRACEPTIVES

$\mathcal{A}$BOUT 90 PERCENT OF THE WOMEN IN THE
United States who engage in sexual intercourse use some form of contraception, yet more than half of all pregnancies are unplanned. One
reason is that many women lack information about contraceptives and
their use. The more you know about your options, the better you can
choose the method that's best for you, and the more effectively you
can use that contraceptive.

The first question most women ask is, "How well does the
method protect against pregnancy?" For each method described
below, there are two effectiveness ratings. Each tells how many times
the method of contraception successfully prevents pregnancy in
100 women in one year. A method with an effectiveness rating of 98
percent prevents pregnancy in 98 of 100 women in one year. The
first rating reflects perfect use, that is when the method is used
correctly every time. The second rating, typical use, takes into account such problems as a condom tearing, a woman forgetting to take
a birth-control pill, or failure to reapply spermicide for repeated intercourse. Only a few contraceptives are not susceptible to this kind
of human error—surgical sterilization, contraceptive injections
(Depo-Provera), and the contraceptive subdermal implant (Norplant).

Beyond effectiveness, there are other important considerations
when choosing your contraception method. Do you need protection
from sexually transmitted diseases (STDs)? Only a male or female
condom protects against STDs. If you are not in a monogamous rela-

tionship with someone who has been tested and found to be free of sexually transmitted diseases, then a condom is the right choice for you. There are other personal considerations too. If you are likely to forget to take pills, then birth-control pills may not be your best choice. If you dislike having to interrupt intercourse or deal with mechanical devices such as diaphragms, then the pill may be better for you. Consider the cost, but also think in terms of the cost per sexual act. Although a method such as an implant (Norplant) has a high up-front cost, in the long run it is much less expensive than most other methods if you are sexually active. If you have sex only occasionally, such methods as condoms, spermicides, or a diaphragm are less expensive. Birth-control pills bring a monthly cost as you purchase each new pack of pills. You must also consider whether you are likely to want to become pregnant in the near future. If so, a barrier method such as a condom or diaphragm rather than a hormonal method may be the right choice for you. Consider all the possibilities and choose a form that's right for you now. As your situation changes, re-evaluate your choice.

Hormonal contraceptives

Hormonal contraceptives include several kinds of birth-control pills as well as implants and injections. They are among the safest and most effective forms of birth control. More women use hormonal methods than any other kind of contraception except surgical sterilization.

Normally, the rising and falling hormonal levels in a woman's body produce the conditions that allow her to become pregnant. The cycle begins when the follicle-stimulating hormone (FSH) stimulates one of the ovaries to begin forming an egg follicle. Meanwhile, rising levels of estrogen cause the uterine lining to thicken and become receptive to an implanted fertilized egg. Midway in the cycle, a surge of leutenizing hormone (LH) causes the fully formed follicle to release an egg. Just before ovulation, hormonal changes alter the consistency of the cervical mucus so that sperm can swim efficiently through it to reach the egg, usually in the fallopian tube. Increasing progesterone further prepares the uterus for pregnancy. If the egg is not fertilized, the egg, along with the cells and blood from the uterine lining, pass out of the body during the menstrual period, and the process starts all over again.

Hormonal contraceptives interfere with this process. Instead of fluctuating hormonal levels, a steady amount of the female hormones estrogen and progesterone are provided by the hormonal contraceptives throughout the menstrual cycle. An unchanging level of estrogen prevents ovulation, while steady levels of progesterone cause the cervical mucus to be inhospitable to the transport of sperm and the uterine lining to inhibit a fertilized egg from implanting itself.

COMBINATION ORAL CONTRACEPTIVES

Effectiveness rating
Perfect use, 99 percent
Typical use, 97 percent

Combination oral contraceptives, often referred to as "the pill," are the most popular hormonal method. The combined pill consists of two hormones, an estrogen (either ethinyl estradiol or mestranol) and a progestin (a synthetic form of the female hormone progesterone). It prevents ovulation and the implantation of a fertilized egg. Progestin also forms a thick cervical mucus that makes it difficult for male sperm to enter the uterus. Combination oral contraceptives have been carefully studied and highly refined since their introduction in the 1960s, and the majority of the products used today are very different from the originals. Probably the most significant refinement has been the decrease in the level of estrogen contained in the pills. This has reduced short-term side effects and long-term health risks associated with estrogen.

There are two main classes of combined oral contraceptives. The high-dose agents containing 50 mcg or greater of estrogen are not used widely today. Lower-dose agents have 35 mcg or less of estrogen per tablet. Today most women start with a low-dose agent to lessen the risks and side effects associated with estrogens. This is important because the bulk of studies showing health risks such as blood clotting, high blood pressure, and liver disease were done on high-dose agents in the 1970s and early '80s.

In the last 10 years, research on combined oral contraceptives has focused on the progestin component. The progestins differ from product to product; most are associated with bothersome side effects such as excess body hair and acne, and some increase blood cholesterol. The researchers strove to determine the optimum dose of a progestin, one that would prevent implantation of an egg while reducing side effects. Based on this research, there are now three kinds of combined oral contraceptives: monophasic, biphasic, and triphasic.

Monophasic (one-phase) pills are used most widely. They provide a steady dose of estrogen and progestin throughout the menstrual cycle. Both high-dose (Ovral) and low-dose (Brevicon, Genora) monophasic products are available.

The biphasic (two-phase) and triphasic (three-phase) pills vary the amount of progestin throughout the menstrual cycle to more closely match the body's natural hormonal cycles. By lowering the progestin dose for at least a phase of the cycle, these pills reduce some of the side effects associated with progestin, including acne, weight gain, headaches, mood changes, and hair growth. The two-phase oral contraceptives (Jenest 28, Ortho-Novum 10/11, Nelova 10/11) have a lower dose of a progestin for the first 10 days of the cycle and a dose of estrogen that remains constant throughout the cycle. The triphasic contraceptives (Ortho-Novum 7/7/7, Tri-Levlen, Triphasil) have varied amounts of a progestin at three points during the cycle and estrogen that either remains constant or varies.

Two new progestins on the market, desogestrel and norgestimate (Desogen, Ortho-Cept, Ortho-Cyclen and Ortho Tri-Cyclen), have substantially fewer side effects than other progestins, including no weight gain, far less body hair growth, and even improvement in acne in some women. They also do not adversely affect cholesterol levels and have no effect on glucose tolerance for diabetics.

Combined oral contraceptives are safe for most women, including nonsmokers over the age of 40. Some studies have suggested that they lower the risk of endometrial cancer, ovarian cancer, and fibrocystic breast disease. In women under 35, they may also increase bone density. Many women find that the pill relieves menstrual cramps.

Do not take a combined oral contraceptive if you are over 35 and smoke cigarettes; the combination will greatly increase your risk of heart attack and stroke. Low-dose pills are safe for women with type 2 diabetes, but not for women with poorly controlled diabetes or peripheral vascular complications from diabetes. Women with high blood pressure can safely use oral contraceptives, but need to be monitored by their doctor. Combination oral contraceptives should not be taken by women with coronary artery disease, cerebrovascular disease, breast cancer, undiagnosed vaginal bleeding, thrombophlebitis or other thrombotic disorders, or active gallbladder disease (estrogen and progestin may promote gallstones, but the new triphasics should have little effect on the gallbladder).

Do not take an oral contraceptive if you think you may be pregnant. If you are breast-feeding, the estrogen in the pill may reduce your milk production and lower the protein component of milk. Although the American Academy of Pediatrics has approved the use of low-dose pills during breast-feeding, progestin-only methods like the minipill are a better choice.

Use

There are two different schedules depending on the product. With one method, you take your first pill the first day of your menstrual period. With the other, you take your first pill the first Sunday after your menstrual period begins. Ask your doctor or pharmacist when you should take your first pill.

Take a pill at the same time each day, preferably at bedtime so that you are less apt to be affected by bothersome side effects such as nausea and breast tenderness. With some prescriptions (21-day), you take no pill during the last week of the cycle. Others (28-day) include a placebo (a pill with no active ingredient) for the last week so that you stay in the habit of taking a pill every day.

Although the pill should protect you from pregnancy even during the first month, many doctors recommend a backup method of birth control for the first month just to be sure. If you are using the Sunday start method, you will need to use a backup method for at least the first seven days of the first month.

If you forget to take a pill, take it as soon as you remember. Carry your pills with you during the day so that if you forget, you can take the pill as soon as you remember. If you miss two pills in a row during the first two weeks of your pack, take two pills the day you remember and two pills the next day. Use a backup method of birth control for the next seven days. If you miss more than two pills in a row, start a new pack of pills and use backup birth control.

If you miss two pills during the third week of your pack and you are a day-one starter, throw out the rest of the pack and start a new pack of pills that day. If you have sex during the first seven days after you missed your pills, use a backup method for those seven days.

If you miss two pills during the third week of your pack and you are a Sunday starter, take one pill every day until Sunday. Then throw out the rest of the pack and start a new pack on Sunday. If you have sex during the first seven days after you missed your pills, use a backup method for those seven days.

If you want to try to become pregnant, finish out your packet of pills. Your periods may be irregular or absent after you stop taking your pills, but you should be fully fertile within three months of stopping.

Side effects

When you first begin taking a combination oral contraceptive, or if you miss a pill, you may have breakthrough bleeding and/or spotting. Breakthrough bleeding is heavier bleeding than spotting and requires use of a tampon or pad. Breakthrough bleeding is a more common side effect than spotting but usually goes away by the third month. If not, talk with your doctor or pharmacist about changing to a different combination oral contraceptive. If breakthrough bleeding occurs during the first 14 days of the cycle, you probably need a product with a higher dose of estrogen. If it occurs during the last 14 days, you probably need a higher dose of the progestin. In the first three months, breakthrough bleeding is not a sign that the contraceptive isn't working, but if it continues beyond three months, seek medical attention.

Combination oral contraceptives can also cause nausea, headaches, bloating, or tender breasts. These side effects may gradually go away or may be reduced by switching to a product with less estrogen. If you experience acne, weight gain, or increased hair growth, it may help to switch to a triphasic product with less progestin or to a product containing low androgenic progestin (norethindrone, desogestrel, norgestimate). Estrogen can cause pigment changes in skin exposed to sunlight, so use a sunscreen with SPF 15 when outdoors.

*W*ARNINGS SIGNS WITH THE PILL

When taking combination oral contraceptives, watch for these symptoms of possible problems. Report them to your doctor. Just remember: ACHES.

A FOR ABDOMINAL PAIN (SEVERE): sign of gallbladder disease, liver problems

C FOR CHEST PAIN: sign of blood clot in lungs

H FOR HEADACHES (SEVERE): sign of stroke, hypertension, migraine

E FOR EYE PROBLEMS (BLURRED VISION): sign of stroke or hypertension

S FOR SEVERE LEG PAIN (CALF OR THIGH): sign of blood clot in legs

MINIPILL

Effectiveness rating
Perfect use, 99 percent
Typical use, 97 percent

The minipill contains only progestin. For breast-feeding women, it is often the best choice because it does not contain estrogen, which can decrease milk production or reduce the protein component of breast milk. The minipill can also be taken by women who have breast cancer or cardiovascular disease, including high blood pressure, by women who smoke, and by those with migraines worsened by estrogen-containing contraceptives. Because it contains only a small dose of progestin (less than that in most combination oral contraceptives), it is slightly less effective than the combination pill (although still highly effective), but its effectiveness does drop quickly if you forget to take a pill. The most common brands of minipill are Ovrette and Nor-Q. D.

The progestin in the minipill prevents pregnancy by producing a thick cervical mucus that blocks the sperm from entering the uterus to fertilize the egg. It also inhibits ovulation and prevents the uterus from building up a thick lining in which a fertilized egg can implant.

MEDICATIONS THAT MAKE BIRTH-CONTROL PILLS LESS EFFECTIVE

Some antibiotics make combination oral contraceptives less effective by decreasing the amount of estrogen available to the body. The amount of interference depends on the dose of the antibiotic, the length of the treatment, and the amount of estrogen you are taking. If you take a low-dose contraceptive, use a backup method of contraceptive (such as a condom or diaphragm) while you are taking the antibiotic. If you are taking a full 10-day course of antibiotics, you must use a second method for the entire monthly cycle. If you have acne and are receiving long-term oral antibiotic therapy, consider using a topical antibiotic product (Topicycline, topical clindamycin gel or lotion, Eryderm) instead of oral antibiotics.

Some anticonvulsants may increase the removal of estrogen by the liver, thereby decreasing the effectiveness of the estrogen. A number of cases of unwanted pregnancy have been reported. A warning sign of this interaction is spotting. If you have seizures and are being treated with one of these anticonvulsants, a better choice may be a progestin-only method, particularly by injection.

antibiotics
  ampicillin
  cephalosporins (Keflex, Ceclor)
  erythromycin
  penicillins (Pen Vee K)
  sulfonamides (Bactrim, Septra)

  tetracyclines
  rifampin
anticonvulsants
  carbamazepine (Tegretol)
  phenytoin (Dilantin)
  phenobarbital

The minipill should not be taken by women with undiagnosed abnormal vaginal bleeding because it may mask the symptoms of a problem.

Use

Take one pill a day, always at the same time of day. For the first two months, use a backup method of birth control. Because the minipill does not consistently suppress ovulation, many medical experts recommend that you use a second method of contraception such as a barrier method for 8 days during each cycle, beginning 4 days before suspected ovulation and ending 4 days after. Ovulation occurs around the day 15 for the average woman with a 28-day cycle.

If you miss taking your pill by more than 3 hours, take it as soon as you remember and use a backup method of birth control, such as a condom and spermicide, for the next 48 hours. If you miss two or more pills in a row, take two pills as soon as you remember and use backup birth control for the rest of the month. To deal with irregular bleeding, use panty liners and carry pads or tampons with you.

If you want to use this method while breast-feeding, wait until breast-feeding is well established, at least six weeks after the birth.

Side effects

Because the minipill contains such a low dose of progestin, typical progestin-related side effects such as tiredness, acne, appetite changes, and mood disturbances are infrequent. But because the dose is so low, there is an increased risk of irregular bleeding. Some women taking the minipill have a longer or shorter menstrual period than usual, and others have spotting at unpredictable times. Some women do not menstruate at all or have as few as two periods a year. If you have no period within 45 days or more, do a pregnancy test. Also watch for the ACHES early warning signs (page 73).

CONTRACEPTIVE IMPLANTS

Effectiveness rating
Perfect use, 99 percent
Typical use, 99 percent

The levonorgestrel implant, sold under the brand name Norplant, is a highly effective method of birth control that provides long-term contraception without the use of pills. A doctor places six rubber capsules (small tubes) filled with a progestin, levonorgestrel, under the skin of your inner arm. Levonorgestrel is released slowly into the body and provides contraception for five years. Similar to other progestin products, levonorgestrel inhibits ovulation, decreases the lining of the uterus, and thickens the cervical mucus, which prevents sperm from reaching the uterus.

Fertility returns within 24 hours of removing the capsules. A disadvantage is that the method becomes less effective after two years in women who weigh more than 150 pounds. The levonorgestrel implant is safe for breast-feeding mothers. Although its manufacturers currently recommend it be inserted six weeks after childbirth to allow for the establishment of breast-feeding, it is often administered immediately postpartum in lactating mothers with no ill effects.

Hormone implants should not be used by women with acute liver disease, active thrombophlebitis, or breast cancer. Similar to the combination oral contraceptives, the levonorgestrel implant can interact with some antiseizure medications (see page 74). Phenytoin, phenobarbital, primidone, and carbamazepine may decrease the effectiveness of the implant and lead to unwanted pregnancy. An alternative method of birth control such as the minipill or medroxyprogesterone (MPS) by injection should be considered if you are receiving one of these seizure medications. The effectiveness of the implants is not affected by antibiotics.

Use

A doctor inserts the implants under the skin of your upper arm. This minor surgical procedure takes 15 to 60 minutes and is usually painless because it is done under local anesthesia. The incision leaves a small scar on your arm. Although the outline of the capsules may be visible to you, the capsules won't break or move around inside the arm. If inserted within the first seven days of the menstrual cycle, the implant will be effective within 24 hours. After five years, the implant must be removed and can be replaced. The implant can be removed sooner if you decide you want to change contraceptive methods or if you want to become pregnant. For removal choose a doctor who is experienced in this technique. Fertility returns within 24 hours. If you are starting a new method of contraception, begin using it the day the implants are removed.

Side effects

Eighty percent of users experience irregular menstrual bleeding. Spotting often stops after a year. Less common side effects are acne, headaches, nervousness, nausea, weight gain, and unwanted hair growth.

Call your doctor if you see any pus or bleeding or feel pain in the area of the implants. These are signs of possible infection.

LONG-ACTING CONTRACEPTIVE INJECTIONS

Effectiveness rating
Perfect use, 99.7 percent
Typical use, 99.7 percent

Medroxyprogesterone acetate (MPA; Depo-Provera) is a safe, highly effective contraceptive that consists of a progestin given by injection every three months. As do minipills and levonorgestrel implants, the injections produce a thick cervical mucus to prevent the sperm from entering the uterus, inhibit ovulation, and decrease the growth of the lining of the uterus.

MPA was approved by the FDA in 1992 after almost two decades of scientific review and is the only injectable contraceptive available in the United States. It is used by 30 million women in over 90 countries. Approval in the United States was delayed by concerns about risk of breast cancer, but a nine-year study of more than 11,000 users found that the risk was comparable to other hormonal contraceptives. The injections were also found to decrease the risk of endometrial cancer.

This method is reliable and doesn't require that you remember to take a pill at the same time each day. MPA may be a good choice for women who have sickle cell disease or who have had epileptic seizures, because it has been shown to reduce the severity of these conditions. Its effectiveness is not affected by the patient's weight or by other drugs.

MPA should not be used by women with acute liver disease, active thrombophlebitis or other thrombotic disorders, or breast cancer. It is safe for breast-feeding mothers and infants but should not be started until breast-feeding is well established, at about six weeks.

Use

The doctor or nurse will inject the recommended dose of 150 mg of MPA into the muscle of your buttocks once every three months. MPA is usually given on day 5 of your menstrual period to ensure that you are not pregnant and to allow for prevention of ovulation during the first month of use. At your appointment, schedule your next injection. If you miss your next appointment, be sure to get your injection within two weeks to ensure continuous contraceptive protection. One injection lasts for 14 weeks, although you will be scheduled for injection every 12 weeks.

To cope with unpredictable menstrual changes during the first few months, wear panty liners and carry pads or tampons with you at all times. Bleeding should lessen, and about 50 percent of women stop menstruating completely after one year. If you experience unusually heavy bleeding, call your doctor.

When you discontinue the injections, you will begin to ovulate again, probably four or five months after the last shot.

Side effects

The side effects of MPA injections are similar to those of other progestin-based birth-control methods. The main side effect is a changed menstrual pattern. Your flow may increase or decrease; the time between periods may be irregular; or you may have spotting. Less common side effects include headaches, acne, abdominal bloating, mood changes, weight gain (2 to 7 pounds), and unwanted hair growth. More women experience headaches, dizziness, depression and mood changes with MPA than with the minipill. If you experience uncomfortable side effects and want to stop using the method, you will have to wait about four or five months after the last shot for your hormone levels to return to normal.

MORNING-AFTER PILL

Effectiveness rating
Perfect use, 99 percent
Typical use, 98 percent

The morning-after pill is a safe and highly effective contraceptive for emergencies, such as sexual assault or failure of your birth-control method (for example, a ripped condom). It is safer than having an abortion at a later date. Morning-after pills contain a high dose of estrogen and progestin. They block the passage of a fertilized egg through the fallopian tube and prevent the growth of the uterine lining.

A number of combination oral contraceptives have been studied for use as morning-after pills. Those most commonly used for this purpose are Ovral, Lo/Ovral, Tri-Levlen, and Triphasil. These pills are available only by prescription. Another drug, mifepristone, may also be used in the future as a form of morning-after contraception. Not yet approved by the FDA, mifepristone (also known as RU-486) blocks the effects of progesterone. A single oral dose has been shown to stop the implantation of a fertilized egg.

Use

If you have had unprotected intercourse, call your doctor or health clinic immediately and ask for morning-after contraception. The pills should be taken as soon as possible after intercourse and must be started within 72 hours.

Side effects

Because of the high dose of estrogen ingested per dose, there is a risk of nausea and vomiting. If you vomit, you must repeat the dose. Side effects include nausea, breast tenderness, and light vaginal bleeding. Also watch for the ACHES danger signs (see page 73).

Barrier contraceptives

Another group of contraceptives place a physical or chemical barrier between the sperm and egg. Often a physical barrier such as a diaphragm or condom must be combined with a chemical spermicide for increased effectiveness. Male and female condoms are the only birth-control methods that protect not only against pregnancy but also against sexually transmitted diseases, including AIDS.

SPERMICIDES

Effectiveness rating
Perfect use, 94 percent
Typical use, 79 percent

Spermicides kill sperm as they enter the vagina. They are available over the counter in several forms—from most to least effective: foam, cream, jelly, gel, films, and vaginal suppository. Some spermicides are designed to be used with diaphragms or cervical caps, and others come with applicators that allow you to insert the product into your vagina. Be sure to check the labeling of the product to determine if it is appropriate for your situation. For example, if you are using a spermicide as the sole method of contraception or with a condom, you should be sure to use a "high concentration" spermicide. Either the lower- or higher-concentration spermicides can be used with cervical caps or diaphragms.

Most spermicide products contain nonoxynol 9, and a few contain octoxynol 9. The two chemicals are similar, but nonoxynol 9 may inhibit a number of organisms associated with STDs, such as chlamydia, genital herpes, syphilis, gonorrhea, and AIDS. For this reason, most people prefer nonoxynol 9.

Used alone, spermicides are less effective in preventing pregnancy than other methods of contraception, but used together with condoms, cervical caps, or diaphragms they can be highly effective. Spermicides offer some, but not sufficient, protection against sexually transmitted disease. Women who are breast-feeding can use spermicides safely.

Use

Pay close attention to the product labeling. Foams, available in aerosol cans, and jellies and creams, available in tubes, all come with applicators. After filling the applicator with the recommended amount of spermicide, insert the applicator high into your vagina and push in the plunger. Foams are effective immediately after insertion and can be applied up to 30 to 60 minutes before intercourse. Jellies and creams should be applied at least 10 minutes but not more than 60 minutes before intercourse for optimal protection (see the package insert for the timing for the particular product).

If you are using a suppository or a spermicidal film, insert it with your finger high into the vagina at least 15 minutes before intercourse to give it time to melt. You must remember to unwrap the suppository before insertion. If you do not give the suppository enough time to melt in the vaginal secretions, you may experience a gritty, irritating feeling during intercourse. Also, you will not have optimal protection.

For all spermicides, insert another dose before repeating intercourse. Most spermicides are effective for one hour; films are effective for two. Do not douche afterward, especially in the first eight hours.

Side effects

Some women and men find that the chemicals in spermicides irritate their skin or genital tissues; if this happens to you, try switching brands.

MALE CONDOM

Effectiveness rating
Perfect use, 97 percent
Typical use, 88 percent
Use with spermicide, 99 percent

Used properly and combined with a spermicide, the male condom is a safe and highly effective method of birth control. A male condom is a thin sheath that is placed on the erect male penis before contact with the vaginal area. It prevents sperm from entering the vagina. In addition to protecting you from pregnancy and sexually transmitted diseases, condoms also provide some protection against cervical cancer and cervical dysplasia. While some men find that using a condom diminishes sensitivity, others find it lengthens the time they can maintain an erection.

Condoms may be made of latex, polyurethane, or animal membrane (lambskin). Latex or polyurethane condoms are the best choices because the animal membrane condoms do not protect against STDs. However, some people are allergic to latex (they have reacted in the past to rubber gloves or a balloon). The irritant may be the spermicide, not the latex.

You can buy lubricated or nonlubricated products. Lubrication reduces the risk of tearing. Condoms are also available with spermicide. Whether or not the condom is prelubricated with spermicide, you should still apply a vaginal dose of spermicide for extra protection.

Use

Condoms are widely available in pharmacies and supermarkets without a prescription. Only male condoms made of latex or polyurethane (and the female condom made of polyurethane) protect against sexually transmitted diseases such as AIDS. To reduce the risk of ripping or breaking, choose a lubricated condom with a reservoir at the tip to collect semen. You can improve the effectiveness of the contraception by choosing a condom with a spermicidal lotion inside and out or by inserting spermicide into your vagina before intercourse.

Make sure your partner is willing to use the condom before you begin to make love. It must be placed on the erect penis before it comes in contact with the vaginal area—pre-ejaculatory secretions may contain sperm. You or your partner places the condom on the erect penis by unrolling the ring down the shaft of the penis to the base. Leave some space at the tip to collect semen; the condom tip should be pinched as it is unrolled to get the air out and to allow for an empty space. If you find it difficult to insert the penis into the vagina, stop so you don't tear the condom. More foreplay may help your vagina lubricate naturally, or use a water-based lubricant (such as K-Y lubricating jelly, Lubrin, or a spermicidal jelly or cream) available from the pharmacy. Do not use an oil-based lubricant like petroleum jelly or baby oil, which can damage the latex. After intercourse, hold the condom at the base while the man withdraws his penis from your vagina so that no semen spills in or near your vagina. Remove the condom from the penis and throw it away.

When using a condom, it is important to have a spermicidal jelly, cream, or foam handy in case the condom breaks. Immediately insert the spermicide into the vagina; don't use a spermicidal suppository or film because they take too long to work. Also, don't use a condom if it is brittle or sticky (these are signs of decomposition). Condoms should be stored away from excessive light or heat; a wallet or glove compartment is not a good storage place for this reason.

DIAPHRAGM

Effectiveness rating
Perfect use, 94 percent
Typical use, 82 percent

A diaphragm is a soft dome of latex or silicone rubber that is coated with spermicide and inserted into the vagina to cover the cervix, preventing sperm from reaching the uterus. It is the spermicide that protects against pregnancy; the diaphragm helps the spermicide do its job by holding the spermicide in place at the opening of the cervix.

When used correctly, a diaphragm is an effective form of birth control, but if the diaphragm does not fit properly, or the woman does not reapply spermicidal jelly each time she has intercourse, the effectiveness drops to about 82 percent, less than the condom and only 3 percent better than spermicide alone.

The diaphragm can be inserted up to six hours before intercourse, so it does not have to interrupt lovemaking. Another advantage is that long-term use may reduce your risk of cervical dysplasia, the abnormal cell changes of the cervix that lead to cervical cancer. Some women, particularly those with several children, may not have strong enough pelvic or vaginal muscles to hold a standard diaphragm firmly in place, but there is a special diaphragm for them.

Use

Diaphragms are between 2 and 4 inches across. Flat-ring diaphragms can be inserted with an applicator. Diaphragms with arcing or coil spring rims can be inserted with your fingers. Both type of diaphragms are available only by prescription and must fit properly to be effective. During a pelvic examination, your doctor will measure you for the correct size and also show you how to insert the device properly. Before leaving the doctor's office, you should also make sure to practice inserting the diaphragm once or twice on your own.

Because tiny holes can develop over time, allowing sperm to leak through, replace your diaphragm once a year. You should be refitted each year too, as your size may have changed. You should also be refitted if you gain or lose 20 or more pounds or if you have given birth or had a miscarriage or abortion.

To use the diaphragm, wash your hands and then squeeze a tablespoonful of spermicidal jelly into the bowl of the diaphragm. Spread a little jelly around the rim to help hold the diaphragm in place. If you are using a coil spring or arcing device, squeeze together two sides of the diaphragm ring and gently insert it into the vagina, pushing it all the way in. Next, push the end nearest the opening of your vagina up above your pelvic bone. Consult the diagram that comes with your diaphragm to make sure you are positioning it correctly. Feel with your finger to make sure the cervix is covered (it feels like a soft mound).

If you are using a flat-spring diaphragm, look for the notches on the applicator that are numbered to match up with the size of the diaphragm. Hold the diaphragm with the dome upward, and hook the rim onto the large notch at the end of the applicator. Then hook the other end of the diaphragm into the notch that has the corresponding number size. The diaphragm should be stretched into a flat oval and the dome should have a number of folds in it. The spermicide should be placed in these folds and be placed around the rim. With the spermicide facing up, the applicator should be inserted into the vagina and angled toward the back. When you have positioned it over your cervix, twist the applicator to release it from the diaphragm. With one finger, push the rim up behind the pubic bone. Consult the directions that come with the device.

Leave the diaphragm in place for at least six hours after intercourse to allow for full protection. If you have intercourse again during that time, or if more than two hours have passed between insertion and intercourse, apply more spermicide into the vagina with an applicator without removing the diaphragm. Do not douche while the diaphragm is in place; douching may dilute the spermicide and reduce its effectiveness. Make sure you remove the diaphragm within 10 hours to avoid the slight risk of toxic shock syndrome.

To remove a diaphragm, wash your hands and reach into your vagina with one finger, hooking the edge of the ring that rests behind your pelvic bone and pulling the ring out. Wash the diaphragm with mild soap, dry it, and store it in its case away from extreme heat or cold. Do not use any dusting powder such as talcum or a perfumed powder on the diaphragm. Check your diaphragm for holes regularly by holding it up to the light. Replace your diaphragm if the rubber shows any signs of deterioration, and replace it every year in any case.

Side effects

The diaphragm is almost completely safe. A few women who use a diaphragm get urinary tract infections. If you have recurring urinary tract infections, tell your doctor that you use a diaphragm. It may be pushing forward near your bladder or urethra, and you may need a smaller size. Any vaginal irritation may be caused by spermicide rather than the diaphragm. Change to another brand. If irritation or urinary infections continue, you may want to switch to a new form of birth control.

CERVICAL CAP

Effectiveness rating
Perfect use, 88.5 percent
Typical use, 82 percent

A cervical cap is a small, thimble-like device that fits over the opening of the cervix and blocks sperm from entering the uterus. It is used with a spermicide. Unlike the diaphragm, it does not rely on vaginal muscles to stay in place—suction holds it in place. Some women find a cervical cap more difficult to insert than a diaphragm because it is smaller and must fit more snugly over the cervix. Unlike the diaphragm, the cap cannot be used during your menstrual period because it will trap menstrual blood and may lead to infection. Menstrual blood flow may also reduce the suction. The cervical cap is less effective in women who have had children because pregnancy and childbirth cause softening of the cervix, so that the suction device is less effective.

Use

Your doctor must fit you with the correct size by measuring your cervix during a pelvic exam. A cervical cap is available only by prescription. A Pap smear is required prior to insertion, three months later, then yearly.

You must insert the cap at least 20 minutes before intercourse to allow a good seal to develop. However, it can be inserted up to 48 hours before intercourse. First wash your hands, then fill one-third of the cap with spermicide. Don't use too much spermicide and don't spread it on the rim. With your finger, feel inside your vagina to locate your cervix, a soft mound. Next squeeze the edges of the cap together with your fingers and push it inside your vagina along the back wall until it reaches your cervix. Push the cap onto your cervix. If you have difficulty reaching your cervix, put one foot up on a chair while inserting the cap.

If the cap is properly placed, you should be able to feel your cervix through it. You should also feel some space in the cup, which will be taken up by cervical secretions. If you have difficulty inserting the cup, ask your pharmacist for a cervical cap "introducer."

After intercourse, feel to make sure the cap remains securely in place. If it has been dislodged, push it back in position and put more spermicide in your vagina without removing the cap. If you have intercourse again, apply more spermicide without removing the cap. Leave the cap in place for at least 8 hours but no longer than 48 hours. Many women notice an unpleasant odor if the cap is in place for more than 24 hours. Do not douche while the cap is in place.

To remove the cap, hook your finger over the rim and pull, or push the cap forward with your middle finger and hook your index finger around the rim and pull. Wash the cap with soap and warm water. A cotton swab should also be used to clean the groove inside the rim of the cap. Do not use dusting powders, oils, or petroleum jelly on the cap. Regularly hold the cap up to the light to check for holes or signs of deterioration. Replace your cap once a year.

FEMALE CONDOM

Effectiveness rating
Perfect use, 95 percent
Typical use, 79 percent

The female condom, if used correctly, protects you and your partner from sexually transmitted diseases as well as pregnancy. Unlike the male condom, the female version also offers some protection against genital herpes and genital warts because it covers your external organs. Unlike a diaphragm or cap, the condom or pouch not only covers your cervix but lines your entire vaginal canal, protecting it from exposure to STDs.

The female condom is available now on a limited basis through clinics but is expected to be available soon over the counter. It consists of two rings connected by a polyurethane sheath that is about 7 inches in length. Polyurethane is thinner and more flexible than latex. It also does not degrade if exposed to oil-based products like petroleum jelly. It comes prelubricated and contains extra lubricant if needed.

Unlike the male condom, which requires the cooperation of the male partner, you control the use of the female condom. However, some women find it cumbersome during lovemaking. If the condom moves with the penis, try using lubricant on the penis or on the part of the condom that extends outside your body. Some men and women also find that the female condom decreases sexual sensitivity.

Use

Keep your condom with you if there is any chance you may have sexual contact. It can be inserted from several hours to minutes before intercourse. To insert the condom, squeeze the sides of the smaller ring together and slide the ring into your vagina, pushing it as far as possible up against your cervix, as if you were inserting a diaphragm. The larger ring remains outside your vagina. You do not have to remove it immediately after sex, but use a new one if you plan to have intercourse again. Before intercourse, you may notice that the condom or pouch has a lot of slack in it; this will be removed during intercourse when the vagina expands. The male should not wear a condom when the female condom is used. If the penis dislodges the condom or if the outer ring is pushed inside the vagina, apply more spermicide.

Other contraceptives

Besides hormonal and barrier methods of contraception, there are a few other choices. One is the most commonly used method of all—

surgical sterilization of the woman or man. Other options are intrauterine devices (IUDs) and natural family planning.

INTRAUTERINE DEVICES

Effectiveness rating, Progestasert
Perfect use, 98.5 percent
Typical use, 97 percent
Effectiveness rating, ParaGard T 380A
Perfect use, 99.4 percent
Typical use, 99.2 percent

An intrauterine device (IUD) is a plastic T-shaped device placed in the uterus to prevent pregnancy. These devices cause an inflammation of the uterus. They may work in part by changing the lining of the uterus so the sperm cannot reach the fallopian tubes to fertilize an egg. Also, the inflammatory response may kill the sperm before they even reach the fallopian tubes.

Because IUDs increase the risk of pelvic inflammatory disease and uterine perforation, which can lead to infertility, they are recommended only for women who have completed their families and are not at high risk of contracting a sexually transmitted disease. The risk of ectopic pregnancy (a pregnancy that lodges outside the uterus) is 10 times greater than for women who take combination oral contraceptives.

IUDs are not recommended for women whose medical history includes thrombosis, problems with blood clotting, anemia, abnormal uterine anatomy, endocarditis, artificial heart valves, or dizziness. They are also not recommended if you live in a rural or remote area far from emergency medical treatment, which would be necessary if you were to bleed excessively or spontaneously expel the IUD.

Two types of IUDs are available. The Progestasert, which must be replaced each year, increases protection by gradually releasing the hormone progesterone. The ParaGard T 380A is covered with a copper wire that intensifies the inflammatory response to the IUD. The Para-Gard T 380A can be worn for eight years and is slightly more effective in preventing pregnancy. The Dalkon Shield, found in the 1970s to cause an unacceptable risk of PID, is no longer on the market.

Use

An IUD is usually inserted during the menstrual period, since there is no chance of pregnancy and the cervix is relaxed. An IUD can be inserted six weeks after childbirth.

You may want to take a mild pain reliever, such as ibuprofen, 20 minutes before the procedure. To insert the IUD, your doctor opens your vagina with a speculum and inserts a slender rod into your cervix to measure it and determine its position. Next, the doctor slides the IUD into your uterus inside a plastic tube, which is then withdrawn, allowing the T-shaped arms of the IUD to unfold. Two strings that hang from the IUD are cut to the proper length inside your vagina. Insertion takes no more than 5 to 10 minutes. You will return to your doctor for a checkup a month later. You may experience mild cramping or discomfort during the procedure and for a few hours afterward. Some people feel dizzy and have a change in blood pressure. Your doctor may prescribe a mild pain reliever and may give you antibiotics to prevent infection. The IUD is effective immediately after insertion. If possible, have someone there to drive you home.

The strings of the IUD should hang inside your vagina where you can feel them with your fingers. For the first few weeks, check them twice a week. After the first few weeks, you should check once a month after your period. If you do not feel the strings or if they are hanging lower or even protruding out of your vagina, call your doctor immediately. The IUD may have slipped from its place and have to be reinserted.

If you want to become pregnant or use a different form of birth control, the IUD must be removed by your doctor. If you become pregnant, have the IUD removed immediately.

Side effects

An IUD may cause heavy vaginal bleeding, spotting, or pain. In particular, your first period after insertion may be heavier and more uncomfortable than usual. These side effects usually lessen with time, but 10 to 15 percent of women have such severe problems that the IUD is removed. In another 5 to 20 percent of women, contractions of the uterus expel the IUD within the first year, usually in the first three months.

Less common complications include infection and injury to the

WARNING SIGNS WITH AN IUD

When using an IUD, watch for these early warning signs. Report them to your doctor. Just remember: PAIN.

P FOR PERIOD LATE: sign of pregnancy

A FOR ABDOMINAL PAIN WITH INTERCOURSE

I FOR INFECTION: fever, discharge

N FOR NOT FEELING RIGHT: string missing, shorter, or longer

wall of the uterus. Watch for signs of ectopic pregnancy (see page 119) and pelvic inflammatory disease (see page 247), both more common among women who use IUDs.

NATURAL FAMILY PLANNING

Effectiveness rating
Typical use, 80 percent

Women who have moral or religious objections to other birth-control methods may choose natural family planning, which attempts to avoid intercourse during fertile times of the menstrual cycle. The woman must first determine the day she ovulates, when the ovary releases a new egg that travels down the fallopian tube to the uterus. The average day of ovulation during a 28-day cycle is day 14, but if you want to use this method, you need to be more exact. There are several ways to pinpoint your ovulation day: an ovulation predictor kit that you can purchase at a pharmacy, the temperature method, or the cervical mucus method. A combination of these methods—rather than one method alone—is the best way to identify your risk-free days. (By the way, many women use these same methods when they are trying to become pregnant and want to find their most fertile time.)

Use

The goal of all three methods is to determine the day you ovulate. The egg can survive for 12 to 24 hours after it is released, but sperm can live for two to seven days inside the fallopian tube. To avoid pregnancy, you must not have intercourse for seven days before ovulation and three days after it.

For the temperature method, take your temperature with a basal thermometer, which measures tenths of a degree, so you can detect a small change in temperature. Your temperature should be taken at the same time each morning before you get out of bed. Any physical activity—even shaking down the thermometer—can influence the temperature reading. (Use a digital thermometer or remember to shake down the thermometer before you go to bed at night.) Record the temperature on a chart. Your temperature usually drops 12 to 24 hours before ovulation and then begins to rise over 24 to 48 hours. The rise is small, only 0.2 to 0.8 degree above your lowest temperature reading. Watch for a temperature elevation that lasts three days. On the fourth day, you can resume intercourse. This method helps you determine that ovulation has occurred, but does not allow you to identify with confidence your preovulatory time, when the risk of fertility is also high; combining this method with the cervical mucus method is a good idea for this reason.

The cervical mucus method monitors the color and texture of your vaginal discharge. As you near ovulation, the mucus from your cervix changes from a whitish-yellow tacky discharge to a more fluid mucus. When you notice a clear, stringy mucus that resembles raw egg white, you are about to ovulate. The last day this thin discharge appears is called the peak day. Ovulation usually occurs on the day after the peak day. You are fertile from the day the thin, clear mucus first appears until four days after the peak day. Your discharge usually becomes thicker after ovulation, and you can consider yourself as infertile from four days after the peak until your period starts. This method does not work if you frequently have vaginal infections. If you combine this method with the temperature method, you have to abstain for 17 days per cycle.

Ovulation predictor tests, available without a prescription, work by detecting a surge in luteinizing hormone. (For more about these tests, see page 125.)

SURGICAL STERILIZATION

Surgical sterilization is a common operation that can be performed on a man or a woman to permanently prevent conception. Couples who do not want to have any more children often choose this method.

The male procedure, vasectomy, is simpler and easier than the female procedure because the male organs are outside the body. The doctor cuts the two tubes (vas deferens) that would otherwise carry sperm manufactured in each testicle to the penis. Afterward, the man has a normal erection and ejaculation, but his semen contains no sperm. Complications of vasectomy are rare but may include hematoma, a painful swelling caused by a leaking blood vessel that lasts a day or two. To reduce the risk of hematoma, the man should stay off his feet for the first 24 hours following the procedure. A couple should use an alternate form of contraception until the man has had two consecutive tests a month apart showing no sperm in his semen.

A woman can be surgically sterilized by a procedure called tubal ligation, which cuts the fallopian tubes so the sperm cannot reach the eggs. The doctor inserts a long, thin tube called a laparoscope through a small incision in the abdomen. Instruments are passed through the tube to cut and clip the two fallopian tubes. Afterward, the woman should rest and recover for several days and may feel discomfort. Complications, which are rare, include infection, internal bleeding, or injury of nearby organs.

chapter 5

HORMONE
REPLACEMENT
THERAPY

$\mathcal{H}$ORMONE REPLACEMENT THERAPY (HRT) IS THE use of hormones, prescribed by your doctor, to replace the drop in hormones, particularly estrogen, that occurs naturally in a woman's body at menopause. Not everyone needs to take hormone replacement therapy, but the health benefits are important enough that every woman should discuss the possibility with her doctor when she approaches or has reached menopause.

To understand what hormone replacement therapy can do for you, you need to understand how a woman's body changes at menopause. Menopause occurs officially when a woman stops menstruating, which happens on average at age 51 but can be earlier or later. It occurs when the eggs a woman is born with are used up. Every woman is born with a set number of ovarian follicles, eggs encased in sacs. At birth, the ovaries contain about 2 million follicles; by puberty, only 300,000 to 400,000 remain. During each menstrual cycle, 6 to 12 of these follicles mature. Each month only one follicle matures enough to release an egg during ovulation, and the rest degenerate. Only about 400 follicles mature and release eggs during a woman's entire reproductive years. At menopause, no viable follicles or eggs are left.

Before menopause, as the follicles mature, they cause the ovaries to produce hormones. There are three estrogens. The most potent is 17-beta estradiol. Half as potent is the next form, estrone. Estrone is broken down into estriol, which is very weak, having only one-eightieth the potency of estradiol. The ovaries also produce progesterone and testosterone during the menstrual cycle. At menopause, the folli-

cles no longer exist to stimulate the production of estrogen and progesterone. However, the ovaries still continue to produce testosterone
for a number of years after menopause.

For several months or years before menopause, a woman's periods
become irregular as less natural hormone is produced. At menopause,
the amount of estradiol produced by the ovaries is close to zero; this
produces symptoms such as hot flashes. The body continues to produce estrone from a testosterone-like product in body fat (which is
why obese women usually have fewer menopausal symptoms than
lean women). At menopause, progesterone levels also fall abruptly to
near zero. Levels of testosterone fall more gradually—about 30 percent less by the fifth year after menopause.

Besides the natural menopause that happens with aging,
menopause can also be caused by the surgical removal of the ovaries.
This causes a drastic change in all the hormones and usually causes
severe symptoms of menopause. Also, premature menopause may occur if the ovaries fail because they are exposed to radiation or cancer
drugs.

While menopause is a natural part of life, not a disease that needs
to be treated, some women find the symptoms uncomfortable and difficult. The decline of estrogen affects not only the reproductive system but also the urinary tract, heart and blood vessels, bones, breasts,
hair, skin, and pelvic muscles. Most dangerously, reduced estrogen
levels raise the risk of heart disease and osteoporosis. Hormone replacement therapy can reduce not only symptoms but also long-term
health risks.

Hormone replacement therapy usually takes the form of a daily
dose of estrogen plus a dose of a synthetic form of progesterone for at
least 13 days of the monthly cycle. Women who have had a hysterectomy can take estrogen alone.

HRT has many benefits, but there are also some unanswered
questions, possible side effects, and for some women, potential risks.
You should base your decision on your symptoms and your personal
and family health histories.

Treating symptoms of menopause

Declining levels of estrogen cause unpleasant symptoms for some, though not all, women. One goal of hormone replacement therapy is to reduce these symptoms.

HOT FLASHES

About three-quarters of women experience hot flashes, which are sudden, intense increases in body temperature lasting one to three minutes. Perspiration and heartbeat may increase. Hot flashes that occur during the night, called night sweats, can lead to insomnia and sleep deprivation. Hot flashes typically begin before the last menstrual period and occur for about five years. A few women have hot flashes much longer, even their whole lives. Hot flashes occur because estrogens stabilize the thermostat in the brain. Without estrogens, the thermostat is more easily influenced by other chemicals in the body. Also, hot flashes may be made worse by drinking hot beverages or alcohol.

Hot flashes are not only uncomfortable but difficult to deal with, particularly in public. One strategy is to dress in layers that you can remove when you feel a hot flash coming on. If night sweats are drenching your night clothes and sheets, keep clean ones close by so you can make yourself comfortable again without disrupting your sleep more than necessary.

Estrogen replacement therapy usually alleviates hot flashes in two to four weeks. An alternative, the blood-pressure-reducing drug clonidine, is sometimes prescribed to relieve menopausal symptoms but is usually less effective and can cause dizziness and fatigue.

If estrogen replacement is not controlling your symptoms, another option is a combination of estrogen with an androgen (methyltestosterone) such as Estratest. This combination has been approved by the FDA only for the treatment of hot flashes that have not been controlled by estrogen replacement.

URINARY INCONTINENCE

Declining estrogen levels often weaken the tissues and muscles of the urinary tract and bladder. The result may be either painful urination or incontinence, the involuntary leaking of urine. Oral hormone replacement therapy can help. Estrogen creams applied to the vagina may also relieve this problem. Estrogens may or may not relieve stress incontinence, the loss of small amounts of urine when coughing, laughing, or jumping.

For mild incontinence, an alternative to HRT is a program of pelvic-floor exercises, known as Kegels, which strengthen the muscles of the pelvic floor and improve bladder control. If Kegel exercises or HRT does not solve the problem, ask your doctor about surgical options.

VAGINAL DRYNESS OR IRRITATION

As estrogen levels decline, the tissues of the vagina become thinner and drier. The vagina may become shorter, narrower, and more prone

PELVIC-FLOOR EXERCISES (KEGELS)

Women of every age benefit from doing pelvic-floor exercises every day to strengthen their pelvic muscles. These simple exercises can prevent or cure many health problems. They can help prevent or reduce urinary incontinence, prepare for and recover from childbirth, increase sexual pleasure, and keep vaginal tissues healthy as a woman ages.

1. To learn how to do Kegels, first locate your pelvic-floor muscles. The easiest way is to stop urinating in midstream. The muscles you used are your pelvic-floor muscles. Stop and start several times to get the feel of the muscle action.
2. Once you have identified the proper muscles, you can do these exercises anywhere, anytime, sitting, standing, or lying down.
3. Flex your pelvic-floor muscles and hold for two to three seconds. Repeat the flex 10 times. Repeat the set of 10 several times during the day.
4. Gradually work up to holding the flex for 8 to 10 seconds. Repeat the flex 10 times. Repeat the set of 10 at least five times a day.

to infection. This condition is called vaginal atrophy. During sexual intercourse, the vagina does not lubricate as easily as it used to, which can make penetration uncomfortable or painful.

Hormone replacement therapy usually relieves vaginal atrophy. An alternative to oral HRT is topical estrogen. Topical estrogen creams are inserted high into the vagina with an applicator and relieve atrophy very well. Since some of the estrogen of a topical cream is absorbed into the system, women who have not had a hysterectomy need to take a progestin to reduce the risk of endometrial cancer caused by taking estrogen alone.

To relieve vaginal dryness, the cream must be applied daily for at least one to three months; then it may be used one to three times a week for symptom control. Possible alternatives to drug therapy are longer foreplay, a water-based lubricant such as K-Y lubricating jelly, and daily Kegel exercises (see box). Regular intercourse, about once a week, will also help keep the vagina healthy.

CHANGES IN BREASTS, SKIN, AND BODY HAIR

After menopause, your breasts may gradually sag as firm breast tissue is replaced by fatty tissues. Exercises cannot improve the firmness of your breasts because there are no muscles in them. Although sagging breasts are not unhealthy, many women find them dismaying. HRT reduces sagging by preserving some breast tissue.

Regardless of whether or not you have hormone replacement therapy, your risk of breast cancer increases as you grow older. It's especially important now to examine your breasts each month and to have regular physical examinations and mammograms.

You may also notice that your body hair grows thicker and darker as you approach menopause. This is caused by the increased influence of the male hormone testosterone. While levels of estrogen are falling abruptly, your ovaries still produce testosterone for some years. Estrogen replacement therapy can prevent this change. An alternative is to remove unwanted hair.

Estrogen loss also makes the skin thinner and less elastic. This contributes to wrinkles, although not nearly as much as sun exposure over the years. Hormone replacement therapy reduces this change. (Because your skin thins as it ages, it is more important than ever to protect your skin from sun exposure; see page 58).

PSYCHOLOGICAL CHANGES

Some women experience sudden mood changes or depression during menopause. It is not known whether or not these psychological changes are directly caused by declining hormone levels.

Estrogen replacement therapy seems to improve emotional well-being for some women, though not as dramatically as it relieves symptoms such as hot flashes. Also, a combination of estrogen and androgen is more likely to improve well-being, energy levels, and mood changes than estrogen alone.

Other changes in a woman's life around the time of menopause can also affect her emotions. During these years, it is common to start a new career, adjust to an empty nest, or cope with divorce or widowhood. Psychotherapy or medications for depression or anxiety (see chapter 15) are more likely to help women than hormones.

Long-term health effects of HRT

While many women first consider hormone replacement therapy because they are having symptoms like hot flashes or vaginal atrophy, an even more important reason to take HRT is protection from two leading health problems of older women: heart disease and osteoporosis. Other health conditions are also affected by the hormones.

Weighing heavily in your decision about HRT should be your personal and family health history. What are the greatest risks to your future health, and how might they be affected by hormone replacement therapy? If you are taking HRT mainly to relieve the symptoms of menopause, then a course of 6 to 12 months will be enough. But if you are seeking the long-term protection from heart disease or osteoporosis, you will need to take the hormones for many years, depending on your family health history.

PROTECTION FROM HEART DISEASE

Heart disease is the number-one killer of women. It is not, as was once thought, a man's problem. However, it does tend to strike women 10 to 15 years later, when estrogen levels drop at menopause.

Most studies show oral estrogen replacement reduces the risk of

WHO SHOULD TAKE HRT?

Your decision about hormones should be based on your personal and family health histories and on your menopausal symptoms.

Reasons to take HRT

- Relief of menopausal symptoms such as hot flashes
- Relief of vaginal dryness, irritation, and pain during intercourse
- Family or personal history of heart disease
- Family or personal history of osteoporosis

Current medical problems that are reasons to not take hormones

- Breast cancer
- Endometrial cancer
- Liver disease
- Thrombophlebitis or thromboembolism
- Vaginal bleeding of unknown cause

Reasons to be cautious about taking hormones

- History of breast cancer
- History of endometrial cancer
- History of liver disease
- Large uterine fibroids
- Endometriosis
- History of thrombophlebitis or thromboembolism
- History of stroke or transient ischemic attack (TIA, mini-strokes)
- Recent heart attack
- Pancreatic disease
- Gallbladder disease
- Fibrocystic breast disease
- High blood pressure
- Migraine headaches

coronary artery disease for women after menopause by about 50 percent. This protection is a major benefit for women at high risk of heart disease. To have these benefits, you have to keep taking the hormones—probably for life.

Oral estrogen replacement therapy raises levels of HDL (good) cholesterol by 12 to 20 percent, which prevents the buildup of the plaque that can clog the arteries. Oral estrogens also reduce LDL (bad) cholesterol by 10 to 15 percent. Estrogens taken by patch, injection, or cream do not have the same benefit because they are not processed by the liver, where these lipoproteins are produced.

New evidence shows that estrogen may also prevent spasms of the walls of blood vessels that contribute to heart attack and stroke. Estrogen replacement has not been linked to high blood pressure or any problems with blood clotting.

One cautionary note is that most of the studies showing that estrogen replacement therapy reduces the risk of heart disease were done with women taking estrogen alone, not the combination estrogen-progestin that is now most common. So far, studies have not shown conclusively whether adding progestin changes the benefits to the cardiovascular system.

PROTECTION FROM OSTEOPOROSIS

Hormone replacement therapy can provide valuable protection from osteoporosis, a devastating bone-thinning disease that leads to debilitating bone fractures in a woman's later years.

Your bones are not the hard, permanent structures they appear to be. Your body is constantly building up and breaking down bone. As a child and young woman, your body builds up more bone than it breaks down. Around age 35, your body begins to break down more bone than it builds. This process continues slowly until your menopause years. Then, when estrogen levels drop, bone loss accelerates dramatically. The brittle, weak bones often break at the hip, wrist, or vertebrae. The last causes a painful humped or curved back.

Estrogen replacement therapy may reverse this process and further prevent bone loss. If begun within three years of menopause, it can actually reverse some of the bone loss that has already occurred and begin building bone again. If started more than three years after menopause, it can prevent further bone loss. If you stop taking the hormones, bone loss begins again. It is never too late to start estrogen replacement therapy to prevent bone loss. Keep in mind that studies have shown a reduction in the rate of fractures in women who began after 65.

While all types of estrogen replacement offer some protection, the oral and patch forms are best for this purpose.

HORMONE REPLACEMENT THERAPY AND CANCER

When estrogen is taken alone, it increases the risk of endometrial cancer (cancer of the lining of the uterus). This risk increases the longer you take estrogen alone. For example, a woman who has taken estrogen for 10 years has twice the risk of endometrial cancer as someone who has taken it only 5 years. This includes all forms of estrogen, including vaginal creams. Adding progestin at least 13 days of a cycle reduces the risk of endometrial cancer to almost zero by blocking the effects of estrogen on the endometrial lining. If you have had a hysterectomy, a procedure that removes the uterus, you do not need this protection.

Less clear is the relationship between hormone replacement therapy and breast cancer. At least 20 studies have looked at the relationship between estrogens and breast cancer, but most have looked at the use of estrogen only, not the combination of estrogen and progestin now commonly prescribed. These studies have had conflicting results ranging from no risk to a 20 to 30 percent increased risk of breast cancer.

One of the largest studies of women, the Nurses Health Study at Harvard, which included nearly 500,000 women, reported significantly more breast cancer among women currently taking estrogen. The same study showed no increased risk among women who had previously taken estrogen replacement therapy but had stopped. Other studies have not shown a link between estrogen and breast cancer. Some experts believe that taking estrogen for a short time (less than 10 years) does not raise a woman's risk of breast cancer, but taking it for 15 or more years does. Though studies are conflicting, women who have a strong family history of breast cancer or who have had breast cancer need to evaluate carefully the pros and cons of the therapy and how long to take it. Women who currently have breast cancer should not take hormone replacement therapy.

The risk of breast cancer with estrogen and progestin, the most common form of hormone replacement, is not known. Studies of the combination of estrogen and progestin are few and have shown conflicting results. Even less well studied is the combination of estrogen with androgen hormones.

INCREASED RISK OF GALLBLADDER DISEASE

Both oral estrogen and progesterone increase the risk of gallstones by stimulating the liver to increase the amount of cholesterol in the bile acids. Transdermal estrogen, administered through a skin patch, does not increase the risk of gallbladder disease because it bypasses the liver. However, women with existing gallbladder disease should use all hormone replacement therapy with caution.

Taking hormone replacement therapy

If you and your doctor choose hormone replacement therapy, the next step is to decide whether you should take estrogen alone or combined with other hormones. There is also a choice of tablet, vaginal cream or suppository, skin patch, or injections.

ESTROGEN ALONE

If you have had a hysterectomy and therefore cannot get endometrial cancer, your doctor will probably prescribe estrogen therapy with no progestin. If your doctor prescribes combination estrogen-progestin therapy, ask why. You probably do not need to take progestin, and you may prefer to avoid its side effects, such as mood disturbances.

The most common prescription is for conjugated estrogens (CEE), a mixture of several estrogens known by the brand name Premarin. It is usually prescribed in a daily dose of 0.625 mg for 25 days of the month (three weeks on/one week off). Estratab, a slightly different combination of estrogens, is available in a similar dosage. Other possible estrogen prescriptions include micronized estradiol (Estrace) and estrone (Ogen), the predominant form of estrogen found naturally in postmenopausal women. All the estrogens on the market are provided in equally effective doses.

If you have trouble remembering to take a tablet every day, you might consider a skin (transdermal) patch that slowly releases estradiol through the skin. The Estraderm patch is applied twice a week (every three days) to the skin. Newer transdermal patches include Vivelle, which is applied twice a week but has the advantage of being smaller and thinner, and Climara, which is applied only once a week.

Another advantage of taking estrogen by patch is that the estrogen bypasses the liver and enters the bloodstream directly, reducing the risk of gallbladder disease. A disadvantage is that the patch does not offer the same protection from heart disease as oral estrogen, though it does protect against osteoporosis.

A third, but much less common, way to take estrogen is by injection. Injected estrogens absorb slowly and circulate through the body for several weeks. Your doctor will administer an estrogen shot, usually into the muscles of the buttocks, once every three or four weeks. Injected estrogens provide no protection against heart disease. Injections are usually used only in women with premature ovarian failure.

Estrogen also comes in a vaginal cream or vaginal suppository. These forms have potent local effects and are primarily intended for use to relieve vaginal dryness and irritation. A cream doesn't offer total hormone replacement, but offers some protection of the bones and can relieve some symptoms like hot flashes.

Side effects

The side effects of estrogen are mild, often nonexistent. A small number of women experience bloating, headaches, or tender breasts. These side effects often subside after several months. For many women, the relief of menopausal symptoms and the long-term benefits far outweigh the mild side effects. The side effects, particularly breast tenderness, are most pronounced in women who have had no estrogen for years, such as women who start taking estrogen 5 to 10 years after menopause. If you are bothered by symptoms, reducing the dose will probably reduce the problem.

ESTROGEN AND PROGESTIN THERAPY

Estrogen combined with a progestin is the best choice for most women who have not had a hysterectomy. Progestin lowers the risk of endometrial cancer. A number of progestins are available for use; the most commonly prescribed progestin is medroxyprogesterone (Provera or Cycrin).

There are several possible regimens. One is a dose of 0.3 to 1.25 mg of conjugated estrogens (or other estrogen equivalent) given daily or for the first 25 days of the cycle (three weeks on/one week off). The dose may vary from woman to woman. A dose of at least 0.625 mg is recommended for prevention of osteoporosis, so this is the usual dose for most women. Medroxyprogesterone (the progestin) is given daily at a dose of 5 to 10 mg for days 14 through 25 of the cycle.

A second approach is estrogen every day or for the first 25 days, and progestin from day 1 through days 12 or 13. A third approach is to take both estrogen and progestin every day for the full month. With a continuous regimen, the dose of medroxyprogesterone is much lower, 2.5 mg daily. Combined estrogen-progestin therapy is available only by oral tablet. One way to take these combinations is in blister packs that list the days so you can easily remember which pill to take when.

You and your doctor can discuss whether to choose a continuous or cyclic regimen. Your choice may be based on two factors: menstrual bleeding and extent of hot flashes on "off days." For example, a woman who has hot flashes on days 25 through 31 (the off days) would be a good candidate for continuous therapy. Also, most women on the continuous therapy stop menstruating after six months to a year. Women on the cyclic regimen usually experience menstrual (with-drawal) bleeding within 10 days after stopping the progestin. These women may eventually stop having a period, but this is less common than with the continuous regimens.

Side effects

The most significant side effect of combination estrogen-progestin is vaginal bleeding. Most women who take progestin for 12 days a month have cyclic bleeding similar to a menstrual period. Women who take progestin every day may initially have menstrual bleeding off and on throughout the month. This irregular bleeding usually stops after a year, but for some women it continues for several years. Compared to a menstrual period before menopause, these periods are lighter, shorter, and less uncomfortable.

Other possible side effects related to addition of a progestin in-clude bloating, irritability, and depression. Side effects may be re-duced by reducing the dosage of progestin or changing the type of progestin prescribed.

ESTROGEN, PROGESTIN, AND ANDROGEN THERAPY

One of the hormones that declines at menopause is testosterone. Although this is a male hormone, a woman's ovaries also produce small amounts. Levels of testosterone in women are about one-fifteenth that of men. At least 25 percent of the total amount of testosterone in a woman's body is produced by the ovaries. Because testosterone increases sexual desire, declining levels cause some women to feel less interested in sex. If you are feeling a lack of sexual interest following menopause, you might want to talk to your doctor about adding androgen in the form of methyltestosterone to the hormone mix. One oral product is currently available that contains estrogen with a relatively low dose of methyltestosterone. The brand name is Estratest.

Estrogen plus androgen has been shown to improve the sense of well-being and energy levels. The combination of estrogen plus androgen is particularly effective for women whose menopause is the result of surgical removal of the ovaries. Testosterone is also FDA approved for treatment of hot flashes that have not responded to estrogen alone.

Side effects

Taking testosterone can cause some side effects, such as an increase in body hair. It has also been shown to increase LDL (bad) cholesterol levels and reduce HDL (good) cholesterol in women, but further studies are needed.

Because testosterone does not protect the endometrium from the effects of estrogen, it is important to take progestin with the combination of estrogen-testosterone if you have a uterus. On a positive note, preliminary studies suggest that adding testosterone may increase bone formation and decrease bone loss.

chapter 6

DRUGS TO TREAT REPRODUCTIVE SYSTEM DISORDERS

*Y*OUR REPRODUCTIVE SYSTEM IS A REMARKABLE SET of organs designed to bring sperm and egg together and then to nurture a fertilized egg inside the uterus for nine months. The reproductive organs include the vagina, cervix, uterus, fallopian tubes, ovaries, and breasts. This chapter covers common disorders of these organs that can cause infertility or pain. Some can be life-threatening, and all should be treated by your doctor.

Endometriosis

Endometriosis is a common condition in which the cells that normally line the uterus (endometrial tissue) grow outside it. Commonly the endometrial tissue grows on the ovaries; on the fallopian tubes; in the lining of the abdominal cavity, bladder, or intestines; and in the space between the uterus and rectum. In some women with this condition, endometrial cells have been found almost everywhere in the body, including the lungs and skin. Endometriosis can cause menstrual pain and infertility. It can occur at any age, but because it often causes infertility, it is usually identified in women in the childbearing ages. The condition usually subsides after menopause.

The cause of endometriosis is not known. What is known is that for 90 percent of menstruating women, some menstrual blood travels up through the uterus and fallopian tubes into the abdominal cavity rather than exiting the body. This is called retrograde menstruation. One theory about endometriosis is that the immune system fails to clear away these renegade endometrial cells. During each menstrual cycle, all endometrial cells inside or outside the uterus follow the cyclic pattern of the female hormones by swelling, shedding, and disintegrating. While cells inside the uterus then pass from the body during menstruation, cells outside the uterus remain after they disintegrate, causing inflammation, internal bleeding, and chronic pain. They may form blood-filled cysts on the ovaries and adhesions between tissues (scar tissue that may interfere with organ function). Adhesions in the pelvic area may interfere with the ability of the fallopian tubes to capture an egg, resulting in infertility.

Symptoms and diagnosis

Many women have endometriosis and don't know it. About one-third of women with endometriosis have no symptoms. Doctors often diagnose the condition after a woman reports menstrual or abdominal pain or when she is having trouble conceiving. If pain is present, it is usually located below the navel and between the hips, starts or worsens a few days before the period, and continues throughout the period. When there are symptoms, they may include:

- Painful or heavy menstruation
- Back pain, particularly before the menstrual period starts
- Pain during intercourse
- Pain during bowel movements, particularly the period
- Diarrhea
- Constipation
- Multiple miscarriages

If your doctor thinks you may have endometriosis, the best way to confirm the diagnosis is through laparoscopy, the insertion of a narrow tube with a "scope," or tiny camera, on the end that allows a surgeon to view the inside of your pelvic cavity. The tube is inserted through an inch-long incision made just above your navel. During laparoscopy, the doctor will determine the number and size of endometriotic cysts or adhesions and will classify your condition as minimal, mild, moderate, or severe.

TREATMENT

Treatment depends on the severity of your condition, your symptoms, your age, and whether you want to have a baby in the future. If you have minimal to moderate endometriosis with few symptoms, your doctor will probably recommend that you wait and see if the problem resolves itself. Most women with minimal to moderate endometriosis are eventually able to conceive with no treatment for the condition.

Surgery

If the condition is causing pain, surgery is usually recommended to remove endometriotic tissues, cysts, and adhesions. There are two types of surgery for endometriosis—conservative and definitive. The conservative approach, which is often chosen by women who want to conceive in the near future, involves surgery under the guidance of a laparoscope. After viewing the endometriotic tissue with the laparoscope, the doctor inserts lasers through the tube to obliterate the tissue. Endometriotic tissues can also be cut and cauterized using the laparoscope as a guide. This procedure is usually done as day surgery and takes 20 minutes to several hours, depending on the extent of endometriotic implants. About half of infertile women who have this procedure are able to conceive. However, this procedure is usually not effective if the lesions are very small, very large, or very dense. Also, endometriosis reappears within five years in about 40 percent of women who have this conservative procedure.

If endometriosis is advanced, the pain is intolerable, and the woman does not want to have any more children, definitive surgery may be advised. Surgery of this type usually involves removal of the uterus, the ovaries, and all endometrial implants, adhesions, and scar tissues. This eliminates pain in at least 90 percent of cases. If you are premenopausal, you need to carefully weigh the benefits and risks of this surgery. If both ovaries are removed, estrogen replacement therapy is usually recommended to treat hot flashes and to lower the risks of heart disease and osteoporosis.

Medications

For mild to moderate pain just before and during your period, NSAIDs such as Advil are effective analgesics. If your pain is not responsive to these analgesics, there are prescription medications that may reduce pain by disrupting the hormonal cycle that causes the painful swelling of the endometriotic tissues. These drugs suppress ovulation and cause either a pseudomenopause or pseudopregnancy. A number of them are also used before surgery to shrink the endometriotic lesions and after surgery to prevent pain from recurrent endometriosis.

- **Combined oral contraceptives.** Oral contraceptives cannot cure the condition, but they can temporarily relieve the pain for about 75 percent of women. Given for six to nine months, they supply a steady dose of estrogen and progestin that inhibits the production of gonadotropin-releasing hormone, GnRH, which normally stimulates the ovary to release an egg. The monthly cycle is stopped, so the endometrial tissue does not swell. (For more about combined birth-control pills, see page 69.)
- **Danazol.** This synthetic male hormone relieves the pain of endometriosis by stopping the monthly hormonal cycle that causes endometrial tissue to swell. It stops the surge of luteinizing hormone (LH), suppresses the secretion of follicle-stimulating hormone (FSH), reduces the production of estrogen and progesterone, and inhibits the growth of endometrial cells. Danazol produces a pseudomenopause, causing the menstrual period to stop. Treatment usually lasts six to nine months. It usually relieves symptoms within two months. Although danazol suppresses ovulation, it should not be used as the only form of contraceptive. Women taking danazol should use a nonhormonal form of contraception such as a condom or diaphragm. Common side effects of danazol include weight gain (10 to 20 pounds), acne, oily skin, growth of excess body hair, hot flashes, muscle soreness or cramps, and skin rash. There is a 20 to 40 percent increase in LDL (bad) cholesterol and a 40 to 50 percent decrease in HDL (good) cholesterol. These adverse effects are reversible, and many women can tolerate them for several months in order to relieve the pain of endometriosis. After a woman stops taking danazol,

fertility returns in two to three months. Danazol may also be given before surgery to shrink the endometriotic implants. Do not take danazol during pregnancy or breast-feeding. For some women, danazol provides permanent relief from symptoms, but symptoms recur in about 5 to 23 percent of women who use it.

- **GnRH agonists.** GnRH agonists (Lupron, Synarel, Zoladex) inhibit the swelling of endometrial tissues by stopping the secretion of FSH and LH and preventing ovulation. Like danazol, these drugs decrease the production of estrogen and cause pseudomenopause. A GnRH agonist may be advised if you do not respond to a combined oral contraceptive or your symptoms persist or recur following surgery. You can take a GnRH agonist by a monthly, intramuscular injection (Lupron), monthly subcutaneous injection (Zoladex), or twice-daily nose spray (Synarel). Treatment lasts for no more than six months. You will stop menstruating during this time. If you are sexually active, you must use a nonhormonal form of contraception such as a condom or diaphragm. Your menstrual period will return about two months after stopping the medication, and fertility usually returns in 30 to 60 days. Do not take this medication during pregnancy or breast-feeding. The side effects include hot flashes, sleep disturbances, headaches, and vaginal dryness. Less common side effects include decreased sex drive, reduced breast size, bloating, and excess hair growth. Unlike danazol, GnRH agonists do not have direct androgenic (male) effects and do not cause changes in cholesterol. However, these agents have been shown to increase bone loss and cause osteoporosis.

- **Progesterone.** Given orally (medroxyprogesterone, Provera) or by injection, progesterone is another common treatment for all stages of endometriosis. Like combination oral contraceptives, the progesterone mimics pregnancy by decreasing the LH surge and decreasing ovulation. Primary side effects are breakthrough bleeding, weight gain, and acne. Many clinicians consider medroxyprogesterone as second-best to either danazol or a GnRH agonist.

$\mathcal{U}$SING NAFARELIN NASAL SPRAY

Nafarelin (Synarel) nasal spray is quickly becoming a widely prescribed medication for treatment of endometriosis. If you are using nafarelin, make sure to use the correct technique as follows:

- Blow your nose gently first.
- After removing the cap, insert the tip of the container into one nostril.
- Tilt your head forward slightly keeping the bottle upright.
- Close the other nostril and squeeze gently while inhaling.
- Keep inhaling for several seconds after you breathe in the medication.
- Any stinging in your nose is not dangerous and should subside shortly.
- Do not use a nasal decongestant within 30 minutes before or after using the spray.
- If you notice hot flashes, report them to your doctor.
- If you notice vaginal dryness, use a water-based lubricant such as K-Y jelly.
- Your menstrual periods will resume five to eight weeks following discontinuation of therapy.

Fibroids

A uterine fibroid is a noncancerous growth that forms inside, outside, or within the walls of the uterus. Other terms for fibroids are myomas, fibromyomas, myofibromas, and leiomyomas. They are the most common pelvic tumor in women 30 to 50 years of age. They are more common among black women, occurring in 50 percent of black women under the age of 30 years, compared to 20 percent of white women of similar age. No one knows the cause of fibroids, but it is known that the female hormone estrogen fuels their growth. Fibroids do not occur before puberty, and their size may be increased by the use of combined oral contraceptives. When estrogen levels drop at menopause, most fibroids shrink or disappear.

A fibroid, which contains smooth muscle held together by fibrous tissue, can be as small as the head of a pin or larger than a grapefruit. Most fibroids are not dangerous or painful and need no treatment, but some cause pain or abnormal vaginal bleeding. They may enlarge over time and alter the shape of the uterus. Fibroids can also cause infertility by blocking sperm from entering the fallopian tube or by preventing a fertilized egg from implanting in the lining of the uterus.

SYMPTOMS AND DIAGNOSIS

Many women with fibroids have no symptoms. Their doctors may discover the condition during a routine pelvic examination or during infertility treatment. Other women with fibroids inside the uterus have painful menstrual periods or lower-back pain. Fibroids can also cause heavier or longer menstrual periods or spotting at other times of the month. If outside the uterus, they may press on nearby organs and cause pain, frequent urination or difficulty with urination, and constipation.

If a fibroid is suspected or discovered, your doctor can examine its size and location with an ultrasound test, a laparoscope (a small tube inserted through your abdomen), a hysteroscope (inserted through the vagina into your uterus), or a special X-ray of the uterus and fallopian tubes called hysterosalpingography.

TREATMENT

If your fibroids are causing no symptoms and are not growing rapidly, you may not need treatment. If you are experiencing symptoms, treatments include surgery and medications. Fibroids usually shrink or disappear after menopause, so before treatment, consider how close you are to menopause.

Surgery

If you are having heavy, painful menstrual periods and have completed your family, one option may be a hysterectomy, the surgical removal of the uterus. Fibroids are the most common reason for a hysterectomy. Another option is a myomectomy, which removes the fibroids but not the uterus. This makes it possible to have a baby in the future, but the surgery is more difficult and complicated than a hysterectomy and may leave scars or adhesions that themselves cause infertility. The fibroids may also recur.

Medications

- **GnRH agonists.** These medications shrink fibroids by inhibiting the body's production of estrogen. When a woman takes GnRH agonists, her menstrual periods stop and she may experience some of the side effects of a natural menopause, such as hot flashes, vaginal dryness, and bone loss. Because of these side effects, these drugs should not be taken longer than six months. Once you stop taking the medication, the fibroids may begin to grow again. GnRH agonists are also used to shrink fibroids and stop heavy bleeding before surgery, making the procedure safer and easier.
- **Danazol.** A synthetic male hormone, danazol shrinks fibroids and stops heavy or painful menstrual bleeding by inhibiting estrogen and progesterone production. It often causes side effects associated with male hormones, such as an increase in body and facial hair. After the drug is stopped, the fibroids often begin to grow again. For more information, see page 109.

Ovarian cysts

A cyst is a tissue sac filled with a fluid, semifluid, or solid substance. Ovarian cysts are not cancerous. They may grow on one or both ovaries. Many kinds of ovarian cysts go away by themselves, but others may require surgery.

Functional cysts, the most common type, are caused by changes in the cells that grow and release an egg during the normal menstrual cycle. Normally a follicle matures each month under the influence of estrogen and ruptures to release an egg. Following ovulation, the remainder of the follicle sac, called the corpus luteum, disintegrates. If the follicle fails to release the egg and instead keeps growing, a follicular cyst can form. After one or more menstrual cycles, the cyst usually disintegrates or ruptures, causing a brief episode of sharp pain. Another problem occurs if a blood-filled cyst forms in the corpus luteum. This kind of cyst can change the length of your menstrual periods and cause more constant, one-sided abdominal pain.

Polycystic disease is many small follicular cysts on the ovaries. These cysts can cause irregular ovulation and irregular periods. The most common cause is an excess of androgen (male) hormones. It is usually treated with a drug with antiandrogen effects, such as the diuretic spironolactone.

Dermoid cysts, also known as teratomas, are formed of skin, hair, bone, or tooth tissues from a woman's own cells. They may cause symptoms by pressing on nearby organs. They are usually removed surgically to prevent rupturing and to rule out cancer. A dermoid cyst may have been on the ovary since birth.

Another common kind of ovarian cyst, called an endometrioma, is a form of endometriosis (see page 106) and is treated similarly to endometriosis.

Symptoms and diagnosis

Ovarian cysts often cause no symptoms and are discovered during a routine pelvic examination; when feeling the abdomen, the doctor discovers that the ovaries are enlarged. Depending on its size, an ovarian cyst can cause the following symptoms.

- Irregular menstrual periods
- Fullness, pressure, aching, or pain in the lower abdomen
- Painful intercourse
- Constipation
- Urge to urinate

If your ovaries are enlarged, your doctor may examine them by ultrasound to see whether there is a cyst and how large it is.

Treatment

If an ovarian cyst is small and you have not reached menopause, a common approach is to wait two or three months to see if it goes away, as most will. If it does not, and the cyst is the functional type, a combination oral contraceptive may be prescribed. By preventing the maturation of the follicle and ovulation, these pills can shrink the functional cyst and prevent the formation of new ones.

If a cyst does not shrink after several weeks of birth-control pills, your doctor may recommend a biopsy (tissue sample) of the mass of cells to determine whether it is cancerous. If it isn't, but it is large or painful, then surgery may be recommended. Surgery is usually recommended for cysts that are greater than 2.5 inches in diameter, which includes most dermoid cysts and endometriomas. If you have not yet reached menopause or would like to maintain your fertility, the surgeon will try to preserve as much of your ovary as possible during the operation. If one ovary is removed, you can still get pregnant.

Past menopause, surgical removal of the cyst is usually recommended because of the increased likelihood of ovarian cancer in this age group.

The most common cause of polycystic ovarian disease is an excess of male hormones (androgens), so treatment includes antiandrogenic drugs.

Premenstrual syndrome

Premenstrual syndrome (PMS) consists of a variety of physical and emotional symptoms that ebb and flow with the menstrual cycle and are severe enough to interfere with the woman's home or work life. Most women have at least one PMS-related symptom, but only a small percent have such severe symptoms.

Levels of estrogen and progesterone are normal in women with PMS. There are many theories regarding the cause of PMS, but none has been proven thus far. Theories include fluctuations in serotonin levels, deficiency in endorphins, deficiency in vitamin B6, and deficiency in prostaglandin E1.

SYMPTOMS AND DIAGNOSIS

PMS symptoms occur during the week preceding the menstrual period, then gradually subside. Symptoms should stop one to four days after the beginning of your period. PMS may occur during most of your menstrual cycles. Some women experience only one symptom; others have several.

Physical symptoms can include:

- Abdominal bloating
- Acne
- Backache
- Breast swelling or tenderness
- Constipation
- Cravings for sweet or salty food
- Diarrhea
- Fatigue
- Headache
- Insomnia
- Joint and muscle pain
- Nausea, vomiting
- Weight gain

Psychological changes can include:

- Anger
- Anxiety
- Crying
- Decreased efficiency or work performance
- Difficulty concentrating
- Feelings of depression, sadness, or hopelessness
- Impaired judgment
- Irritability
- Loneliness or social withdrawal
- Restlessness or agitation
- Tension

When you report your symptoms to your doctor, it is important to include the time during your menstrual cycle that you experience each one. This will help the doctor determine whether you have premenstrual syndrome or whether your symptoms suggest endometriosis, thyroid dysfunction, clinical depression, or pelvic infection. Many doctors recommend keeping a chart or calendar of physical or psychological symptoms for each day of your menstrual cycle. Each day, grade the intensity of your symptoms using a scale (1 to 10, with 10 being most severe) and a symptom code such as A for anger, B for bloating, C for cravings, and D for depression. A record of two or three months will tell you and your doctor whether or not these symptoms tend to recur at the same time and whether they point to PMS.

TREATMENT

Self-help techniques

Changes in your diet or habits may help relieve some of your symptoms.

- If you feel anxious or nervous or are having trouble sleeping, reduce your intake of caffeine.
- Reduce your consumption of tobacco and alcohol, which, like caffeine, can magnify PMS symptoms.
- If your breasts or abdomen swell, cut down on salt, which causes your body to retain water.
- Exercise regularly. Women who get regular aerobic exercise, such as 20 to 30 minutes of brisk walking per day, are less likely to experience PMS symptoms.
- Use stress management techniques, such as meditation, to help cope with moodiness or anxiety.

Medications

Although no specific drug has ever been approved by the FDA to treat PMS, doctors use a variety of medications to treat different symptoms. These treatments may be appropriate if symptoms are severe and if self-help techniques have not produced results. Talk to your doctor before taking any of the many over-the-counter medications being marketed as treatments for PMS, as none is yet considered generally safe and effective. Prescription drugs to treat the symptoms of PMS may include:

- **Alprazolam.** A benzodiazepine (page 319), alprazolam can relieve some of the emotional or psychological symptoms of PMS. It improves mental function, mood, and pain levels but has little or no effect on physical complaints. It is best taken only during the second half of your menstrual cycle, and the dose should be tapered down after your period begins.

- **Antidepressants.** When taken daily for about three months, antidepressants such as fluoxetine (Prozac) and clomipramine (Anafranil) may relieve some of the mood swings and psychological symptoms of PMS, particularly tension, depression, anger, fatigue, irritability, anxiety, and confusion.
- **Bromocriptine.** This drug, which is used to suppress lactation after childbirth, is sometimes prescribed to relieve breast pain and tenderness. Your doctor will prescribe a low dose to be taken for part of each cycle (from the time of ovulation until the start of your period). The dose may be gradually increased or decreased based on whether your symptoms are subsiding and whether you have side effects such as nausea, vomiting, and headaches.
- **Diuretics.** If you experience uncomfortable bloating or swelling of your abdomen or breasts, diuretics may be prescribed in low doses and for a limited number of days of each cycle (days 18 through 26). They should be used cautiously because of possible dangerous side effects, including the loss of potassium. The preferred diuretic for PMS is spironolactone (Aldactone), which is relatively weak and does not cause potassium loss.
- **GnRH agonists.** Given daily by nasal inhalation or by monthly injection, GnRH agonists may alleviate many of the physical symptoms of PMS, including swelling, breast tenderness, and the psychological symptoms of anxiety and tension. Symptoms sometimes worsen the first two weeks. This "flare response" is a reaction to the increase in estrogen level. After the initial month of treatment, PMS symptoms are reduced. Treatment with these agents for PMS should be short term because of the risks associated with an artificial menopause. Side effects, which usually start in the second or third month, are hot flashes, weight gain, acne, and bone loss. (For more on GnRH agonists, see page 110.)
- **Combination birth-control pills.** Oral contraceptives are sometimes prescribed to relieve breast pain and bloating and mood swings. The use of oral contraceptives for this purpose is controversial. They relieve symptoms in only a small number of women and often worsen depression, irritability, breast tenderness, and

abdominal bloating. (For more about combination birth-control pills, see page 69.)

- **Progesterone.** Although this synthetic hormone has been widely prescribed as a rectal or vaginal suppository for a variety of PMS symptoms including mood swings, studies have failed to prove that it works. Considered ineffective by many clinicians, progesterone is still prescribed widely for the alleviation of swelling and breast tenderness. It can cause mood disturbances, weight gain, and breakthrough bleeding.

Other drugs have been tried to treat PMS with varying success. Vitamin B6 (also known as pyridoxine) is often found in multivitamins called "PMS formulas." The high dose of vitamin B6 that has been advocated (100 to 200 mg) causes more problems than it cures. Many cases of nerve damage, with numb or tingling limbs, have been reported in people taking high doses of B6. Other substances that are sometimes sold as PMS remedies but that have no proven effectiveness include atenolol and evening primrose oil.

On the other hand, at least one study has shown that calcium supplementation (1,000 mg elemental calcium per day) improves mood, anxiety level, back pain, and fluid retention. Calcium plays a role in muscle contraction and in hormone regulation.

Ectopic pregnancy

Ectopic pregnancy, also called tubal pregnancy, occurs when a fertilized egg lodges in a fallopian tube instead of implanting in the uterine lining where it can grow normally. An ectopic pregnancy cannot result in a live birth. Most often the ectopic pregnancy occurs in a fallopian tube that has been narrowed by scar tissue or damaged by infection or surgery. The risk of ectopic pregnancy is greater for women who have had a sexually transmitted disease (see page 241), pelvic inflammatory disease (see page 247), tubal sterilization, or fertility treatments that induce ovulation. Your risk is also increased if your mother took diethylstilbestrol (DES) during pregnancy.

An ectopic pregnancy is dangerous and can be life-threatening. If the fertilized egg lodges in a fallopian tube, it continues to grow until it ruptures the tube, causing pain and bleeding.

SYMPTOMS AND DIAGNOSIS

Pain is one of the major symptoms associated with ectopic pregnancy. It is usually one-sided in the lower abdomen or pelvis and lasts for several hours. Because ectopic pregnancy can be life-threatening, call your doctor immediately if you experience:

- Missed menstrual period
- Abdominal pain on one side
- Abnormal vaginal bleeding

Occasionally, there are no symptoms until the tube ruptures.

To determine if you have an ectopic pregnancy, your doctor will administer a pregnancy test and find out when your last menstrual period began. About two weeks after your next period was due, an ultrasound examination can reveal whether there is a pregnancy in your uterus. If the ultrasound does not show a pregnancy, more tests will be needed, including a follow-up ultrasound and blood hormone tests. Your doctor may also look for an ectopic pregnancy with a laparoscope, a long tube with a camera at the end that is inserted through a small incision in your abdomen.

TREATMENT

Treatment depends on the location of the ectopic pregnancy and whether or not a fallopian tube has ruptured.

Surgery

If the ectopic pregnancy is in a fallopian tube, the developing fetus, placenta, and surrounding tissues can be removed through laparoscopic surgery. If the tube has already ruptured, it may have to be surgically removed as well. In this case, your remaining fallopian tube will still function normally, allowing further, normal pregnancy if that tube is healthy.

Medication

An ectopic pregnancy that is diagnosed early and has not ruptured may be treated with methotrexate, which kills rapidly dividing cells such as those in a newly fertilized egg. Most women are still able to conceive normally following methotrexate therapy. Methotrexate is taken as one or two injections deep into muscle tissue, usually into your buttocks. The drug gradually disintegrates the tissue of the ectopic pregnancy, and the body absorbs it. Some women experience pelvic pain for several hours following the injections. This pain can be treated with medication and gradually subsides by itself. Your doctor will monitor your condition carefully in the hours and days following methotrexate therapy, watching for signs of rupture or other complications. The most common side effect is gastrointestinal pain for several days. Side effects are less common in single-dose therapy, but multi-dose therapy eliminates the pregnancy faster.

Fibrocystic breast changes

You may have noticed lumps or bumps in your breasts that become larger or more tender just before menstruation and then recede again after your period. Most women have felt such lumps at one time or another. Lumpy breasts, known medically as fibrocystic breast changes, usually do not need treatment unless the swelling is uncomfortable or painful. However, it is important to have all lumps examined by your doctor to make sure they are not cancerous. Fibrocystic breast changes are uncommon after menopause.

SYMPTOMS AND DIAGNOSIS

The most common symptoms of fibrocystic breast changes are pain and tenderness, particularly for several days before your menstrual period. The lumps or pain may occur in one or both breasts and may be in only one area of the breast or distributed throughout. Occasionally there is some discharge from the nipple; be sure to tell your doctor if you see this, as it is sometimes a symptom of breast cancer.

If your doctor is not sure whether a lump is due to fibrocystic breast disease or cancer, you will have a biopsy so that a tissue sample can be examined.

TREATMENT

Fibrocystic breast changes do not have to be treated unless the swelling is painful for you. Sometimes it helps to wear a support bra around the clock. For some women, reducing caffeine consumption may help reduce swelling or tenderness.

Some women with fibrocystic breasts develop fluid-filled cysts. Cysts are treated with a simple procedure called needle aspiration, in which your doctor draws out the fluid with a needle.

Medications

A variety of drug treatments can relieve the discomfort of fibrocystic breast changes.

- **Danazol.** This synthetic male hormone is often used to treat severe cases. Treatment, which lasts three to six months, usually reduces pain and other symptoms. Danazol (see page 109) reduces production of estrogen, which can swell fibrocystic tissues.
- **Hormonal contraceptives.** Contraceptives containing progestin (combined birth-control pills, the minipill, implants, and injections) can reduce the pain and swelling. (For more about hormonal contraceptives, see page 68.)
- **Diuretics.** Also known as water pills, diuretics can reduce the swelling and pain of fibrocystic changes. They help the body eliminate excess fluid through the kidneys. At first, diuretics can cause unusual fatigue and increased urine flow. It is best to take diuretics early in the day so that you aren't wakened during the night by a need to go to the bathroom. Diuretics can have other side effects, including dizziness, increased sensitivity to sun exposure, and deficiencies of potassium and calcium.

Infertility

Infertility is defined medically as a failure to conceive after one year of trying. Often the problem is simply that the couple is not having intercourse during the most fertile days in the woman's menstrual cycle. If that is not the case, a fertility specialist can look for other possible reasons. Infertility is caused by female factors in 40 percent of cases, male factors in 40 percent of cases and a combination of factors in 20 percent of cases. Your partner may have a low sperm count or his sperm may not be able to swim adequately through the cervical mucus to reach the egg. In women, the most common problems are a blocked fallopian tube or failure of the ovary to release an egg. Infertility can also be caused by endometriosis (see page 106) or scars caused by pelvic inflammatory disease (PID, see page 247) or sexually transmitted infections. Some causes of infertility can be treated quickly and easily, but other treatments are expensive and emotionally draining. Infertility treatment is not always successful; about half of couples with infertility eventually conceive.

DIAGNOSIS

Diagnosis is not always easy. Among the tests you may have are a pelvic examination, an ovulation test, a postcoital test (of cervical mucus and sperm activity), an ultrasound of the fallopian tubes and uterus, or a hysteroscopic or laparoscopic examination of your pelvic cavity. Your partner will also need to have a thorough physical exam and submit a semen sample for testing. The goal of testing is to find out if you are ovulating regularly and, if so, whether the man's sperm can successfully reach the egg released each month from the ovary.

TREATMENT

Treatment of infertility depends on the cause. If your doctor determines that endometriosis (see page 106), fibroids (see page 111), or ovarian cysts (see page 113) are the cause, then you will be treated for these conditions.

Ovulation drugs

One of the most frequent causes of infertility is failure to ovulate regularly. To establish that this is the cause of infertility, you may be asked to chart your basal body temperature for two months, use an ovulation prediction test, or have a transvaginal ultrasound 12 to 16 days before your next period.

If lack of ovulation or inconsistent ovulation is identified by tests, your doctor may prescribe a drug to stimulate your ovaries to produce eggs each month. A variety of hormones stimulate ovulation. If you are considering treatment for infertility, be aware that many of these drugs are very expensive and that a growing number of health-care plans are not including coverage for fertility drugs. Among the drugs available to supplement natural hormones in this process are:

- **Clomiphene.** If a woman is not ovulating and has infrequent periods or long menstrual cycles, Clomiphene (Clomid, Milophene, Serophene) is often the first drug prescribed. It binds to estrogen receptors and blocks the effects of your natural estrogen, estradiol. When the body senses a reduction in estrogen, it secretes follicle-stimulating hormone to increase estrogen production. This triggers ovulation. You may need to visit your doctor once each month just before you begin the five-day clomiphene treatment to check for excessive stimulation of the ovaries and to make sure you have not already conceived. Clomiphene causes ovulation in 60 to 80 percent of cases; pregnancy results in 25 to 50 percent of these women. Treatment usually lasts six to nine months, or until conception occurs. Clomiphene increases the chance of multiple births by less than 10 percent. Do not take the medication if there is a chance you are already pregnant, because there is a slight risk of fetal abnormalities.

- **Human menopausal gonadotropins.** If clomiphene does not cause you to ovulate, injections of human menopausal gonadotropins (HMG, Pergonal) may work. HMG contains the hormones FSH and LH. These hormones cause the ovarian follicle to mature and grow. HMG must be given with human chorionic gonadotropin (HCG), a hormone that mimics the LH surge and causes ovulation. The dose of HMG has to be very precise to minimize the chance of multiple pregnancies and to avoid swollen ovaries (a painful condition called hyperstimulation). You will need close medical supervision and frequent examinations while using this medication. When used with HCG, HMG (Pergonal) induces ovulation in 90 percent of women treated, but causes high rates of multiple pregnancies, miscarriages, and premature births. Do not take this medication if you suspect you are already pregnant, if you have undiagnosed abnormal vaginal bleeding, if you have enlarged ovaries or ovarian cysts, or if you have a pituitary gland tumor. You may experience some swelling or rash at the site of the injections. Other side effects include bloating, breast tenderness, mood swings, and abdominal pain.

- **Gonadotropin-releasing hormone pump.** When clomiphene treatment fails, another alternative is a pump that injects GnRH agonist hormone through a tiny catheter placed in a vein just under the skin of the forearm. To mimic the natural release pattern of GnRH, the pump releases a small surge of GnRH hormone once every 90 minutes to stimulate production of the pituitary hormones necessary for ovulation. The pump is about the size of a small portable radio and can be worn under clothing. You carry it with you around the clock through all normal activities. Your doctor will closely monitor your dose and the status of your ovaries with ultrasound exams. The risks of this treatment include infection and inflammation at the injection site.

- **Bromocriptine.** If you are not ovulating because your pituitary

HOW TO USE AN OVULATION PREDICTOR KIT

Ovulation predictor kits are a good but not totally reliable way to find out whether you are ovulating and when. They are available without a prescription. You test your urine once a day to check for a surge in LH (luteinizing hormone), which triggers ovulation.

You perform the test by urinating once a day at the same time each day on a test stick. Choose the first day of your testing by subtracting 17 days from the total number of days of your monthly cycle. If you normally have a 28-day cycle, you would start the test on day 11. If you normally have a 35-day cycle, you would start the test on day 18. Hold the absorbent tip of the tester in your urine stream for at least five seconds, wait five minutes, then read the test results. When you get a positive reading, you've detected the LH surge and you will ovulate in the next 24 to 36 hours. LH usually appears in the urine 8 to 40 hours before you ovulate. You can stop testing when you see the positive reading.

When used as natural birth control (see page 90), these kits are not completely reliable. If you attempt to use them for this purpose, keep in mind that sperm stay viable for 72 hours.

gland is secreting too much prolactin, the hormone that stimulates production of breast milk, bromocriptine therapy may be successful. Bromocriptine (Parlodel) inhibits secretion of prolactin. As your prolactin levels return to normal, your pituitary gland begins to function normally again, and ovulation can begin. Before beginning bromocriptine therapy, your doctor may take an X-ray of your pituitary gland (in your head) to make sure it contains no tumor. If a tumor is found, your doctor may recommend postponing pregnancy until the tumor is treated. This drug does not increase the likelihood of multiple births. For most women, ovulation begins within two months. If not, your doctor may prescribe a combination of bromocriptine and clomiphene.

Hormone treatments for men

Supplemental hormones can treat thyroid or adrenal conditions that can affect sperm quality. A problem with the adrenal gland can be treated with bromocriptine (see above). If no specific cause for poor-quality semen can be found, and other causes such as exposure to toxic substances or excess heat have been eliminated, some doctors recommend treatment with a stimulating hormone such as clomiphene, human menopausal gonadotropin, human chorionic gonadotropin, or testosterone.

TREATING OTHER CAUSES OF INFERTILITY

Surgery can repair damage or obstruction caused by endometriosis, fibroids, or adhesions. These procedures are difficult and have long recovery periods, but are often effective. When there is a problem with the cervical mucus, the usual cause is infection. Oral antibiotics such as a tetracycline or erythromycin (see page 233) will be prescribed for both partners for 10 to 14 days of the cycle. If the cause is a scarred or narrowed cervical canal, the doctor can do a dilation procedure. If the cervical mucus is too acidic, the treatment may be a douche of bicarbonate solution just prior to intercourse.

If other treatments fail, some couples try assisted reproductive technology, which tries to bring sperm and egg together to produce a successful pregnancy. These techniques are costly, time-consuming, stressful, and often not successful, but they do offer hope to couples who have not been helped by traditional fertility treatments. The techniques currently available include artificial insemination using donated sperm, intrauterine insemination, in-vitro fertilization (sperm and egg combined outside the body, then implanted in the uterus), gamete intrafallopian transfer (GIFT; egg and sperm placed together in the fallopian tube before fertilization), zygote intrafallopian transfer (ZIFT; fertilized eggs placed in fallopian tube), and surrogate motherhood.

chapter 7

MEDICATIONS DURING PREGNANCY AND CHILDBIRTH

Q UESTIONS ABOUT DRUG SAFETY BECOME MORE urgent when you are pregnant because most drugs will pass through the placenta and into the developing fetus. When you are pregnant, and also when you trying to become pregnant, take no prescription or nonprescription medication without first talking to your doctor.

Can you take the headache or cold pills you usually rely on? What if you develop an infection or high blood pressure? And how safe are the drugs often used to relieve pain during labor and childbirth? This chapter will help you answer important questions like these.

Steps toward a healthy pregnancy

The best time to begin a healthy pregnancy is before you even become pregnant. Then and in the nine months to come, you need to consider your health, genetic factors, the food you eat, and the medications you take.

NUTRITION AND VITAMIN SUPPLEMENTS

Even before you become pregnant, start eating a balanced diet with lots of fresh vegetables and fruits, whole grains, and low-fat dairy products. Most women already eat plenty of protein from meats, fish, and cheese. Vegetarians normally get as much protein as they need, but if necessary can increase their protein by eating more beans. To

TAKING A HOME PREGNANCY TEST

If you suspect you may be pregnant, a home pregnancy test is an accurate way to find out. Several brands are available in most pharmacies and are easy to use.

The first day that you can use the test is the first day of your missed period. If you don't know which day your period should have started, take the test at least 34 days after the beginning of your last period (almost all women have monthly menstrual cycles shorter than 34 days). You can also use the test any day after that. The test takes between 3 and 30 minutes to complete, depending on the product.

These tests work by detecting a hormone called human chorionic gonadotropin (HCG) in the urine. This hormone is produced by cells that eventually make up the placenta. The level of HCG peaks approximately 60 to 70 days after fertilization of the egg, then decreases and remains constant throughout pregnancy. Home pregnancy tests can detect low levels of HCG and have an accuracy rate of 95 percent or better. However, the instructions on the package must be carefully followed.

If the test confirms your pregnancy, see your doctor to begin your prenatal medical care. If the test results are negative, first make sure that you did the test correctly. If you did, wait the number of days specified by the manufacturer (usually 3 to 7 days) and repeat the test. If the second test is negative, contact your physician. An underlying medical problem may be the reason for your missed period.

avoid gaining too much weight early on, limit fatty and sugary foods, which add calories without nutrition.

If you are trying to become pregnant, or even if you are sexually active and may become accidentally pregnant, it is a good idea to take a multivitamin each day. Make sure it contains 0.4 mg (400 mcg) of folic acid, which can help prevent birth defects (see box). If you are already pregnant, most doctors recommend taking a multivitamin supplement that is formulated specially for pregnant women.

Megadoses of vitamin A during pregnancy (prolonged high doses over 25,000 IU daily) can lead to a number of fetal deformities, including cleft palate and lip, limb reductions, and heart defects.

FOLIC ACID

A lack of folic acid (folate) in the diet may cause a neural tube defect in the fetus. Because the problem happens in the first weeks of pregnancy, perhaps before you even know you are pregnant, start taking a multivitamin supplement containing 0.4 mg of folic acid as soon as you start trying to become pregnant. All women of childbearing age should meet the recommended daily allowance of 0.4 mg of folic acid each day by eating fortified cereals, green vegetables, citrus fruits, and liver. If you think you may not be getting this amount, take a vitamin supplement, particularly if you are trying to get pregnant.

Women who have had a baby with neural tube defect and are trying to conceive again should take a higher dose of folic acid. The recommendation for women who have already had a baby with a neural tube defect is 4 mg per day of folic acid for at least one month before conception, then for the first three months of pregnancy. This amount should be prescribed by your doctor as a separate vitamin. Do not attempt to take in 4 mg of folic acid from multivitamins, as you may ingest toxic doses of vitamins A and D, which are also in these multivitamins.

MEDICAL CARE

If you are planning a pregnancy, visit your doctor for a checkup and a discussion of any difficulties in previous pregnancies, your birth control method, and your use of prescription, over-the-counter, social, and recreational drugs.

If you suspect you may be pregnant, see a doctor immediately to begin your prenatal care. Besides confirming that you are pregnant and calculating your due date, your doctor will identify any existing health problems that could cause problems during pregnancy. You will visit your doctor regularly throughout your pregnancy—probably once a month at first, then once every two or three weeks until week 36, then weekly.

Throughout pregnancy, your doctor will perform a variety of tests ranging from listening to the fetal heartbeat to viewing the fetus with an ultrasound machine. Some women, particularly those over age 35, may choose to have an amniocentesis test in which a sample of amniotic fluid, taken with a long needle inserted into the abdomen, is examined for possible chromosomal abnormalities such as Down syndrome. You may also have blood pressure tests, blood tests, an alpha-fetoprotein test for neural tube defects, urine tests, and a glucose tolerance test for gestational diabetes (see page 144).

EXERCISE

It's best to start getting in shape with a regular program of aerobic exercise, such as brisk walking or aerobic dance, before you become pregnant. Exercise at least three times a week for a minimum of 20 to 30 minutes. If you exercise before you are pregnant, you can keep exercising at that level throughout your pregnancy or until it begins to feel uncomfortable near your final weeks.

If you did not exercise before you became pregnant, you may start a moderate walking program now. However, don't do intensive exercise if you were not already in good aerobic condition before you became pregnant. When your blood rushes to your unconditioned muscles to supply oxygen, the fetus may be deprived of oxygen. Unaccustomed exercise may also raise your core body temperature to a level that is unhealthy for the fetus.

Take your pulse periodically during exercise to make sure it does not exceed 140 beats per minute. Avoid sports in which you might take a fall, such as horseback riding, downhill skiing, or snowboarding. Don't exercise at high elevations without consulting with your doctor first.

Particularly useful during pregnancy are pelvic-floor exercises, known as Kegels (see page 96). These easy exercises will help you carry your baby to term, push it out during labor, and heal after childbirth.

STOPPING HARMFUL RECREATIONAL DRUGS

When you are pregnant or trying to become pregnant, you need to rethink all your habits regarding alcohol, tobacco, and illegal drugs. These drugs cross the placenta and may harm the developing fetus.

CAFFEINE

Many beverages contain caffeine, including coffee, tea, and soda pop. A variety of over-the-counter medications also contain caffeine. Studies are conflicting, but heavy caffeine consumption (more than three cups of coffee a day) may be associated with a higher rate of miscarriage and infertility. It is best to limit yourself to one cup of coffee or other caffeinated beverage a day.

- **Alcohol.** Drinking during pregnancy can cause fetal alcohol syndrome, which includes physical defects of the eye, ears, mouth, nose, heart, and brain as well as mental retardation. No one knows the level of alcohol that is safe, so it is best to abstain altogether.
- **Tobacco.** Smoking or taking tobacco in any form increases the risk of miscarriage, stillbirth, or a baby with a low birth weight and medical problems. Babies of mothers who smoked during pregnancy are also more likely to die from sudden infant death syndrome. If you smoke, quit now.
- **Illegal drugs.** Illegal drugs can cause birth defects and other serious problems. Many babies born to mothers who used drugs must go through a painful physical withdrawal after birth and are left with devastating health problems.

Prescription and nonprescription drugs during pregnancy

You are probably accustomed to taking over-the-counter medications or prescription drugs whenever you need them. If you have a headache, you may take a pain reliever. If you have asthma, you may routinely use a bronchodilator. But once you are pregnant or even considering becoming pregnant, you and your doctor must determine whether you should continue these drugs.

Almost every substance, including drugs, can cross from your blood to the developing fetus via the placenta. Starting during the fifth week of life, the placenta allows nutrients and oxygen to pass from the mother's blood to the fetus, and wastes from the fetus to pass back into the mother's blood for removal. The walls of the placenta, which separate your circulation from that of the fetus, are very permeable and allow drugs and chemicals to pass through. If a drug is present in your bloodstream, it is very likely to cross into the fetus's circulatory system. Upon reaching the fetus, the drug may interfere with organ development or may pass out again without having any negative effects. The molecules of some drugs (including heparin and insulin) are too large to cross the placental membrane.

There are common drugs that increase the risk of birth defects or even death of the fetus. While a number of drugs have a clear history of harming fetal development, far more have never been studied in pregnant women, so doctors are reluctant to prescribe most drugs during pregnancy. Too little is known about which drugs are and are not safe. Before a drug is marketed, the FDA requires that it be tested in animals to see whether it interferes with normal fetal development. Although animal studies can identify drugs that cause gross abnormalities in a developing fetus, the results of animal testing often cannot be applied to humans. Animals such as rabbits and rodents remove drugs from their bodies differently than humans do. Also, they often receive a test dose 50 to 100 times that intended for use in humans. The best approach is to avoid taking any drug, over the counter or prescription, unless it is specifically recommended by a doctor who is aware that you are pregnant.

Despite risks, women with serious health conditions, such as epilepsy or high blood pressure, may need to continue medication during all or part of their pregnancies. Other drugs, such as the common pain reliever acetaminophen, are considered safe in small doses.

In making the decision to take a drug during pregnancy, you and your doctor must carefully consider:

- **Your health.** Do you have a health condition that threatens your health or that of the fetus if left untreated? Do you have a liver or kidney disease that could interfere with your body's ability to remove the drug from your system? Have you already taken the drug during early pregnancy or shortly before pregnancy, so that it may have already affected the fetus?
- **The drug.** Does the drug cross the placenta? How long must you use the drug for it to be effective? Might its effects on your body

PUTTING DRUG RISKS IN PERSPECTIVE

Drugs cause only a tiny fraction of all birth defects. With or without drugs, the risk of having a baby with a birth defect is 2 to 3 percent. The cause of 50 to 65 percent of these birth defects is unknown. Genetic factors account for 12 to 26 percent of birth defects and chromosomal abnormalities for 5 to 6 percent. About 5 to 10 percent of birth defects are caused by environmental factors, including maternal infections (rubella, cytomegalovirus) and exposure to chemicals. Drugs account for only 3 percent of the birth defects caused by environmental factors. However, drugs also can cause infertility, miscarriage, slow growth of a fetus, and drug addiction in the newborn.

harm the fetus; for example, would it raise your blood pressure, cause uterine contractions, or reduce blood flow to the uterus? Does the drug have a history of causing fetal abnormalities? Has the drug been studied during pregnancy? Are there safer treatment alternatives, both drug and other?

- **The timing.** How far along are you in your pregnancy? The fetus is most vulnerable during the first trimester, particularly days 18 to 60, when the vital organs are developing. Also, if the drug is known to cause a birth defect, it usually has a specific "window" when it is most likely to cause the problem. Some drugs are more likely to cause problems later in pregnancy. For example, if the antibiotic tetracycline is taken after the teeth begin to calcify (month 5), it can interfere with the buildup of calcium and permanently stain or discolor the baby's teeth. Aspirin and other drugs that reduce the blood's ability to clot can be dangerous in late pregnancy, causing excess bleeding during labor.

DRUGS THAT MAY BE HARMFUL AND SHOULD BE USED WITH CAUTION

- **Aspirin.** Studies are conflicting, but high doses of aspirin taken for long periods during pregnancy have caused stillbirth and fatal birth defects. Occasional use of aspirin for headache or minor aches and pains appears to be safe during the first two trimesters of pregnancy, but a safer analgesic is acetaminophen (Tylenol). During the last trimester, avoid taking aspirin because it can prolong labor and cause excessive bleeding during delivery. Low-dose aspirin (40 to 150 mg daily) is recommended for some women during the first and second trimesters to reduce the risk of pregnancy-induced high blood pressure (preeclampsia).

- **Antithyroid drugs.** Hyperthyroidism (an excess of thyroid hormone) occasionally develops during pregnancy. Antithyroid drugs are sometimes administered to treat hyperthyroid conditions during pregnancy, but they may affect development of the fetus's thyroid gland, causing a potentially dangerous goiter. Of the two antithyroid drugs, propylthiouracil is usually preferred over methimazole because it crosses the placenta less effectively. To prevent goiter and suppression of the fetal thyroid gland, these drugs are used in the lowest doses possible. (For more about hyperthyroidism, see page 286.)

- **Propranolol.** This beta-blocker has been used during pregnancy to treat a variety of conditions, including hyperthyroidism, high blood pressure, and irregular fetal heart rhythms. Possible effects on the newborn include slow heartbeat, hypoglycemia, growth retardation, and lethargy. Other beta-blockers can have the same effect—it may be that propranolol is more often linked to these problems because it is used most widely. If a beta-blocker is used near term, after birth the baby's heart rate and blood pressure must be monitored closely for at least 48 hours.

- **Phenytoin.** This antiseizure medication taken by epileptic mothers puts an infant at risk for fetal hydantoin syndrome, which includes an abnormally small head, low-set hairline, broad nasal bridge, short neck, and other abnormalities. Although this risk is well known, phenytoin (Dilantin) is often continued during pregnancy if it has controlled the woman's seizures well in the past. The risk of fetal hydantoin syndrome, 5 to 10 percent, is less than the danger posed by a seizure.

- **Theophylline.** Commonly used as a bronchodilator by people with asthma and other lung diseases, in high concentrations theophylline can cause the newborn to have rapid heartbeat, irritability, and vomiting. Infants may also experience withdrawal symptoms that must be treated with theophylline therapy.

DRUGS TO STOP WHEN PLANNING A PREGNANCY

Some drugs that are harmful to a developing fetus do not clear from your system for several weeks. If you are taking any drugs for a health condition, do not stop taking them without the advice of your doctor, but make sure your doctor knows you are planning a pregnancy. These are some of the commonly prescribed drugs that remain in the body for days to weeks after stopping the drug:

antidepressants (particularly the SSRIs—Prozac, Paxil, etc.)

antipsychotics

barbiturates (phenobarbital)

benzodiazepines (Valium)

estradiol (oral contraceptives)

isotretinoin (Accutane, for acne)

lithium

nonsedating antihistamines (astemizole, terfenadine)—these take months to clear

methotrexate

warfarin

DRUGS THAT SHOULD NOT BE USED DURING PREGNANCY

The following drugs should not be used during pregnancy because they increase the risk of birth defects.

- **Methotrexate.** This folic acid antagonist, used for chemotherapy and sometimes to treat ectopic pregnancy or arthritis, has been linked to brain and facial deformities, missing fingers and toes, malformed ribs, and growth retardation. If you have undergone treatment with methotrexate, you should wait at least 12 weeks before attempting to become pregnant.
- **Tetracycline antibiotics.** This common antibiotic drug class, which includes demeclocycline, doxycycline, tetracycline, mino-

cycline, and oxytetracycline, can stain the child's teeth when taken anytime after the fourth or fifth month of pregnancy. These drugs can also interfere with bone growth and should be avoided throughout pregnancy.

- **Warfarin.** Taken in the first trimester, the anticoagulant warfarin (Coumadin) has been associated with fetal warfarin syndrome, which can include low birth weight, eye defects, nasal defects, hearing loss, heart disease, impaired mental development, or fetal death. Taken during the second or third trimester, it can cause mental retardation, seizures, deafness, or fetal death. During the final trimester it can cause severe bleeding in mother or fetus. Warfarin should not be taken at any time during pregnancy. Heparin is the alternative anticoagulant for women with clotting disorders that require treatment during pregnancy.
- **Diethylstilbestrol.** Used commonly during the 1950s to prevent miscarriage, diethylstilbestrol (DES) has been shown to deform the reproductive system of the fetus. It is no longer used during pregnancy.
- **Lithium.** Widely used to treat manic depressive disorder, lithium is not recommended during pregnancy, particularly during the first trimester, due to possible congenital heart defects and other effects.
- **Inorganic iodides.** These drugs, which include Lugol's solution and super-saturated solution of potassium iodide (SSKI), are sometimes used to treat hyperthyroidism or respiratory disorders. Iodide therapy is not recommended during pregnancy because it can cause fetal hypothyroidism or goiter. The enlarged fetal thyroid gland, or goiter, may compress the trachea (windpipe), leading to fetal death.
- **Vitamin A derivatives (Accutane, Etretinate, Retin A).** Taken orally to treat severe acne, isotretinoin (Accutane) can cause a variety of brain, facial, and heart defects and miscarriage. The critical period of exposure is early in pregnancy. Effective contraception must be used for at least one month before beginning Accutane, during treatment, and for one month after stopping treatment. Etretinate, a vitamin A derivative used to treat psoriasis, carries similar risks; since the drug has been found in the body two years after treatment stops, effective contraception must be used indefinitely after the medication is taken. Retin A

and retinoic acid creams used to reduce skin wrinkling are minimally absorbed and present a lower risk to the developing fetus, but they should also not be used during pregnancy.

- **Other drugs.** Other drugs that should not be taken during pregnancy because they raise the risk of physical deformities include ACE inhibitors, clomiphene, danazol, estradiol, leuprolide, misoprostol, and valproic acid.

DRUGS THAT CAN BE TAKEN SAFELY DURING PREGNANCY

All medications taken by a pregnant woman pose a potential risk to the fetus and should be avoided if possible. But some medications can be used safely when taken in correct dosage and overseen by a doctor. They include:

acetaminophen (pain relief)
antibiotics (infections)
  ampicillin
  cephalexin
  erythromycin
  penicillin
antiemetics (for severe nausea)
  chlorpromazine
  meclizine
  prochlorperazine
  promethazine
  trimethobenzamide
antihistamines
  chlorpheniramine
  diphenhydramine
antihypertensives (for high blood
    pressure)

hydralazine
  labetalol
  methyldopa
bronchodilators
  albuterol
bitolterol
  metaproterenol
  salmeterol
  terbutaline
cold medications
  guaifenesin
phenylephrine nasal spray
steroids
prednisone

DRUGS THAT CAUSE WITHDRAWAL SYMPTOMS

If the fetus becomes addicted to a drug used during pregnancy, it will go through withdrawal when the drug stops suddenly at birth. The infant may be jittery, tremble, and have a shrill, high-pitched cry. It may be inconsolable and have a difficult time sucking and swallowing.

Withdrawal often occurs when a mother has been using recreational drugs such as alcohol, cocaine, or amphetamines. Withdrawal can also occur when the mother has been using certain drugs for treatment of illness, including codeine, phenobarbital as an anticonvulsant, and benzodiazepines such as clonazepam for anxiety disorders. Drugs that may cause neonatal withdrawal syndrome include:

alcohol
amphetamines
barbiturates
benzodiazepines
 alprazolam
 chlordiazepoxide
 clonazepam
 diazepam
cocaine

codeine
ethchlorvynol
heroin
meperidine
methadone
morphine
pentazocine
propoxyphene HCl

Treating common medical problems during pregnancy

It is safest to avoid taking any medication during pregnancy. Many of the health problems associated with pregnancy can be treated with simple remedies that do not involve medications. However, some mothers have severe symptoms or a pre-existing health condition that requires medical treatment. Medication during pregnancy can be safe when taken with a doctor's supervision. Virtually all drugs cross the placenta and reach the developing fetus, but not all have been found to harm the fetus. Here are some common problems and recommended treatments.

FDA RATINGS

Although it is best to avoid any medications during pregnancy, some conditions require treatment. To guide doctors and their patients, the Food and Drug Administration has given drugs the following ratings:

- Category A: Studies in humans show no risk to fetus. Possibility of fetal harm is remote.
- Category B: Animal studies show no risk to the fetus, but no studies have been done in humans. *Or* animal studies have shown a risk, but these risks have not been confirmed in studies of humans.
- Category C: Risk cannot be ruled out, as human studies are lacking, but potential benefits may justify the risk. Animal studies have revealed adverse effects on the fetus, but there are no studies in humans. The drug should be given only if the potential benefits outweigh the potential risks. It is better to treat a condition with a nondrug therapy or use a category A or B drug instead.
- Category D: Results of studies in women show a risk to the fetus but the benefits from the use of the drug may be acceptable despite the risk. For example, it may be best to control epileptic seizures with phenytoin and face a 5 to 10 percent risk of fetal hydantoin syndrome (page 137) rather than the death of the fetus due to an uncontrolled seizure.
- Category X: Do not use during pregnancy. Studies show clear fetal risk.

ASTHMA

During pregnancy, asthma may improve, worsen, or stay the same. An asthma attack decreases the oxygen in the mother's blood, which in turns reduces the oxygen reaching the fetus. Because asthma increases the risk of hemorrhage, miscarriage, premature birth, and stillbirth, the benefits of treatment outweigh the risks to the mother and baby. In general, a pregnant woman with asthma is treated in the same way as anyone with asthma.

FDA RATINGS FOR COMMON DRUGS

asthma
 albuterol C
 bitolterol C
 theophylline C
 cromolyn B
 metaproterenol C
 nedocromil B
 corticosteroids (inhaled) B
 salmeterol C
allergies
 chlorpheniramine C
 diphenhydramine C
diabetes
 insulin B
 oral sulfonylureas D
epilepsy
 carbamazepine C
 phenobarbital D
 phenytoin D
 valproic acid X
gastrointestinal disorders
 antacids (magnesium,
  aluminum and calcium-
  containing) B
 cisapride C
 H2-antagonists B

metoclopramide B
sucralfate B
high blood pressure
 ACE inhibitors D
 beta-blockers C
 clonidine C
 diltiazem C
 furosemide C
 hydralazine C
 hydrochlorothiazide D
 labetalol C
 methyldopa C
 nifedipine C
 prazosin C
 verapamil D
headache
 acetaminophen B
 sumatriptan B
nausea
 dimenhydrinate (Dramamine)
  B
 doxylamine (Unisom) B
 meclizine B
thromboembolic disease
 heparin C
 warfarin D

- **Bronchodilators.** A woman with asthma may use an inhaler containing a beta-2-agonist bronchodilator during pregnancy. Beta-2-agonists such as albuterol, bitolterol, metaproterenol, and salmeterol are delivered primarily to the lungs and achieve low levels in the blood. The oral beta-agonist terbutaline is also safe during pregnancy, but it is more likely to cause an increase in heart rate. Fetal heart rate can be monitored throughout pregnancy in women treated with terbutaline.
- **Anti-inflammatory drugs.** If you have wheezing, coughing, or

shortness of breath more than three times a week, talk with your doctor about using an anti-inflammatory drug to shrink swollen air passages and ease breathing. Anti-inflammatory therapy can include inhaled corticosteroids or a mast-cell inhibitor such as cromolyn sodium or nedocromil. The full results of anti-inflammatory therapy often do not appear for two to four weeks, so resist any temptation to use more than the prescribed dosage.

- **Theophylline.** This therapy should be used in pregnancy only if your asthma is not controlled by a combination of bronchodilator and corticosteroid therapy. In the most severe cases, a once-a-day dose of theophylline in the evening can help treat nighttime asthma. Newborn babies who were exposed to theophylline in the uterus have shown jitteriness, vomiting, and irregular heartbeat.

COLDS, FLU, AND ALLERGIES

When a cold or flu strikes, don't reach for the over-the-counter medicine you usually take. Instead, try some other methods first. A humidifier can loosen congestion, make breathing easier, and soothe your throat. Instead of a decongestant, try saline nasal sprays (Ocean Spray), which deliver water directly to the respiratory tissues.

During pregnancy, some women who have never before had allergies develop vasomotor rhinitis and sinusitis, a harmless but annoying nasal stuffiness and postnasal drip. The cause is unknown but may be hormonal. Allergies that existed before pregnancy can lessen or worsen.

Medications

- **Nasal decongestants.** Instead of decongestant pills, use a nasal spray. Less medication will circulate throughout your body, and more will go directly where it's needed. A nasal spray containing phenylephrine is a safe choice. Use it only when needed and no longer than three days in a row. Don't use oral decongestants containing phenylpropanolamine or pseudoephedrine. The oral agents are less effective than the nasal sprays in contracting the smaller blood vessels of the nasal passages to reduce congestion, and they may raise blood pressure and possibly reduce the flow of blood and oxygen to your uterus.

- **Cough medicines.** For a dry, hacking cough, some over-the-counter cough suppressants containing dextromethorphan are relatively safe. For a productive cough, increasing your intake of fluids is the best way to loosen respiratory secretions. If an over-the-counter cough preparation is warranted, those containing guaifenesin are also relatively safe. Make sure to take a guaifenesin containing product with an 8-ounce glass of water. Also, before using any cough syrup, check the labeling for the alcohol content.
- **Antihistamine.** Most doctors believe it is safe to use certain antihistamines occasionally to treat allergies. The safest choice is chlorpheniramine (Chlor-Trimeton allergy pills). The antihistamine diphenhydramine (Benadryl) is probably safe; however, there are some reports of it causing cleft palate when taken during the first trimester of pregnancy. Although the risk is considered low, it is best to avoid the use of diphenhydramine during the first trimester. Brompheniramine should be avoided during pregnancy because it has been associated with fetal malformations. Overall, an antihistamine should be used only when necessary. Long-term use should be avoided. Newer antihistamines such as terfenadine (Seldane), which have become popular because they do not cause drowsiness, cannot be safely recommended because of a lack of studies during pregnancy.

CONSTIPATION, HEMORRHOIDS

Constipation and hemorrhoids are common complaints during pregnancy. Constipation develops because progesterone, a hormone released in high quantities during pregnancy, relaxes the muscles of the intestines, so the bowel does not evacuate as efficiently as usual. Also, as the uterus grows, it presses on the intestine, causing discomfort and difficulty in passing stool. Iron supplements used to treat anemia during pregnancy also contribute to the development of constipation. Hemorrhoids often occur because the enlarged uterus presses on the blood vessels in the anal area. The increased pressure leads to hemorrhoids with itching, burning, swelling, pain, and occasionally bleeding.

You can usually prevent constipation with these steps:

- Drink six 8-ounce glasses of water every day (unless another medical condition dictates otherwise).
- Exercise daily.
- Increase fiber in your diet by eating whole-grain breads and cereals and plenty of fresh fruits and vegetables.

Preventing constipation can relieve and prevent hemorrhoids. If you do develop hemorrhoids, clean the area regularly with a mild soap and water and pat dry after every bowel movement. A sitz bath (available over the counter) two or three times a day will also relieve swelling and pain.

Medications

If your constipation is severe and will not go away, do not take a chemical stimulant laxative such as castor oil, which can cause uterine contractions, or a saline cathartic, which can contain a high quantity of sodium. Instead, use a fiber-based bulk laxative (Metamucil) or a mild laxative such as milk of magnesia. Stool softeners taken orally are safe throughout pregnancy. (For more on laxatives and how they work, see page 54.)

For hemorrhoids, pregnant women can use over-the-counter creams or ointments containing astringents or the local anesthetics benzocaine or pramoxine (Americaine ointment, Anusol ointment). They should avoid products containing hydrocortisone. Although corticosteroids such as hydrocortisone and prednisone are relatively safe during pregnancy, there is no need to add the risk of these agents to the treatment of hemorrhoids, which are usually a relatively minor condition.

DIABETES

Two to three percent of women who have never had diabetes develop "gestational diabetes" during pregnancy, and some women are diabetic before they become pregnant. Either condition must be monitored carefully. Some cases of diabetes can be controlled with diet and exercise and require no drug treatment. In other cases, a woman must control her blood sugar with insulin injections. Fortunately, insulin is a safe and effective way to control diabetes during pregnancy and does not harm the fetus.

A natural substance manufactured by the body, insulin allows sugar (glucose) to be converted into energy in the body's cells. People with diabetes cannot make insulin, or their bodies cannot use the insulin efficiently, so the level of sugar in their blood may get too high. (For more on diabetes, see page 291.) If diabetes is not controlled during pregnancy, the high blood sugar may cause birth defects (neural tube defects, heart defects, cystic kidneys) and will increase the mother's risk of miscarriage, high blood pressure, hydramnios (excess fluid in the amniotic sac), and cesarean delivery (the last because the baby is likely to be large).

If you do not have diabetes before you become pregnant, your doctor will test your blood sugar levels between weeks 24 and 28, when the risk of developing gestational diabetes is highest. You have a greater than average risk of developing gestational diabetes if you have a family history of diabetes, have had gestational diabetes during a previous pregnancy, are overweight, are over age 35, have had a stillbirth or given birth to a child with birth defects, or have given birth to a large infant. Women of African, Asian, or Hispanic descent are also at higher risk.

If you have diabetes before you become pregnant, you and your doctor will carefully monitor your blood sugar during pregnancy. Whether your diabetes is new or pre-existing, you will need to follow a special program of diet and exercise. Blood tests will show whether you need to take insulin to control your blood sugar levels. (For information on insulin, see page 299.) Oral antidiabetic agents (sulfonylureas) such as glipizide and glyburide are not recommended during pregnancy. Because they stimulate the release of insulin from the pancreas, they may increase the secretion of insulin from the fetal pancreas and cause hypoglycemia. If you have type 2 diabetes and your condition cannot be controlled by diet alone during pregnancy, insulin will be used instead of an oral antidiabetic drug. The newer oral agents, acarbose and metformin, are also not recommended because their safety during pregnancy has not yet been established.

EPILEPSY

Epilepsy presents a difficult dilemma during pregnancy. The medications normally used to prevent seizures pose a significant risk to the fetus, but discontinuing medication may lead to seizures that produce even more risk for the fetus and the pregnant woman. The usual strategy is to maintain the medication regimen that has successfully controlled seizures before pregnancy and, when possible, stick with a single anticonvulsant drug during pregnancy.

Medications

- **Carbamazepine.** Until 1989 carbamazepine was the first choice for controlling seizures during pregnancy. Although it crosses the placenta rapidly, it appeared to present less risk to the fetus than other medications. Early reports of the use of this drug showed that exposed newborns had a smaller head circumference than other infants but that the difference disappeared after about six months. More recently, though, case reports have linked the drug to the fetal hydantoin syndrome formerly associated only with phenytoin (see below). Currently the use of carbamazepine during pregnancy is controversial. Carbamazepine should be continued during pregnancy if it has controlled seizures well in the past. Switching to another anticonvulsant may lead to seizures. Discuss your options with your doctor if you have epilepsy and become pregnant. Do not discontinue your medication without consulting your doctor.

- **Phenytoin.** Phenytoin (Dilantin), the most commonly prescribed anticonvulsant, is associated with a high risk of abnormalities of the face, skull, and limbs as well as mental retardation, called fetal hydantoin syndrome. About 5 to 10 percent of exposed babies develop this syndrome, and another 30 percent develop some of the abnormal features. The symptoms may be subtle and difficult to diagnose. There is some debate over whether this syndrome results from phenytoin itself or from a deficiency in folic acid. Phenytoin decreases the absorption of folic acid, so you will be advised to take a vitamin supplement with at least 0.4 mg of folate throughout your pregnancy if you are taking phenytoin. Phenytoin also causes a deficiency in clotting factors in the fetus, and it may cause a condition called hemorrhagic disease of the newborn. Within 24 hours after birth, infants born to mothers who took phenytoin during pregnancy often require an injection of vitamin K, which stimulates the production of clotting factors.

- **Ethosuximide.** Ethosuximide (Zarontin) is the preferred drug for treating absence (formerly known as petit mal) epileptic seizures in the first trimester of pregnancy. Although there have been a few reports of fetal abnormalities, most experts believe this drug is safer than others used for this purpose during pregnancy.

- **Valproic acid.** Valproic acid (Depakene) should never be used in pregnancy. Typically prescribed at other times to treat both generalized and absence seizures, valproic acid can cross the placenta to the fetus and cause congenital abnormalities, jaundice, fetal distress, and neural tube defects.

- **Phenobarbital.** This anticonvulsant is not routinely used as a single drug but is combined with phenytoin to treat refractory seizures. Like phenytoin, phenobarbital can decrease the absorption of folic acid and can cause a deficiency in clotting factors in the newborn. Phenobarbital may cause some of the minor features of fetal hydantoin syndrome, but it has not been associated with the full fetal hydantoin syndrome. However, an additional concern with phenobarbital is withdrawal symptoms in the exposed infant.

HEARTBURN

Heartburn, known medically as reflux esophagitis, is irritation and pain caused by the backwash of stomach acids into the esophagus (the tube that carries food from your throat to your stomach). Heartburn occurs in 25 percent of pregnant women, most often during the third trimester of pregnancy as the enlarging uterus puts pressure on the stomach. Progesterone also contributes by relaxing the lower esophageal muscle, allowing intestinal contents to flow back up through the esophagus. Symptoms may worsen when you bend over, lie down, or lift heavy objects. You can reduce the chance of heartburn by avoiding:

- Big meals (eat smaller meals, more frequently)
- Eating near bedtime
- Products that irritate the stomach, including caffeinated beverages, aspirin and ibuprofen, alcohol, nicotine, and acidic foods such as tomato sauce
- Lifting heavy objects
- Lying down immediately after eating

If your symptoms are severe, choose an over-the-counter antacid such as Maalox, Mylanta, Tums, or Rolaids. These antacids can be used safely during pregnancy. Too little research is available to recommend the use of H2-antagonists during pregnancy; these drugs include cimetidine (Tagamet), ranitidine (Zantac), famotidine (Pepsid), and nizatidine (Axid).

HEART DISEASE

Heart disease is uncommon among women of childbearing age, except for congenital or rheumatic disorders. Because pregnancy increases the workload of the heart, women with heart problems must be closely monitored during pregnancy and may need to take medications. Your doctor will be watching for any signs of declining heart function or inadequate blood supply for the placenta and fetus. Because blood circulation to the fetus is often less than normal, women with heart conditions often give birth to smaller babies. They are also at higher risk of miscarriage.

Medications

For more on medications to treat heart disease, see page 188. Among the heart medications that have a long history of use during pregnancy and have not been found to harm the fetus are:

- **Digoxin.** Digoxin is used to treat heart failure and abnormal heart rhythms. Although it readily crosses the placenta to the fetus, it has not been found to cause abnormalities or disease.
- **Quinidine.** Commonly prescribed to treat abnormal heart rhythms in pregnant women, quinidine has not been linked with any adverse effects on the fetus.
- **Disopyramide.** Although disopyramide, which is used to treat abnormal heart rhythms, has not been widely prescribed during pregnancy, it has not been linked with any adverse effects in the fetus.
- **Lidocaine.** Sometimes administered intravenously when a problem with heart rhythm is life-threatening, lidocaine presents minimal risk to the fetus when administered in the usual doses, although one study linked it with low muscle strength in newborns.

- **Mexiletine.** Although experience with mexiletine during pregnancy is limited, this antiarrhythmic agent has not been linked with any adverse effects on the fetus.

HIGH BLOOD PRESSURE

High blood pressure (hypertension) is one of the most common complications of pregnancy, affecting about 7 percent of pregnant women. Some women have high blood pressure before they become pregnant or early in pregnancy. Others develop it later. High blood pressure that occurs after week 20 of pregnancy is called toxemia or pregnancy-induced hypertension. When there is also fluid retention or the presence of protein in the urine, the condition is called preeclampsia. Monitoring your blood pressure is one of the most important reasons you need to see your doctor regularly throughout your pregnancy.

High blood pressure can cause a variety of health problems for the fetus, including slower growth and premature birth. Very high blood pressure can interfere with blood flow to the fetus, depriving it of oxygen and nutrients. The higher your blood pressure, the more likely it is that complications will occur. Preeclampsia can lead to eclampsia, which involves seizures in the mother. Also, uncontrolled high blood pressure can lead to stroke or diseases of the kidneys, eyes, and liver.

You are more likely to have high blood pressure during pregnancy if you are over age 35, have a family history of high blood pressure, have poor nutrition, have diabetes, or are obese. You are considered to have high blood pressure during pregnancy if your systolic reading (the top number) is more than 30 points above your reading before you were pregnant and if your diastolic reading (the bottom number) is more than 15 points higher.

Medications

If your diastolic pressure reaches 100, treatment with medication is likely. Some medications used to treat high blood pressure at other times are not safe during pregnancy. If you are taking medication for high blood pressure and are considering pregnancy, consult your doctor about appropriate medication. ACE inhibitors are particularly dangerous to the fetus.

If your blood pressure cannot be controlled with oral medications, your doctor may recommend intravenous medication, bed rest, or hospitalization. Your doctor will also perform ultrasound exams and other tests to determine whether your fetus is healthy. Early delivery may be necessary if your baby is close to full term. In most cases, a woman's blood pressure returns to normal after the baby is delivered, unless she has chronic high blood pressure.

- **Methyldopa.** The most commonly used and probably safest choice, Methyldopa is the only antihypertensive medication whose long-term effects on the child have been studied. In one study, children whose mothers took methyldopa during pregnancy were found to have normal development at ages 4 and 7. If used during pregnancy, methyldopa often causes tiredness and mild dizziness.
- **Beta-blockers.** After methyldopa, one of the beta-blockers, labetalol, is the second choice for treating high blood pressure in pregnant women. Labetalol is a unique beta-blocker that also has alpha-blocking properties (see page 197). During pregnancy it is preferred over the other beta-blockers because it does not decrease heart rate or impair blood flow to the fetus. Other beta-blockers (propranolol, atenolol, metoprolol) may slow the baby's heart rate after birth, so the heart rate will be monitored for the first 24 to 72 hours after birth. A lower heart rate in an infant may require treatment because not enough blood and nutrients are being delivered to the baby's organs. This is an uncommon problem and is treated with intravenous fluids and possibly drugs. The use of beta-blockers in the mother, particularly propranolol, has also been associated with slower growth of the fetus and hypoglycemia in the newborn. There have been no studies of the effects of exposure to beta-blockers in infants past age 1.
- **Calcium channel blockers.** This is another type of drug commonly used to treat hypertension. Calcium channel blockers have not been well studied in pregnancy and are not routinely used then. However, in some women with preeclampsia, the calcium channel antagonist nifedipine has been found to be very effective.
- **Diuretics.** Diuretics are occasionally prescribed for high blood pressure, particularly if they were successfully used before pregnancy. They reduce blood volume, which may reduce the amount of blood reaching the fetus.

- **ACE inhibitors.** This type of vasodilator, used to treat high blood pressure and heart failure, has been shown to cause kidney damage in the fetus or fetal death if administered during the second or third trimester. ACE inhibitors can be used preceding pregnancy but should be discontinued as soon as possible once you discover you are pregnant.

INFECTIONS

During your pregnancy, you are more vulnerable than usual to some infections. Also, the effects of an infection can be more serious than usual. The good news is that there are antibiotics that are safe during pregnancy, including the oldest antibiotic, penicillin. Some antibiotics can harm the fetus and must be avoided.

If you see signs of an infection, see your doctor, because it can be dangerous not to treat an infection. For example, toxoplasmosis, caused by a parasite that lives in raw meat and in the feces of some mammals, including cats, can cause the fetus to have neurological problems or partial blindness. Cytomegalovirus, a virus that causes mild, if any, symptoms in adults, if passed to the fetus can cause severe illness, birth defects and mental retardation, blindness, or death.

To avoid infections during pregnancy:

- Practice good hygiene, especially by washing your hands frequently.
- Avoid sexually transmitted diseases by using a condom during intercourse.
- If you have not had the childhood diseases chicken pox, rubella, and fifth disease, take extra care to avoid infection when coming in contact with infected individuals. Early in the pregnancy, talk with your doctor about previous immunizations and childhood illnesses. Rubella vaccine is not recommended during pregnancy. To boost immunity against chicken pox, the varicella immune globulin can be taken. If you are unsure about your history of childhood illnesses, your physician can test you for rubella.
- If you are prone to the flu based on your past history, or if you have a chronic disease, such as pulmonary disease or a cardiac condition, it may be wise to get a flu shot when pregnant. However, pregnancy alone is not a reason to get the flu shot.

- To avoid toxoplasmosis, have someone else change the kitty litter. Also, use gloves while gardening. Do not eat raw meat, and wash your hands thoroughly after handling it.
- Reduce your chance of a urinary tract infection, which is common during pregnancy, by drinking several large glasses of water a day, urinating frequently, urinating after intercourse, and washing your genital and anal area daily with mild soap and water.

Medications

There are several antibiotics considered safe during pregnancy, some considered unsafe, and many for which too little information is available. Antibiotics kill bacteria but have no effect on infections caused by viruses such as cold and flu. (For more about antibiotics, see page 233.)

- **Penicillin.** Penicillin and its synthetic versions (ampicillin, amoxicillin) are safe for pregnant women. They can treat a variety of infections, including respiratory infections and some sexually transmitted diseases.
- **Sulfonamides.** A common choice for treating urinary tract infections, sulfonamides (sulfisoxazole or Gantrisin; trimethoprim-sulfamethoxazole or Bactrim) readily cross the placenta to the fetus during all stages of pregnancy. They appear, however, to have no adverse effect on the fetus during the first two trimesters. Do not take sulfonamides during the third trimester because they increase the risk of kernicterus, a rare disorder that damages the fetus's brain.
- **Erythromycin.** Often prescribed for people allergic to penicillin, erythromycin is relatively safe throughout pregnancy. It crosses the placenta but only in small amounts and has not been associated with any fetal abnormality or illness. Erythromycin is not safe for women who have had liver disease.
- **Tetracycline.** The popular antibiotic tetracycline should not be used during pregnancy, particularly anytime after month 3, when the fetal teeth and bones are forming. It may cause staining of the teeth, underdeveloped tooth enamel, and poor development of the long bones.

NAUSEA AND VOMITING

Many pregnant women experience some nausea or vomiting, especially during the first trimester. Although sometimes referred to as morning sickness, these symptoms can appear at any time of day. Nausea usually disappears by the end of the fourth month.

To prevent and relieve nausea:

- Eat smaller, more frequent meals throughout the day.
- When you feel nauseated, eat dry carbohydrate snacks like crackers or toast.
- Avoid eating or even smelling foods that trigger nausea.
- Avoid foods that are greasy or fried, very hot or very cold, or very spicy.
- Drink plenty of liquids between meals.
- Dairy products sometimes trigger nausea. If you must avoid dairy products, ask your doctor about taking a calcium supplement.

A deficiency of vitamin B6 (pyridoxine) sometimes causes nausea and vomiting during the second trimester. If your doctor determines you have a B6 deficiency, you can safely take a dose of 10 to 30 mg a day. Other symptoms of B6 deficiency include mental depression, lethargy, fatigue, impaired glucose and insulin metabolism, numbness and tingling of the arms and legs, loss of balance, and anemia.

Medications

If self-help techniques don't work, and you can't keep down any foods or liquids for three or more days, medication may be appropriate to prevent nutritional deficiencies for you and the fetus. Unfortunately, nausea typically occurs during the first trimester, when the fetus is most likely to be harmed by a drug. Before taking any medication for nausea or vomiting during pregnancy, talk to your doctor.

- **Meclizine.** The drug prescribed most often to relieve severe nausea during pregnancy is meclizine. Relatively large studies have shown no increase in fetal defects. Take the medication with food or a glass of water to lessen stomach irritation. The side effects of meclizine, particularly drowsiness, may gradually go away after your body becomes accustomed to the medication.

- **Dimenhydrinate.** Dimenhydrinate (Dramamine) relieves nausea effectively and has a low potential for harming the fetus. It should not be taken near term because it has been reported to stimulate uterine contractions, causing premature labor.
- **Pyridoxine.** Also known as vitamin B6, pyridoxine does not relieve nausea during pregnancy in women who are not deficient in the vitamin. However, when combined with the antihistamine doxylamine (Unisom), vitamin B6 in low doses (25 to 100 mg per day) can effectively relieve nausea and vomiting of pregnancy. Doxylamine appears to be safe and has not been associated with congenital malformations or inadequate fetal weight gain. Excessive doses of vitamin B6, particularly greater than 100 mg per day, should be avoided. Deficiencies and excessive quantities of vitamin B6 are associated with nerve disorders and can cause tingling and numbness in the lower limbs.
- **Phenothiazines.** When used in low doses, phenothiazines (including promethazine, prochlorperazine, and chlorpromazine) appear to be safe. They are used when other drugs have failed.

PAIN

At times during your pregnancy, you may experience a headache, backache, or other aches and pains. More serious and painful conditions can also occur. As with most conditions during pregnancy, it is best to try other approaches before you try a medication.

For headaches, try the following techniques:

- Eat regularly; hunger can trigger a headache.
- Get enough sleep.
- If you get a headache, find a quiet, darkened place to sit or lie down with your eyes closed.
- Get a breath of fresh air and avoid stuffy, smoky rooms.
- Lie down and try this stress reliever. First tense, then relax each set of muscles in your body, starting with your toes and working up to your torso, shoulders, head, and down through your arms and hands.

As your pregnancy progresses, you may feel lower-back pain. The increased weight in your abdomen can lead you to arch your spine into a "swayback" position that strains your vertebrae. Try these techniques to avoid or relieve lower-back pain:

- To pick something up, bend your knees instead of leaning over from the waist.
- Wear low-heeled shoes.
- Do pelvic-tilt exercises regularly. Stand with your back against a wall. Squeeze your buttocks together and tilt your pelvis forward to flatten your spine against the wall. Hold for 5 seconds. Release gently and repeat 10 times.

Medications

Some pain relievers are safe during pregnancy, others not. (For more on pain relief medications, see chapter 10.)

- **Acetaminophen.** When nondrug methods do not relieve your pain, the best choice is acetaminophen (Tylenol). Acetaminophen is safe at any stage of pregnancy. Take acetaminophen as directed and do not exceed the recommended dose.
- **Aspirin.** Avoid aspirin during pregnancy, particularly during the last trimester, when it can prolong labor and cause excess bleeding during delivery.
- **Ibuprofen.** Avoid ibuprofen (Advil, Motrin, Nuprin) particularly during the third trimester. Like aspirin, it inhibits blood clotting and can cause excessive bleeding. All drugs in this class, known as the NSAIDs (see page 211), carry this same precaution—including naproxen sodium (Aleve).
- **Opiates.** When more severe pain must be treated, such as after an accident or emergency surgery, opiates work well. If they are used longer than two days, however, the fetus can become dependent on the drug and experience painful withdrawal.

Drugs during labor and delivery

Many women give birth without medications, but others need or want the pain relief that medication can bring. A medical condition may also dictate the need for drugs. A premature or late delivery is more likely to involve medications. Even if you are planning a natural childbirth, it is a good idea to learn about drugs that may be needed if complications should develop.

SUPPRESSING-PREMATURE LABOR

A normal pregnancy lasts about 40 weeks. Labor is considered premature if before week 37 there are regular, painful uterine contractions every 10 minutes or less that last at least 30 seconds each, and if the cervix has thinned (effaced) at least 80 percent and opened (dilated) by at least 2 centimeters.

Complications that increase the risk of premature labor are multiple fetuses (twins, triplets, etc.), kidney infections, bleeding during pregnancy, two or more previous abortions during the second trimester, excess amniotic fluid, and an abnormal uterus or cervix. Premature rupture of the membranes is also a cause of preterm labor. Premature infants are more likely to have low birth weight and a variety of disorders, including immature lungs. Because of this, doctors often try to prevent premature labor and allow the fetus to continue to develop normally in the uterus for as long as possible.

If you experience contractions before week 37, call your doctor immediately. The sooner attempts are made to stop the contractions, the more likely they are to succeed. Your doctor will want to observe you for 30 minutes to an hour and will perform a pelvic exam to see if your cervix is dilated. You may also have an ultrasound to determine the size and position of the baby. Depending on the health of the fetus, including its estimated weight and lung maturity, your doctor may simply allow labor to take its course. Also, if you have signs of an infection such as fever or an increased white blood cell count, or if the membranes have ruptured, labor will usually be encouraged.

If the fetal lungs are immature and labor is not already too far along, steps may be taken to suppress it. The first step is sedation and rest. Many women carry the fetus for another two weeks with this therapy. If this fails, the labor may be suppressed with drugs. Labor should not be suppressed if your membranes are ruptured or bulging, if your cervix is dilated more than 4 centimeters, or if you or the fetus has severely high blood pressure or heart disease.

WHEN PREMATURE LABOR SHOULD NOT BE SUPPRESSED

conditions in the mother
  eclampsia
  diabetes (uncontrolled)
  heart disease
  high blood pressure (severe)
  vaginal bleeding
conditions in the fetus
  intrauterine fetal death
  fetal distress

intrauterine infection
retarded growth
progression of labor
  ruptured membranes
  bulging membranes
  cervical dilation over 4
    centimeters
inaccurate due date

Medications

- **Magnesium sulfate.** Used for many years to suppress premature labor, magnesium sulfate is administered intravenously in a gradually increasing dose until the contractions stop. It is less likely to cause side effects than the most common alternative therapy, the beta-agonists. The side effects of magnesium sulfate include lethargy, flushing, and nausea. Levels of magnesium in the blood can easily be monitored to prevent toxicity. Rarely, chest pain and excess liquid in the lungs (pulmonary edema) occur. A drawback is that magnesium must be taken intravenously. Although magnesium is available in tablet form for oral use, its absorption from the intestines is highly variable and not reliable. After contractions have stopped during IV magnesium therapy, doctors usually prescribe ritodrine (see below) in an oral form as a follow-up.

- **Ritodrine.** The beta-agonist ritodrine suppresses labor by slowing the uterine contractions. Related drugs such as terbutaline, isoxuprine, albuterol, and metaproterenol have also been used for this purpose. Your doctor will begin treatment with a small intravenous dose of the drug, which is gradually increased until the drug stops the contractions. You will continue with the drug at the lowest effective dose for 12 to 24 hours after the contractions cease. You may then receive periodic injections of the drug and take oral doses until you deliver. If your contractions start again, you may resume injections of the drug. The disadvantage to the beta agents is that their effects are not limited to the uterine muscle. They can stimulate the heart, causing an increased heart rate and possibly chest pain. These drugs may also increase your serum glucose (sugar), which may require the use of insulin. Although expensive, terbutaline has been used by injection through a subcutaneous pump for home use. Because the dose of terbutaline used by subcutaneous pump is lower than that used orally or by IV injection, the side effects of terbutaline by this route of administration are minimal.

RELIEVING PAIN DURING LABOR AND CHILDBIRTH

As during the rest of pregnancy, during labor and childbirth most drugs will reach the fetus. At this stage of pregnancy, the placenta and fetal circulation are particularly permeable to drugs. In a vaginal birth with no complications, it is safest to use few or no drugs.

Natural childbirth techniques

Natural childbirth is a vaginal delivery without pain relief drugs. Many women choose this option so that their babies will be free of any residual effects of drugs and so that they themselves can have the greatest control, mobility, and participation during the delivery. Whether you are in a hospital or a birthing center, whether you have an obstetrician or a nurse midwife, there are a number of nondrug ways to make labor and childbirth easier and more comfortable:

- Before the birth, take classes to learn and practice breathing techniques.
- To speed up labor, try sitting, standing, walking, and squatting.
- Concentrate on only one contraction at a time.
- Relax between contractions by taking a few deep breaths.
- Get a lower-back rub from your partner; learn the proper techniques beforehand.
- Drink plenty of fluids during early labor, and suck on ice chips throughout labor.

Medications

There are two kinds of pain relief medications available during child-birth—analgesics and anesthetics. Analgesics are given by injection, while anesthetics can be given topically to a small area of the skin, regionally, or by inhalation. Regional anesthesia is the most common method of providing pain relief during labor and delivery. It completely eliminates pain by blocking the conduction of pain impulses in a specific region of the body, such as from the waist down.

- **Analgesics.** An analgesic, which is usually a narcotic, is injected into a muscle or vein and circulates through the blood system. Some of the analgesics used during childbirth include meperidine (Demerol), fentanyl (Sublimaze), nalbuphine (Nubain), butorphanol (Stadol), and morphine. The pain relief will last about one hour, after which you can try to go without medication for a while. The goal of injectable analgesic therapy is to make you comfortable rather than to make you pain-free. The analgesic will make you and the baby feel somewhat "drugged" and sedated. If a narcotic medication is given too early in labor, it can slow progress. If it is given too close to delivery, the baby may be sedated at birth. In particular, meperidine (Demerol) may interfere with the baby's ability to suckle at the breast. If you are considering breast-feeding, you may want to avoid injectable narcotic analgesics, particularly meperidine (Demerol).
- **Epidural.** The most common form of regional anesthesia during childbirth, epidural anesthesia numbs you from the waist down, though you can still move your legs. An anesthetic, usually bupivacaine, is injected into a small space between your spinal cord and vertebrae. The drug can be administered as a one-time dose or given continuously, after the needle is removed, through a tube left attached to your back. Placement of a catheter allows more drug to be administered at a later time when pain increases or in the case of a cesarean birth. An epidural anesthetic takes effect in about 20 minutes, and the duration of pain relief depends on the anesthetic used. An epidural allows you to remain alert during labor, although you will not be able to walk around while the epidural is working (a common way to speed up labor). The epidural may also make it more difficult to push the baby out.

Epidurals are used for uncomplicated labor and may also be used for cesarean section. Adverse effects are minimal, but some women develop a headache after the anesthetic wears off. Rarely, epidural anesthesia temporarily numbs the lower legs.

- **Paracervical block.** A form of regional anesthesia, paracervical block can decrease the pain caused by the stretching of the cervix during labor. It is administered by injection into your cervix. This anesthesia does not interfere with your ability or urge to push. It must be repeated every hour to remain effective and is used infrequently.

- **Pudenal block.** A pudenal block is an injection of anesthetic through the vaginal wall during the second stage of labor to relieve pain in the area between the vagina and rectum caused by stretching. This anesthesia does not interfere with the urge or ability to push and is often given to relieve the pain of episiotomy, an incision to enlarge the vaginal opening.

- **Spinal anesthesia.** The spinal form of regional anesthesia is rarely used except for cesarean section. The anesthetic is injected into the spinal fluid, numbing the complete abdominal and perineal area and completely removing the urge to push. For uncomplicated labor, epidural anesthesia has virtually replaced spinals because epidurals allow you to still feel the pressure of the contraction so you can be involved in the labor. Spinals may also cause severe headaches and can cause blood pressure to fall.

- **General anesthesia.** Drugs given by inhalation or injection for general anesthesia cause complete loss of consciousness. They are rarely used except for emergency cesarean delivery.

- **Postpartum pain relief.** If you have delivered your baby by cesarean section, you will be given pain relief in the form of injections of morphine or ketorolac. (See page 217 for descriptions of these drugs commonly used for postoperative pain.)

INDUCING LABOR

There are drugs that can start or speed up uterine contractions. Drugs may be used to induce labor if:

- There is a vaginal or uterine infection.
- The pregnancy is more than two weeks past the due date.

- The mother's blood pressure is dangerously high.
- There is too little amniotic fluid around the baby.
- The baby is unusually small and not growing.
- There is vaginal bleeding.
- The membranes rupture after the 36th week.

Your doctor may first try to bring on labor by breaking the amniotic sac and allowing the liquid to flow out. Breaking the membranes stimulates prostaglandin production, which can start uterine contractions. If labor contractions do not start 12 to 24 hours after your membranes break, your doctor may use medication. Low doses of prostaglandin (dinoprostone) in the form of a vaginal suppository may be administered to your cervix to prepare it for labor.

Medication

- **Oxytocin.** The synthetic hormone Oxytocin (Pitocin) is used to bring on labor. It is given intravenously in a continuous stream, increasing every 15 to 20 minutes until contractions begin. The goal is to induce contractions that come every 2 to 3 minutes and last 45 to 60 seconds. A monitor will track the baby's heart rate. Clinicians will monitor your contractions, blood pressure, and heart rate. All of this monitoring will alert the doctor to any complications. The most common, though still rare, complication is a ruptured uterus. Oxytocin can reduce blood flow to the baby, resulting in decreased heart rate, oxygen deficiency, and fluid retention. Oxytocin produces more intense and painful contractions than a woman might experience without the medication, and increases the chances that some form of pain reliever will be used. Oxytocin should not be used when vaginal delivery is not recommended. It is also used to decrease bleeding after childbirth.

chapter 8

DRUGS DURING BREAST-FEEDING

*A*FTER REACHING AN ALL-TIME LOW IN THE EARLY 1970s, breast-feeding has surged in popularity because of evidence that breast milk is the ideal food for an infant. Breast-feeding is one of the best choices you can make for your child, but, it does give you some additional responsibilities, among them the need to consider the potential impact on your baby of any drug you take. Small amounts of any food or drug are likely to reach your breast milk and your baby. Also, a few drugs can reduce your milk supply.

Drugs in breast milk

Because most drugs that enter your body also enter your breast milk, it is best to take no drug, including medications, alcohol, tobacco, or street drugs, while breast-feeding. If you do need a drug for a medical condition, however, the baby is less likely to be affected now than during the pregnancy. In general, the amount of a drug that passes from your blood into breast milk is far lower than that which reaches the fetus through the placenta. The amount of a drug that reaches breast milk depends on the drug's chemistry. There may be only 1 or 2 percent as much drug in the breast milk as in the mother's bloodstream. Also good news is that in many cases, the timing of a drug can be controlled to reduce the amount the baby receives.

On the negative side, there is not much solid information about whether individual drugs accumulate in breast milk or harm the baby, because the Food and Drug Administration does not require pharmaceutical companies to do these studies. The American Academy of Pediatrics (AAP), however, periodically reviews the studies that have been published on drug use and breast-feeding and recommends which drugs are or are not compatible with breast-feeding. This chapter incorporates these recommendations.

Since the response to drugs is very individual, one baby may react to a particular drug while another does not. For this reason, watch your baby for signs of a reaction when you or the baby is taking any drug. Some symptoms are subtle, but others are obvious if you know what to look for. For example, antibiotics (which are prescribed often during breast-feeding) may pass in only minimal amounts into the milk, but most infants develop diarrhea (which can be dangerous at this age) and diaper rash. Antihistamines can cause irritability. Drugs such as codeine, oxycodone, or morphine may cause sedation or changes in sleep patterns. Even if a drug is considered safe to use during breast-feeding, it is wise to monitor your baby for any signs of drug exposure.

Your baby's response to medication you take is influenced by:

- Age—a younger baby's stomach and intestines are less able to absorb a drug, and its kidneys and liver can't remove it from the body as well
- Weight
- Amount of milk consumed
- Prematurity
- Drug dosage—larger dosages increase the baby's exposure to the drug
- Frequency—more frequent use increases the baby's exposure

Make sure that your doctor knows that you are breast-feeding before prescribing any drug. Tell your doctor your feeding schedule and the baby's age and overall health.

Because studies are lacking, it is best to play it safe and avoid drugs unless you really need them. This advice applies to prescription medications and over-the-counter medications as well as vitamin supplements, herbs, and any other forms of medicine unless specifically recommended by a doctor who knows you are breast-feeding.

Concerns about drugs, however, should not discourage you from breast-feeding. Breast-feeding will benefit both your baby and you. It is rare that a drug or substance is so dangerous to your infant that you will be advised to stop breast-feeding.

ADVANTAGES OF BREAST-FEEDING

Breast-feeding your child, particularly in the first few months, brings benefits to both you and your baby. It:

- Provides the ideal nourishment for your baby.
- Reduces the chance of infections for your baby (particularly respiratory and ear).
- Reduces your baby's risk of allergies and digestive disorders such as inflammatory bowel disease.
- Provides a sense of closeness and interdependence for you and your child.
- Eliminates the chore—and the expense—of mixing formulas and washing bottles.
- Stimulates hormones that encourage your uterus to shrink back to its normal size.
- Improves tooth and mouth development in your child.

Alcohol, smoking, and recreational drugs

Almost everything you put into your body will come out in small quantities in your breast milk, including alcohol, tobacco, caffeine, or street drugs.

*I*F YOU HAVE TAKEN A HARMFUL SUBSTANCE

If you have ingested some substance that you think might be harmful to your baby, contact your pediatrician and/or pharmacist. Depending on the substance and the time that it takes for your body to absorb and remove it, you may be advised to give your baby formula for the next feeding or two and to discard your milk during this time. During this waiting time, the harmful substance will pass from the milk back into your blood for removal by your liver or kidneys. Pumping your milk and throwing it away does not speed up the process of drug removal, though it will keep up your milk supply and may make you more comfortable.

ALCOHOL

Alcohol is one of a few drugs that crosses freely into milk. The amount of alcohol in the milk is the same as the amount in the mother's blood. Research is lacking, but one study has shown that as little as one drink a day has a small but measurable effect on motor development. It may also slow the baby's response to outside stimuli. Alcohol can also suppress milk production; the more you drink, the less milk you will produce.

Heavy drinking will make the baby lethargic and drowsy. If you drink, look for these and other symptoms, including deep sleep from which the baby cannot be aroused, deep breathing, no reaction to pain, inability to suck, excessive perspiration, and feeble pulse. Call your child's doctor immediately if you notice these symptoms.

Although heavy drinking has long been discouraged during breast-feeding, women were once encouraged to take a single beer or glass of wine to help them and their babies relax. Now doctors discourage alcohol consumption and advise that if you drink, you limit yourself to a single drink within a 24-hour period.

If you have had some alcohol, wait one to two hours per drink before breast-feeding your child. Feed your baby formula during this time if she is hungry.

If you are planning to go out to a party and expect to have several drinks, you can express your milk and refrigerate it ahead of time, leaving it for the sitter to give to the baby. You may also want to have another bottle of expressed milk available if the baby wakens after you come home. If your breasts are uncomfortably full, you can express milk to relieve the discomfort and discard the milk.

CAFFEINE

Caffeine enters breast milk in small amounts. Up to two cups of coffee a day appear to be safe. With large amounts—four or five cups of coffee a day or eight 12-ounce bottles of a caffeine-containing soft drink (cola, Mountain Dew)—caffeine accumulates in the breast milk and may make the infant jittery and wakeful. Many women who want to encourage their infants to sleep well switch to decaffeinated beverages. Their infants begin to sleep better a day or two later. Symptoms are more likely to appear in premature infants and newborns (less than four months of age), who are less able to metabolize the caffeine.

TOBACCO

Smoking harms a nursing infant in several ways. Nicotine, the addictive substance in tobacco smoke, passes into breast milk when you smoke. Symptoms of elevated nicotine levels in an infant include vomiting, diarrhea, colic, rapid heart rate, and restlessness. Call your infant's doctor immediately if you notice any of these symptoms. Smoking also reduces breast milk production, making it more likely that the mother will supplement breast milk with formula and discontinue breast-feeding. Smoking has another unpleasant effect: the baby is more likely to be colicky, fussy, and irritable than other babies. Smoking also can reduce the rate at which your baby gains weight.

Being exposed to your smoking secondhand also harms your baby. Babies who live with smokers are six times more likely to develop pneumonia, bronchitis, and ear infections during the first two years of life. Also, they have more colds and are more likely to develop asthma and other health problems. And children who grow up in homes where someone smokes are more likely to become smokers themselves.

If you smoke, here are some ways to reduce your baby's exposure to cigarette smoke.

- It's best to quit. If you've tried in the past and have failed, ask your doctor for help. Knowing you're helping your child may be just the motivation you need to make it stick this time.
- Never smoke in the same room with the baby. Go outside to smoke or at least to another room with an open window. Ask others who smoke to do the same.
- Nurse your infant before you have a cigarette, when your nicotine levels are lower.
- Switch to low-nicotine cigarettes.

RECREATIONAL DRUGS

It is important to use no street drugs while you are breast-feeding. Cocaine will give your baby the same symptoms you might experience, including irritability, tremors, and high blood pressure. Because an infant's body can't break down the cocaine, it will accumulate. Speed, uppers, or amphetamines will make your infant over-stimulated or excessively drowsy. Amphetamines can also reduce your milk supply. Marijuana has not been well studied, but one study showed a decrease in motor developments at age 1. If you are a heavy marijuana user, you should not breast-feed your infant. If you use occasionally, avoid breast-feeding for several hours following the use of the drug. Also, avoid exposure of the child to the smoke, as you would with cigarettes.

Any woman who uses needles to shoot street drugs should not breast-feed for at least two reasons: the risks associated with the drug itself and the risk of transmission of HIV, the virus that causes AIDS. Needles put you at high risk of the deadly AIDS virus, which you can transmit to your baby through the milk. In the United States, both the Centers for Disease Control and the Department of Public Health do not recommend breast-feeding for HIV-positive women.

Prescription and nonprescription drugs

If you have a condition that requires medication, evaluate any drug carefully with your doctor or pharmacist. It is still best to avoid taking medication if you can, but you probably don't need to stop breast-feeding your infant. Some medications are safer than others—including some common over-the-counter drugs.

QUESTIONS TO ASK

When considering a medication while breast-feeding, the first question should not be, Should I stop nursing? The first question should be, Do I really need this medication? You and your doctor will need to answer this and the following questions about a drug you might take.

- Is the drug medically necessary? Are there nondrug alternatives?
- Is this the safest drug for my condition? Is there a better choice—perhaps a less-common drug that will not accumulate as much in the breast milk?
- Can I take the drug in a topical form or a nasal spray instead of orally (this lowers the amount in the milk)?
- Is there a chance this drug could pose a risk to my infant? Some drugs are known to be harmful (see page 170).
- Would it be safer to delay the drug therapy? The younger the baby, the more vulnerable. Immature kidneys and liver cannot eliminate drugs well, so they may build up in the small body. Premature infants are particularly at risk. In some cases, the use of a drug can be delayed for a week or two after the baby is born. When you first arrive home from the hospital with your newborn, do not take any drugs without first consulting your doctor.
- Should the levels of drug in my infant's blood be monitored while I am taking this drug? This is necessary with some drugs, such as antidepressants.
- How should I monitor my baby for excessive drug exposure? Should I look for side effects such as diarrhea, rash, or changes in behavior?
- Can I time the doses to lessen the effect on my baby? Often a mother can time her doses of medication and breast-feeding schedule so that the infant gets little, if any, of the drug through the breast milk. See below for instructions on timing your nursing.
- Does the drug interfere with lactation? A small number of drugs can suppress milk production. Bromocriptine and some others can

increase the body's responsiveness to the brain chemical dopamine. The drugs amantadine and flumandine, sometimes prescribed to help prevent the flu, can have a similar effect (but a flu vaccine does not). Birth-control pills containing estrogen also reduce milk production. Make sure your doctor knows you are breast-feeding before prescribing any of these medications.

• Should I consider discontinuing breast-feeding? In a few cases, a drug that might harm the nursing infant is necessary for your own health.

TIMING YOUR MEDICATIONS

If you take a drug occasionally—for example, for a headache or allergy—it may be possible to time your medication and breast-feeding so that your infant receives as little of the drug as possible. When you take a drug chronically (every day)—such as for an infection, high blood pressure, depression, diabetes, or chronic allergies—the drug achieves a constant level in the blood and other body tissues and fluids, and it is not possible to time your breast-feeding to prevent ex-

BEFORE YOU HAVE A MEDICAL TEST

Some diagnostic tests involve drugs too. If any medical test is suggested, always tell your doctor you are breast-feeding. It is particularly important to avoid exposing the baby to radioactive drugs, which are used in a variety of imaging tests such as thyroid gland tests. After a radioactive test, you will need to avoid breast-feeding for some period, depending on the radioactive substance used. If made aware ahead of time that you are breast-feeding, a nuclear medicine physician may be able to choose a substance that will leave the body as quickly as possible. Before the test is done, find out how long you will need to avoid breast-feeding. Then pump and freeze enough milk to cover this period. After taking the test, pump your breasts to maintain milk production but discard all of the milk for the designated time period. Your milk can be sampled for radioactivity before you resume feeding.

DRUGS YOU SHOULD NOT TAKE WHILE BREAST-FEEDING

Drug	Cause for concern
amphetamines	irritability, poor sleeping pattern
bromocriptine	suppresses lactation, may be hazardous to the mother
cocaine	cocaine intoxication
cyclophosphamide	may suppress immune system, possible carcinogen
cyclosporine	may suppress immune system, possible carcinogen
doxorubicin	may suppress immune system, possible carcinogen
ergotamine	vomiting, diarrhea, convulsions
heroin	tremors, restlessness, vomiting, poor feeding
levodopa	suppresses lactation, may be hazardous to mother
lithium	high concentrations found in infants; long-term effects on development are unknown but of concern
methotrexate	may suppress immune system, possible carcinogen
monoamine oxidase inhibitors (MAOIs)	inhibit lactation
nicotine	may cause shock, vomiting, diarrhea, rapid heart rate, restlessness, decreased milk production
phencyclidine	unknown effects, but potential hallucinogen in all exposed

posure to the drug by your infant. A drug taken only when needed, however, does not reach a constant amount in the blood. The drug reaches an effective amount in the bloodstream and in the areas of the body where it works (such as painful joints or other body tissues). Your liver and kidneys then gradually remove the drug from your body over a period of hours. If you don't take the drug in a continu-

*D*RUGS THAT MAY BE HARMFUL OR INTERFERE WITH BABY'S DEVELOPMENT

The effects of these medications depend on the doses and length of treatment.

antianxiety medications
  diazepam
  lorazepam
  midazolam
  prazepam
  quazepam
  temazepam
antidepressants
  amitriptyline
  amoxapine
  desipramine
  dothiepin
  doxepin
  fluoxetine
  fluvoxamine
  imipramine
  paroxetine

  sertraline
  trazodone
antipsychotic medications
  chlorpromazine
  perphenazine
  clozapine
  fluphenazine
  haloperidol
  mesoridazine
  perphenazine
  risperidone
  thioridazine
antibiotics
  chloramphenicol
  metronidazole

ous regimen, it will not reach the "steady state," at which the same amount of drug enters and leaves the body.

When you take a medication as needed—for example, an analgesic for acute pain such as headache—the level of the drug in your bloodstream is not constant. You can try to breast-feed when the level of the drug in your body is lowest. The time depends on the drug. For example, peak concentration of oral codeine occurs after two hours. If you take a codeine-containing product for acute pain from a dental procedure, minor surgery, or severe migraine, you should try to avoid breast-feeding approximately two hours after taking the drug. At this time, the amount in your blood and in your milk is greatest. Avoiding nursing at this time lowers the risk of exposure to the baby and lowers the risk of symptoms such as excessive drowsiness and poor responsiveness.

If you are taking a drug for a short time, ask your pharmacist if it is advisable to change your "medication administration time" to lower the risk of drug exposure to the baby. This technique is possible for short-term, "as needed" use of antihistamines, analgesics containing codeine or oxycodone (Tylenol with Codeine, Percocet), and orally administered nasal decongestants (Sudafed). Also, if you are taking a drug "as needed," such as an antihistamine, try to avoid long-acting products that are described as extended release, delayed release, sustained release, or timed release, since these remain in the body for a prolonged time. Use a prompt-release product if available.

Timing the feeding to your medication schedule may be more difficult with a newborn who feeds every few hours on demand or has an unpredictable schedule, but it is often possible with an older baby who has a regular feeding schedule.

Another approach is to take your medication just before your infant's longest sleep period (any time of the day), in the late evening, for example. If the drug has a short-term effect and is readily removed from the body, such as a codeine-containing product, Tylenol, Advil, Benadryl, or Sudafed, take it before the baby's longest period of uninterrupted sleep. By the time you resume breast-feeding, much of the short-acting drug will have been removed from your body and from the milk. Ask your pharmacist if the drug is short-acting and would be advised for use before the baby's longest period of sleep.

Safe treatments for common health problems

Before reaching for a medication, always ask yourself if you really need it. Next, think about using remedies other than drugs; for example, if you are congested, try a humidifier. If you do choose a medication, find out if it can be taken in a topical cream or nasal spray instead of a pill; in these forms, less medication enters the bloodstream and the milk.

ALLERGIES

Nose sprays and eye drops containing decongestants are better choices than oral drugs because little if any drug enters your bloodstream. The amount that is accessible to the milk is extremely low. Unfortunately, there have been no studies of most antihistamines during breast-feeding. When possible, use a product such as saline nasal spray (Ocean Spray), which reduces nasal congestion but does not contain an antihistamine.

If you need an oral antihistamine, avoid any long-acting products designated as sustained release or timed release. Choose instead a short-acting product such as diphenhydramine (Benadryl) or chlorpheniramine (Chlor-Trimeton) after breast-feeding and before the baby's longest period of uninterrupted sleep. Try to avoid combination products containing antihistamines, decongestants, and analgesics because they increase the risk of drug exposure to the baby. Make sure to watch the baby for signs of exposure to the antihistamine, such as irritability or a change in sleep pattern. Information on long-acting, nonsedating antihistamines such as Seldane and Hismanal is lacking. Based on their chemistry, they may reach high, sustained levels in the breast milk. Talk to your doctor about the use of an intranasal product such as fluticasone (Flonase) or flunisolide (Nasalide), anti-inflammatory drugs that effectively reduce allergic symptoms but are minimally absorbed in the blood.

ASTHMA

Inhaled corticosteroids (Beclovent, Azmacort) and bronchodilators (Ventolin, Serevent) are the drugs of choice for asthma treatment during breast-feeding. They reach only minimal concentrations in the blood and milk. When used at the recommended doses and frequency, inhaled steroids and bronchodilators can be used safely during breast-feeding. Inhaled products containing either cromolyn (Nasalcrom) or nedocromil (Tilade) have not been studied during breast-feeding; however, they reach negligible levels in the blood. Also, women who have asthma can safely use the bronchodilator theophylline. This medication can occasionally cause irritability and fretful sleep in infants, so the dose should be kept as low as possible.

CONTRACEPTION

Although breast-feeding suppresses ovulation for several months, it is not a reliable form of contraception. You may ovulate before your period resumes and not know it. Unless you're interested in becoming pregnant again right away, use contraception while you are breast-feeding, particularly after five weeks postpartum.

The best choices are the barrier methods, including condoms and diaphragms. To use a diaphragm you must be fitted properly by your health-care provider. If you were using a diaphragm before you became pregnant, you must be refitted now. Condoms are available in most pharmacies and have the advantage of protecting against sexually transmitted diseases. (For more on barrier methods and their use, see page 79.)

If you prefer a hormonal contraceptive, the American Academy of Pediatrics considers all of the following as compatible with breast-feeding: combined oral contraceptives containing estrogen and a progestin, the progesterone-only pill (minipill), levonorgestrel implant (Norplant), or medroxyprogesterone by injection (Depo-Provera). The estrogen in a combined birth-control pill can interfere with your milk production and decrease the amount of protein in the milk. A low dose containing 35 mcg or less of estrogen should be used when possible.

Because progestins do not interfere with milk production or content, progestin-only contraceptives are a better choice. Progestin-containing contraceptives have been well studied in breast-feeding and have not been shown to interfere with normal growth and development of the baby. However, because these agents have not been studied in breast-feeding women before six weeks postpartum, they are currently not recommended for use until that time. (For more on hormone-based contraceptives, see page 68.)

DEPRESSION

Most antidepressants and antipsychotic medications are best avoided during breast-feeding because their long-term effects are unknown. This can present a problem for a woman who has a history of depression, since the condition may worsen after pregnancy. Also, about 10 percent of new mothers develop postpartum depression. This condition, which begins from one to eight weeks after delivery and may last over a year, is characterized by sleep disturbances, poor concentration, and hostility.

Postpartum depression should not be confused with the "baby blues" experienced by as many as 80 percent of new mothers. The baby blues are periodic short episodes of anxiety, mood changes, and weeping. The episodes usually occur two to three days after delivery and are gone within two weeks. The baby blues can be helped by getting out of the house or joining an activity that involves social contact, such as a new mother's group or other activity, particularly one that provides babysitting. Participating in these activities can relieve the feelings of isolation that sometimes accompany new motherhood.

Postpartum depression and other depression cannot be helped by psychological support alone. They have serious implications for both the mother and her baby and need to be treated with antidepressants and psychotherapy, usually for at least a year. Unfortunately, most drugs used to treat depression and other mental disorders have been inadequately studied during breast-feeding. According to the American Academy of Pediatrics, these drugs may be used during breast-feeding, but their effects on the baby are unknown and may be of concern. Before starting an antidepressant, the following factors should be considered:

- The overall health of the baby
- Whether the baby was already exposed to the antidepressant before birth
- The mother's overall physical and mental health

Some women with depression have been successfully treated with the tricyclic antidepressants, such as desipramine, nortriptyline, and imipramine. If one of these antidepressants is prescribed for use during breast-feeding, the dose may be given once daily before the baby's longest period of uninterrupted sleep. Also, the baby should be watched closely for signs of drug exposure during the initial month or two after starting the medication. Signs and symptoms of drug exposure include changes in sleep pattern, decreased response to stimuli, excessive crankiness or irritability, and change in weight gain or feeding habits. Periodic sampling of the baby's blood may also be advised. Also, in a few cases, these drugs have reduced the milk supply.

Lithium, commonly prescribed for manic-depressive disorder, should not be used during breast-feeding because it causes poor responsiveness. For anxiety, a mood disorder that is often worse after delivery, the usual drug treatments are benzodiazepines, but the effects on infants have not been studied well. Some benzodiazepines, including Valium, have been associated with poor suckling and drowsiness. If you have difficulty sleeping, zolpidem (Ambien) is considered compatible with breast-feeding.

DIGESTIVE DISCOMFORTS

Digestive problems like heartburn and constipation should be relieved with nondrug methods when possible. For constipation and hemorrhoids, try a high-fiber diet and plenty of water. The nonabsorbed bulk laxatives, such as Metamucil, and stool softeners are also considered safe. The stimulant laxative bisacodyl (Dulcolax) is also considered safe. (For more on treating constipation, see page 54.)

For heartburn, avoid eating just before bedtime. Also avoid acidic foods such as tomato sauce and take a nonsystemic antacid (Mylanta, Maalox) for immediate relief. The use of an H2-antagonist during breast-feeding is controversial. Initially the AAP considered cimetidine (Tagamet) incompatible with breast-feeding because of the high concentrations achieved in breast milk and the potential for the drug to alter the baby's stomach chemistry. Recently the AAP reclassified cimetidine as compatible with breast-feeding. Of the three H2-antagonists available over the counter, famotidine (Pepcid AC) appears to reach the lowest level in the breast milk and is considered by most to be preferable to cimetidine (Tagamet HB) or ranitidine (Zantac 75) during breast-feeding. If an H2-antagonist is used for heartburn, take it in the smallest recommended dose. As an added precaution, try to take it as a single nighttime dose before the baby's longest period of sleep.

HIGH BLOOD PRESSURE

If you have high blood pressure, consult with your doctor. Depending on how high it is, you may be able to control it with diet and exercise alone. Certain antihypertensive drugs are considered safe for a breast-feeding mother: methyldopa, captopril, diltiazem, hydrochlorothiazide, verapamil, nifedipine, propranolol, labetalol, and metoprolol. Other common antihypertensives, including clonidine, reach high concentrations in breast milk. Clonidine and guanfacine may also decrease your milk supply. Reserpine may cause nasal stuffiness and increased lung secretions in your infant. Talk with your doctor about which medication to use.

INFECTIONS

Some antibiotics and other drugs that fight infections are considered safe during breast-feeding to treat vaginal infections, mastitis, urinary infections, pneumonia, and conjunctivitis.

Avoid chloramphenicol, the fluoroquinolones (Cipro, Floxin), and metronidazole (Flagyl). If metronidazole is indicated for treatment of trichomoniasis (a sexually transmitted disease), a single 2-gram oral dose can be administered. You should avoid breast-feeding for at least 24 hours after the dose and discard the milk. Sulfa antibiotics (Bactrim, Septra, Gantrisin) should be used with caution, and should not be used if the infant is less than one month old. Although considered as compatible with breast-feeding by the American Academy of Pediatrics (because they are poorly absorbed from the milk), tetracyclines should be avoided when there is an alternative medication because they may stain the baby's teeth. All antibiotics, even the penicillins and cephalosporins, which are considered safe, can cause diarrhea or a skin rash. Monitor the baby closely.

Mastitis is an infection of the milk ducts of the breast which, if left untreated, can become chronic and may last for months. Symptoms include a wedge-shaped area of the breast that is tender, hot, very painful, and swollen, and a sudden fever or flu-like symptoms. Mastitis can be caused by poor drainage of a duct, and fatigue or stress can make you more vulnerable. Mastitis is not the same as engorgement, a condition in which both breasts become gradually swollen immediately after childbirth but with no fever or flu symptoms. It is also not a plugged duct, which makes the breast feel tender after feedings but causes milder pain, little or no heat sensation, and no fever or flu-like symptoms. A plugged duct may lead to mastitis if not recognized early and treated with moist heat, massage, and rest.

Mastitis requires antibiotics. If you have mastitis, you should continue nursing on both breasts but start the infant on the unaffected side while the affected side "lets down." The organism causing the infection is normally present in a baby's mouth, so continued nursing doesn't transmit the infection to the baby. Make sure that you empty the affected side by feeding or pumping. It is very important to get bed rest. Take an antibiotic (usually a penicillin, cephalosporin, or erythromycin) for at least 10 to 14 days. Take all of the antibiotic, even if you feel better on day 3, to prevent a relapse. Use ice packs or warm compresses, whichever gives you relief from pain and inflammation. Take Tylenol, Advil, or aspirin as needed for pain. Drink plenty of fluids.

If mastitis recurs, you may need to be treated with a low-dose antibiotic for the duration of lactation. Because antibiotics change the normal way the body controls the growth of yeast, you may develop a yeast infection (sometimes referred to as thrush) after treatment for mastitis. This usually causes severe, fiery pain when the baby nurses. It is treated by massaging an antifungal cream such as nystatin (Mycostatin) on the nipples and areola after each feeding. The baby also needs treatment with an antifungal medicine such as nystatin oral suspension to protect you from reinfection. If the yeast infection doesn't respond to topical therapy, you may need an oral antifungal such as fluconazole or ketoconazole.

NIPPLE SORENESS

Topical creams or ointments (such as A and D ointment) and vitamin E oil do not relieve sore nipples and may be ingested by your infant. Instead, properly position your infant, make sure the full areola is in the baby's mouth, and air your nipples frequently for 15 minutes at a time to promote drying and healing.

PAIN RELIEF

For pain relief, acetaminophen (Tylenol) is the drug of choice because the infant's body can tolerate and remove it well. Of the NSAIDs, ibuprofen (Advil, Motrin, Nuprin) has been studied most extensively. Doses up to 1.2 grams a day (six doses of 200 mg or three doses of 400 mg) do not reach measurable amounts in the milk. At this daily dose, the infant is exposed to less than 1 mg of ibuprofen per day. Occasional use of aspirin (single dose for headache) is okay, but Tylenol is preferable. If you take a single dose of aspirin, try to avoid breast-feeding for two hours afterward.

Narcotics such as codeine, oxycodone, and morphine should be used only on a limited basis while breast-feeding. Try to avoid feeding the baby for at least two hours after a dose and also monitor the baby for changes in sleep pattern, responsiveness, or stool.

COMMON DRUGS CONSIDERED SAFE WHILE BREAST-FEEDING

While the best choice is to do without drugs whenever possible, the following drugs are considered safe when taken in the correct dosage.

analgesics (for pain)
  acetaminophen
  codeine
  ibuprofen
  ketorolac
  naproxen
antibiotics (for infection)
  ampicillin
  cefaclor
  cephalexin
  clindamycin
  erythromycin
  penicillins
  sulfisoxazole
  trimethoprim-
    sulfamethoxazole
anticonvulsants (for seizures)
  carbamazepine
  phenytoin
antihypertensives (for high blood pressure—ACE inhibitors, beta-blockers, diuretics, beta-blockers and calcium channel antagonists)
  atenolol
  captopril
  diltiazem
  enalapril

hydrochlorothiazide
metoprolol
methyldopa
nifedipine
propranolol
cardiac drugs
  digoxin
  heparin
  quinidine
  warfarin
diuretics
  hydrochlorothiazide
laxatives
  senna
tuberculosis medications
  isoniazid
  rifampin
other medications
  cimetidine
  cisapride
  insulin
  magnesium sulfate
  methimazole (doses less than 10 mg/day preferred)
  prednisone
  propylthiouracil
  pseudoephedrine (preferably by nasal spray)
  rubella vaccine

part three

DRUGS TO TREAT DISEASE

chapter 9

DRUGS FOR CARDIOVASCULAR DISORDERS

*C*ARDIOVASCULAR DISORDERS INCLUDE CORONARY artery disease, high blood pressure, angina, arteriosclerosis, abnormal heart rhythms, and stroke.

What most people call "heart disease" is coronary artery disease, the result of gradual clogging (arteriosclerosis) of the coronary arteries. These blood vessels, which supply oxygen-rich blood and nourishment to the heart muscle, may become clogged and scarred over the years from the buildup of fat and cholesterol. Arteriosclerosis doesn't cause symptoms, but it can lead to coronary artery disease, a condition that causes chest pain or angina and can ultimately cause a heart attack. If arteriosclerosis blocks arteries that supply blood to the brain, it can cause a stroke.

Some people think of heart disease as a men's health problem, but it is the number-one killer of women. The American Heart Association reports that nearly half of the approximately 500,000 people who die of heart attack each year are women. The difference is that women tend to develop heart disease about 10 or 15 years later than men, after they lose the protection of the female hormone estrogen at menopause.

In recent decades, scientists have pinpointed the causes of cardiovascular diseases and have discovered that lifestyle changes can help prevent and reverse them. Tremendous progress has also been made in developing drugs to treat heart disease and stroke. Medications can prevent or dissolve blood clots, relax the arteries to increase the flow of blood, and reduce blood cholesterol levels to slow the gradual buildup of fatty plaque in the arteries.

Coronary artery disease and heart attack

About 5 million Americans have coronary artery disease. When a coronary artery narrowed by years of plaque buildup is suddenly blocked, usually by a blood clot, the result is a heart attack. The blood can no longer reach part of the heart muscle, bringing oxygen. Often that part dies. If enough of the heart muscle dies, the patient may also die. Women are more likely to die from their first heart attack than men are. Women also tend to stay in the hospital longer and are more likely to die within a year of a heart attack. These findings may be explained by women's smaller body size and frame or by the fact that women are more likely than men to also have other illnesses.

SYMPTOMS

A common symptom of coronary artery disease is the chest pain called angina. Women are more likely than men to have this warning sign. Angina is usually triggered by exercise, exposure to cold, or stress, all of which increase the heart's need for oxygen. Another type of angina, called Prinzmetal's or variant angina, can occur when you are resting. It is triggered by a temporary spasm of the coronary artery rather than by a blockage or buildup of plaque. Variant angina is more common in women than men. Whether your angina occurs at rest or with exercise, the type of pain is the same. It often feels like pressure or heaviness in the center of the chest and may radiate to the neck, shoulder, arm, or lower jaw, particularly on the left side of the body. An attack usually lasts for 5 to 15 minutes. Angina often occurs off and on for weeks before a heart attack and is a critical warning sign you should not ignore. See your doctor at once.

Not every woman experiences angina before a heart attack. Although more frequent in men than women, sudden cardiac death from a heart attack can occur without warning. The symptoms of a heart attack may resemble angina but may be more severe. If symptoms last for 20 minutes or more, calling 911 or an ambulance immediately can save your life. Many people survive a heart attack, but the longer the delay in getting help, the more damage your heart muscle may suffer. Once part of the heart muscle is damaged, it will never fully function again. It is important to know the warning signs of a heart attack and to get help quickly. You may experience one or more of these signs:

- Chest pain or pressure that radiates to your neck, shoulder, arm, or jaw
- Uncomfortable squeezing, tightness, or pressure in the center of your chest, or across your chest
- Pain in your neck, jaw, arms, or back
- Dizziness, perspiration, fainting, nausea, or weakness
- Heartburn or indigestion that does not disappear after taking antacids
- Chest pain or angina that does not disappear when you take sublingual nitroglycerin tablets as directed

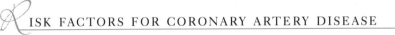

RISK FACTORS FOR CORONARY ARTERY DISEASE

Some women are more likely to have coronary disease than others. The following factors increase your risk of this disease. If you have some risk factors that cannot be controlled, it's particularly important that you make changes in your life that will reduce those factors you can control.

- High blood pressure
- Diabetes
- Smoking
- LDL cholesterol above 160
- Family history of heart attack before age 55
- Obesity
- Sedentary lifestyle
- Over age 55
- Premature menopause without hormone replacement
- High waist-to-hip ratio (above 0.85). Calculate by dividing your waist measurement by your hip measurement (for example, 28 inches divided by 38 inches is .73).

IS YOUR CHOLESTEROL TOO HIGH?

If your blood cholesterol is too high, fatty plaque deposits can form in your arteries, eventually blocking the flow of blood and causing a heart attack or stroke. Most women who are nonsmokers and do not have high blood pressure or diabetes have normal cholesterol levels until menopause. The female hormone estrogen boosts HDL (the good, high-density lipoprotein) and suppresses LDL (the bad, low-density lipoprotein). After menopause, the protective effects of estrogen are lost, so over the next 5 to 10 years, a woman's risk of heart disease gradually rises. This is one of the main reasons that doctors often recommend oral hormone replacement therapy (HRT), which includes estrogen, for postmenopausal women at risk of heart disease.

Before menopause, most women's cholesterol levels are normal. Your doctor may recommend a first, baseline cholesterol level by the age of 35 and then one every five years until menopause. After menopause, have an annual cholesterol level. A technician will draw a small vial of blood from a vein in your arm and send it to a laboratory for analysis. Your doctor may also measure the blood for triglycerides, another form of fat that has not yet been shown to directly increase your risk of heart disease.

A normal level is total cholesterol under 200, HDL above 50, and LDL under 130. In assessing your risk of heart disease, the LDL and HDL levels are more important than the total. Sixty to 70 percent of cholesterol is carried in the LDL form. In this form, cholesterol can be taken up by the arteries and form plaque. HDL transports cholesterol from the arteries to the liver for removal from the body.

If your cholesterol levels are normal, you can maintain them by eating a low-fat diet and getting regular aerobic exercise. If your cholesterol levels are too high, your doctor may first advise improving your diet and losing weight. People have reduced their total cholesterol 10 to 20 percent by reducing the amount of saturated fats and cholesterol in their diets. Exercise also increases HDL cholesterol.

Cholesterol-lowering drugs are now widely prescribed for people who have elevated cholesterol levels and heart disease, high blood pressure, or a family history of heart disease or stroke. (For more on these medications and how they work, see page 204.)

TREATMENT

Depending on the severity of your condition, your doctor may recommend lifestyle changes, drug therapies, or surgery.

Lifestyle changes

Whether you already have coronary artery disease or are at risk because of a family history of the disease or high cholesterol levels (see page 186) or high blood pressure (see page 191), talk with your doctor about the following lifestyle changes:

- **Quit smoking.** If you smoke, this is the most important change you can make. Smoking increases your risk of forming blood clots, and nicotine can constrict the coronary arteries, increasing the risk of angina. If you smoke while taking a combination oral contraceptive, you increase your risk of developing heart disease or stroke by 20 times. If you quit smoking now, your risk of a heart attack will return to that of a nonsmoker within three to five years.
- **Reduce the saturated fat in your diet.** Cut down on meats (particularly beef, pork, and chicken skin), full-fat dairy products, eggs, and butter. Eat more fruits, vegetables, whole grains, and fish. Remove fat and skin from meat and poultry and blot or drain off fat. Cook with monounsaturated fats (olive and canola oils) whenever possible.
- **Exercise regularly.** Almost any kind of repetitive exercise (walking, swimming, bicycling, rowing), three or more days a week, can strengthen your entire cardiovascular system and lower your blood pressure. If you have angina, talk with your doctor about precautions—for example, avoiding exertion after a heavy meal when blood tends to pool in your gut, away from your heart. Under such circumstances, mild exertion may trigger a heart attack.
- **Reduce your weight.** If you are more than 20 percent over your ideal weight, talk to your doctor about a weight-reduction plan. Eating fewer calories than you burn each day is the key to a successful weight-loss program.
- **Consider hormone replacement therapy.** If you have reached menopause, the estrogen in oral hormone replacement therapy will improve your blood cholesterol levels and provide long-term protection against heart disease.

Medications

Many different medications are available to treat coronary artery disease. Often several are combined. Your doctor may prescribe one drug, determine the correct dosage, then add another drug. Some drugs deliver more blood to your heart or reduce your heart's workload and thus its need for oxygen. Some drugs, like sublingual nitrates, can be taken as needed to relieve angina by improving the elasticity of your blood vessels and increasing blood flow to your heart. People with severe angina may take a combination of nitrates, beta-blockers (see page 200), and calcium channel blockers (see page 202). Aspirin reduces the chance that a blood clot will form and lodge in an already narrowed artery, causing a heart attack; it is given both as a preventive measure and after a heart attack. (For a full description of drugs that treat coronary artery disease, see page 196.)

Surgery

If you have had angina or a heart attack, or if diagnostic tests have revealed blocked coronary arteries, your doctor may recommend surgery to increase the blood flow to your heart.

Coronary artery bypass surgery is a widely used and highly successful surgical procedure in which the blocked section of an artery is replaced by a "bypass" blood vessel. It is usually reserved for those with angina who do not respond to drug therapy and for those who have substantial blockage (greater than 70 percent) in the major coronary artery that feeds the heart (the left anterior descending artery) or in at least three coronary arteries. Part of a blood vessel is removed from a healthy part of the body, usually the leg, and a short piece is sewn onto the blocked vessel to redirect the blood around the blockage. The chest must be opened, general anesthesia is required, and recovery time is long. Fewer women than men undergo this operation, and women are more likely to die afterward. The reasons are not fully understood but may be because women's blood vessels are smaller or because women tend to be older when they are first diagnosed with coronary artery disease.

Following bypass surgery, most people can be more active and are free of pain for at least five years. However, bypass surgery does not prevent arteriosclerosis from developing in the new bypass vessels, so you need to continue diet restrictions and lifestyle modifications.

Angioplasty is a procedure that opens a blocked artery. A long, thin catheter is threaded through the arteries to the blockage. Through the tube, the surgeon passes either a tiny cutting device to scrape away the blockage or a tiny balloon that inflates and increases the opening of the artery. Angioplasty is less invasive than a bypass operation, does not involve opening the chest, and recovery lasts only a few days, but the artery is less likely to remain open than with a bypass. To increase the likelihood that the artery stays open, the surgeon may insert a stainless steel tube, called a stent, into the artery during angioplasty. The stent prevents the blood vessel from collapsing and can be left in place after the balloon is removed. As with bypass surgery, women have lower success rates with angioplasty and higher complication rates. Women are more likely to receive drug therapy than surgical procedures for cardiac disease.

Arrhythmia

An abnormal heart rhythm, which can be too slow or too fast, is called an arrhythmia. If you occasionally feel your heart flutter, pound, or even miss a beat, do not be alarmed. Almost everyone's heartbeat has some irregularities. Your heartbeat or pulse is supposed to speed up when you exercise or are suddenly alarmed. If you have an arrhythmia, though, you will feel your heart sometimes beating irregularly at unexpected times, such as at rest. Your heart should normally beat between 60 and 100 times a minute, except when you are exercising, when it often exceeds 100.

Your heartbeat is governed by electrical signals sent by the sinus node at the top of the right atrium (pumping chamber) of your heart. The electrical signals pass through the heart in an intricate system involving the sinus node, the upper and lower pumping chambers of the heart, and a node between these chambers (atrioventricular node). When something interferes at any point with the transmission of signals within this system, the result may be arrhythmia. Coronary artery disease (see page 184) is the most common cause. Other causes include high blood pressure, hyperthyroidism, pregnancy, cigarette smoking, alcohol use, cocaine use, and scarring from a heart attack.

Symptoms

You may have no symptoms of an arrhythmia, but if you do, they will reflect the degree of abnormality in both the rate and rhythm of your heartbeat. If your heartbeat is too slow, you have a bradycardia and your heart may not be pumping enough blood to your brain or other organs. You may often feel tired or lightheaded and may lose consciousness. If your heart is beating too fast, you have tachycardia; this may be caused by excessive caffeine ingestion, smoking, stimulant drugs, and strenuous exercise. The most common symptoms are racing of the heart, dizziness, shortness of breath, and fainting. If the rhythm is both erratic and too fast, as with atrial fibrillation, the pumping chambers of your heart do not have enough time to fill with blood before each contraction. With each contraction, your heart ejects spurts of blood that are insufficient to supply oxygen to your organs. With this common arrhythmia, the symptoms are a fluttering feeling in the chest, palpitations, dizziness, fainting, chest pain, and shortness of breath.

People are often most aware of irregular rhythms when they go to bed at night, particularly while lying on the left side. While some people ignore heart palpitations, dizziness and fainting are hard to ignore. Fainting may occur because the heart is beating so slowly or irregularly that too little blood reaches the brain. If you experience any of these symptoms, particularly more than once, see your doctor.

Treatment

Arrhythmias may not require treatment, but highly erratic rhythms that result in symptoms require medication or a device like a pacemaker. An abnormal rhythm is usually diagnosed by using a simple, painless test called an electrocardiogram (ECG) performed in the doctor's office or at home with a portable machine. The home test, called the Holter monitor, monitors your heart rhythms for 24 hours at a time with a purse-sized device worn on a belt.

Beta-blockers, calcium channel blockers, and digoxin have all been used to regulate and slow the heart rhythm. Your doctor may prescribe a combination of these medications to treat a rapid, irregular heart rhythm such as atrial fibrillation, as well as related disorders such as angina or high blood pressure. Other commonly prescribed antiarrhythmiacs include quinidine, procainamide, lidocaine, and mexiletine. (For a description of these drugs and how they work, see page 198.)

In some cases, an electronic device to control your heartbeat may be necessary. A pacemaker can speed up the heartbeat. An implantable defibrillator controls an irregular rhythm originating from the ventricle, such as ventricular tachycardia or ventricular fibrillation. With this automatic device, an electrical shock is generated to restore the normal rhythm.

High blood pressure

High blood pressure is called the "silent killer" because it usually has no symptoms. You won't know you have it unless you are tested, but it can cause heart attack, stroke, and kidney damage. High blood pressure involves the circulatory system. By increasing the pressure in the blood vessels, high blood pressure makes the heart work harder and contributes to heart disease. All stages of high blood pressure, including mild or stage I high blood pressure, increase your risk of nonfatal and fatal cardiovascular disease (heart attack, coronary artery disease) and kidney disease. High blood pressure is also the most significant risk factor for stroke and is the most common health problem in the United States, affecting 50 million Americans. It is more common among men before age 60; then the risk for men and women is about the same. African-Americans are at greater risk at all ages.

Your blood pressure is a measurement of the pressure or force of your blood against the walls of your blood vessels. Your blood pressure reading has two numbers. The top number, the systolic, measures the pressure in your arteries while your heart is beating. This number should not exceed 140. The second number, the diastolic, measures the pressure when your heart is resting between beats. The diastolic reading should not exceed 90. If either the systolic or diastolic readings exceed normal levels and stay elevated, you have high blood pressure. These normal levels do not increase with age. For pregnant women, high blood pressure is defined as an increase in systolic by at least 30 points or an increase in diastolic by at least 15 points. Your blood pressure reading can vary depending on the time of day that it is taken, whether you have recently had a cigarette, or if you have recently drunk a caffeine-containing beverage. For an accurate reading, your pressure needs to be taken several times on different days.

TREATMENT

High blood pressure can be treated with lifestyle changes and medications. In the vast majority of cases, the cause of high blood pressure is unknown, and you will probably require lifelong treatment. In a small number of cases, high blood pressure is caused by a treatable condition such as hyperthyroidism, pheochromocytoma (a rare tumor on the adrenal glands), or drug reaction. To determine whether your condition is reversible, a complete physical examination, drug history, and family history are required.

Lifestyle changes

If you have high blood pressure, there are several steps you can take to help control it.

- Lose weight. If you are more than 10 percent above your ideal body weight or you have a waist-to-hip ratio higher than 0.85 (page 185), then losing as little as 9 pounds can significantly lower your blood pressure.
- Exercise regularly. Regular aerobic exercise such as walking, biking, or swimming can lower your blood pressure and help you lose weight.
- Eat less salt. For some, but not all, people with high blood pressure, decreased salt intake can reduce blood pressure. Keep your salt intake below 6 grams a day (sodium below 2.3 grams).
- Eat a low-fat, low-cholesterol diet to reduce the buildup of fatty plaque in your arteries.
- Reduce your alcohol intake—no more than two drinks a day.

Medications

There are many effective drugs for high blood pressure. It is very important to continue taking medication that has been prescribed. Because high blood pressure has no symptoms, you may get lax about taking your pills or may even think your condition is cured. Remember that high blood pressure is "the silent killer."

The five most commonly prescribed drugs for high blood pressure are diuretics (water pills), beta-blockers, angiotensin-converting enzyme (ACE) inhibitors, calcium channel blockers, and alpha-blockers. Diuretics and beta-blockers are preferred because in large, well-designed studies they increased survival in people with high blood pressure. However, diuretics and beta-blockers may not be most appropriate for everyone. For example, people with asthma should not receive a beta-blocker, diuretics may worsen gout; and both diuretics and beta-blockers may increase triglyceride levels.

Stroke

A stroke occurs when an artery that delivers blood to the brain bursts (hemorrhagic stroke) or is blocked (ischemic stroke). Part of the brain does not get the flow of oxygen-rich blood it needs to function. A severe stroke kills nerve cells, often leading to difficulty with speech, memory loss, and paralysis on one side of the body.

Women are more likely to have a stroke than men. After age 35, the risk of stroke in women doubles each decade. African-American women are twice as likely to have a stroke as white women.

An ischemic stroke, which accounts for 80 percent of strokes, is usually caused by the gradual buildup of fatty plaque in the arteries that deliver blood to the brain. When a blood clot lodges in an artery that is already clogged with plaque, it shuts off blood to part of the brain. These strokes occur most often at night or in the early morning when blood pressure is low.

Some people have smaller warning strokes called transient ischemic attacks (TIAs), ministrokes that cause dizziness or fainting. TIAs, which last from 2 to 15 minutes per episode, serve as an early warning sign that a stroke is coming in a matter of days, weeks, or months.

A hemorrhagic stroke occurs when a blood vessel in the brain bursts, flooding the surrounding tissue with blood. This causes a loss of normal blood flow to tissues of the brain. The accumulating blood from the burst artery also puts pressure on surrounding tissues, causing further damage. Severe, untreated high blood pressure is a primary cause of hemorrhagic stroke.

Prevention includes most of the same steps that are recom-

TAKING YOUR OWN BLOOD PRESSURE

You should have your blood pressure checked during regular checkups. Between checkups, or to monitor the effectiveness of their treatment program, many people take their own pressure. If you or a family member takes your blood pressure, follow these steps to get an accurate reading.

- Do not smoke or drink caffeine less than 30 minutes before.
- Rest for at least 5 minutes before taking your reading.
- Sit with your arm bared, supported, and at heart level.
- Make sure the cuff size of the blood pressure device is the correct size for your arm. The portion of the cuff that is inflated is called the bladder. In order to have an accurate reading, the bladder must circle at least 80 percent of your arm.
- During one sitting, take two or more readings separated by at least 2 minutes. Average the two readings by adding them together and dividing by two.
- Home devices (manual or semiautomatic) should be calibrated at least yearly. The place where you purchased the device can often perform this service.

mended for preventing coronary artery disease. (For more details on these preventive steps, see page 187.)

- Quit smoking.
- Control your blood pressure with medication and/or diet and exercise.
- Eat a diet low in saturated fats.
- Do regular, aerobic exercise.
- If you have passed menopause and are at risk for cardiovascular disease (see page 185), consider hormone replacement therapy.

SYMPTOMS

A stroke is a medical emergency. The longer you wait to get medical help, the more damage you may suffer. Calling 911 or an ambulance quickly can mean the difference between the continuation of a normal life and permanent disability or death. The warning signs of stroke can be subtle. Watch for:

- Sudden weakness or numbness of the face, arm, or leg on one side of the body
- Sudden dimness or loss of vision, particularly in one eye
- Loss of speech or trouble understanding speech
- Sudden severe headache with no known cause
- Unexplained dizziness, unsteadiness, or sudden falls

TREATMENT

The goal of treatment can be to prevent a stroke or to minimize its damage.

Medication

If you are at risk of stroke, your doctor may prescribe an anticoagulant drug such as warfarin (see page 201) or an antiplatelet drug such as aspirin to prevent blood clots from forming and blocking your blood vessels. A daily dose of aspirin is the most common preventative agent, but other drugs are also available.

If you are having a stroke, doctors must first determine which type. For an ischemic stroke, you may be given drugs to dissolve a clot that is blocking your artery. Once your condition stabilizes, you may take drugs to prevent future clots from forming. For a hemorrhagic stroke, the goal is to limit the amount of damage to the brain by controlling your blood pressure with medication and to reduce swelling in the brain with medication.

Surgery

If you are having ministrokes (TIAs) and tests show a narrowed carotid artery, one of two in the neck that deliver blood to the brain, your doctor may recommend surgery to improve blood flow and prevent stroke. A carotid endarterectomy is an increasingly common procedure performed through an incision in the side of the neck. The artery is opened, the fatty plaque is scraped out, and the artery and incision are closed. Endarterectomy may also involve balloon angioplasty to press the plaque into the wall of the vessel. The artery some-times narrows again. Aspirin can help prevent recurrence.

If you have had a hemorrhagic stroke, immediate surgery may be necessary to repair the ruptured blood vessel. In some cases, blood clots in the brain are surrounded by swollen, bruised brain tissue. The swelling presses on surrounding brain tissues and can cause further damage. Surgery may be necessary to drain the area.

After a stroke, long-term treatment depends on the extent and the nature of the damage. Most women who have a stroke regain most of their functioning within a few days or weeks. Others must learn to live with disabilities such as loss of speech, inability to understand language, vision loss in one eye, and paralysis on one side of the body. Physical therapy and speech therapy are important parts of a treatment program for people who have these disabilities. Depression is also common after a stroke. Treatment for depression helps some women make more progress in regaining speech and physical abilities.

Drugs to treat cardiovascular diseases

Many of the same drugs are used to treat all cardiovascular diseases. There are drugs to treat blood pressure, angina, high cholesterol, abnormal heart rhythms, and blood clotting. Often several are prescribed together.

ACE INHIBITORS

ACE inhibitors (angiotensin-converting enzyme inhibitors) are used to treat high blood pressure and also heart failure, a condition in which the heart pumps inefficiently. ACE inhibitors are vasodilators, drugs that relax the blood vessels so that blood flows more freely. They reduce the body's production of the hormone angiotensin II, which constricts blood vessels. ACE inhibitors not only lower blood pressure but also reduce the workload on the heart. They are costly but are often the best choice for people who have a combination of problems including high blood pressure and diabetes. ACE inhibitors have also been shown to improve patient survival following heart attack by reducing the likelihood of heart failure and the progression of heart failure.

COMMON ACE INHIBITORS

benazepril (Lotensin)   lisinopril (Prinivil, Zestril)
captopril (Capoten)   quinapril (Accupril)
enalapril (Vasotec)   ramipril (Altace)
fosinopril (Monopril)

Side effects

A common side effect of ACE inhibitors, which appears to occur more frequently in women, is a dry, hacking cough. This chronic cough may go away on its own or may be alleviated only by stopping the drug. All ACE inhibitors cause this side effect; switching from one ACE inhibitor to another usually results in return of the cough. Other side effects include dizziness, weakness, disturbance in taste (with captopril), rash, and itching.

Because ACE inhibitors may increase your potassium level, they should not be taken with potassium-sparing diuretics such as spironolactone (Aldactone). If you are also taking lithium, have your blood levels of lithium checked, as ACE inhibitors reduce your body's ability to eliminate lithium. ACE inhibitors should be used with caution in people with kidney disorders. If you have a kidney disorder, ACE inhibitors can help if diabetes is the cause, or they may worsen bilateral renal artery stenosis. ACE inhibitors should not be taken during the second and third trimesters of pregnancy. One advantage of ACE inhibitors is that, unlike other blood pressure medications, they do not raise cholesterol levels.

ALPHA-BLOCKERS

Alpha-blockers (alpha-adrenergic blocking drugs) reduce blood pressure by dilating the blood vessels. These drugs block the nerve receptors, called "alpha receptors," which, when stimulated, constrict blood vessels. By relaxing or dilating both the veins and the arteries, alpha-blockers make it easier for the heart to pump blood. They are taken orally on a daily basis.

COMMON ALPHA-BLOCKERS

doxazosin (Cardura)   terazosin (Hytrin)
prazosin (Minipres)

Side effects

The most prominent side effect, which is most evident for the first few days, is an abrupt drop in blood pressure when you stand up. This can cause dizziness and fainting. This effect usually occurs within the first few hours after taking a dose of the drug (within one hour with prazocin and up to six hours after a dose of doxazocin) and lessens over time. To prevent this effect, the first dose of the drug should be taken at bedtime. You may also be aware that you may become light-headed if you drink alcohol, remain standing for a long time, exercise, or experience hot weather. If you are taking this drug, take care to change positions slowly, not abruptly, particularly during the first few days of drug therapy. Remain in air-conditioned rooms during hot spells as much as possible. Avoid drinking alcohol. Less common side effects include nausea, headache, and heart palpitations.

ANTIARRHYTHMIC DRUGS

This diverse group of drugs speeds up, slows down, or otherwise regulates abnormal heart rhythms (arrhythmias). Be particularly careful to take these drugs exactly as prescribed by the doctor. Never take more than prescribed.

Usually the antiarrhythmic drug improves an abnormal heart rhythm, but sometimes it worsens the situation by causing another arrhythmia. Because of this, antiarrhythmic drugs are usually first prescribed during a hospital stay so that the heart rhythm can be carefully monitored. The drug can then be continued safely at home.

Your heart's response to the drug may change over time. It is essential that your doctor monitor your heart regularly. You will need to have blood drawn periodically to determine the level of drug in your system, and you will need to have an ECG routinely. The drugs may be administered by oral dose or by injection.

Digoxin directly strengthens the pumping action of the heart muscle and reduces the heart rate. It is used to treat heart failure and to control the fluttering of the heart known as atrial fibrillation. Originally obtained from the foxglove plant, digoxin has been used for more than 200 years. It increases the amount of calcium supplied to the heart muscle, which boosts the strength of the contractions. Over the years, its use has declined in the treatment of heart failure because of the availability of newer drugs such as the ACE inhibitors, which are very effective and safer. Digoxin may interact with a number of other drugs, including antacids, bile acid binding agents, and quinidine. Levels of digoxin in the blood must be measured periodically, and you should watch for signs of drug excess such as nausea, loss of appetite, and tiredness. Do not discontinue this medication suddenly because it may cause a serious change in heart function. Digoxin can be taken in tablet or liquid form or by injection.

COMMON ANTIARRHYTHMIC DRUGS

amiodarone (Cordarone)
digoxin (Lanoxin)
disopyramide (Norpace)
flecainide (Tambocor)
lidocaine (Xylocaine)
mexiletine (Mexitil)
procainamide (Procan SR,
    Pronestyl, Pronestyl SR)

quinidine gluconate (Duraquin,
    Quinaglute Dura-Tabs,
    Quinalan)
quinidine sulfate (Quinora,
    Quinidex Extentabs)

Side effects

The side effects of antiarrhythmic drugs vary widely depending on the drug. The commonly prescribed quinidine often causes stomach upset and diarrhea. Lidocaine, mexiletine, and tocainide are more likely to cause lightheadedness, dizziness, headache, and blurred vision. Amiodarone, the most potent antiarrhythmic drug, can cause lung inflammation, thyroid abnormalities, and photosensitivity reactions.

Drug interactions are common with this group of drugs, so it is important to tell any doctor who prescribes a new medication which specific antiarrhythmic you are taking. Quinidine and digoxin are often taken together, particularly by people with atrial fibrillation, but the levels of these drugs need to be watched closely to prevent digoxin toxicity. Also, amiodarone can significantly decrease the elimination of both digoxin and warfarin, two common drugs.

BETA-BLOCKERS

Beta-blockers are sometimes prescribed alone or in combination with other drugs to treat high blood pressure. They may also help protect against migraine headaches and thyroid disease. Beta-blockers lower the heart rate and reduce the force of heart contractions.

The beta-blockers are a complex group of drugs that include selective agents (beta-blockers that block only certain beta receptors on the cells of the body), nonselective agents such as propranolol (Inderal), and beta-blockers that also have alpha-blocking properties (labetalol). In the treatment of high blood pressure, beta-blockers generally tend to be more effective in people under age 50. They are generally not recommended for people with circulation problems in the hands, legs, or feet because they tend to constrict the blood vessels in these limbs. People with asthma or other bronchial diseases should not take any of these drugs because they can cause spasms in the bronchial tubes. Beta-blockers should generally be used with caution by people with diabetes because they may interfere with the control of blood sugar.

Do not stop taking these medications suddenly. Sudden withdrawal may increase your angina and increase the chance of heart attack.

Side effects

Side effects are common with beta-blockers. Because they block the effects of norepinephrine and epinephrine, substances that help you respond to physical challenges, all beta-blockers cause lethargy and fatigue. They may also cause depression, cold hands and feet, nausea, or nightmares. The drug may decrease HDL cholesterol and increase your triglycerides (see page 186).

COMMON BETA-BLOCKERS

acebutalol (Sectral)
atenolol (Tenormin)
betaxolol (Kerlone)
Esmolol (Brevibloc)
labetalol (Normodyne, Trandate)

metoprolol (Lopressor, Toprol-XL)
nadolol (Corgard)
penbutalol (Levatol)
propranolol (Inderal)

BLOOD THINNERS

Blood thinners prevent blood clots from forming or growing. This is important because a blood clot can lodge in an already narrowed artery and cause heart attack and stroke. There are three groups of blood thinners: anticoagulants, antiplatelets, and thrombolytics. Each has a specific use.

An example of an anticoagulant is heparin, used in the hospital during open-heart surgery to prevent clots from forming while the blood is being oxygenated by the heart-lung machine. Heparin is also used to treat deep-vein thrombosis, a condition in which blood clots form in veins of the legs and may travel to the lungs. Many doctors prescribe heparin during an ischemic stroke to prevent extension of the clot and further clot formation. Because heparin can be given only by injection, most people who require long-term prevention of clot formation are switched from heparin to warfarin (Coumadin), an oral anticoagulant. Warfarin is widely used to prevent clots in people who have had an ischemic stroke or a heart attack and in those with atrial fibrillation, artificial heart valves, and rheumatic heart disease.

Antiplatelet medications inhibit the clumping together of platelets, cells that help blood clot. If you have had a heart attack or stroke, your doctor may prescribe a low dose of aspirin (one 80 mg baby aspirin or one 325-mg aspirin) to prevent further blood clots.

Aspirin is probably the single most important drug for prevention of stroke. Many people with angina or a family history of heart disease who have not had a heart attack or stroke take aspirin daily for prevention. However, aspirin is not for everyone. It can cause gastrointestinal bleeding. Research has shown that men age 50 and older who have some risk factors for heart disease may benefit from taking aspirin. The benefits are thought to be similar in women, although research is lacking. If you are at risk of heart attack or stroke, discuss with your doctor the possibility of taking aspirin.

Thrombolytic drugs are used in emergency treatment of a heart attack or stroke. Streptokinase, t-PA, and APSAC are three common thrombolytics used to dissolve a clot that is blocking an artery during a heart attack or ischemic stroke. These drugs are given intravenously during an attack or as soon as possible afterward. Unlike anticoagulants and antiplatelet drugs, thrombolytics can dissolve the clot and open the artery before permanent damage to the heart or brain can be done.

COMMON BLOOD THINNERS

anticoagulants
  heparin
  low molecular weight heparin
    (enoxaparin, Lovenox)
  warfarin (Coumadin)
antiplatelets
  aspirin

ticlopidine (Ticlid)
thrombolytics
  alteplase (t-PA, Activase)
  anistreplase (APSAC,
    Eminase)
  streptokinase (Streptase,
    Kabikinase)

CALCIUM CHANNEL BLOCKERS

The mineral calcium is necessary for the activation of your heart's natural pacemaker, the sinus node, and it is involved in the transmission of electrical impulses from the upper to lower chambers of the heart.

By blocking the flow of calcium in these two areas of the heart, the calcium channel blockers lower heart rate and regulate abnormal heart rhythms.

Calcium has another role in circulation. It allows the muscles of the blood vessels to contract, which constricts or narrows them. By blocking the passage of calcium into the muscles that regulate artery tone, these drugs lower blood pressure and lower the workload of the heart.

Calcium channel blockers can also prevent spasms of coronary arteries. For this reason, and because they reduce the workload of the heart, they are used for angina.

Side effects

Calcium channel blockers are well tolerated by most people. Some side effects include dizziness, headache, swelling of ankles, constipation (especially with verapamil), redness of the face and neck, palpitations, nausea, and low blood pressure. Calcium channel blockers have no adverse effects on cholesterol.

COMMON CALCIUM CHANNEL BLOCKERS

amlodipine (Norvasc)	nicardipine (Cardene)
bepridil (Vascor)	nifedipine (Adalat, Procardia,
diltiazem (Cardizem SR,	Procardia XL)
Cardizem CD, Dilacor XR)	verapamil (Calan, Isoptin,
felodipine (Plendil)	Verelan)
isradipine (Dynacirc)	

CENTRALLY ACTING DRUGS

Centrally acting drugs act on receptors in the brain to cause blood vessels throughout the body to open up. This reduces blood pressure.

The centrally acting drug clonidine is also used to minimize withdrawal symptoms for people quitting smoking or drinking and to relieve hot flashes during menopause. Methyldopa, another centrally acting drug, is the drug of choice for treating high blood pressure in pregnant women (see page 150).

Side effects

Many people taking these drugs experience drowsiness, sedation, fatigue, depression, dry mouth, dizziness, constipation, stuffy nose, swollen ankles or feet, or fever. If you experience some of these symptoms, talk with your doctor or pharmacist about the possibility of changing your dosage or your medication. These drugs should not be stopped suddenly, as this causes a rapid rise in blood pressure.

COMMON CENTRALLY ACTING DRUGS

clonidine (Catapres)	guanfacine (Tenex)
guanabenz (Wytensin)	methyldopa (Aldomet)

CHOLESTEROL-LOWERING DRUGS

Not all cases of elevated cholesterol need treatment with drugs. Cholesterol-lowering drugs are usually recommended only after several months of dietary therapy and weight loss have failed. Even if you begin drug therapy, you will need to continue your dietary and other lifestyle changes. There are a number of drugs in this class, and they have variable effects on total cholesterol, LDL, HDL, and triglyceride levels. Depending on your cholesterol profile, you may need to be treated with a combination of agents.

Cholestyramine (Questran) and colestipol (Colestid) reduce total and LDL cholesterol by binding bile acids in the intestine. Bile acids are formed from cholesterol and are essential for the digestion of fatty foods. As bile acids are removed from the body by these binding agents, the liver acts by forming more bile acids from cholesterol. The amount of cholesterol in the body, including LDL-cholesterol, subsequently falls. These medications come in powder form and must be mixed with a liquid such as water, apple juice, or orange juice. To avoid the gritty taste, drink the mixture through a straw. These drugs can also be taken in tablet form. Their side effects are minimal but may include constipation, bloating, heartburn, nausea, vomiting, and headache. These drugs may also interfere with the absorption of other drugs, such as warfarin, digoxin, and thyroid hormone, so it is best to take them at least four hours before or after such drugs.

The statin drugs, such as lovastatin (Mevacor), decrease the production of cholesterol and increase the liver's removal of LDL cholesterol. This class of drugs can also reduce triglycerides and raise HDL. Possible side effects are headache, constipation, flatulence, rash, muscle ache, weakness, dizziness, lightheadedness, or liver dysfunction. Depending on the statin agent prescribed, you may need to take the drug with food (as with lovastatin), and it may interact with other drugs, such as warfarin.

The vitamin nicotinic acid, also known as niacin (Nia-Bid, Niacels, Niacor, Nicolar, Nicobid, Slo-Niacin) lowers triglycerides and LDL cholesterol and raises HDL cholesterol. Though it is available over the counter, talk with your doctor before using it. Niacin causes a number of bothersome side effects, including itching, rash, gastrointestinal distress, dizziness, lightheadedness, and rapid heartbeat. Niacin should be taken with food to prevent stomach upset. Also, if you experience skin flushing or warmth, this effect can be lessened by taking an aspirin (325 mg) 30 minutes before the morning dose of niacin. The flushing reaction usually occurs during the first few days to a week of drug therapy and it lessens over time. Niacin should be used with caution by people with diabetes and gout. Also, niacin can cause a liver abnormality accompanied by flu-like symptoms. Call your doctor immediately if you develop flu-like symptoms such as fever, nausea, and muscle aches.

Probucol (Lorelco) increases the removal of LDL cholesterol from the blood, but it causes only a modest reduction in LDL compared to the other cholesterol-lowering agents. It may also lower the HDL. Probucol has no effects on triglycerides. It may cause indigestion, diarrhea, headache, rash, and insomnia.

COMMON CHOLESTEROL-LOWERING DRUGS

cholestyramine (Questran)
colestipol (Colestid)
fluvastatin (Lescol)
gemfibrozil (Lopid)
lovastatin (Mevacor)
niacin, nicotinic acid (Nia-Bid,

Niacels, Niacor, Nicolar,
Nicobid, Slo-Niacin)
pravastatin (Pravachol)
probucol (Lorelco)
simvastatin (Zocor)

DIURETICS

Commonly known as water pills, diuretics lower blood pressure by increasing the kidney's removal of water and sodium. There are many types of diuretics, and they differ in the area of the kidney in which they work, in potency, and in side effects.

Thiazide diuretics lower blood pressure most effectively. They not only increase the kidney's removal of water and sodium, but also relax the tone of the arteries.

The loop diuretics, including furosemide or Lasix, are the most potent, and they are usually reserved for treatment of congestive heart failure. By reducing the amount of fluid or blood that the heart has to pump through the body, they lessen workload and relieve symptoms of congestion (shortness of breath, fatigue). Loop diuretics are also used for the treatment of high blood pressure in people who have poor kidney function.

The weakest diuretics are the potassium-sparing agents such as spironolactone (Aldactone) and triamterene (Dyrenium). These are available in combination with the thiazides (e.g., Dyazide, Maxzide) for treatment of high blood pressure. They are used alone in the treatment of premenstrual syndrome and water retention due to liver disease. Diuretics are often combined with other drugs to lower blood pressure or treat heart failure.

Side effects

Side effects are uncommon but may include lethargy and leg cramps. These effects may be the result of potassium loss, which most commonly occurs with loop diuretics. Potassium loss can be relieved with

COMMON DIURETICS

amiloride (Midamor)

bendroflumethiazide
(Naturetin)

benzthiazide (Exna)

bumetanide (Bumex)

chlorthalidone (Hygroton)

furosemide (Lasix)

hydrochlorothiazide (Esidrix)

methylclothiazide (Enduron)

metolazone (Zaroxolyn,
Mykrox)

polythiazide (Renese)

spironolactone (Aldactone)

trichlormethiazide (Naqua)

triamterene (Dyrenium)

combination diuretics
hydrochlorothiazide and
spironolactone
(Aldactazide)

hydrochlorothiazide and
amiloride (Moduretic)

hydrochlorothiazide and
triamterene (Dyazide,
Maxzide)

---

potassium supplements or by taking a combination diuretic containing a potassium-sparing agent. Many of the diuretics are sulfas; they
can cause a skin rash if you have allergy to sulfa drugs. Also, all diuretics may aggravate gout, and some may interfere with the control
of blood sugar.

NITRATES

Nitrates are among the oldest and most common drugs used to treat
angina, prevent angina, and prevent heart attack. They dilate the
coronary arteries that supply oxygen to the heart. They also relax the
tone of the large veins that return blood to the heart. By regulating the
amount of blood presented to the heart, they reduce the workload, so
that blood is more effectively pumped to the body's organs. Although
nitrates reduce blood pressure, they are not used to treat high blood
pressure because this effect does not last. They also increase heart
rate.

Nitrates can be taken several ways. To treat an attack of angina, nitrates are most commonly taken as a sublingual tablet placed under
the tongue, where it is allowed to dissolve. To prevent angina on a
daily basis, nitrates are also taken as a tablet to be swallowed and as a
skin patch. All forms of preventive therapy for angina (skin patch,

COMMON NITRATES

isosorbide dinitrate (Isordil, Sorbitrate)
isosorbide mononitrate (ISMO)
nitroglycerin (Minitran, Nitro-Bid, Nitrodur, Nitrodisc, Nitrogard, Nitroglyn, Nitrol, Nitrolingual, Nitrong, Nitrostat, Transderm-Nitro)

ointment, and oral tablets) must be used intermittently throughout the day to avoid the development of tolerance. Your doctor may tell you to remove the patch for at least 10 hours of the day (usually at night) or to take the oral tablet at specific times of the day to prevent tolerance.

Side effects

Most people tolerate nitrates well. When you begin nitrate therapy, side effects are common and usually include headaches, flushing, and dizziness. To limit dizziness and fainting, it is best to take the drug, particularly the sublingual form, while sitting.

COMBINATION MEDICATIONS

Some drugs that are often prescribed together can come in a single tablet. Many people prefer the convenience of a combination tablet. Treatment usually begins with several separate medications so that your doctor can determine which combination is right for you. A combination tablet may be prescribed later for long-term use. The side effects of combination tablets will be similar to those of the individual medications they contain.

COMMON COMBINATION DRUGS

atenolol/chlorthalidone (Tenoretic): beta blocker/diuretic

benazepril 5 /hydrochlorothiazide (Lotensin HCT): ACE inhibitor/diuretic

bisoprolol/ hydrochlorothiazide (Ziac): beta blocker/diuretic

captopril/hydrochlorothiazide (Capozide): ACE inhibitor/diuretic

nadolol/bendroflumethiazide (Corzide): beta blocker/diuretic

propranolol/hydrochlorothiazide (Inderide): beta blocker/diuretic

timolol/hydrochlorothiazide (Timolide): beta blocker/diuretic

chapter 10

D R U G S   F O R   P A I N

*P*AIN IS AN UNPLEASANT SENSATION THAT MAY DISTURB your comfort, thoughts, emotions, daily activity, and sleep. Pain is not a disease, but rather the symptom of an underlying disease or condition. It often alerts you to danger—for example, when you touch something hot or overexert yourself playing a sport. Pain may also help you and your doctor discover medical disorders so they can be treated.

Pain that occurs immediately after a body injury is known as acute pain. When body tissues are damaged by surgery, accident, or a burn, they release chemicals called mediators (including substance P, histamine, and prostaglandins) that stimulate nerves in the skin, muscles, or joints. These nerves send signals through the spinal cord to the brain. The brain interprets the signals as pain, and you then feel pain in the area of body injury. Acute pain may be local and confined to one area or can be more diffuse and difficult to locate. In some cases, for example, a heart attack, acute pain is caused by reduced blood flow to an organ or tissue. With this type of pain, a number of nerves in the area of reduced blood flow are stimulated, and pain is interpreted by the brain as coming from many places. This is "referred pain." For example, a heart attack may cause pain referred to the back, the jaw, and the left arm.

Pain that lingers or a painful condition that cannot be cured is called chronic pain and may require long-term treatment. Chronic pain can be caused by cancer, shingles, a back problem, or nerve conditions. Like acute pain, chronic pain can be either local (for example, back pain) or diffuse (cancer pain).

Some kinds of pain, for example, a mild headache, can be treated with nonprescription medications and forgotten once they go away. But severe or recurring pain should be evaluated by your doctor both for treatment and to rule out possible disorders.

Whether your pain is minor and temporary or more serious and chronic, it is important to know that you need not suffer. Medications and a variety of nondrug pain management techniques can relieve most pain. If you are in pain, tell your doctor. Be persistent until you get the level of pain relief that allows you to enjoy life as fully as possible.

Analgesic drugs

Drugs that relieve pain are called analgesics. Nonprescription nonnarcotic pain relievers such as aspirin, acetaminophen (Tylenol), and ibuprofen (Advil, Motrin) are the best choice for most kinds of pain, particularly muscle pain. Over-the-counter NSAIDs (nonsteroidal anti-inflammatory drugs), including ibuprofen, aspirin, naproxin sodium (Aleve), and ketoprofen (Actron), are also effective for pain associated with inflammation (headache, dental pain, sprains, menstrual pain).

The next level of potency is a nonnarcotic pain reliever available by prescription. Prescription medications include NSAIDs at higher doses and corticosteroids such as prednisone for inflammatory pain conditions (such as severe rheumatoid arthritis). The prescription NSAIDs can treat the local pain of chronic headaches, arthritis, and bone-related pain associated with cancer.

The third level is a prescription drug combining a nonnarcotic pain reliever (acetaminophen, aspirin) with a narcotic pain reliever (codeine, oxycodone). Commonly prescribed combination medications are Percocet, Percodan, and Tylenol with Codeine. They are primarily used for moderate to severe pain that will last a short time, such as the pain following tooth extraction or the pain associated with minor surgery.

The most potent drugs are pure narcotics, like morphine, which are available for severe acute or chronic pain. Narcotic drugs are most useful for the diffuse pain associated with cancer, heart attack, or major surgery.

Special categories of pain, including nerve pain and migraines, may call for drugs that are not ordinarily used as pain relievers, including antidepressant medication.

ASPIRIN

Aspirin is the common name for acetylsalicylic acid. It is a specific type of NSAID known as a salicylate. Aspirin relieves mild to moderate musculoskeletal pain, reduces fever, is an anti-inflammatory drug, and acts on the platelets in the blood to prevent clotting. Aspirin relieves pain by inhibiting the production of prostaglandins, chemical mediators of pain and inflammation.

Of the NSAIDs, aspirin best prevents blood clots. It is recommended for people who have had angina, a heart attack, or ministrokes. A low dose (325 mg every other day) decreases the risk of first heart attack in both women and men over the age of 50.

Because aspirin reduces blood clotting, it should be discontinued a week before any surgery and should not be used to relieve pain following tooth extraction.

Side effects

Aspirin can irritate the lining of the stomach, leading to discomfort, bleeding, or ulcers. Coated and buffered forms reduce this irritation. Alcohol increases it. Effervescent aspirin preparations (Alka-Seltzer) may also reduce irritation. They are high in sodium, however, and should not be used by people on sodium-restricted diets or people with high blood pressure, heart disease, or renal disease.

Aspirin should be avoided during the third trimester of pregnancy. It increases the risk of unnecessary, prolonged bleeding during labor. It also may prolong labor by inhibiting prostaglandins responsible for uterine contractions.

About 1 million people in the United States have aspirin intolerance, a condition that is often inappropriately called aspirin allergy. The symptoms are very fast or difficult breathing, difficulty swallowing, swollen tongue, gasping for breath, wheezing, dizziness, fainting, hives, puffy eyelids, change in face color, or fast, irregular heartbeat. If you notice any of these symptoms, get emergency help immediately. Aspirin intolerance is more likely among people with chronic hives, asthma, or chronic rhinitis. It usually occurs in people in their thirties and forties, including people who have used aspirin in the past with no adverse effect. If you have been diagnosed with aspirin intolerance, you should avoid aspirin and other drugs known to have similar effects, including all NSAIDs, particularly ibuprofen, naproxen, and indomethacin.

People who can't tolerate aspirin can take acetaminophen (see be-

---

BUYING A NONPRESCRIPTION PAIN RELIEVER

Despite the mind-boggling array of brand names, all over-the-counter oral pain relievers contain either acetaminophen (see below) or one of the NSAID drugs (see below): aspirin, ibuprofen, ketoprofen, or naproxen sodium.

Some medications also include caffeine, which may boost effectiveness but can keep you awake or cause illness. Routine use of caffeine-containing pain relievers may lead to withdrawal headaches (the same as stopping the routine use of coffee or another caffeine-containing beverage). Some medications include an antihistamine. This medication affects histamine, which is one of the chemical mediators of pain. The addition of an antihistamine may increase pain relief and may help you sleep.

"Extra strength" pain relievers usually contain a higher dosage of the medication than the regular strength drug. Some drugs have the initials IB or PM after them. "IB" simply means they contain ibuprofen. "PM" means they contain an over-the-counter sleep aid, usually diphenhydramine, an antihistamine that makes you drowsy.

All nonprescription pain relievers except naproxen sodium are available in generic form. Ask your doctor or pharmacist if you can take the generic equivalent, which will save you money.

It may be useful to know the comparable doses of these over-the-counter pain relievers. These dosages of different drugs provide a comparable amount of pain relief:

- 650 mg of aspirin or Tylenol equals 200 mg of ibuprofen
- 25 mg of ketoprofen or 440 mg of naproxen equals 400 mg of ibuprofen

low) or a nonacetylated salicylate such as choline salicylate and magnesium salicylate. The nonacetylated salicylates do not irritate the stomach as much as aspirin, but they do not reduce fever or treat pain as effectively.

ACETAMINOPHEN

Acetaminophen reduces fever and relieves pain. It probably works by acting on the brain. Unlike aspirin and the NSAIDs (see below), it does not reduce inflammation. Acetaminophen can be used for everyday aches and pains like headaches and toothaches. Brand names include Tylenol, Aspirin-free Anacin, and Aspirin-free Excedrin. It is safe to use while pregnant or breast-feeding.

Because it does not reduce blood clotting, acetaminophen is a good treatment for the pain associated with tonsillectomy and dental surgery.

Side effects

Unlike aspirin and the NSAID drugs, acetaminophen does not cause gastric irritation or bleeding. It can be used safely by people with aspirin intolerance, asthma, and gout. If you have heartburn or ulcers, or if you have had intolerance to one of the other pain relievers, reach for the acetaminophen first.

Taking excessive amounts or taking the drug for an extended period can cause liver damage. Drinking alcohol while taking the drug can also damage the liver.

NONSTEROIDAL ANTI-INFLAMMATORY DRUGS (NSAIDS)

The drug group NSAIDs includes ibuprofen, ketoprofen, naproxen sodium, and prescription drugs. NSAIDs reduce swelling or minor inflammation by interfering with the pain-inducing chemicals called prostaglandins at the site of the pain.

NSAIDs are the best choice for any pain caused by inflammation, such as backache, rheumatoid arthritis, sprains, bruises, sunburns, and minor toothaches. Ibuprofen works better than acetaminophen or aspirin for menstrual pain and for the pain related to episiotomy and gout. Naproxen sodium relieves pain longer than ibuprofen, which is good for long-lasting pain such as arthritis. If you need quick relief from pain, try ibuprofen rather than naproxen.

In addition to the over-the-counter pain relievers, there is a long list of similar NSAID medications available by prescription only. Your doctor may prescribe a prescription NSAID if the over-the-counter drug fails or if you have a condition that is known to respond to a specific drug. The NSAID drugs differ in terms of their potency, speed, effects on blood clotting, duration of pain relief, frequency of dosing (once daily to four times a day), adverse effects (particularly on the digestive tract), their potential to cause drug interactions, and cost. No one NSAID is superior to all others. Although your pain may respond poorly to one NSAID, you may have excellent relief with another.

Side effects

By far the most common and troubling side effect of these drugs is stomach irritation. If the drug irritates your stomach, it may be best to take it with food, although food or antacids may slow down or reduce the drug's effectiveness. For quickest action, take the first several doses 30 minutes before or two hours after eating. Do not take a protective-coated product with food or antacids; the coating will be removed and the risk of stomach ulcers will be increased. Do not drink alcohol while taking an NSAID drug, as it will increase stomach irritation.

NSAID drugs can also cause gastric bleeding. The symptoms are severe abdominal cramps, pain or burning in the stomach or abdomen, diarrhea or black tarry stools, continuing nausea, heartburn or indigestion, or vomiting of blood or material that looks like coffee grounds. If you notice any of these symptoms, stop taking the medication and call your doctor immediately.

If you need to continue NSAID therapy for arthritis pain or a chronic inflammatory pain condition, at least two NSAIDs, nabumetone and etodolac, have a very low risk of stomach irritation. Also, if you are predisposed to gastric ulcers and have a high risk of gastric bleeding, you may be a candidate for misoprostol (Cytotec) therapy. Misoprostol supplies the body with a prostaglandin that normally prevents gastric irritation. Misoprostol is FDA approved for the preven-

COMMON NONSTEROIDAL ANTI-INFLAMMATORY DRUGS (NSAIDS)

nonprescription
 aspirin
 ibuprofen (Advil, Genpril,
  Motrin IB, Nuprin)
 ketoprofen (Orudis KT,
  Actron)
 naproxen sodium (Aleve)
prescription
 choline salicylate (Arthropan)
 choline magnesium salicylate
  (Trilisate)
 diclofenac (Cataflam,
  Voltaren)
 diflunisal (Dolobid)
 etodolac (Lodine)
 fenoprofen (Nalfon)
 flurbiprofen (Ansaid)
 ibuprofen (Motrin, Rufen)

indomethacin (Indocin)
ketoprofen (Orudis, Oruvail)
ketorolac (Toradol)
magnesium salicylate (Magan,
 Mobidin)
meclofenamate sodium
 (Meclomen)
mefenamic acid (Ponstel)
nabumetone (Relafen)
naproxen sodium (Anaprox)
naproxen (Naprosyn,
 Naprelan)
oxaprozin (Daypro)
piroxicam (Feldene)
sodium salicylate
salsalate (Disalcid)
sulindac (Clinoril)
tolmetin (Tolectin)

tion of gastric ulcers induced by NSAIDs (including aspirin) in people at high risk (the elderly, those with history of gastric ulcers). To protect against NSAID-related gastric irritation, misoprostol must be given for the length of NSAID therapy. Do not use misoprostol during pregnancy because it may cause uterine contractions and miscarriage.

In people with aspirin intolerance (see page 212), NSAIDs can cause similar symptoms of very fast or difficult breathing, difficulty swallowing, swollen tongue, gasping for breath, wheezing, dizziness, fainting, hives, puffy eyelids, change in face color, or fast, irregular heart-beat. If you notice any of these symptoms, get emergency help immediately. Rarely, NSAIDs can cause allergic reactions in people with no history of aspirin intolerance.

Rare side effects include sore throat or fever; swelling fingers, hands, or feet; weight gain, and decreased or painful urination. Some NSAIDS, including ibuprofen, can interfere with blood pressure control in people taking either diuretics or beta-blockers. Most NSAIDs can also decrease blood flow to the kidneys in people who have heart failure, high blood pressure, or liver disease. NSAIDs should be used with caution if you have any of these conditions.

OPIATES

When other pain relievers don't work and pain is moderate to severe, a group of narcotic analgesics called the opiates may be the next choice. Opiates such as morphine are derived from the opium poppy plant or synthetic versions. They mimic the pain-suppressing chemicals found naturally in the body, such as endorphins. Opiates are particularly effective for pain caused by surgery, labor and delivery, burns, kidney stones, and cancer.

Opium, an ancient drug, has also been a drug of abuse and can be addictive when used for purposes other than treating pain. Because of this problem, doctors have sometimes been reluctant to prescribe opi-

PATIENT-CONTROLLED PAIN RELIEF

When you are in pain, it can be difficult to wait for a nurse or doctor to bring you your next dose of pain reliever. A relatively new technique allows the patient to control her own pain medication with a small computerized pump. The pump is most commonly used for patients with pain from cancer, trauma, or following surgery (including cesarean section).

The small pump, about the size of a personal cassette player, can hang from a belt or clothing. Each time the patient feels a need for a dose, she pushes a button and the pump dispenses a preset dosage of pain reliever (usually morphine or another opiate) through a tiny catheter and an intravenous needle.

Some patients worry that they might give themselves too much of the drug and overdose, but the pump is programmed to determine the dose and the maximum doses per hour. In many cases, the lock-out (time between available doses) is 10 to 15 minutes. In fact, patients who dose themselves tend to use less drug than those who receive pain relief by injection.

OPIATES

alfentanil (Alfenta)	methadone (Dolophine)
codeine	morphine (various; MS Contin)
fentanyl (Sublimaze, Duragesic)	oxycodone (Percocet, Percodan,
hydrocodone (Vicodin, Lorcet,	Tylox)
Lortab)	oxymorphone (Numorphan)
hydromorphone (Dilaudid)	propoxyphenene (Darvon)
levorphanol (Levo-Dromoran)	sufentanil (Sufenta)
meperidine (Demerol)	

ate pain relievers or to increase a dosage when a patient develops a tolerance to the current dosage. However, recent research has shown that most people have no problem stopping the medication once they have no further medical need for it. Because of this, health professionals have been increasingly willing to help people relieve their pain with these effective drugs. Opiate medications are often prescribed in combination with a nonnarcotic pain reliever such as ibuprofen, aspirin, or acetaminophen.

Opiate medications can be administered by injection into the muscle, through an epidural catheter, in tablets or oral solutions, in a skin patch, or via a patient-controlled intravenous pump. Your doctor will have to adjust your dose until it is right. When you first begin taking opiate medications, your doctor should assess your response within the first few hours. If your pain does not subside, report it immediately. Large doses given to patients unaccustomed to these drugs can dangerously slow down breathing, so the person must be closely monitored.

If you need chronic pain therapy, it is common to build up a tolerance to an opiate after a week. Your doctor may increase your dose or may prescribe a different opiate medication. Though people with long-term severe pain, such as cancer pain, may need increasing dosages, it is rare that no dose is high enough to relieve all their pain.

Short-term use of an opiate for acute pain does not cause dependence or the potential for abuse. If you need short-term pain therapy following surgery, for a severe burn or for another severe painful condition, you shouldn't fear addiction.

If you need to take an opiate on a chronic basis, take the medication on a regular schedule. If you wait until the pain reappears, it will be harder to treat. If you take an opiate drug for several weeks and stop suddenly, you may experience withdrawal symptoms. Instead, your doctor will gradually reduce the dosage for several weeks.

Side effects

Common side effects are constipation, nausea, and sedation. If you need to take an opiate for a week or more, you should consider starting a stool softener on the day that the opiate is started. If you are prone to constipation, the use of a stimulant laxative such as Senokot is also advised.

Another common side effect of the morphine-like opiates is itching. Itching without the presence of a skin rash or shortness of breath is not a sign of allergy. Instead, it is caused by the release of histamine from cells in the skin and stomach. Antihistamines such as diphenhydramine (Benadryl) can control the itching. If you experience upset stomach, take the opiate with food. Rarely, the opiates may cause true allergy, with such symptoms as hives, facial edema, difficulty swal-

COMBINATION DRUGS

If a nonnarcotic pain reliever is not enough, it may be combined with an opiate. The opiate interferes with the transmission of pain in the spinal cord and the brain, while the nonnarcotic drug acts at the site of tissue injury. The combination is one of the most effective ways to relieve pain. The major disadvantage of these combination drugs is that they are not long acting and therefore are useful only in treating acute pain, not chronic pain. These combinations must usually be taken every three or four hours.

hydrocodone/acetaminophen   oxycodone/aspirin (Percodan)
   (Vicodin)   oxycodone/acetaminophen
codeine/acetaminophen   (Percocet)
   (Tylenol with Codeine)

lowing, and shortness of breath; if you experience any of these symptoms, seek medical attention immediately.

Back pain

Back pain is one of the most common types of chronic pain. It can be dull, nagging, occasional pain; constant and disabling pain; or an acute, sharp pain that comes on suddenly, often the result of a seemingly harmless movement such as swinging a tennis racket or even bending over to tie your shoe. Back pain often starts around age 30 and can continue, off and on, for years. Bouts of back pain often gradually disappear as a person ages. Lower-back pain can be normal if you are pregnant, are having your period, or in the week before your period. It can also be a sign of osteoarthritis or endometriosis.

The backbone is not one bone. It consists of 24 separate bones, the vertebrae, held together by muscles and ligaments The cushioning between the vertebrae is a spongy disc. The backbone's function is to support the body's upright carriage and to protect the spinal cord. Because of the complexity of the backbone's structure and its many parts, it is susceptible to a variety of problems that can cause pain. There are three main categories of lower-back pain: strains and sprains, herniated disc syndromes, and lumbar dysfunctions (including nonspecific lower-back pain). Rarely, lumbar spine stenosis, an overgrowth of bone that compresses the spinal cord, is the cause of lower-back pain.

While some back pain is not serious and can be controlled with over-the-counter medication, exercise, and proper posture, some back pain is a symptom of a serious condition. See your doctor if your back pain is combined with any of the following symptoms or problems.

- Weak or numb legs
- Intense pain in the lower spine for more than two weeks
- Recent fall or accident
- Fever or chills

TREATMENT

For acute pain caused by sprain or strain, bed rest is helpful only for the first day or two. Then you should get back on your feet and live your life as normally as possible. Moderate movement will keep your joints flexible.

Surgery provides no or little help for most types of back pain. The spinal manipulation practiced by chiropractors is often effective for the relief of nonspecific lower-back pain.

The best drug treatment for back pain caused by sprain or strain is a nonprescription nonnarcotic pain reliever, such as aspirin, ibuprofen (Advil, Motrin), or naproxen (Aleve). Ibuprofen may be the most effective. Naproxen (Aleve) lasts somewhat longer for the same dosage. If a drug does not help, ask your doctor whether you should increase the dose or try a different pain reliever.

Cancer pain

Many people who have cancer fear they will experience pain. However, some cancer patients, even those with advanced cancer, have no or very little pain. And if you do feel pain, it can and should be treated. There is no reason to suffer untreated cancer pain.

Cancer pain tends to be chronic, that is, to continue over a period of days, weeks, or months. There may also be episodes of acute pain following surgery for cancer, after chemotherapy, or if you have a growing tumor. Cancer causes pain because it invades and injures the tissues of the body. Both opiate drugs and nonnarcotic pain relievers such as aspirin and ibuprofen can relieve pain by suppressing signals in the nerves, spinal cord, and brain that result from tissue injury.

Describe to your doctor the type, intensity, and location of the pain. Some kinds of cancer pain include:

- Chemotherapy pain: painful numbness and tingling caused by damage to the nerves
- Postmastectomy pain: tight, constricting burning pain in the arm and chest wall
- Radiation-induced nerve tumors: painful, enlarging tumor in the area that was radiated

- Tumor infiltration of a nerve: constant burning pain and an area of numbness

Pain treatment often starts with a nonnarcotic pain reliever. If the pain persists or increases, you may then receive a combination non-narcotic/narcotic pain reliever. If this combination fails to relieve your pain, your doctor may increase the dosage of the narcotic pain reliever. The nonnarcotic may be discontinued or continued at this time. Patients with severe cancer pain are usually treated effectively with opiate medications. If drug tolerance develops, your dose may be increased regularly. NSAID drugs are often combined with opiates, particularly for bone pain. Amphetamines may be prescribed for enhancement of mood or alertness, and antidepressants are used for nerve pain. A short course of a corticosteroid (dexamethasone) may decrease spinal pain.

Nondrug pain relief techniques are also useful for cancer patients. You can find many self-help books on these topics or ask your health-care professionals about them. One nondrug method, transcutaneous electrical nerve stimulation (TENS), is a low-voltage electrical stimulation that inhibits mild pain in some cases, although its effectiveness is mainly attributed to the placebo effect. Acupuncture treats pain by inserting small needles into specific places in the skin. Simple relaxation techniques and imagery can help with brief episodes of pain, for example, during procedures. If your pain is persistent and difficult to treat, short-term psychotherapy may help, particularly if you are depressed.

Menstrual pain

Some women have painful menstrual periods, a condition known to doctors as primary dysmenorrhea and to many women as cramps. During each menstrual period, the menstrual fluid is removed from the uterus by contractions caused by prostaglandins. Women with primary dysmenorrhea have high levels of prostaglandins, which cause the uterus to contract more forcefully and at an increased rate. This may lead to poor oxygen delivery to the area and sharp, abdominal pain. Some young women feel similar cramps when their cervix stretches open to release the monthly menstrual flow. Menstrual pain is the most common cause of absence from work or school in women from age 20 to 24, but it tends to decrease as a woman ages.

Menstrual pain usually starts on or about the first day of your menstrual period and gradually subsides over the next 72 hours. Other symptoms that often accompany dysmenorrhea include nausea, headache, backache, constipation, or diarrhea.

TREATMENT

Your doctor will first try to rule out other causes of menstrual pain, including pelvic inflammatory disease or endometriosis. If these or other causes seem unlikely, your doctor may prescribe medication. Exercises such as leg lifts and partial sit-ups also help relieve menstrual cramps by decreasing the release of prostaglandins and by increasing your natural production of endorphins.

The medications most commonly prescribed to relieve menstrual pain are:

- **NSAIDs.** Menstrual pain caused by the release of prostaglandins during menstruation can often be relieved with NSAIDs. Because prostaglandin release is highest in the first 48 hours of your period, treatment for dysmenorrhea should be started on the first day of your period and continued for three days. Ibuprofen is the most effective choice. If ibuprofen does not relieve the pain, ask your doctor about increasing the dosage. Prescription NSAIDs

---

NSAIDS FOR MENSTRUAL PAIN

nonprescription
  ibuprofen (Advil, Motrin IB,
    Nuprin)
  naproxen (Aleve)
  ketoprofen (Orudis KT)
prescription
  diclofenac (Cataflam,
    Voltaren)

ketoprofen (Actron, Orudis)
meclofenamate sodium
  (Meclomen)
mefenamic acid (Ponstel)
naproxen sodium (Anaprox)
naproxen (Naprosyn)

are also available, the most effective being mefenamic acid (Pon-stel). A study showed that 80 to 85 percent of women with dys-menorrhea were helped by one of the NSAIDs.

- **Combination birth-control pills.** If NSAIDs do not substan-tially relieve the pain, or if you cannot tolerate them, your doctor may prescribe a combination birth-control pill, which relieves menstrual pain in about 90 percent of women. Contraceptive pills reduce menstrual pain by suppressing ovulation and reducing the prostaglandin levels.

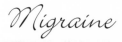

Migraine

Headaches are probably the most common source of pain reported to doctors. They are not usually a sign of an underlying health problem, although your doctor may perform tests to rule out serious problems such as a tumor.

Tension-type headaches (also called muscle contraction, tension, or stress headaches) are believed to be caused by muscle contractions. They produce a dull, aching pain in a band across the head. Unlike migraine, they affect both sides of the head and can usually be treated by nonprescription pain relievers.

A migraine headache is a less common disorder that appears mainly in women of childbearing age. Migraines tend to run in fami-lies. This type of headache comes on rapidly. The pain usually pul-sates, often on one side of the head, and may be preceded by flashing lights or accompanied by nausea and vomiting. You may also be sen-sitive to light and sound and need to seek out a quiet, dark place to rest. Migraines can last 4 to 48 hours.

The cause of migraines is unclear, although there may be a lack of natural pain-relieving brain chemicals such as serotonin. There is some evidence that migraines are associated with the changing estro-gen levels of the menstrual cycle. Many women find that their mi-graines disappear completely during pregnancy. Most headaches, including migraine headaches, become less frequent with age and di-minish following menopause.

Many things can trigger a migraine, including certain foods, alco-hol, exposure to bright sunshine, intense emotional stress, irregular sleeping patterns, and fluctuations in estrogen levels.

TREATMENT

The best treatment for migraine is prevention. To avoid this kind of headache:

- Identify and avoid triggers such as alcohol, sun exposure, or certain foods (common culprits are red wine, aged cheese, chocolate, nuts, caffeine, and foods containing monosodium glutamates or nitrites).
- Go to bed and get up at the same time every day to establish a regular sleeping pattern.
- Review any medications you are taking with your doctor to determine if one or more might be contributing to your headaches. Headaches are a common side effect of drugs used to treat high blood pressure, some antibiotics, and combination oral contraceptives.
- Reduce stress with meditation, relaxation exercises, or biofeedback.

If these measures do not substantially reduce the frequency and intensity of your migraines, talk with your doctor about treatment with medication. Over-the-counter analgesics such as aspirin, acetaminophen, or ibuprofen may reduce the pain of mild attacks. There are also prescription alternatives for treatment. Often prescribed for

COMMON DRUGS FOR MIGRAINES

acetaminophen (Tylenol)	butorphanol (Stadol)
aspirin	methylsergide (Sansert)
aspirin with caffeine and	dihydroergotamine (DHE)
butalbital (Fiorinal)	divalproex (Depakote)
acetaminophen with	ergotamine (Cafergot)
isometheptene and	sumatriptan (Imitrex)
dichloralphenazone	
(Midrin)	

mild to moderate migraine are combination pain relievers such as Fiorinal (aspirin in combination with caffeine and a weak barbiturate, butalbital) or Midrin (acetaminophen; isometheptene, a drug that constricts the cerebral vessels; and dichloralphenazone, a mild sedative). Also, for mild to moderate migraine, prescription NSAIDs may be recommended by your doctor.

For more severe migraine, drugs known as ergots used to be commonly prescribed, but a newer drug, sumatriptan, is now prescribed more widely because it has fewer side effects.

Drugs prescribed to *treat* migraine include:

- **Sumatriptan.** Taken when symptoms first appear, sumatriptan (Imitrex) is administered by tablet or auto-injector. Most people choose the later method, which brings relief in 10 to 30 minutes; the tablets work in about 2 hours. Sumatriptan constricts blood vessels in the brain. The most common side effect is pain at the site of the injection. Sumatriptan may cause a rise in blood pressure and angina-type chest pain. It should not be used by people with heart disease, and it should be used with extreme caution by people who have risk factors for heart disease (diabetics, smokers, postmenopausal women, and people with high blood pressure). Because of the risk of excessive constriction of blood vessels, sumatriptan should not be used within 24 hours after taking an ergot drug.
- **Ergotamine.** When over-the-counter analgesics fail, ergotamine (Cafergot) can be taken orally or by inhaler or suppositories. Ergotamine can abort an oncoming migraine headache by constricting the cranial blood vessels. It is usually less effective than sumatriptan. Ergotamine may cause a variety of unpleasant side effects, including nausea, vomiting, muscle aches, tremor, and tingling hands or feet. A rare but serious complication is gangrene of the bowel or limbs, which is more likely to occur if you take excessive doses. If ergotamine is used for an extended time, you may build up a tolerance to the drug, so that larger doses are required. Carefully follow instructions for taking ergotamine and do not exceed the recommended dosage. Dihydroergotamine (DHE), a derivative of ergotamine, has had success similar to ergotamine in treating migraines that do not respond to over-the-counter analgesics. It can be injected and may soon be

available in nasal spray. DHE has fewer side effects than ergotamine.

- **Butorphanol.** Butorphanol (Stadol) is an opiate nasal spray that may be effective for moderate to severe migraine but causes drowsiness and mood swings.

Drugs prescribed to *prevent* migraine include:

- **Beta-blockers (see page 199), calcium channel blockers (see page 202), and tricyclic antidepressants (see page 306).** These drugs may be prescribed for daily use by people with frequent or severe migraines.
- **Methylsergide.** An ergot product, methylsergide (Sansert) may help prevent severe migraine. Side effects may include weight gain, edema, and vascular spasm.
- **Divalproex.** The anticonvulsant divalproex (Depakote) decreases the frequency and severity of migraine headache.

Nerve pain

Nerve pain is often more difficult to treat than other kinds of pain. Nerves can be damaged by injury, cancer, diabetes, alcoholism, vitamin deficiencies, and the herpes zoster virus (commonly known as shingles).

TREATMENT

Nerve pain responds poorly to conventional pain medications, including opiates. Instead, nerve pain often responds to "adjuvant" drugs that were originally developed for another purpose. Some of these medications include tricyclic antidepressants, anticonvulsants, and clonidine.

- **Tricyclic antidepressants.** These antidepressants were widely used before the newer antidepressants such as Prozac were developed. They can treat dull, aching, burning pain such as peripheral neuropathy, a painful, tingling numbness in the legs and arms caused by nerve damage from diabetes, vitamin B12 deficiency, cancer, alcoholism, and shingles. Your doctor may begin with a low dosage and increase it slowly until you reach a dose that effectively quiets your pain. You may not experience the full pain-relieving effects of the drug for several days or weeks. Don't stop taking your medication if you don't experience immediate relief. The dosage you will be taking is often lower than that which might be prescribed for depression. If you experience side effects such as dry mouth, blurred vision, sedation, or insomnia, report them to your doctor. (For more on antidepressants, see page 305.)

- **Anticonvulsants.** Normally prescribed to treat epilepsy and other seizure disorders, anticonvulsants may also help with brief, sharp pain in the peripheral nerves (arms, legs). Pain relief is not immediate with these drugs. The most effective drugs in this group are carbamazepine (Tegretol) and clonazepam (Klonopin). Some anticonvulsants have dangerous interactions with other drugs, including the anticoagulant warfarin and antidepressants, so make sure your doctor knows about any other medications you are taking. Be particularly careful not to exceed the prescribed dosage because of the dangerous effects of overdose. Some of the more common effects of these anticonvulsant medications include blurred vision and rapid eye movements, clumsiness, dizziness, lightheadedness, nausea, or vomiting.

- **Capsaicin.** A product derived from red peppers, capsaicin

ADJUVANT DRUGS FOR NERVE PAIN

tricyclic antidepressants	clonazepam (Klonopin)
amitriptyline (Elavil)	gabapentin (Neurontin)
desipramine (Norpramin)	phenytoin (Dilantin)
doxepin (Sinequan)	valproic acid (Depakene)
imipramine (Tofranil)	capsaicin
nortriptyline (Aventyl,	centrally acting
Pamelor)	antihypertensives
anticonvulsants	clonidine (Catapres)
carbamazepine (Tegretol)	

(Zostrix) is available over the counter and approved for use in the treatment of neuralgic pain associated with shingles and diabetic neuropathy. It works by depleting the amount of substance P, a pain mediator, at the peripheral nerves. Capsaicin is also effective for temporary relief from rheumatoid arthritis, osteoarthritis, and neuralgia (shingles, diabetic neuropathy, and HIV neuropathy). It is applied topically to the affected areas three to four times a day. The side effects are burning at the application site, stinging, and redness. These usually go away with continued dosing.

- **Clonidine.** This centrally acting antihypertensive medication may relieve some forms of nerve pain that cannot be helped by opiate medications or other adjuvant pain medications.

Osteoarthritis

Osteoarthritis, also known as "wear and tear" arthritis, affects almost everyone over age 60 to some degree. It occurs when the cartilage that normally cushions the joints thins and breaks down, causing the ends of the bones to rub against each other. It can develop from injury, overuse, or just many years of normal use. Osteoarthritis is usually not curable, but its symptoms can be managed with a combination of medications and self-help techniques. There are many types of arthritis, but osteoarthritis is by far the most common. Other types include rheumatoid arthritis (caused by inflammation of the connective tissue), psoriatic arthritis, and lupus arthritis. The treatment below applies to osteoarthritis.

SYMPTOMS

Osteoarthritis most commonly affects the joints in the hands, hips, knees, neck, spine, and feet. Its symptoms include:

- Dull ache or soreness in a joint, especially when you move
- Stiffness and loss of range of motion in a joint
- Sound of grating or rubbing of bones
- Bumps (bone spurs) on joints, particularly the hands or feet

TREATMENT

The first choice for treatment of osteoarthritis is acetaminophen (Tylenol) because it is an effective analgesic and has few side effects. Acetaminophen is less likely than other analgesics to cause discomfort or bleeding in the intestinal system, which is a concern for older people. The anti-inflammatory properties of other analgesics are not needed for osteoarthritis. If acetaminophen does not relieve the pain, the next choice is a nonacetylated salicylate (page 214), and the third choice is a nonsteroidal anti-inflammatory drug (NSAID) such as aspirin, ibuprofen, naproxen, or ketoprofen. There is also a variety of prescription NSAIDs available to treat osteoarthritis. Other agents sometimes prescribed for osteoarthritis are topical products such as methyl salicylate or capsaicin cream.

Nondrug techniques that can supplement your medication are massage, heat packs, and especially range-of-motion exercises. Special exercises move the joint through its full range of motion, bathing the cartilage in rejuvenating fluid. Ask your doctor or physical therapist for a set of range-of-motion exercises for your joints.

Postoperative pain

After surgery, tissues that have been disrupted or cut will release pain mediators, but there are drugs to relieve this pain. Pain relief after surgery is important for recovery. Not only can persistent pain impede recovery, but pain stimulates the output of the stress hormones, adrenaline and cortisol, while the body should be resting. Pain discourages coughing and deep breathing, which help prevent pneumonia. It reduces a patient's ability to be mobile, increasing the chance of blood clots forming and lodging in the heart, lung, or brain.

TREATMENT

It is better to use drugs to prevent pain from surfacing than to treat it later, which requires a higher dose. Because of this, you should receive drugs for pain relief on a regular schedule, every few hours, not as needed when the pain occurs.

When planning for surgery, discuss the postoperative pain relief regimen with your surgeon. Ask what steps will be taken if you need additional pain relief. If you experience pain after your operation, speak up. Don't assume your doctor and nurses know how much pain you are feeling.

Ask your doctor about patient-controlled pain relief (see page 217). At the first tinge of pain, the patient controls the flow of intravenous pain medication with the touch of a button. This method has resulted in less pain for patients and shorter hospital stays.

The drug of choice for relief of postoperative pain is usually morphine. Morphine is usually administered intravenously at first rather than in oral form. After the most acute pain has passed and you are able to drink and swallow, you can switch to oral medication. Your doctor may continue the morphine or choose another opiate such as codeine. Meperidine (Demerol) is a commonly prescribed medication for postoperative pain, but in larger doses, its side effects can include irritability, nausea, and vomiting. Ketorolac (Toradol), the only injectable NSAID, is approved for the short-term treatment of pain. It is commonly used for relief of moderate to severe postoperative pain, including that associated with abdominal, gynecologic, oral, orthopedic, or urologic surgery. Ketorolac may also be combined with an opiate drug, which reduces the dose of the opiate. Like the other NSAIDs, ketorolac may cause stomach irritation or bleeding and reduces the ability of the blood to form clots. Ketorolac should not be used during labor because it can increase bleeding, but it can be used after a birth. If a person has a history of stomach ulcers, an opiate is a better choice.

COMMON DRUGS FOR POSTOPERATIVE PAIN

codeine	morphine
hydromorphone (Dilaudid)	oxycodone/acetaminophen
ketorolac (Toradol)	(Percocet)
meperidine (Demerol)	oxycodone/aspirin (Percodan)

chapter 11

DRUGS FOR INFECTIONS

TINY LIVING ORGANISMS ARE EVERYWHERE—IN THE air, water, and soil as well as on your skin and in your lungs, digestive tract, and reproductive organs. These microscopic organisms include bacteria, viruses, fungi, and the single-celled organisms called protozoa. Infections caused by microorganisms are contagious; we catch them from other people, animals, contaminated water, or even ourselves—as when bacteria from the colon or vagina invade the urinary tract. Normally your immune system protects your body from these invaders. If it can't, the result is an illness called an infection. Some infections affect your whole body; for example, a flu virus causes fever, muscle aches, and joint pain. Other infections—for example, a vaginal infection or a head cold—affect only part of the body. The symptoms and treatment depend on the organism and the location of the infection.

Drugs used to treat infection

Drugs for infections are grouped by the organisms they attack. Antibiotics are for bacterial infections, antiviral drugs for viral infections, and antifungal drugs for fungal infections.

ANTIBIOTICS

Antibiotics, which kill or inhibit the growth of bacteria, are among the most commonly prescribed of all drugs. They are used to treat a wide range of disorders from minor infections to life-threatening conditions like pneumonia. Antibiotics are not effective against viral infections, including most colds and flu. Since the discovery of the first antibiotic, penicillin, in 1941, many types have been developed.

Antibiotics work either by killing the bacteria directly or by halting their reproduction so that the body's natural defenses are able to overcome them. Some antibiotics are effective against only a limited number of microorganisms, while others, known as broad-spectrum antibiotics (cephalosporins, fluoroquinolones), can destroy an array of organisms. Because they may interfere with the normal bacterial environment in the stomach, intestines, and vaginal tract, most antibiotics can have side effects such as nausea, diarrhea, and yeast infection. Some antibiotics make hormonal contraceptives less effective (see page 38), and others increase sensitivity to sunlight (see page 34).

An additional risk with some types of antibiotics, particularly the penicillins, is allergy. Although allergic reactions are uncommon, they can cause severe skin rashes all over the body, shortness of breath, or a change in blood pressure. If you are allergic to penicillin or related drugs, tell your doctor whenever a new medication is prescribed. If you have had a reaction to a penicillin in the past, your physician will probably not choose to prescribe one to you in the future. This decision is based on the severity of your reaction to penicillin and the length of time since you were last exposed (1 year versus 20 years ago). The sulfa drugs, which are another type of antibacterial drug and include the combination drug sulfamethoxazole-trimethoprim (Bactrim, Septra), may also cause allergic skin reactions, but the risk of a reaction is low.

The choice of antibiotic for the treatment of your infection will depend on a number of factors besides allergy, including your age, the function of your liver and kidneys, other drugs you are taking, the results of any cultures that were taken from the site of your infection (throat, sputum, urine, blood), and whether you are pregnant or breast-feeding.

Some antibiotics have been used so widely that the bacteria they

DANGEROUS COMBINATIONS WITH SELDANE AND HISMANAL

It is toxic and may be fatal to combine the popular antihistamines terfenadine (Seldane) or astemizole (Hismanal) with the commonly prescribed antibiotic erythromycin or the antifungal drug ketoconazole. Erythromycin and ketoconazole interfere with the body's ability to metabolize both terfenadine and astemizole. High levels build up, leading to an abnormal heartbeat, which has resulted in fatal heart arrhythmias (irregular heart rhythms).

Despite repeated warnings from the government and pharmaceutical companies, these drugs are sometimes prescribed at the same time. If you take either terfenadine or astemizole for allergies, be extra careful when receiving antibiotic or antifungal treatment, for example, for a yeast infection. Make sure your prescription is not for erythromycin or ketoconazole. If it is, talk with your doctor or pharmacist about discontinuing terfenadine or astemizole. The interaction is most severe with erythromycin and ketoconazole, but it may also occur with clarithromycin, itraconazole, fluconazole, and miconazole. The package information extends the warning to each of these antibiotics and antifungal drugs. Erythromycin and clarithromycin are commonly used for bronchial infections. Antifungals such as ketoconazole, itraconazole, fluconazole, and miconazole are used for a variety of infections, including nail infections and yeast infections.

target have developed new ways to grow and reproduce. These "resistant" bacteria can no longer be killed by those antibiotics. Like other organisms, resistant forms can be passed from one person to another. The problem of drug resistance can be somewhat reduced by following some general principles of infection control.

- Use antibiotics only when necessary for treatment of an infection. Overuse, such as for prevention of a suspected infection, contributes to the development of resistance.
- Take the full course of medication. If you stop sooner, any leftover bacteria are more likely to develop drug resistance.
- Practice good hygiene. Organisms, including ones that are resis-

ANTIBIOTIC DRUGS

aminoglycosides
  gentamicin
  neomycin
  netilmicin
  streptomycin
  tobramycin
cephalosporins
  cefaclor (Ceclor)
  cefadroxil (Duricef)
  cefazolin (Ancef, Kefzol)
  cefepime (Maxipime)
  cefixime (Suprax)
  cefoxitin (Mefoxin)
  cefpodoxime (Vantin)
  ceftriaxone (Rocephin)
  cephalexin (Keflex, Keftab)
  cephalothin (Keflin)
fluoroquinolones
  ciprofloxacin (Cipro)
  lomefloxacin (Maxaquin)
  norfloxacin (Noroxin)
macrolides
  azithromycin (Zithromax)
  erythromycin
  clarithromycin (Biaxin)
penicillins and related drugs
  amoxicillin
  amoxicillin-clavulanate
    (Augmentin)
  ampicillin
  aztreonam (Azactam)
  dicloxacillin

imipenem (Primaxin)
penicillin G
penicillin V
ticarcillin (Ticar)
ticarcillin-clavulanate
    (Timentin)
sulfonamides
  sulfamethoxazole (Gantanol)
  sulfamethoxazole-
    trimethoprim (Bactrim,
    Septra)
  sulfisoxazole (Gantrisin)
tetracyclines
  demeclocycline
  doxycycline (Vibramycin)
  minocycline (Minocin)
  oxytetracycline
  tetracycline
urinary antiseptics
  methenamine (Mandelamine,
    Hiprex)
  nalidixic acid (NegGram)
  nitrofurantoin (Furadantin)
other antibacterial drugs
  bacitracin
  chloramphenicol
  clindamycin (Cleocin)
  colistin
  dapsone
  metronidazole (Flagyl)
  trimethoprim (Trimpex)
  vancomycin

tant to commonly prescribed antibiotics, are routinely spread from person to person through hand-to-hand contact and by coughing and sneezing. Wash your hands frequently, and cover your mouth when you cough or sneeze.

Use

- Take the full prescription. Not all antibiotics are prescribed for 7 days. Depending on the infection, you may be prescribed a single dose, a 3- to 5-day course, or a 14-day course.
- If you have leftover antibiotics, do not use them later or give them to someone else. Specific antibiotics are effective only against specific bacteria, so use only the antibiotic prescribed by your doctor for your particular infection.
- Take your antibiotic at the same time each day. Some antibiotics are taken three or four times a day, others once a day. Follow your doctor's instructions carefully.
- Report any side effects or allergic reactions. Watch for nausea, vomiting, or diarrhea and for signs and symptoms of allergy, including itching or burning skin, rash, shortness of breath, or difficulty swallowing.
- Before taking the antibiotic with other prescribed or over-the-counter medications, talk to your pharmacist about the potential for drug interactions. Some antibiotics (tetracyclines, fluoroquinolones) should not be taken directly with antacids, iron preparations, or bismuth products (Pepto-Bismol). The fluoroquinolones interact with theophylline, a prescription drug used for bronchial conditions, and may cause a toxic reaction. The commonly prescribed antibiotic trimethoprim-sulfamethoxazole (Bactrim, Septra) can block the breakdown of warfarin, an anticoagulant, causing serious bleeding episodes.

ANTIVIRAL DRUGS

To survive, a virus has to penetrate the cells of the body. Unlike bacteria, which can reproduce independently, viruses can reproduce only by using the enzymes and metabolism of your cells. As the result, a drug that can effectively damage a virus will also damage the host cells—your cells. This makes it difficult to develop antiviral drugs. Fortunately, the body's immune system can eliminate most viruses by itself. A good example is the common cold, which is caused by a virus. There is no drug cure, but the body can normally get rid of the virus within 10 days. However, some viruses produce serious, even life-threatening infections for which no drug is completely effective. One

ANTIVIRAL DRUGS

antiretroviral (AIDS) drugs
  didanosine (ddI, Videx)
  indinavir (Crixivan)
  lamivudine (3TC, Epivir)
  ritonavir (Norvir)
  stavudine (d4T, Zerit)
  zalcitabine (ddC, Hivid)
  zidovudine (AZT, Retrovir)
anti-influenza drugs
  amantadine (Symmetrel)
  rimantadine (Flumadine)

other antiviral drugs
  acyclovir (Zovirax)
  famciclovir (Famvir)
  flucytosine
  foscarnet (Foscavir)
  ganciclovir (Cytovene)
  idoxuridine
  ribavirin (Virazole)
  trifluridine
  valacyclovir (Valtrex)
  vidarabine

example of a drug that is available to curb viral infections is acyclovir, which can curb a genital herpes infection but cannot cure it. A few drugs can slow the progress of the human immunodeficiency virus (HIV), which causes AIDS, but there is currently no cure.

ANTIFUNGAL DRUGS

The fungus known as candida causes the common vaginal infections known as yeast infections. It also causes thrush, which can infect the mouths and digestive tracts of breast-feeding babies and the nipples of breast-feeding mothers. Another common fungal infection is athlete's foot. Ordinarily your immune system and the bacteria normally present in your mouth, intestines, and vaginal tract prevent fungal overgrowth. If either of these defenses is disturbed, you may develop a fungal infection; possible causes are antibiotics, chemotherapy, major surgery or transplantation, or an immunodeficiency disease (AIDS).

Antifungal drugs either kill or inhibit the growth of the fungus. Some bind to the cell wall of the fungus and punch a hole in it. Essential parts of the cell leak out and the fungus dies. Other drugs penetrate the fungus cells and kill them by interfering with key metabolic processes.

ANTIFUNGAL DRUGS

amphotericin B	ketoconazole (Nizoral)
clotrimazole	itraconazole (Sporanox)
fluconazole (Diflucan)	miconazole (Monistat)
flucytosine (Ancobon)	nystatin (Mycostatin)
griseofulvin (Gris-PEG, Fulvicin P/G)	tolnaftate (Tinactin)

Colds and flu

Colds and the flu are caused by viruses. More than 120 viral strains that may cause a cold have been identified.

The viral infection of a cold is usually limited to the nose but may extend to the throat, larynx, and lungs. The hallmark sign of a cold is a clear, watery fluid from the nose that may change to a thicker, yellow-tinged secretion over days. There is usually no fever. A dry cough may appear and change to a more productive, congested cough a few days later. Sneezing is common. Unlike the flu, most colds are not associated with headache, joint pain, muscle aches, extreme fatigue, or fever.

Cold medicines do not cure colds—your body's natural immunity does, over days or weeks. Cold medications only treat symptoms, so choose one that addresses the symptoms you have and avoid those intended for symptoms you *don't* have. If you have a single symptom such as a stuffy nose, use a product that contains a single drug—a nasal decongestant. Unnecessary use of combination products will only increase your chance of experiencing bothersome side effects.

Since colds are not caused by bacteria, they can't be treated with antibiotics. However, the cold may inflame and obstruct certain parts of the body, leading to a bacterial infection that can be treated with antibiotics. The most common bacterial complications of a cold are infections of the sinuses (sinusitis), ear (otitis media), lungs (pneumonia), and tonsils (tonsillitis). The major sign of a bacterial infection is fever. If you develop a fever after having a cold for five to seven days, see a doctor for possible treatment with antibiotics. Your doctor will also probably recommend an over-the-counter pain reliever to reduce aches and fever. A fever does not work in your favor, so it is best to reduce it with medication. Headache can be another sign of bacterial infection.

Influenza, or flu, is a viral infection of the air passages that causes fever, headache, muscle ache, and weakness. These symptoms are often followed by a cough, sore throat, and runny nose. After a day or two, fever and other symptoms tend to subside, and they usually disappear after five days. The respiratory symptoms may linger.

Although the infection usually clears up after 7 to 10 days, it sometimes takes a more severe turn, and thousands of people die from its complications each year. Because of this risk, annual flu shots are recommended for people over 65 and anyone with a chronic respiratory condition (including asthma), diabetes, heart disease, kidney disease, or AIDS. Each fall's vaccine contains the viral strains that are most likely to prevail during the coming season.

There are two drugs that can prevent flu if you have been exposed and may lessen the symptoms if you already have it. These drugs—amantadine and rimantadine— are started before you contract the flu or as soon as possible after exposure. They are not to be used during breast-feeding because both can interfere with milk production and secretion.

If you are generally in good health, a flu will generally cure itself. Take an over-the-counter pain reliever to reduce fever, aches, and pains. Rest in bed. Gradually return to normal activities once the fever subsides.

The most common active ingredients in nonprescription cold and flu medications are antihistamines, decongestants, and cough medicines. Many cold and flu medications add a pain reliever (such as acetaminophen or ibuprofen), but this extra ingredient is not necessary if you do not have pain (for example, a headache or body aches). A nonprescription drug labeled for allergy and sinus can have exactly the same ingredients as one labeled for cold and flu. Instead of looking at the front of the package, look at the ingredients.

ANTIHISTAMINES

Antihistamines are best used for the runny nose and sneezing caused by allergies, not the common cold or flu. However, they are often in-

ANTIHISTAMINES

brompheniramine	phenindamine
chlorpheniramine	pyrilamine
diphenhydramine	triprolidine

cluded in cold and flu medications, and they do help a small number of people who have a cold or flu. Antihistamines may make you drowsy or sleepy. If you notice this effect, do not drive a car or do other activities that may be dangerous.

DECONGESTANTS

Decongestants are the best choice if your nose is stuffy. They constrict the swollen blood vessels that are blocking the airways in your nose and sinuses. Sprays and drops work faster than oral decongestants, and they cause fewer side effects because less drug enters the body. Nasal sprays are easier to use than drops, and they work better because they spread the decongestant over a larger surface area in the nasal canal.

Oral decongestants may make you jittery. Avoid caffeine, which exaggerates this side effect. Do not use the more potent nasal decongestants (oxymetazoline and xylometazoline) longer than three days, to avoid sinus irritation that causes further congestion, a problem called "rebound congestion." Oral decongestants, particularly those

DECONGESTANTS

Sprays and drops	Oral decongestants
ephedrine	phenylephrine
naphazoline	phenylpropanolamine
oxymetazoline	pseudoephedrine
xylometazoline	

containing phenylpropanolamine, should be used cautiously by people with hyperthyroidism, hypertension, and arrhythmias.

COUGH MEDICINES

If you have a dry, hacking cough (rather than one caused by runny postnasal drip), a cough suppressant (antitussive) may help, particularly at night to help you sleep. An expectorant is sometimes added to a cough suppressant to thin the sinus secretions, making it easier to breathe.

If you have a productive, congested cough, the best treatment is to drink more fluids (not alcohol or caffeine) and use a humidifier. Drinking six to eight glasses of water per day is the best expectorant. It will thin the mucus and make breathing easier. If fluids alone are not effective, then a product containing guaifenesin may help.

COUGH MEDICINES

Cough suppressants	Expectorants
codeine or hydrocodone	guaifenesin
(prescription only)	iodinated glycerol
dextromethorphan	(prescription only)
diphenhydramine	

Sexually transmitted diseases

If you are sexually active, it is very important to protect yourself from sexually transmitted diseases (STDs). As a woman, you are particularly vulnerable because the warm, moist environment of the vagina encourages the growth of bacteria, fungi, and viruses. STDs are much more common than you might think, and they can have serious consequences, including pain, infertility, and even death.

For safer sex, use a latex condom correctly every time you have sexual contact with a partner, unless you are certain you are in a mutually exclusive monogamous relationship in which both of you have been tested and found free of disease. A male or female condom is the only form of contraception that can protect you from STDs.

STDs caused by bacterial infection (chlamydia, gonorrhea, syphilis) can usually be cured with antibiotics. Those caused by viruses (herpes) are not curable, but their symptoms can be treated.

AIDS

AIDS (acquired immunodeficiency syndrome) is caused by the human immunodeficiency virus (HIV). AIDS is now the fourth most common cause of death among young women in America. It can be contracted through sexual contact with an infected partner, through a contaminated needle shared when injecting drugs, and from mother to child during pregnancy or breast-feeding.

In the early stage, an HIV-infected person may have no symptoms or may develop flu-like symptoms such as fever, night sweats, muscle aches, tiredness, and swollen lymph nodes. Some people have no symptoms for many years, yet they can still transmit the virus to other people. You can contract the virus from someone who has no idea he has it.

In the later stages, a person with HIV develops a wide array of symptoms and infectious diseases. The impaired immune system cannot fight off organisms that are commonly found in the environment and can normally be warded off. These organisms, such as candida, herpes, and *Pneumocystis carinii*, cause severe infections that require rapid, high-dose drug treatment followed by long-term, lower-

ANTIRETROVIRAL DRUGS FOR HIV AND AIDS

didanosine (ddI, Videx)	stavudine (d4T, Zerit)
indinavir (Crixivan)	zalcitabine (ddC, Hivid)
lamivudine (3TC, Epivir)	zidovudine (AZT, Retrovir)
ritonavir (Norvir)	

dose prevention therapy with drugs. Antiretroviral drugs can slow the progress of the underlying virus (HIV), and other antiviral drugs are used to treat and suppress opportunistic viral infections such as cytomegalovirus and herpes viruses. Antibiotics are used to treat and control bacterial infections, and antifungal drugs are used to control candida and other fungal infections. However, there is no cure for this fatal disease.

CHLAMYDIA

Chlamydia is the most common sexually transmitted disease caused by bacteria. The infection can spread beyond the vagina and cervix to the uterus and fallopian tubes. It is the most common cause of pelvic inflammatory disease (PID, see page 247), which can lead to pain and infertility. The bacteria is passed back and forth between sexual partners. Men frequently have discharge and pain during urination. Three-quarters of women infected with chlamydia have no symptoms, and others have increased yellow-colored vaginal discharge, a burning sensation during urination, or pain or pressure in the pelvic area.

Chlamydia is treated with antibiotic drugs. Make sure your partner is treated for the same condition, or he is likely to pass the infection back to you. During treatment, you should not have sexual intercourse. Later, to lower your risk of future infection, use a latex condom. Certain contraceptive methods, including spermicides, the diaphragm, and the cervical cap, somewhat lower the risk of acquiring chlamydia infections.

The currently recommended drugs for this infection are azithromycin or doxycycline. Alternative drugs are ofloxacin or erythromycin. For pregnant women, the choices are erythromycin or amoxicillin.

DRUGS FOR CHLAMYDIA

azithromycin	erythromycin
doxycycline	ofloxacin

GENITAL WARTS

Genital warts are a sexually transmitted disease caused by the human papillomavirus. In women, they are tiny, painless, flat or raised, pink or white areas on the vulva, vagina, cervix, or anus or inside the throat. If not treated, they can grow quite large, but in early stages they can be too small to see. The bumps may first appear two or three months after contact with a sexual partner who has the infection. Because the warts are caused by a virus, they cannot be cured, but they can be treated. After treatment, they can recur.

Some kinds of genital warts increase the risk of cancer of the cervix, vulva, vagina, and anus in women and the penis and anus in men. If you have been diagnosed with genital warts, be sure to have a Pap smear every year to screen for cervical cancer.

In a quarter of cases, genital warts clear up on their own. When treatment is required, the warts can be removed by cryosurgery (freezing with liquid nitrogen), laser surgery, conventional surgery, or a topical drug, podophyllin. All treatments involve some soreness or pain. The method depends on the size and location of the warts. In many cases, cryotherapy is the most effective treatment.

If the wart is small and external, you may be able to have it treated with podophyllin. A doctor or nurse applies the drug to the wart with a cotton-tipped swab. Extreme care must be taken that the drug not touch the normal tissue around the wart, as this can cause burning or irritation. Usually the skin around the wart is first covered with a protectant, such as petroleum jelly. Within one to four hours after podophyllin treatment, the areas of application must be thoroughly washed off. An over-the-counter preparation of podophyllin is available for home use. Although it contains a lower concentration of podophyllin than the prescription drug, it should be used with similar precautions. A podophyllin product should never be used on large

DRUGS FOR GENITAL WARTS

podophyllin
podophyllotoxin 0.5% (Podofilox, Condylox)

skin surfaces because it can be absorbed through the skin and cause a toxic reaction.

GENITAL HERPES

Genital herpes is a viral infection that causes repeated outbreaks of painful sores and blisters on the vulva, in or around the vagina, in the anus, or on the cervix. Herpes is incurable and is easily transmitted to sexual partners. Genital herpes is caused by the herpes simplex virus 2. A related virus, herpes simplex virus 1, which causes cold sores and fever blisters around the mouth, can be transmitted to the genitals during oral sex.

The herpes virus can be transmitted to a partner during sexual contact even when there is no outbreak of sores. Once you transmit herpes, the virus becomes housed in nerve cells. The virus comes out of the nerves and sheds particles on the skin in the genital area. Although you or your partner may not have sores at the time, the viral particles may be shedding on the skin and the virus may be transmitted. Herpes comes out of the nerves on a sporadic basis, following an illness, during stress, or following a change in your normal diet. During a time of viral shedding, it can be transmitted during skin-to-skin, vaginal, anal, or oral contact. Genital herpes can also be transmitted to an infant during childbirth. If you are pregnant and have been diagnosed with herpes or suspect you may have it, make sure to tell your doctor so that precautions can be taken during childbirth. Herpes infection can increase the risk of miscarriage, premature labor, and delivery. A herpes-infected baby is at increased risk of blindness and brain damage.

Although herpes cannot be cured, antiviral drugs can be taken during an outbreak to relieve symptoms and help the blisters heal more quickly. The first episode of genital herpes is usually the most severe, can last for 12 days, and may be associated with fever, swollen glands, and headache. Use of an oral antiviral drug such as acyclovir can decrease the duration of viral shedding from 10 days to 2 days and reduce the duration of symptoms by from 10 days to 5 days. If your outbreaks are frequent or severe, taking suppressive drug therapy—medication every day for several months—may help.

DRUGS FOR GENITAL HERPES

acyclovir (oral)   valacyclovir
famciclovir

GONORRHEA

Even though gonorrhea may have no symptoms, it can cause pelvic inflammatory disease (see page 247) and can damage the joints, heart, or brain. It is the second most commonly acquired STD and is transmitted by sexual intercourse, oral sex, or anal sex. The infection may appear in the vagina, cervix, urinary tract, rectum, or throat.

Although some women have no symptoms, others have a green or yellow discharge from the vagina or rectum and a burning or itching during urination. Men have symptoms more often than women, including a dripping discharge from the penis and burning or itching during urination. If your sexual partner has these symptoms, tell your doctor. To determine if you have gonorrhea, your doctor will examine cells taken from your cervix.

Gonorrhea can be treated with antibiotics. Penicillin is no longer effective because of resistant bacteria. Both partners must be treated at the same time. Your doctor may recommend a follow-up test about two weeks after treatment to make sure the infection is completely gone. Half of women who have gonorrhea also have the bacterial infection chlamydia (see page 243).

ANTIBIOTICS FOR GONORRHEA

If chlamydia is also present
  ceftriaxone and doxycycline or
    tetracycline
  ceftriaxone and azithromycin
  cefixime and doxycycline or
    azithromycin

If chlamydia is not present
  ceftriaxone
  cefixime
  ciprofloxacin
  ofloxacin
  spectinomycin

PELVIC INFLAMMATORY DISEASE

Pelvic inflammatory disease (PID) is an infection in the upper female reproductive tract (often several bacterial infections), most commonly the uterus, fallopian tubes, or ovaries. About 85 percent of PID cases are caused by sexually transmitted diseases such as chlamydia or gonorrhea. Because women often have no symptoms from chlamydia, it is not discovered until it has spread and caused PID.

Symptoms may include mild or severe pelvic pain, back pain, a change in vaginal discharge, fever, or chills. If the cause is chlamydia, the symptoms will be mild. Untreated PID can scar and block the reproductive organs, causing infertility or ectopic pregnancy, a potentially life-threatening condition (page 119).

Because PID is usually caused by a number of organisms, a combination of antibiotics is the usual treatment. There may be a single injection of antibiotic followed by an oral antibiotic for 7 to 10 days. For more severe cases, one or more intravenous antibiotics may need to be administered in the hospital. If the condition does not respond to antibiotics, a laparoscopic tube may be inserted through the abdomen to locate an abscess (infected fluid-filled sac) in the pelvic area and drain it.

ANTIBIOTICS FOR PELVIC INFLAMMATORY DISEASE

ceftriaxone and doxycycline	cefotetan and probenecid
cefoxitin and probenecid and doxycycline	ofloxacin and clindamycin
	ofloxacin and metronidazole

SYPHILIS

Syphilis is a bacterial infection. Left untreated, it damages the heart, brain, eyes, nervous system, bones, and joints. It can be transmitted through sexual intercourse, oral or anal sex, or contact with the skin sores of an infected person. Syphilis can also be transmitted to a fetus during pregnancy. If the baby survives the infection, he or she may be born deaf or have permanently damaged bones or liver.

The early symptoms of syphilis (stage 1) appear 10 days to three months after exposure to the bacteria. The primary symptom is a round, smooth, raised, painless sore on the genitals, inside the vagina, or anywhere on the body where there has been sexual contact (tongue, rectum). Because the sore is painless, it often is not noticed. If left untreated, the sore goes away after a few weeks, but the bacteria remain in the body. In some cases, the disease goes dormant and no further symptoms ever appear. In other cases, the infection progresses to stage 2, in which syphilis in the blood causes the development of symptoms all over the body. Three to six months after the infection is acquired, a nonitchy rash may develop and spread over the body, including the palms and soles. Large, flat, light gray patches may appear on the genitals. Other symptoms may include fever, fatigue, sore throat, hair loss, and swollen glands. If left untreated, these symptoms may disappear entirely or come and go. In the final, potentially fatal stage 3, the disease damages the heart, brain, eyes, nervous system, and joints.

Syphilis is identified by taking a sample from a sore and looking for the bacteria under a microscope. At all stages, syphilis is treated with the antibiotic penicillin. If you are allergic to penicillin, you may take tetracycline, doxycycline, or ceftriaxone instead. You will have a follow-up examination and tests 3, 6, and 12 months after therapy to make sure the disease is fully cured. If you are diagnosed with syphilis, your sexual partner should be told so he can also be treated.

DRUGS FOR SYPHILIS

benzathine penicillin G	doxycycline
ceftriaxone	tetracycline

Urinary tract infections

A urinary tract infection occurs when bacteria find their way into the urinary tract, including the bladder, urethra (tube connecting the bladder to the outside of the body), ureters (tubes that bring urine from the kidneys to the bladder), and kidneys. Normally no bacteria live there (as they do in your digestive tract and vagina).

Almost all women get a urinary infection at some time in their lives. Women get these infections much more often than men because the urethra is much shorter (1 inch in a woman, 6 inches in a man), so the microorganisms have a shorter road to travel from the outside of the body to the bladder. Also, a woman's urethral opening is much closer to the anus, a source of bacteria. Sexual contact can push bacteria into the urinary tract. Pregnancy and childbirth increase the risk of urinary infections.

Urinary tract infections are easily treated with a variety of antibiotics. The first choice for women is usually trimethoprim-sulfamethoxazole (Bactrim, Septra), a fluoroquinolone such as Cipro, doxycycline, or a cephalosporin.

PREVENTING URINARY TRACT INFECTIONS

- After a bowel movement, wipe yourself from front to back.
- Empty your bladder before sexual intercourse and within 10 minutes afterward.
- If you use a diaphragm, make sure that it fits appropriately. If it is too big, the rim may put pressure on the bladder, which makes a urinary tract infection more likely.
- *Don't* douche routinely with substances other than diluted vinegar.
- During your period, change your tampon or pad frequently.

DRUGS FOR URINARY TRACT INFECTIONS

amoxicillin	norfloxacin
ampicillin	ofloxacin
cefadroxil	sulfamethoxazole
cephradine	sulfamethoxazole-trimethoprim
cephalexin	sulfisoxazole
ciprofloxacin	tetracycline
doxycycline	trimethoprim
nitrofurantoin	

CYSTITIS AND URETHRITIS

Cystitis is a bacterial infection of the bladder. Urethritis is a bacterial infection of the urethra, the tube that carries urine from the bladder out of the body. Bacteria from the vagina or the rectum can easily enter the urethra and spread into the bladder.

The symptoms of cystitis and urethritis are similar in women, including pain or burning sensation during urination, frequent urination of a small amount, and sometimes blood in the urine. To confirm the diagnosis, your doctor may examine a urine sample under the microscope for the presence of the bacteria. The most common cause of a urinary tract infection is the bacteria *E. coli*, found in most people's digestive tracts. Often antibiotics will be started immediately. Penicillins and tetracyclines have become less useful over the years because bacteria have developed some resistance to these drugs, but other antibiotics are effective. If you have recurring urinary tract infections, your doctor may prescribe an antibiotic that you take before intercourse to help prevent the infection.

KIDNEY INFECTION

Sometimes a urinary infection may go untreated, either because no symptoms appear or because the symptoms are attributed to something else such as a vaginal infection. If left untreated, a minor infection can move into the kidneys. This serious condition, called pyelonephritis, can cause permanent kidney damage or kidney failure.

The symptoms of a kidney infection include a burning sensation during urination and a frequent need to urinate. A fever, chills, vomiting, and lower-back pain are additional symptoms. The infection is treated with antibiotics for two or three weeks. Some severe cases require hospitalization and intravenous antibiotics.

Vaginitis

Vaginitis makes the tissues of the vagina irritated, red, and swollen. It is often caused by an overgrowth of bacteria or fungus. These organisms normally occur in a healthy vagina, but the acidic environment there keeps their growth in check. If the vagina's chemical balance is changed by birth-control pills, antibiotics, obesity, uncontrolled diabetes, douching, pregnancy, or recent childbirth, the organisms can multiply and cause an infection. Other cases of vaginitis are sexually transmitted.

BACTERIAL VAGINOSIS

Bacterial vaginosis involves the excess growth of a number of different bacteria normally present in a healthy vagina. The symptom is a thin, gray discharge with a fishy odor. The condition is often, but not always, sexually transmitted. The drug used for its treatment depends on the extent of your symptoms and whether or not you are pregnant. In women who are not pregnant, bacterial vaginosis is routinely treated with the oral antibacterial medication metronidazole (Flagyl) or a vaginal gel or cream containing metronidazole. Your sexual partner may also need to be treated so he won't reinfect you.

TRICHOMONIASIS

Trichomoniasis ("trick") is a sexually transmitted vaginitis caused by a protozoan, *T. vaginalis*. The infection may appear in a woman's vagina or in a man's urethra (the tube that carries urine from the bladder). During pregnancy, the infection can cause premature delivery or low birth weight. The best way to prevent trichomoniasis is by using a latex condom during sexual intercourse.

Some women have no symptoms from this infection, but others

notice a yellowish-green, malodorous, foamy discharge from the vagina and vaginal itching or irritation. Some women have discomfort during intercourse and pain when urinating. Many cases are discovered through a routine Pap smear. Men may have a clear discharge from the penis and discomfort during urination.

Trichomoniasis is treated with the antibacterial drug metronidazole. Your partner must be treated at the same time.

YEAST INFECTION

A vaginal yeast infection (also known as candidiasis or moniliasis) is an overgrowth of the fungus candida. Yeast infections, the most common vaginal infections, can be difficult to cure and can occur repeatedly. The symptoms are itching, burning, and redness in the vaginal area. There is often a white discharge that looks like cottage cheese.

Yeast infections can be treated with nonprescription antifungal medications, including clotrimazole and miconazole nitrate. A vaginal cream, suppository, or tablet is placed high in the vaginal canal every day for either three or seven days. Some products are also available with a cream to be used externally on the vulva to relieve itching. Similar antifungal medications are also available by prescription, including vaginal preparations and fluconazole (Diflucan), an orally administered tablet that can be taken as a single dose.

If you have been diagnosed previously with a yeast infection, been treated by a doctor, and recognize the same symptoms again,

DRUGS FOR YEAST INFECTIONS

nonprescription	prescription
clotrimazole (FemCare, Femstat-3, Gyne-Lotrimin, Mycelex-7)	butoconazole (Femstat)
	clotrimazole (Femcare, Gyne-Lotrimin, Mycelex-G)
miconazole (Monistat 3, Monistat 7, Monistat Dual Pak)	terconazole (Terazol 3, Terazol 7)
	tioconazole (Vagistat-1)

you can try a nonprescription medication. You should continue to use the vaginal product for the three- to seven-day treatment course, even if you start your period. If the preparation leaks from the vagina, use a sanitary napkin to prevent staining of your undergarments. If your symptoms do not respond in a day or two, see a doctor immediately, because you may have a more serious infection that must be treated with antibiotics or other medications. If you have never been treated for a yeast infection before, see a doctor for a diagnosis.

chapter 12

DRUGS FOR CANCER

ANCER IS THE UNCONTROLLED GROWTH OF AB-
normal cells in normal tissue. The abnormal cells form a tumor that
can destroy the tissues of vital body organs. In some cases, the cells
spread, or metastasize, from the site of the tumor to other parts of the
body, such as the liver or bones, and damage these organs. If you have
been diagnosed with cancer, read as much as you can about your disease and its possible treatments. Take a list of questions to your doctor, and write down the answers so you can refer to them later. Ask
your family, friends, and organized cancer groups for their help; there
is evidence that emotional support can play an important role in re-
covering from cancer.

Treating cancer with drugs

In many cases, the first treatment for cancer is surgery to remove the
tumor. Next, radiation treatments may be used to kill any remaining
cancer cells in a local area surrounding the tumor site. Many cancers
are cured with a combination of surgery and radiation, but sometimes
these treatments do not do the job. Drug therapy, called chemotherapy, may then be used to kill cancer cells throughout the body. Hormone therapy, another form of drug therapy, can help fight cancers
that are fueled by hormones.

Many new anticancer drugs are currently undergoing the large
clinical trials that are required before FDA approval. Some have

shown success in treating cancer. If you are interested in finding out about experimental drugs, ask your doctor about clinical trials in your area.

CHEMOTHERAPY

Chemotherapy is drug therapy for cancer. Its goal is to prevent the return of the cancer and its spread to locations other than the original tumor site. Unlike surgery and radiation, chemotherapy reaches and destroys cancer cells in nearly every part of the body.

Chemotherapy may be given by mouth or by injection into veins or muscles. Dozens of drugs are used to treat cancer. They are often prescribed in combination. By interfering with the cancer cells at different stages in their growth, the combination drug regimens are usually more effective than any single drug. Common single and combination drugs are listed under individual cancers later in this chapter.

Side effects

Chemotherapy drugs attack and kill rapidly dividing cells throughout the body, both normal and cancerous. Because chemotherapy is toxic to some of the body's healthy cells as well as the cancer cells, it often causes side effects. It is most likely to harm normal cells that rapidly divide and reproduce, such as the blood-producing cells in the bone, cells lining the digestive tract, and hair follicles. Some women have few effects, while others are severely affected.

Dealing with the side effects of chemotherapy is more difficult if you don't fully understand why your doctor has prescribed the drug and what it can do for you. If you have concerns or fears about the therapy, talk about them. Many side effects can be lessened, either by steps you can take or by other drugs. Make sure to ask your doctor the following questions if you are considering chemotherapy:

- Why is the doctor suggesting it?
- What are the success rates?
- What are the goals of the chemotherapy treatment in your specific case? To further reduce the size of a tumor? To prevent spread of cancer or recurrence of cancer in the same area?
- How long will the treatment take?
- What specific drugs and regimen will be prescribed and why?

- What side effects should you expect?
- Is there anything that can be done to prevent the side effects?
- When are the side effects most likely to occur? Immediately after the treatment or days to weeks later?

Different chemotherapy drugs have different side effects. For example, some drugs nearly always cause hair loss, while others don't affect the hair at all. Among the most common side effects of chemotherapy are:

- **Hair loss.** Chemotherapy drugs may cause thinning or loss of hair not only on your head but also on your eyebrows, eyelashes, arms, legs, and pubic area. Hair loss usually begins 7 to 10 days after a single treatment of chemotherapy. Hair always grows back about three months after the end of treatment, and most insurance plans now cover the cost of a good wig. It is best to buy a wig beforehand. Your hairdresser can style it for you. You can also purchase a variety of scarves and turbans. Not all drugs cause hair loss. Doxorubicin, one of the most powerful drugs used to treat breast cancer and several other forms of cancer, nearly always causes hair loss, but another potent breast cancer drug, cisplatin, does not. Other drugs that cause hair loss are cyclophosphamide, ifosfamide, 5-FU, dactinomycin, daunorubicin, bleomycin, paclitaxel, and vindesine.

- **Infections.** Many chemotherapeutic drugs kill the cells of the bone marrow that produce blood cells. When white blood cells are not formed in the bone marrow, the body loses a major defense against infections. The massive fall in the number of white blood cells usually occurs within 7 to 10 days after starting chemotherapy, and the count does not recover for another 14 days. During this time, you can reduce your risk of infections by washing your hands frequently and avoiding crowds and sick people. Try to avoid cutting yourself, and if you do, bandage the cut right away. Watch for any signs or symptoms of infection, particularly fever. If you have a fever, call your doctor immediately so you can start antibiotics. A major breakthrough in the prevention of infection is the development of colony-stimulating factors that can be injected at home to increase the recovery of the white blood cells.

- **Anemia.** Chemotherapy may reduce your red blood cell count, making you feel tired, dizzy, cold, or short of breath. If your anemia becomes severe, your doctor may recommend a blood transfusion or an injection of erythropoietin to increase your production of red blood cells.

- **Abnormal bleeding.** Platelets, the blood cells that initiate normal clotting of blood, are formed in the bone marrow. Chemotherapy may reduce your platelet count, causing you to bleed more easily. To prevent unnecessary bleeding, use an electric shaver and a soft toothbrush. Unless specifically recommended by your doctor, avoid taking aspirin and other painkillers that further reduce blood clotting. Acetaminophen (Tylenol) does not affect blood clotting and is safe to take at this time. Report any unusual bleeding or bruising to your doctor. If bleeding is severe, a transfusion of platelets may be needed.

- **Nausea and vomiting.** Most chemotherapy drugs cause some nausea, depending on the drug, the dose, and your individual reaction. However, there are better medicines than there used to be to reduce this side effect. To prevent nausea and vomiting, you will take antiemetic drugs before you begin the treatment and continue them for 24 to 48 hours. Nausea often starts 1 to 2 hours after a chemotherapy injection, but usually does not last more than 24 hours. To help prevent nausea, do not eat any solid foods, only liquids, for several hours before chemotherapy. After chemotherapy, eat light, bland foods for several days. When you feel nauseated, take an antiemetic, eat some dry crackers, and stay in bed for an hour or so to prevent vomiting. Avoid odors that make you nauseated. If the antiemetic drug regimen is not effective, ask your doctor for a different drug or combination of drugs that may work better for you. Some of these drugs may cause their own side effects, such as headaches, constipation, and restlessness.

DRUGS TO PREVENT NAUSEA AND VOMITING

dexamethasone (Decadron)	ondansetron (Zofran)
granisetron (Kytril)	metoclopramide (Reglan)
lorazepam (Ativan)	prochlorperazine (Compazine)

- **Diarrhea.** Chemotherapy drugs often cause temporary mild diarrhea. If you experience severe diarrhea or intestinal cramps for more than 24 hours, call your doctor who may prescribe an antidiarrheal drug and who will want to make sure the symptoms are not caused by a gallbladder or kidney problem. Avoid foods that typically cause loose bowels, gas, or cramps, including greasy fried foods, beans, cabbage, bran cereal, and spicy foods. Dairy products also cause cramps and diarrhea in some people.
- **Sore mouth.** Because the cells of the mouth reproduce rapidly, they are a target for many chemotherapeutic drugs. Some chemotherapy drugs cause a sore mouth and throat for about five days after treatment. If you experience irritation or pain in your mouth or throat, avoid acidic foods such as tomatoes and tomato sauce, citrus fruits, and spicy or rough food. Because the mouth contains many organisms and the tissues are inflamed and damaged, there is a risk of infection. If your mouth becomes so sore you cannot eat, call your doctor, who can prescribe a painkiller and a mouthwash that will alleviate the problem. If you tend to get cold sores, an antiviral medication may help. If your tongue develops a white covering, you may have a yeast infection (mouth thrush), which can cause soreness and difficulty eating. An antifungal drug such as nystatin may be prescribed to be used as a mouthwash or taken orally to treat the infection.
- **Irregular menstruation and infertility.** Your menstrual period may become irregular or stop during therapy, but should return to normal after therapy is complete. Chemotherapy drugs can damage the ovaries and cause infertility. The infertility may be temporary or permanent depending on the drug or the dosage. Although pregnancy may be possible for some women during chemotherapy treatment, it is not recommended because the drugs can cause birth defects. For this reason, it is important to use birth control throughout your treatment. If a woman is pregnant when cancer is discovered, it may be possible to delay treatment until the baby is born. For women who need treatment sooner, it may be possible to delay treatment until week 12 of the pregnancy, when risk to the fetus will be less.
- **Sexuality.** Chemotherapy drugs do not directly affect your libido or sexual desire, but the fatigue and stress of cancer therapy may do so. The drugs may also cause the tissues lining the vagina to

become dry and sore. If you want to have sex, a water-based lubricant found in the drugstore will make intercourse more comfortable. If your desire for sex is reduced, discuss this openly with your partner. It is a normal and often temporary situation. Your partner's fears about cancer may also affect your physical relationship. Reassure your partner that sexual activity will not harm you, nor will the chemotherapy drugs harm your partner.

- **Other side effects.** Chemotherapy drugs can cause a variety of skin problems, such as dryness, spots, rashes, and sensitivity to the sun. Protect your skin with a sunscreen (see page 58), clothing, and a hat. If your eyes become dry, try eye drops or artificial tears. If you see any changes in urine, such as color, frequency, or pain, contact your doctor. You may encounter other side effects, including muscle aches and pains, fatigue, flu-like feelings, tingling in your fingers and toes, loss of muscle strength, and disrupted balance. Most of these side effects are temporary. Ask your doctor for help if they cause you excessive discomfort.

Other considerations during chemotherapy

Ask your doctor what you can eat during treatment. Usually there are no diet restrictions. If you are taking other medications for other conditions, ask your doctor whether you should continue them. Some physicians recommend total abstinence from alcohol, but others believe that an occasional glass of wine or beer is not harmful. Check with your doctor.

You will need extra rest during this time. Some women are able to continue their normal routines, but others must take time off from work and other activities. Expect that you will have some low-energy days when you will not be able to keep up with your usual responsibilities.

HORMONE THERAPY

Some forms of cancer, particularly breast and uterine, are stimulated by certain hormones. By removing or limiting the amount of the hormone in the body, doctors can slow the growth of cancer cells. Hormone therapy can be used to prevent recurrence of cancer that has been treated with surgery and radiation or to slow the growth of cancer that has recurred.

Surgery or radiation treatment is sometimes used to stop the body from producing hormones. In a woman with breast cancer, the ovaries may be surgically removed or radiated to stop the production of estrogen.

Antiestrogen drugs

Forms of breast cancer that are fueled by the female hormone estrogen are often treated with drugs that decrease the production of estrogen or alter the cancer cells' ability to be stimulated by estrogen. Not all forms of breast cancer respond to hormone therapy. To find out whether the therapy may help, a test is done to count the number of estrogen receptors, the sites on the cancer cells that respond to estrogen.

The most widely used antiestrogen drug is tamoxifen. A number of new antiestrogen medications have been developed, including toremifene. Like tamoxifen, these drugs inhibit the effects of estrogen on the multiplying cancer cells. (For more about tamoxifen and other antiestrogens, see page 265.)

Progestins

Progestins, which are synthetic versions of the female hormone progesterone, can help treat breast cancer that has spread to other parts of the body, as well as endometrial cancer. The options are megestrol and high doses of medroxyprogesterone acetate.

Aminoglutethimide

Aminoglutethimide is used to treat cancer that has spread to the bone or lymph nodes. Aminoglutethimide decreases the production of body hormones, including estrogen. It is used primarily by postmenopausal women with advanced breast cancer.

Anastrozole

A recently approved medication, anastrozole, decreases estrogen production without affecting the adrenal glands, making toxic reactions minimal. It is considered an exciting new development in the treatment of advanced breast cancer in women past menopause.

Androgens

Androgens are male hormones that may be used to treat cancer that has spread to other parts of the body. In particular, testolactone has been used to treat advanced breast cancer in postmenopausal women. This androgen works by decreasing the production of estrone, the primary estrogen in postmenopausal women. The side effects include growth of facial and body hair, lowering of the voice, and an increase in the size of the clitoris. The extent of these side effects depends on the dose and the duration of treatment.

Inhibitors of pituitary hormone

The most effective of these drugs interfere with FSH (follicular stimulating hormone) and LH (luteinizing hormone), the hormones made by the pituitary gland that control the ovaries. They decrease estrogen secretion and are used to treat not only breast cancer but also ovarian and endometrial cancer.

Breast cancer

Breast cancer is the formation of cancer cells in tissues of the breast, which extend into the armpit and collar area. The number of cases of breast cancer has risen dramatically during the past 20 years. Some of the increase is due to better detection with self-examinations and mammograms, but not all has been explained. The good news is that earlier detection and better treatment have reduced cancer deaths. The vast majority of women who are diagnosed with early-stage breast cancer (stage 1) are free of cancer five years later and never experience a recurrence.

Too little is known about the causes of breast cancer to provide women with a clear set of prevention guidelines. It is known that risk is greater for women who:

- Have a mother, sister, or daughter who had or has breast cancer
- Had an early puberty (before age 12)

- Had a late menopause (after age 50)
- Have a history of benign breast disease
- Had a first pregnancy after age 30
- Have passed menopause

Factors that may raise the risk of breast cancer include:

- High-fat diet
- Obesity
- Drinking more than three alcoholic beverages per week
- Estrogen replacement therapy

SYMPTOMS AND DIAGNOSIS

Because so little is known about prevention of breast cancer, early detection remains the best defense. Early diagnosis is crucial for successful treatment. The most common symptoms of breast cancer are:

- Lump in the breast; can occur anywhere, but is most common at the top of the breast on the side nearest the armpit
- Discharge from a nipple (clear, bloodied, or colored)
- Breast discomfort (described as a pulling sensation); change in the size or shape of the breast
- Nipple retraction
- Painful or red skin

Breast self-examination

You should examine your breasts every month. More cases of breast cancer are discovered by the woman herself than by any other method. Here are the steps:

1. Examine your breasts at the same time each month after you have had your period; if you do not have periods, do the examination on the same day each month.
2. Look in the mirror. Examine your breasts with your arms down at your sides and then with your hands clasped over your head. Look for any lumps, dimpling, puckering or retraction of nipple, discharge from nipple, bleeding, swelling, or changes in the skin of the nipple or difference in size between your two breasts.

3. Squeeze both nipples between your fingers and watch for any discharge.

4. Put both hands on your hips and push your elbows forward to heighten chest muscles while looking for any puckering or changes in skin texture or color.

5. In the shower, when your breasts are wet and soapy, raise your right arm above your head and begin feeling your right breast with the soft pads of the fingers of your left hand. Move outward in ever-larger circles from the nipple, covering the entire breast area up to your armpit and collarbone. Repeat three times using light, medium, and deep pressure to examine the entire depth of the breast. Repeat with the other breast.

6. Lie down to flatten your breasts. With your right arm raised and tucked behind your head, press firmly against your breast with your left hand, making a series of three circles around your breast, starting with a small one around the nipple and growing larger with each circle. Using light, medium, and deep pressure, cover the entire breast area, including the armpit and chest up to your collarbone. Repeat on the opposite breast.

In addition to monthly self-examinations, you should have an examination by your doctor regularly (see box for schedule).

Mammogram

A mammogram is a low-level X-ray that reveals changes in breast tissues. It can detect a lump that is too small for you to feel yourself, and it can be used to verify the location of a known lump. Get a baseline mammogram when you are between the ages of 35 and 40. Breast cancer is less common before 40, and a mammogram is less effective because the breast tissues are denser and less revealing.

Before having a mammogram, do not use talcum powder, lotion, or deodorant. You will be asked to remove your clothes from the waist up. A technician will help you place your breast on a platform on the mammogram machine, then will slowly lower a compression plate to spread out your breast tissue as much as possible. The technician will take the X-ray. There may be more than one view of each breast. Later a radiologist will examine the X-ray for signs of breast cancer, which can take the form of a dense white mass with radiating arms or

BREAST CANCER SCREENING

The American Cancer Society recommends the following schedule of breast cancer screening.

Age 20 to 39	Breast self-exam monthly
	Breast exam by physician every 3 years
	Base line mammogram at age 35 to 40
Age 40 to 49	Breast self-exam monthly
	Breast exam by physician every year
	Mammogram every 1 to 2 years
Age 50 and up	Breast self-exam monthly
	Breast exam by physician every year
	Mammogram every year

a cluster of tiny white spots. Scattered, isolated white dots, known as calcifications, are not cancerous.

If you, your doctor, or the radiologist detects a suspicious lump or mass of cells in your breast, the next step may be a biopsy, a procedure that involves taking a tissue sample. The cells obtained from the tissue sample are then examined under a microscope to determine whether you have cancer. The simplest method, which takes only minutes to perform, is a needle biopsy. A needle is inserted into the lump, and fluid containing tissue cells is removed. Other methods of biopsy are used if the lump is difficult to feel, if the tumor is large, or if the entire lump needs to be removed.

TREATMENT

If a biopsy shows you have breast cancer, further tests will be performed to help you and your doctor choose the best treatment. Blood and urine tests and a bone scan can help determine whether or not the cancer cells have spread beyond the identified tumor. A hormone-receptor test shows whether estrogen is "feeding" the cancer. The type of treatment will depend on the size of the tumor, your age, menopausal status, and the stage of the disease.

If your cancer is in the early stage (stage 1) and has not spread, your treatment is likely to be surgery and possibly radiation. If there is any indication that the lymph nodes in the area of the tumor or elsewhere in the body contain cancer cells (stage 2 or 3), you will be advised to have drug therapy with either hormones or chemotherapy following surgery and radiation. Late-stage disease (stage 4) is usually incurable because the cancer has spread beyond the breast tissue to vital organs, such as the bone, liver, brain, or lungs.

Surgery

Instead of removing the entire breast (mastectomy), surgeons today are more likely to recommend removing only the tumor (lumpectomy) or the tumor and a portion of the surrounding tissue (partial or segmental mastectomy). These more conservative approaches have been found to be as effective as mastectomy, particularly in women with stage 1 or 2 disease.

Radiation treatment

Surgery is almost always followed by radiation treatment to help prevent local spreading or recurrence of the disease. Radiation works best on a small area, such as around the tumor site to kill any cells not removed by surgery, and it cannot treat cancer that has moved to other sites in the body. A high-powered X-ray machine directs a beam of radiation at the affected area once a day, five days a week, for five weeks. Each treatment lasts only a few minutes. Another method uses radioactive implants. In addition to preventing tumor recurrence, radiation can also be used to shrink a large tumor before surgery or to slow the growth of an inoperable tumor.

Hormone therapy

Estrogen fuels the growth of some breast cancers. Hormone therapy can reduce the effects of estrogen on the cancer cell. It is used primarily when the cancer has spread beyond the breast and an estrogen-receptor test has shown that the cancer cells are the type that are stimulated by estrogen.

Tamoxifen, which blocks the binding of estrogen to receptors in the breast, is often recommended in premenopausal women with stage 1 or 2 cancer as an alternative to surgically removing the ovaries. Tamoxifen is usually taken for two or more years. The effects of hormone therapy are often not apparent for 12 weeks. A new approach called "total estrogen blockade" combines tamoxifen with another hormone therapy called LH-RH analogs, which prevents the ovaries from releasing estrogen.

Most women have no side effects from tamoxifen. Some experience hot flashes, which are usually temporary and are more pronounced in premenopausal women. Tamoxifen may cause hair loss and can increase HDL (the good cholesterol) and bone density. A slight weight gain of a few pounds is common. Other, rare side effects include nausea, vomiting, loss of appetite, rash, headache, depression, fatigue, hair loss, and high calcium levels in the blood. Though tamoxifen does not usually cause side effects, it may increase a woman's risk of endometrial cancer.

If the cancer returns after tamoxifen therapy, and the woman is past menopause, another option is the synthetic hormone progestin. Progestin and tamoxifen are equally effective, but tamoxifen is usually chosen because it has fewer side effects and has been used longer for this purpose. Progestins like megestrol (Megace) may increase appetite and thus weight, which is dangerous because added body fat can fuel tumor growth.

Tamoxifen is also being tested as a preventive medication for women at high risk of developing breast cancer.

Chemotherapy

Chemotherapy is used three ways to treat breast cancer: as an additional therapy to surgery and radiation to prevent recurrence, as the main treatment for advanced cancers, and to relieve symptoms from cancer that has spread. Chemotherapy is not given routinely to everyone because it causes a variety of side effects. It is not used for early-stage cancer that has not spread to the lymph nodes.

After surgery and radiation, when examination of the lymph nodes and other tests indicate that there is a risk of cancer appearing in other parts of the body, chemotherapy may be advised to eliminate cancer cells that cannot be detected but are thought to be still in the body. This approach is usually recommended for women who are under 65, have a tumor more than 2 centimeters in diameter, and have cancer cells in the blood vessels of the breast or lymph nodes.

Chemotherapy may also be used as the first line of treatment when there is a tumor larger than 5 centimeters, a tumor too firmly attached to the chest wall or rib cage to be easily removed, or a cancer that has spread to the lymph nodes. In this case, chemotherapy is usually combined with radiation treatments. Once the tumor has shrunk, surgery may follow.

If the cancer has already spread to other parts of the body, chemotherapy may slow its growth, alleviate symptoms caused by the cancer, and improve quality of life.

Chemotherapy is usually prescribed for three to six months. A common regimen is intravenous administration followed by a 21-day rest period before the next dose. Another pattern is a combination of oral and intravenous drugs followed by a two-week rest.

DRUGS FOR BREAST CANCER

cyclophosphamide/doxorubicin/
   fluorouracil
cyclophosphamide/
   methotrexate/fluorouracil
cyclophosphamide/
   mitoxantrone/fluorouracil

methotrexate/fluorouracil/
   leucovorin
mitomycin-C/vinblastine
paclitaxel (Taxol)
vinblastine/doxorubicin/
   thiotepa/fluoxymesterone

Cancer of the cervix

In recent decades, more women have been diagnosed with cervical cancer, but deaths have declined dramatically. The reason is that routine Pap smears are detecting this cancer early enough to be completely cured in most cases.

The cervix is the doughnut-shaped opening between the vagina and the uterus. Cancer of the cervix develops very slowly. Before it appears, some of the cells change; the abnormal cells are called cervical dysplasia. Later these cells spread throughout the cervix and into surrounding areas.

Women are more likely to get cancer of the cervix if they:

- Had sexual intercourse before age 20
- Have had more than one sexual partner
- Have had genital warts
- Have had a sexually transmitted disease
- Smoked for a long time

To reduce your risk, practice safer sex by using a condom every time you have sex or by having a mutually monogamous sexual relationship with someone who is free of disease. The female condom is even better than the male condom because it covers the woman's external genitals, protecting them from genital warts from papillomavirus, which increase the risk of cervical cancer.

Symptoms and diagnosis

Cervical cancer and its precursor, cervical dysplasia, can be easily detected with a Pap smear. Since cervical cancer usually has no symptoms in its early stages, it's important for all women to have a Pap smear every year, starting when they are 18 or first become sexually active. A Pap smear is performed by your doctor or health-care practitioner during a pelvic exam. A small brush or scraper takes a sample of cells to be examined under a microscope. If your Pap smear shows abnormal cells, your doctor may take a tissue sample (biopsy) to check for the presence of cancer cells. If cancer is present, your doctor will perform a complete exam and take blood and urine samples to determine how far it has spread.

The symptoms of later stages can include painful intercourse, vaginal bleeding after intercourse or between periods, and abnormal vaginal discharge usually observed after intercourse.

Treatment

The type of treatment depends on the size and stage of the tumor and your age and medical condition. If the cancer has not spread beyond the cervix, the usual treatment is a hysterectomy to remove the cervix

DRUGS FOR CANCER OF THE CERVIX

bleomycin	doxorubicin
carboplatin	ifosfamide
cisplatin	

and uterus. If a woman with early-stage cancer wants to retain her fertility, she may choose a cone biopsy, in which a cone of tissue is surgically removed from the cervix.

Radiation therapy is used when the cancer has moved beyond the cervix and the upper part of the vagina to the uterus, vulva, lower third of the vagina, rectum, or bladder. Depending on the extent of cancer spread, external radiation, internal radiation, or a combination of both may be used. For external radiation, beams are directed to the pelvic area to kill any remaining cancer cells. For internal radiation, the doctor places radioactive implants inside the uterus and vagina to kill any cancer cells in this area. One of the side effects of internal radiation is diarrhea, which can be treated with diphenoxylate with atropine (Lomotil) or loperamide hydrochloride (Imodium).

Surgery or radiation therapy often causes the body to produce less estrogen. Hormone replacement therapy is usually prescribed to reduce any symptoms this causes.

Although cervical cancer rarely recurs after radiation therapy, when it does, treatment may not be successful. A possible treatment for recurrent cervical cancer is total pelvic exenteration, the removal of the reproductive organs, bladder, rectum, and vagina.

Chemotherapy may also be used to treat recurrent cancer or cancer that has spread beyond the uterus. The drugs used to treat cervical cancer may cause a variety of side effects, including nausea, vomiting, weight loss, diarrhea, hair loss, suppression of bone marrow production, and various dysfunctions of the kidneys, nervous system, and ears. (For more on chemotherapy and coping with its side effects, see page 255.)

Lung cancer

Since 1987 lung cancer has surpassed breast cancer as the leading cause of cancer death among women. The reason is that over the past several decades, the number of women smoking has increased greatly. Although the number of women smokers has been declining recently, the cancer cases of today are the result of several decades of increased smoking. The American Cancer Society estimates that cigarette smoking is responsible for about 85 percent of all lung cancer cases. A woman's risk of lung cancer increases with age. The most likely age to be diagnosed with lung cancer is between 55 and 70.

The single most important step you can take to prevent lung cancer is to quit smoking. Even reducing smoking will help. The more you smoke, the more likely you are to get cancer and to get it sooner. Even if you don't smoke, you may be at risk of developing lung cancer if you are often exposed to secondhand smoke. Risk is also increased by exposure to radioactive materials, asbestos, and high levels of air pollution.

SYMPTOMS AND DIAGNOSIS

The signs and symptoms of lung cancer depend on the location of the tumor in the lung and the extent to which the cancer cells have spread to other parts of the body. A cough is often the first symptom. See your doctor for a chest X-ray if you develop a cough that won't go away. Lung cancer can spread to other parts of the body, especially the brain, bones, and liver, and pain may occur in those areas. In later stages, possible symptoms are:

- Coughing up blood
- Shortness of breath
- Wheezing, hoarseness, difficulty swallowing
- Chest pain
- Back pain
- Weight loss
- Swollen neck or face
- Weak shoulder, arm, or hand

DRUGS FOR LUNG CANCER

cisplatin	mitomycin
cyclophosphamide	paclitaxel
doxorubicin	vinblastine
etoposide	vindesine
ifosfamide	vinorelbine

If there is a characteristic shadow on your X-ray, the diagnosis can be confirmed with a biopsy. A tissue sample can be taken with a bronchoscope, a long, thin tube inserted through the mouth or nose and into the lung, or with a needle inserted through the chest wall. Lymph nodes may also be removed surgically and biopsied to determine whether the cancer has spread to them.

Treatment

Treatment depends on the type of lung cancer, the size and location of the tumor, and whether the cancer has spread to the lymph nodes or other parts of the body.

The type of lung cancer called "small cell" is a rapid-growing, quickly spreading disease that responds to radiation and chemotherapy. Chemotherapy is usually given for one to five days and repeated about once a month depending on the drug regimen. After two courses, your doctor will evaluate the response. (For information about coping with the side effects of chemotherapy, see page 255.)

Nonsmall cell lung cancer, a slower-growing cancer, is usually treated with surgery if the cancer is limited to one lung or the nearby lymph nodes. If you cannot undergo surgery because of other health problems such as heart disease, radiation is an alternative. Radiation may also be used if the tumor's position makes removal difficult or impossible—for example, if it is attached to a major blood vessel or the esophagus or trachea (windpipe). Chemotherapy has not been widely successful, but it has helped some people, particularly if the tumor is inoperable or the disease is advanced. You and your doctor can discuss whether you are likely to respond to drug treatment.

Cancer of the ovary

The ovaries are two small organs that release an egg each month into the fallopian tubes. The ovaries are susceptible to cancer because the ovarian cells are continually dividing. Constantly reproducing cells are more likely to produce cells with mutations that can lead to cancer.

Cancer of the ovary is the second most common reproductive cancer among women (after endometrial cancer) and is one of the most deadly cancers because it is often not detected until it is far advanced.

Family health history is the most important risk factor. Some women with a strong family history of the disease may choose to have their ovaries removed after they have finished childbearing and are approaching menopause. Women in their fifties and sixties are at the highest risk of developing ovarian cancer, while premenopausal women are more likely to develop noncancerous cysts rather than cancer. Your risk is also greater if you:

- Never took oral contraceptives
- Never had children
- Had children later than age 30
- Reached menopause after age 55
- Have a family history of other cancers

SYMPTOMS AND DIAGNOSIS

Symptoms are often missing or vague. Possibilities include:

- Swollen, bloated, or painful abdomen
- Feeling full after a light meal
- Lack of appetite
- Nausea or vomiting
- Gas or indigestion
- Unexplained weight loss or gain
- Constant need to urinate
- Diarrhea or constipation
- Abnormal vaginal bleeding

Unfortunately, there is no completely accurate screening test for cancer of the ovary. During a routine annual pelvic examination, your

DRUGS FOR OVARIAN CANCER

carboplatin	cisplatin and paclitaxel (Taxol)
cisplatin	doxorubicin, cisplatin,
carboplatin and	cyclophosphamide, and
cyclophosphamide	hexamethylmelamine
cisplatin and cyclophosphamide	

doctor checks for abnormalities. Putting one hand inside your vagina and one hand on your abdomen, the doctor feels the size and shape of the ovaries. If an abnormality is found, you may have a blood test called CA 125. This test looks for a protein that a cancerous ovary sheds into the blood. Although useful in making the diagnosis, the CA 125 sometimes fails to detect an existing cancer, particularly in the early stage. A transvaginal ultrasound exam of the ovaries may reveal abnormalities. Ultimately, exploratory abdominal surgery may be necessary to conclusively diagnose the cancer and to discover whether it has spread beyond the ovaries. Because ovarian cancer is hard to detect early, it is often discovered at an advanced stage.

TREATMENT

Surgery is the most common treatment. Because the goal is to remove as much of the cancer as possible, other tissues near the ovaries in the pelvic cavity may be removed as well. Your doctor may remove your ovaries as well as your fallopian tubes, uterus, and tissues connecting the intestines to nearby organs in the abdomen (the omentum). To kill any cancer that may have been too small to remove surgically, you may have radiation therapy (see page 269).

If the cancer has spread beyond the ovaries to the fallopian tubes, intestines, or lymph nodes, further treatment with radiation (internal or external) or chemotherapy is necessary. The choice is made based on the stage of your disease and the findings of your surgery. If the disease is advanced, chemotherapy is used to kill all remaining cancer cells in the body. Chemotherapy may be taken in pill form, intravenously, or by needle directly through the abdominal wall into the cavity containing the pelvic organs (the peritoneum).

The most common drug is cisplatin, used alone or combined with other drugs. Its side effects include nausea and vomiting, numb hands and feet, suppressed immunity, anemia, and hearing loss. (For more on coping with the effects of chemotherapy, see page 255.)

Recently paclitaxel (Taxol), a drug also used to treat breast cancer, has been incorporated into chemotherapy for ovarian cancer. It can effectively treat cancer that has spread to other organs. Paclitaxel may cause an allergic reaction or a variety of side effects, including abnormal heart rhythms, numb and tingling hands and feet, inflamed mucous membranes, and nausea and vomiting.

Regardless of the treatment plan chosen, a repeat biopsy will be done to determine your response to therapy.

Endometrial cancer

Endometrial cancer is located in the lining of the uterus. It is usually curable, particularly when diagnosed early. It is a different disorder than sarcoma, a less common cancer of the muscle wall of the uterus, and is treated differently. Fibroids (see page 111) are a different kind of tumor in the uterus, but they are not cancerous.

Like breast cancer, endometrial cancer is more likely to occur if a woman has been exposed to high levels of estrogen over her lifetime. Endometrial cancer most often occurs around or following menopause. The following factors increase your risk:

- Obesity
- Irregular menstruation or ovulation
- History of infertility
- Early menstruation
- Late menopause

DRUGS FOR UTERINE CANCER

carboplatin	cyclophosphamide
cisplatin	doxorubicin

- History of polycystic ovarian disease
- History of endometrial hyperplasia
- History of cancer of the breast, ovary, or colon
- Estrogen replacement therapy without progestin
- Use of the drug tamoxifen to treat or prevent breast cancer

SYMPTOMS AND DIAGNOSIS

Because endometrial cancer can spread, it is important to identify and treat it as early as possible. The warning signs include:

- Abnormal vaginal bleeding or discharge (from a blood-tinged discharge to bleeding)
- Difficult or painful urination
- Pain during intercourse
- Pain in the abdominal or pelvic area

If your doctor suspects endometrial cancer, the first test will be a pelvic examination to feel for any lumps or changes in the shape of your uterus. The next step is a biopsy to take a sample of the lining of the uterus. A small amount of tissue can be removed during a pelvic examination. Another way to take a tissue sample and also look for signs of cancer, is to insert a small tube with a camera into the uterus through the vagina (hysteroscopy).

TREATMENT

If you have cancer but it has not spread beyond the uterus, you will have a hysterectomy to remove the uterus, fallopian tubes, and ovaries. Surgery is usually followed by radiation treatment. Radiation may also be used if the cancer has spread beyond the organs removed or if you are suspected to have a high risk of recurrence.

If the cancer has spread or recurred after radiation, hormone therapy or chemotherapy may be used to control the cancer, though they cannot cure it. Hormone treatment with progesterone controls the growth of the endometrial cancer cells. Hormonal drugs used to treat uterine cancer include medroxyprogesterone and megestrol acetate. If hormone therapy fails to contain the spread of cancer, chemotherapy may be considered. Drug therapies may halt the progression of the cancer for several months.

chapter 13

DRUGS TO TREAT OSTEOPOROSIS

OSTEOPOROSIS IS A DISEASE IN WHICH THE BONES gradually become porous and weak. Far more common among women than men, it is the primary cause of the fractures of the hip, wrist, and vertebrae that often cause disability among older women.

Building strong bones throughout life

While treatments for osteoporosis have improved, it is difficult and sometimes impossible to rebuild bones that have been weakened over many years. By far the best treatment is prevention, ideally starting in childhood, but preventive efforts are helpful at any age.

Bones appear to be hard, permanent structures, but they are not. Instead, your bones undergo a constant process of breaking down and rebuilding. About one-quarter of your bone mass is broken down and rebuilt every year. Bone density is regulated by a number of hormones and growth factors. Vital to the rebuilding is calcium, a mineral found in dairy products and some other foods. Calcium is also needed in the bloodstream for nerve cell activity and for the contraction of muscles, including the heart. If there is not enough calcium in the diet to maintain adequate levels in the blood, the bone will release calcium into the blood to maintain these important body functions. For women, the hormone estrogen plays a key role in preserving bone mass, by preventing the breakdown of bone and the release of calcium into the blood.

In childhood, more bone is formed than broken down. In early adulthood, the processes are about equal. Starting in a woman's thirties, a gradual loss in bone density begins. Tiny pores in the structure of the bone grow larger. When estrogen levels drop at menopause, the loss of bone increases alarmingly, as much as 2 percent of bone each year for the next five years. Bone loss then tapers off to 0.5 to 1 percent a year and continues at that pace.

Besides menopause, other conditions that lower estrogen cause bone loss at any age. They include excessive exercise or the eating disorder anorexia nervosa, both of which decrease body fat, a source of estrogen. Stopping menstruating is a sign that estrogen levels are low.

If you have some of the following risk factors for osteoporosis, it is particularly important that you take steps to keep your bones strong.

- White or Asian ancestry
- Family history of osteoporosis
- Small or narrow body frame
- Smoking
- Inactivity
- Never having children
- Excessive exercise (causing menstrual period to stop)
- Anorexia nervosa (causing menstrual period to stop)
- Late puberty
- Early menopause (natural or caused by surgical removal of both ovaries)
- Low lifetime calcium consumption
- Excessive alcohol consumption
- Lactose (milk) intolerance
- Consistently high animal protein intake
- Drinking more than three cups of coffee daily

Obviously, you can't change your ancestry or some of the other factors on this list, but you can make a big difference by addressing those factors you do control. The sooner in life you start, the better.

- **Get enough calcium in your diet.** The best source of calcium is food (see page 279), but you should take a calcium supplement if you can't fulfill the daily requirements (see box below) through food alone. The best supplement is calcium carbonate. It provides the most calcium per dose, is inexpensive, and is well absorbed. Common brand names include Tums and Oscal 500.

- **Get enough vitamin D in your diet.** Vitamin D helps your body absorb calcium from food. Your body manufactures some vitamin D every time your skin is exposed to sunlight, but probably not enough to meet the daily requirement of 400 IU (international units). Good sources of vitamin D are dairy products, eggs, and oily fish like salmon and bluefish. If you aren't sure you are getting enough, take a daily multivitamin containing 400 IU vitamin D. Milk is a good source of both vitamin D and calcium.

- **Exercise regularly.** The right kind of exercise to ward off osteoporosis puts weight or stress on your bones. Walk, run, hike, lift weights, use a stair climber, or do aerobic dance rather than swim, row, or bicycle—activities in which your weight is supported. Do weight-bearing exercise for 30 minutes three times a week.

- **Don't smoke.** If you haven't quit already, doing so will lower your risk of osteoporosis while preventing life-threatening diseases like lung cancer and emphysema. Women who smoke one pack per day throughout their lives lose 5 to 15 percent of their bone density by the time of menopause.

RECOMMENDED DAILY CALCIUM

The National Institutes of Health recommend that women get the following amounts of calcium every day.

Girls and young women under 24: 1,200 to 1,500 mg

Age 25 to 50: 1,000 mg

Age 50 to 65, taking estrogen: 1,000 mg

Age 50 to 65, not taking estrogen: 1,500 mg

Over 65: 1,500 mg

Pregnant or breast-feeding: 1,200 mg

GOOD SOURCES OF CALCIUM

Food	Calcium (mg)
low-fat or nonfat yogurt (1 cup)	350–420
skim milk (1 cup)	300
2 percent milk (1 cup)	295
frozen low-fat yogurt ($^1/_2$ cup)	60–100
frozen nonfat yogurt ($^1/_2$ cup)	80–150
cheese: Cheddar, Swiss, mozzarella, American (1 ounce)	180–270
broccoli, cooked (1 cup)	135
kale, cooked (1 cup)	180
spinach, cooked (1 cup)	250
dried beans, cooked (1 cup)	90
salmon, canned (3 ounces)	170

- **Cut back on alcohol.** Alcohol suppresses the bone cells that stimulate bone formation. Moderate consumption of alcohol (one glass a day or less) is probably safe.

DRUGS THAT CAUSE BONE LOSS

If you take any of these drugs, you may increase your risk of osteoporosis. Ask your doctor about changing, reducing, or discontinuing your medication, but do not stop taking it without consulting your doctor first.

antacids with aluminum
    (if used excessively)
chemotherapy (methotrexate)
corticosteroid drugs (long-term)
furosemide (Lasix)
GnRH agonist therapy
    (Lupron, Synarel)

heparin (long-term, dose over
    15,000 u per day)
phenytoin (Dilantin)
thyroid replacement drugs
    (levothyroxine doses over
    0.15 mg per day)

- **Control caffeine consumption.** Two cups of coffee a day or less is probably safe. If you drink at least one 8-ounce glass of milk per day, you can counteract the adverse effects of the two cups of caffeine on the bone.
- **Don't diet or exercise excessively.** If your menstrual periods stop, it's a sign that your estrogen is too low to protect your bones.

Osteoporosis

Osteoporosis is a disorder in which the bones are porous, weak, and prone to fracture.

SYMPTOMS AND DIAGNOSIS

Osteoporosis often has no symptoms until a bone breaks. The most common sites are the hip, wrist, and spine.

Chronic pain in the spine is a symptom of tiny, hairline fractures in the vertebrae. As the number of small fractures grows, the back curves and the woman's height shrinks. Some women also experience muscle spasms in the back. Spinal fractures usually occur in women between the ages of 51 and 75. In women with premature menopause following surgical removal of both ovaries, a spinal fracture may occur at an earlier age, usually within three to six years after surgical menopause.

A wrist fracture often occurs when a woman with osteoporosis tries to break a fall by putting out her hand. A wrist fracture is sometimes mistaken for a sprain. If you injure your wrist and the pain persists, talk to your doctor.

Hip fractures, which are about half as common as spinal fractures, usually occur later in life. Recovery from a hip fracture takes many months and may never be complete. Sometimes it is necessary to have hip-replacement surgery. Some women never regain their ability to walk without assistance. About one-third of women who live to the age of 90 have a hip fracture, and one-half are permanently disabled. A large percentage of women also develop complications from surgery (blood clots, pneumonia) and depression.

Bone scans

If you are at high risk of osteoporosis or have symptoms such as a bone fracture, ask for a bone density test. A test can also help you decide whether you should start hormone replacement therapy to help maintain your bone density (for more about hormone replacement and osteoporosis, see page 100). If you have previously been diagnosed with osteoporosis, a bone density test can help your doctor evaluate whether your treatment for osteoporosis is working.

Dual energy X-ray absorptiometry (DEXA) is the fastest, safest, and most precise way to measure the bone density of the hips, spine, forearm, or entire body. The test takes three to seven minutes and uses a low dose of radiation. It can accurately detect even small amounts of bone loss.

Dual photon absorptiometry measures bone density in the spine, neck, and hips with two beams of low-dose radiation. Because the test takes 20 to 40 minutes and delivers more radiation than DEXA, it has largely been replaced by DEXA. Single photon absorptiometry is an imaging technique that uses a single beam of low-dose radiation to detect bone loss in the wrist or heel. A computed tomography (CT) scan is a good way to assess bone loss in the lower spine, and it provides the earliest indication of postmenopausal bone loss. A CT scan delivers more radiation than other methods, however, and is more expensive and time-consuming.

TREATMENT

While osteoporosis is much easier to prevent than to reverse, there are vitamins, hormones, and medications that can help prevent further bone loss.

Pain relief

Back aches or muscle spasms may be treated with heat, massage, and orthopedic supports. The pain-relieving drugs most commonly recommended for osteoporosis are the NSAID drugs, such as aspirin, ibuprofen, and others. (For more on NSAIDs, see page 223.)

Surgery

When a fracture occurs, surgery may be necessary to set the bone or place pins to support the bony structures while they heal. A badly broken hip may be replaced with an artificial one. Physical therapy can help with recovery from a fracture or surgery.

Vitamin and calcium supplements

If you have been diagnosed with osteoporosis or are at high risk, you should take a calcium supplement daily (see doses in box on page 278) and a multivitamin containing 400 IU of vitamin D.

Even if you already have osteoporosis, calcium prevents resorption of bone and can slow or prevent further bone loss. Calcium is probably not effective in preventing bone loss in the first five years after menopause, but it can delay bone loss later on. Calcium is best used in combination with estrogen replacement therapy and with the other drugs to prevent further loss.

Hormone replacement therapy

Replacing the estrogen lost at menopause through hormone replacement therapy is the most effective way to keep an older woman's bones strong. Estrogen replacement therapy works best when started as soon as possible after menopause, before a great deal of bone is lost. However, if started in women who are 10 to 15 years past menopause, it can also help prevent further bone loss. Estrogen has been shown to prevent spinal and hip fractures in women after menopause.

Menopausal women who have had a hysterectomy can take estrogen alone. Women who still have their uterus take a combination of estrogen and another female hormone, progestin, to protect against endometrial cancer. (For more on hormone replacement, see chapter 5.)

The benefits of the estrogen will continue as long as you take the hormones, but when you stop, bone loss begins again. For long-term benefits, you must take the hormones for at least seven years. Lifelong use is currently advocated. The level of benefit appears to be related to the dose. Besides an oral medication, a transdermal system (skin patch), although not studied as extensively as the oral estrogen in women with osteoporosis, is also effective in preventing osteoporosis. Premenopausal women will not gain any benefit from estrogen replacement unless they have had their ovaries surgically removed or have a disorder that is causing them to lose bone.

Bisphosphonates

These drugs can prevent bone loss and can actually build up bone in some women who have already suffered severe bone loss due to osteoporosis.

Avoiding Falls

Because falls are the main source of fractures, women who have osteoporosis should take these preventive steps.

- Many falls occur because inactivity has weakened the muscles. You can keep your muscles strong by taking regular walks and lifting weights. Talk with your doctor, then start an exercise program.
- Reduce or eliminate alcohol consumption so you won't become unsteady on your feet.
- Many medications cause drowsiness, which can lead to stumbling and falling. Ask your doctor or pharmacist whether any of the prescription or nonprescription drugs you take has this side effect.
- Make sure your home is well lit so you won't trip or stumble over unnoticed cords, rugs, or furniture.
- Tack down loose rugs. Keep electrical cords away from walking areas. Remove small objects from the floor.
- Move unstable furniture away from heavily traveled areas so you won't be tempted to lean on it for support.
- Put supportive railings in stairway and bathroom areas.
- Use nonskid mats and strips, in colors that stand out from the surrounding floors, in your bathroom and kitchen.
- Outdoors, maintain a clear, dry pathway to and from your car or other common destinations.

- **Etidronate (Didronel).** Etidronate is approved to treat Paget's disease and other conditions that break down bone. Although it is not currently FDA approved for osteoporosis, it has recently been found useful in treating this condition. Studies show it increases the density of vertebrae and reduces the risk of spinal fractures when taken orally for two weeks every three months for two years. This intermittent schedule—two weeks every three months—is needed because etidronate can prevent minerals from entering bone, thus weakening it. Etidronate is not without side effects, however, including nausea, upset stomach, diarrhea, and a temporary increase in bone pain. Etidronate must be taken with calcium and vitamin D supplements.

- **Alendronate (Fosamax).** By increasing bone density, alendronate reduces fractures in the vertebrae. Approved for use in osteoporosis, it is taken orally once daily for up to three years by postmenopausal women. Alendronate is more effective than etidronate in preventing further fractures of the vertebrae, and at currently recommended doses, it is less likely to interfere with bone mineralization. Side effects are less common than with etidronate but may include headache, flatulence, and diarrhea. Food can interfere with its absorption, so it must be taken with a full glass of water the first thing in the morning, at least 30 minutes before the first food, drink, or other medication. After taking the drug, you need to remain in the upright position for at least 30 minutes. Calcium and vitamin D supplements must be taken if you are using alendronate.

Calcitonin

Like estrogen and the bisphosphonate drugs, calcitonin inhibits the release of calcium from the bone into the bloodstream and has been shown to increase spinal bone density. As a preventive medication, it is recommended for women who are at least five years postmenopause, have low bone mass, and cannot take estrogens. In women with established osteoporosis, calcitonin also relieves pain both at rest and with motion. Following a fracture, women who have received injections of calcitonin require fewer analgesics for pain and are not confined to bed as long.

Formerly available only in injection form, calcitonin now comes in an easily used nasal spray (Miacalcin). Women taking calcitonin by injection or by nasal spray need to supplement their diet with 1,000 mg of calcium and a multivitamin containing 400 IU of vitamin D each day to prevent the development of hyperparathyroidism, a condition that leads to kidney stones, fatigue, indigestion, and increased thirst and urination. Allergic reactions and side effects with the injected calcitonin, including facial flushing, nausea, and dizziness, occur far less frequently in women receiving the nasal product. The spray can cause nasal dryness, redness, crusting, itching, or irritation.

chapter 14

DRUGS FOR ENDOCRINE DISORDERS

*T*HE GLANDS OF THE ENDOCRINE SYSTEM PRODUCE powerful chemicals called hormones that regulate metabolism, growth, menstrual cycle, and other body functions. When a gland produces too little or too much of a hormone, this affects the body organs it regulates.

Hyperthyroidism

The thyroid gland wraps around the windpipe at the base of the neck. The hormones it produces help maintain the normal function of nearly all body organs, regulate growth and metabolism, and control the expenditure of energy.

Hyperthyroidism occurs when the level of thyroid hormone in the blood is too high. Eight times more women than men have this condition. The most common cause is Graves' disease (diffuse toxic goiter), in which an abnormal antibody stimulates the thyroid to secrete excessive amounts of hormone. Graves' disease may occur at any age, but it is most likely to be diagnosed during a woman's twenties or thirties. Another cause of hyperthyroidism is toxic nodules (lumps) in the thyroid gland. Toxic nodules most commonly occur in women over 60. Other causes of the condition are deQuervain's thyroiditis and silent thyroiditis. These autoimmune diseases can destroy part of the thyroid gland, releasing large amounts of hormone into the blood. DeQuervain's thyroiditis often follows a viral respiratory infection. Silent thyroiditis can occur in the period following childbirth.

SYMPTOMS AND DIAGNOSIS

Because the symptoms of hyperthyroidism vary widely, the condition is difficult to diagnose. Older people are particularly apt to have no symptoms. See your doctor if you notice any combination of these signs and symptoms:

- Unexplained weight loss despite increased appetite
- Heart palpitations (often the only symptom in older women)
- Mood swings, irritability, nervousness
- Heat intolerance
- Fatigue
- Weak muscles
- Diarrhea
- Protruding or bulging eyes
- Increased sweating
- Hair loss
- Increased nail growth
- Insomnia
- Irregular or skipped periods

A definite diagnosis can be made through a blood test that measures the amount of thyroid stimulating hormone (TSH), a pituitary hormone that stimulates the thyroid to produce thyroid hormone. When the thyroid gland is producing too much hormone, the pituitary gland releases less TSH, so a low TSH level indicates a high thyroid hormone level.

TREATMENT

There are three primary approaches to the treatment of hyperthyroidism: medications, surgery, or radiation. The choice is based on future plans for pregnancy, size of the goiter, presence of other disease (particularly heart disease), and the possibility of a remission. With Graves' disease, there is a 25 to 30 percent chance of remission with the use of antithyroid medications. Toxic nodules are far less likely to go into remission with medication use, so they are usually treated with surgery or radiation.

Medications

- **Thioamides.** The most common treatment is an antithyroid drug, methimazole (Tapazole) or propylthiouracil (PTU). These drugs prevent the thyroid from getting the iodine it needs to produce the hormone. Symptoms usually improve in a few days, and the drug will have its full effect in four to six weeks. Because the effects of these drugs are delayed, additional drugs such as iodides and beta-blockers (see below) are taken initially to control symptoms. Thioamide use may continue for six months to two years or until remission occurs. Afterward, the doctor monitors the blood for signs that the disease is returning. While taking thioamides, report any rash, fever, sore throat, or flu-like symptoms because they may be symptoms of agranulocytosis, a condition caused by a drop in white blood cells. While taking this medication, tell your doctor if you become pregnant or want to become pregnant. Thioamides should not be used during the first trimester of pregnancy; however, PTU can be used safely during the second trimester of pregnancy and during breast-feeding. To avoid problems with drug interactions, tell all your health care professionals that you are taking medication for hyperthyroidism, particularly when you receive a prescription for a new medication.
- **Iodides.** Iodides (Lugol's solution, supersaturated potassium iodide—SSKI) are used for short-term management of hyperthyroidism, for example, before surgery or during the initial week of thioamide therapy. They inhibit the production and release of thyroid hormone. They work in 2 to 7 days, but the effect does not last longer than 14 days. Iodides can cause skin rashes, conjunctivitis, burning mouth, sore throat, and symptoms of a head cold. Iodides are considered as an additional, rather than primary, therapy for hyperthyroidism. When used two weeks before thyroid surgery, they make the gland smaller and firmer, so that the procedure is easier and safer.
- **Beta-blockers.** Beta-blockers (propranolol and nadolol) are sometimes prescribed in conjunction with other drug therapies to

control cardiovascular symptoms, including heart palpitations and abnormal heart rhythm, as well as high blood pressure, anxiety, tremor, and heat intolerance. They are used to control symptoms before the gland is removed surgically and also to treat deQuervain's thyroiditis.

Surgery and radiation

If the thyroid has become inflamed and enlarged, occasionally part will be surgically removed. Surgery may be indicated if the enlarged gland is obstructing the esophagus or if cancer is suspected. Following gland removal, thyroid hormone replacement therapy is needed.

If drug therapy is ineffective and surgery is not indicated, radiation treatments are sometimes used. Radiation is usually suggested for older people, for whom surgery is riskier, and for cases in which hyperthyroidism returns after surgery. Radiation is not recommended during pregnancy. Radioactive iodine treatments are given as a single dose of liquid or capsule. The radiation accumulates in the thyroid gland and kills some of the tissue. During the first few days, the radiation will be present in your saliva and other body fluids and may harm other people, particularly small children and pregnant women. During this time it is best to avoid kissing and other intimate contact with other people and to use disposable plates and eating utensils. If a second dose of radiation is needed, it should be separated from the first dose by at least three months.

Hypothyroidism

Hypothyroidism occurs when the thyroid gland produces too little thyroid hormone. It is the most common thyroid disorder, occurring in about 6 percent of women over the age of 60. Hypothyroidism is usually the result of Hashimoto's disease, an autoimmune disorder in which antibodies destroy thyroid cells, decreasing or blocking the production of thyroid hormone. Hashimoto's disease is four times more common in women than men, and it tends to run in families. Hypothyroidism can also be caused by treatment for hyperthyroidism or by long-term lithium therapy.

Symptoms and diagnosis

Symptoms of hypothyroidism develop slowly and may not be noticeable for years. See your doctor if you experience any combination of these signs and symptoms:

- Goiter (a swelling on the side of the neck)
- Fatigue
- Lack of energy
- Unexplained weight gain
- Depression
- Intolerance of cold temperatures
- Muscle cramps, stiffness, or weakness
- Anemia
- Unusually heavy menstrual periods
- Infertility
- Constipation
- Dry skin and hair

If your doctor suspects hypothyroidism, a simple blood test can confirm the diagnosis. High blood levels of TSH indicate a lack of thyroid hormone in your body.

Treatment

Hypothyroidism can be treated but cannot be cured. Drug therapy often needs to continue for the rest of the patient's life.

The usual treatment is thyroid replacement hormones, taken in tablet form. Most are synthetic versions of the thyroid hormone naturally manufactured by the body. The most commonly used is levothyroxine (Synthroid, Levothroid, Levoxine), which is inexpensive and is taken once a day. Other drugs include liothyronine (Cytomel) and liotrix (Thyrolar). These hormone replacement drugs are not interchangeable, however, and the best course of therapy is to chose one and stick with it. Each of these hormones interacts with a number of drugs that lower their absorption. They should not be taken within six hours after taking a bile acid binding drug (cholestyramine or colestipol). Aluminum-containing antacids and sucralfate substantially reduce their absorption and they should not be taken with any of these hormone replacements. Relief of symptoms begins within two weeks. Symptoms such as weight gain and facial puffiness subside within two to three days. Skin temperature, mental alertness, and physical activity may improve as well. TSH levels begin to fall within hours of starting drug treatment but will not be in the normal range for six to eight weeks. You will see your doctor about once a month until your thyroid hormone levels are normal and any side effects or symptoms are resolved.

Your doctor will try to keep your dose of the hormone as low as possible because higher doses (greater than 0.15 mg levothyroxine) may contribute to osteoporosis. You will continue treatment for the rest of your life. Side effects are rare, but tell your doctor if you experience unusual sweating, headache, or diarrhea. Excessive doses may cause abnormal heart rhythm, sweating, weight loss, angina, heart attack, or heart failure.

Women taking estrogen replacement therapy or contraceptives containing estrogen may need to take a slightly higher dose of thyroid hormone. Larger doses of thyroid hormone are also needed during pregnancy. Diabetics may need to increase insulin dosages. Heart patients taking anticoagulant drugs may need to increase their dosage of anticoagulant because thyroid hormones increase blood clotting.

Type 2 diabetes

Diabetes is a group of conditions caused by excess levels of glucose in the blood. Glucose is the sugar that is the primary fuel of the cells of the body. Diabetes occurs when the pancreas does not produce enough insulin, the hormone that allows glucose to pass into the body's cells, or when the body's cells resist using the insulin that is available. Normally, two hours after a meal, the glucose from the food has passed into the tissues and muscles. In a person with diabetes, blood glucose levels remain high all day. Eating sugar does not cause diabetes, although people who are already diabetic must carefully control their diet, including their intake of sugar.

About 90 percent of people with diabetes have type 2, or noninsulin-dependent, diabetes, in which the body's cells resist insulin. This condition usually begins after age 40 and is more common in people who are overweight or obese. The information about symptoms and treatment that follows pertains to this type of diabetes.

Another kind of diabetes—type 1, or juvenile, diabetes—usually begins in childhood. Treatment includes insulin injections and a controlled diet.

There is also a form of diabetes called gestational diabetes (page 144), which occurs only during pregnancy. All pregnant women are screened for this condition between weeks 24 to 28. Although glucose levels usually return to normal after pregnancy, women who have gestational diabetes have a higher risk of developing type 2 diabetes later in life.

Diabetes is so dangerous that twice as many women die from its complications as from breast cancer. People with diabetes have an increased risk of stroke, heart disease, high blood cholesterol, kidney failure, nerve damage in their hands and feet, foot infections, and an eye disease called diabetic retinopathy, which can lead to blindness. Carefully controlling the condition can prevent many of these problems. Unfortunately, early diabetes has few, if any, symptoms, and therefore many people do not know they have it.

SYMPTOMS AND DIAGNOSIS

Type 2 diabetes may have no symptoms, particularly in its early years. In some cases, the following symptoms, which are usually mild, appear.

- Excess appetite
- Weight gain
- Weight loss despite an increased appetite (more common in type 1)
- Increased thirst
- Increased urination
- Wounds, cuts, or infections (including vaginal infections) that recur or will not heal
- Fatigue
- Blurred vision
- Tingling or numbness in hands or feet
- Itchy skin

Diabetes is diagnosed by a blood glucose test. Usually the test is done after you have fasted overnight (for about 12 hours). After fasting, results greater than 140 mg/dL indicate diabetes.

TREATMENT

Once you are diagnosed, your doctor and nutritionist will set up a treatment plan that includes diet, exercise, and regular tests to monitor your condition. For type 2 diabetes, oral medication and, in some cases, daily insulin injections may also be prescribed. Weight control is extremely important. In some people with type 2 diabetes, a return to healthy body weight brings blood glucose levels back to normal.

The goals of treatment are based on your age and the presence of other conditions or diseases. Experts in diabetes management recommend maintaining a fasting glucose of 70 to 140 mg/dL and a hemoglobin A1c of less than or equal to 7 percent. These levels reflect "tight control." Most people with type 2 diabetes test their blood glucose levels several times a day and are well aware of their "numbers."

Recent studies have shown that many people with diabetes are not getting the care they need to reduce the likelihood and severity of complications, particularly cardiovascular disease, which causes about 75 percent of related deaths. If you have been diagnosed with diabetes, you should see your doctor at least twice a year. More visits may be necessary if you have complications.

Monitoring tests

Good diabetic care involves regular tests and monitoring. The following techniques are used for both types 1 and 2 diabetes.

- **Hemoglobin A1c.** A blood test for glycosylated hemoglobin (HbA1c) will show how well your blood sugar levels have been controlled during the preceding two to three months. It is the only test that can indicate your glucose control over a period of time rather than at an isolated time. The better your glucose levels are controlled, the less likely you are to have the health problems associated with diabetes. An elevated test result shows poor glucose control. You should have this test every six months, or every three months if you are taking insulin. It does not require fasting.

- **Home blood glucose monitoring (HBGM).** This testing method, which is often called finger-stick testing, allows you to test your own blood sugar levels at home. Several systems are available for purchase, and they differ in meter size, volume of blood required, size of the readout, sensitivity to light and moisture, and availability of technical support. To use any of these systems, you must first take a sample of blood by lightly pricking the end of your finger. The drop of blood is put on a paper strip, then the strip is placed into a small machine. After a minute, your blood glucose level appears on the machine. As a backup to the machine, some systems allow you to read the strips directly to determine your glucose level. Home glucose monitoring is usually performed about four times a day, before meals and at bedtime. The machines need to be periodically recalibrated and cleaned, and the strips have to be stored carefully so they don't deteriorate. The results of home testing can be evaluated by your doctor at your next visit.

- **Fasting blood glucose test.** A blood sample is drawn in the doctor's office following a fast of about 12 hours. This test is often required when the HbA1c test is abnormal or when finger-stick records show that blood sugar is being poorly controlled. It can also evaluate the accuracy of finger-stick tests.

- **Blood cholesterol testing.** Elevated blood cholesterol should be treated aggressively with cholesterol-lowering drugs (page 204) to lower your risk of heart attack and stroke. Most people diagnosed with diabetes have a high risk of these life-threatening occurrences. You should have regular blood tests of your triglycerides, total cholesterol, and HDL (good) and LDL (bad) cholesterol levels.

- **Urine testing.** With the availability of home blood glucose monitoring, urine testing for glucose is not routinely advised. Urine glucose tests measure only the glucose that spills from the kidneys into the urine. They are recommended only for people who cannot or will not use home blood glucose testing. In the doctor's office, you may be asked to provide a urine sample to test for albumin, a protein. Increased levels may indicate early kidney damage. Patients who have had diabetes for less than five years can have the test done with a standard urine sample. Those who have had diabetes for more than five years should collect all their urine for 24 hours to be tested.

Diet

To keep your blood-sugar levels steady, you should eat small meals and snacks on a regular schedule. Also, you need to limit your calories so you can lose weight. The best diet is low in fat and high in fiber, particularly the soluble fiber in oatmeal, oat bran, and beans, which helps lower cholesterol. To delay the complications of diabetes, a diet low in cholesterol (less than 300 mg per day) and in sodium (less than 3 grams a day) is also advocated. Simple sugars (refined sugars, sucrose) can be eaten in limited amounts. Both no-calorie sweeteners (aspartame, saccharin) and sweeteners like fructose and sorbitol are acceptable. Overall, carbohydrates should constitute no more than 60 percent of your total calories.

Although it is best to avoid alcohol because it can alter blood sugar levels, the American Diabetes Association currently says that small amounts (no more than 2 ounces per day once or twice a week) are acceptable. Alcohol should never be ingested on an empty stomach because it can cause a rapid decline in blood sugar.

Exercise

Talk with your doctor about establishing a regular exercise program. The recommended program is usually daily aerobic exercise, like brisk walking or riding an exercise bicycle. Exercise helps control your weight and improves your cardiovascular health, which can be damaged by diabetes over time. To keep your blood sugar level stable, about 30 minutes before exercising, eat a light snack with a carbohydrate, such as crackers and a glass of skim milk.

Medications

Many people will need no medication if they follow their diet and exercise program carefully. Others need to control blood sugar with antidiabetic or hypoglycemic drugs or with insulin injections. New drugs are allowing much better control of type 2 diabetes than in the past.

DRUGS TO CONTROL BLOOD GLUCOSE

sulfonylureas (first generation)
  acetohexamide (Dymelor)
  chlorpropamide (Diabinese)
  tolazamide (Tolinase)
  tolbutamide (Orinase)
sulfonylureas (second
    generation)
  glipizide (Glucotrol, Glucotrol
    XL)

glyburide (DiaBeta,
  Micronase, Glynase
  Prestab)
biguanide
  metformin (Glucophage)
nonsystemic therapy
  Acarbose (Precose)

- **Sulfonylureas.** At one time, sulfonylurea drugs were the only oral medications for controlling blood glucose, and they remain the first choice. Sulfonylurea drugs stimulate the release of insulin from the pancreas, decrease the breakdown of glycogen in the liver, and increase the response of the body's cells to insulin. There are two classes of sulfonylureas, the first- and second-generation agents. Although the second-generation agents (glipizide and glyburide) are about 100 times more potent, there is no evidence that they are more effective in the treatment of type 2 diabetes. Compared to many of the first-generation agents, glipizide and glyburide offer more convenient dosing, and they are less likely to accumulate in the body if there is liver or kidney disease. Not all of the sulfonylureas are appropriate for people with type 1 diabetes, and they should not be used during pregnancy. Side effects differ with each medication and most commonly include nausea, abdominal fullness, and heartburn. These sulfa drugs may cause allergic skin reactions in people with sulfa allergy. Most importantly when taking sulfonylureas, watch for signs and symptoms of low blood sugar, or hypoglycemia (see box).
- **Metformin (Glucophage).** Approved in the United States in 1995, metformin decreases glucose production in the liver and increases glucose uptake by the body's cells. It may be used with diet alone or in combination with a sulfonylurea or insulin. It does not cause weight gain as the sulfonylureas do, an important benefit because many diabetic people are overweight, and it improves

HYPOGLYCEMIA

Hypoglycemia is low blood sugar. The number-one cause of hypoglycemia among older people is a sulfonylurea drug taken for type 2 diabetes. If you are taking a sulfonylurea drug, watch for these signs and symptoms of low blood sugar.

- Blood glucose level of less than 50 mg/dL
- Blurred vision
- Sweating
- Hand tremor
- Intense hunger
- Feeling cold
- Headache
- Confusion
- Palpitations

If hypoglycemia is occurring during the night, you may wake up with a headache in the morning (similar to a hangover) or be awakened by sweating. When hypoglycemia is developing, some people experience a warning sign of tingling of the lips or tongue. At the first sign of symptoms, you should ingest 10 to 20 grams of a rapidly absorbed carbohydrate, such as orange juice or a nondiet soda ($^1/_2$ cup), apple juice ($^1/_3$ cup), grape juice ($^1/_4$ cup), table sugar (2 teaspoonfuls or 2 cubes), or small hard candies (5 to 6 pieces). If you still have symptoms 15 to 20 minutes later, take another 10 to 20 grams of rapidly absorbed sugar. Try not to overdo it with carbohydrates; you may get hyperglycemia. After your symptoms have stabilized, you should have a small snack consisting of a complex carbohydrate and a protein to provide a continued source of glucose.

cholesterol levels. But it has side effects that may include a metallic taste in the mouth, diarrhea, nausea, vomiting, and other gastrointestinal symptoms. The side effects can be prevented by starting at a low dose and slowly increasing the dose to the desired level. When side effects do appear, they can often be lessened by taking the dose with meals. Metformin may decrease the body's ability to absorb vitamin B12 and folic acid, causing deficiency in these vitamins. Unlike phenformin, a similar drug taken off the market in 1977, metformin rarely causes the fatal condition lactic acidosis, but you should watch for the warning signs of weakness and labored breathing. Because alcohol may interfere with lactate metabolism, it should not be used when you are on metformin.

- **Acarbose (Precose).** A recently approved medication called acarbose acts on the intestine to delay the digestion of carbohydrates and inhibit the absorption of glucose. In order for it to be effective, it must be taken with the first bite of a meal. Unlike the other oral agents for treatment of type 2 diabetes, acarbose does not affect the release of insulin from the pancreas or the body's response to insulin. It has fewer side effects than other hypoglycemic drugs, but can cause flatulence and diarrhea. It can be combined with dietary control of diabetes or with other oral antidiabetic drugs. Do not take acarbose if you have inflammatory bowel disease, ulceration of the colon, or partial obstruction of the colon. It is taken three times a day at the start of each main meal.

- **Insulin.** If diet and oral drugs fail to control your blood sugar levels, your doctor may recommend daily insulin injections. Some people with type 2 diabetes may be treated with the combination of a sulfonylurea and insulin. You can give yourself insulin shots at home each day (see box). Most people who take insulin do so for the rest of their lives. You will adjust your dosage regularly according to the results of finger-stick tests (page 294) several times a day. Some women require more insulin at certain stages in their monthly cycles because of changing hormone levels. Some women find they need less insulin at menopause.

Treatment of complications of diabetes

- **Urinary tract infections and vaginal yeast infections.** When the level of glucose in the urine and vaginal secretions is high, microorganisms thrive. If you have diabetes and develop a urinary tract infection or vaginal yeast infection, treatment should be for the full seven days (not the abbreviated three- to five-day course) to make sure you prevent spread of the infection into the kidneys. (See page 249 for more on urinary tract infections and page 252 for more on yeast infections.)

- **Neuropathy.** This common complication makes the legs and feet feel numb, tingly, and in severe cases, painful. Careful con-

TAKING INSULIN

- Check the expiration date on the insulin bottle to make sure the medication has not expired.
- Inspect your insulin carefully before each use. Do not use it if its appearance has changed (become cloudy if normally clear) or if it contains unusual particles.
- Store unused vials of insulin in the refrigerator. The vial currently being used can be stored at room temperature (cold insulin is much more painful on injection). Vials of insulin that have not been completely used should be discarded after one month if they have been left at room temperature. Extreme temperatures of more than 100 degrees can lead to a loss of insulin potency.
- Before injecting insulin, agitate the product by rolling it between the palms of your hands. Do not shake the product, to prevent foaming.
- Give your shot at the same time each day.
- Choose a spot for your morning injection (abdomen, for example) and continue to use that area, although not the exact spot, for each morning injection. Chose a different site (thigh, for example) for your afternoon injection and continue to use that same area each afternoon.
- After injecting the dose, release your hold on the skin before the syringe is withdrawn. After removing the needle, apply pressure to the injection area with your finger to avoid leakage of the insulin from the injection site. Do not massage the injection area after removal of the needle because this may lead to faster action of the drug.
- Write down the time and dose daily.
- Never skip a shot unless your doctor tells you to.

trol of diabetes reduces the chance this will develop. Neuropathy is thought to be caused by poor blood flow to the nerves and an increase in platelet aggregation in the blood. The condition is usually helped by nonprescription drugs, including NSAIDs (see page 214), but prescription drugs may be needed. The most commonly used prescription drugs are antidepressants (amitriptyline and imipramine, see page 305) and the anticonvulsant carbamazepine. The topical nonprescription cream called capsaicin (Zostrix) can relieve the pain and make it easier to walk and to get a restful night of sleep. It takes several weeks before you see the effects of Zostrix.

- **Gastroparesis.** Diabetes may cause the stomach to work more slowly than normally, causing nausea, vomiting, and abdominal pain. The drug of choice to stimulate the stomach muscles into action is metoclopramide (Reglan). Cisapride (Propulsid) or erythromycin works for some people.

chapter 15

DRUGS TO TREAT ANXIETY, DEPRESSION, AND INSOMNIA

CHANGES IN MOODS AND EMOTIONS ARE A NORMAL and important part of life. But sometimes mood changes or anxieties gradually begin to interfere with the ability to carry on normal daily activities and to enjoy life. If you experience any of these problems, help is available.

Many mood or emotional disorders can be effectively treated with psychotherapy, also called "talk therapy," medications, or a combination of the two. If you take a medication, it may treat either the disorder itself or symptoms such as insomnia. A growing number of new drugs, including the well-known fluoxetine (Prozac), treat chemical imbalances in the brain that cause disorders such as depression and anxiety. Interestingly, women take more sedatives, antidepressants, antipsychotic agents, and other psychiatric drugs than men do. One reason is that women are more likely to report emotional symptoms to their doctors and get the help they need.

Any physician can prescribe drugs for mental disorders, but because of the complexity of the medications, it is often best to see a doctor who is trained in treating mental disorders—a psychiatrist. You may also work with a psychotherapist for counseling or behavioral therapy.

Depression

Depression is a state of feeling hopeless, empty, despondent, gloomy, and pessimistic. You may lose your usual energy and all your hope for the future. Each day may seem worse than the last. At night, you may not sleep well. You may take little pleasure in activities you formerly enjoyed and may have difficulty carrying out your responsibilities and activities. Getting out of bed each morning may take a major effort. You may lose your appetite and lose weight. You may be unable to concentrate. These feelings may grow until you feel like giving up on life.

Such signs of depression may go away by themselves after a few days or weeks, or they can last for months or even years if untreated. Depression triggered by an event such as job loss, divorce, or loss of spouse usually lessens with the passage of time and the support of family, friends, or psychotherapy. Depression that occurs every day for at least two weeks, that may or may not have a known cause, and that interferes with normal daily activities is called a major depressive disorder and may need to be treated with a combination of medication and psychotherapy.

Depression is extremely common and is diagnosed at least twice as often in women as in men, particularly during the ages of 25 through 45. One in three women becomes depressed at some point in her life. Depression occurs as a single episode in 30 to 50 percent of people and as a recurring condition in 50 to 70 percent of people.

SYMPTOMS AND DIAGNOSIS

Depression can take many forms and has a variety of emotional, physical, and cognitive symptoms. If any combination of the following symptoms does not diminish with time, see your doctor.

- Feelings of sadness, hopelessness
- Feelings of guilt or worthlessness
- Inability to concentrate
- Irritability
- Loss of pleasure in activities you used to enjoy

- Difficulty sleeping
- Fatigue and loss of energy
- Loss of appetite
- Weight loss
- Weight gain
- Thoughts of ending your own life

If the symptoms are mild, the depression can go on for years without ever being diagnosed. Nevertheless, symptoms such as sleep problems, low energy, and low self-esteem can cause problems in relationships and on the job. Depression, even if mild, can and should be treated.

More severe symptoms point to major depression, a disabling disease that saps a person of all strength and will to live. A person with major depression may exhibit a complete lack of interest in all of her usual activities and relationships. Major depression includes at least five of the following symptoms for at least two weeks.

- Depressed mood or loss of interest or pleasure
- Sleeplessness
- Loss of appetite or weight gain
- Lack of energy
- Irritability
- Difficulty concentrating
- Guilt and feelings of worthlessness
- Decreased sexual desire
- Thoughts of suicide

The most dangerous symptom of major depression is thoughts of suicide. Suicide is a very real threat to anyone suffering from major depression. All thoughts of suicide or suicide attempts should be taken seriously. Some attempts at suicide may be indirect—for example, eating so little that the person becomes malnourished. A suicide attempt should never be dismissed as merely an attempt to get attention. Immediately after emergency medical treatment, the person should talk with a mental health professional.

MANIC DEPRESSIVE DISORDER

Manic depressive disorder (bipolar disorder) is a mood disorder that is quite different from depression, although it may include depression. A person with manic depressive disorder experiences disruptive, wide mood swings between deep depression and extreme elation. The symptoms of manic depressive disorder, which tends to run in families, can vary widely. Some people have more frequent and prolonged bouts of depression, while others have more manic episodes. The initial signs of mania are being talkative, with flight of ideas from one unrelated topic to another, staying awake all night, and bursts of energy. During a manic episode, the person often must be in the hospital for protection and for treatment.

Manic depressive disorder is caused by a chemical imbalance that can often be effectively treated with medication. The condition is usually chronic and must be treated over the long term, usually for life. The most common and effective treatment is lithium carbonate. For the small percentage of people who are not helped by lithium, some alternative drugs are available including the anticonvulsant drug carbamazepine (Tegretol) or valproate (Depakote), which was recently approved by the FDA for the treatment of this disorder.

TREATMENT

Many people believe that someone who is depressed can "snap out of it," "shake it off," or "pull themselves together," but the reality is that people with depression are not able to cure themselves.

People who are depressed sometimes attempt to treat themselves by taking nonprescription sleeping pills or antianxiety pills. Instead of helping, these medications can make the symptoms worse. Some people turn to alcohol, which is itself a depressant and can deepen depression. Many people turn to pills and alcohol not knowing that their real problem is a depression that could be successfully treated with antidepressant medication and counseling.

Your treatment will begin with a medical examination to look for any physical problems that may mimic depression, for example, hypothyroidism or diabetes. If medical causes are ruled out, you should

DRUGS THAT CAN CAUSE DEPRESSION

Sometimes depression can be caused by a medication you are taking. The following prescription and nonprescription drugs most commonly contribute to depression. Some of them (stimulants, corticosteroids), cause depression when they are discontinued. Depression can be an uncommon side effect of other medications as well, so talk to your doctor if it occurs while you are taking any medication.

alcohol
amphetamines and
    other stimulants
barbiturates
benzodiazepines
carbamazepine
clonidine
cocaine
estrogens (including
    contraceptives and
    hormone replacement
    therapy)

hydralazine
indomethacin
levodopa
methyldopa
propanolol
steroids

make an appointment with a psychiatrist or psychologist who is trained in treating depression.

Depression triggered by an event, such as a death, is often effectively treated with psychotherapy or a support group of other people experiencing a similar situation. Major depression is more likely to be treated with a combination of medication and psychotherapy. The support of friends, family, a support group, or a therapist is an important part of treating depression. People with depression tend to isolate themselves from other people, but social support is an important part of both prevention and cure.

Medications

Antidepressant drugs are not stimulants, nor are they addictive. They work by altering brain chemicals that control mood. There are four categories of antidepressants: tricyclic agents, selective seritonergic agents, cyclic antidepressants (bupropion, nefazodone), and mono-amine oxidase inhibitors. They differ in side effects, drug interactions, and the brain chemicals affected. All of the antidepressants can take several weeks to fully relieve depression, but they usually help with insomnia, anxiety, and appetite within a week. After six to eight weeks, your doctor will evaluate whether the medication and dose are right for you. Because people respond to drugs in different ways, you may have to try several medications before you find one that works well and does not cause unpleasant side effects. Once you find an antidepressant that works for you, you may need to continue it for at least six months. When you are ready to stop treatment, your dosage must be lowered gradually.

- **Tricyclic antidepressants.** Tricyclics have been used for decades and continue to be used successfully to treat depression. They increase the levels of both norepinephrine and serotonin in the brain and also inhibit the effects of histamine and acetyl-choline. Tricyclics can have a sedating effect, so they are usually taken at bedtime. They are particularly useful for people who have depression associated with difficulty sleeping. Your doctor will start you with a low dose to help prevent side effects and will gradually increase your dosage to a level that effectively treats depression. Other side effects include dry mouth, weight gain, blurred vision, constipation, and increased heartbeat. Some tricyclics (imipramine, clomipramine, amitriptyline) may also cause a drop in blood pressure upon standing, which can lead to fainting spells or dizziness. This side effect can be lessened by rising slowly from a sitting or reclining position. Tricyclics also cause a decrease in sexual drive or desire in about a quarter of women. They can interact with a number of drugs, including the antiarrhythmic drugs quinidine and procainamide and the MAOIs. Make sure that you speak with your doctor or pharmacist before taking any other nonprescription or prescription drug.
- **Selective serotonin reuptake inhibitors (SSRIs).** SSRIs (including Prozac) raise the level in the brain of serotonin, a chemical messenger associated with mood changes. Because they have a specific effect on only one chemical messenger, they have fewer side effects than other antidepressant drugs. As a result, they are

now widely used for depression, anxiety, and other emotional and mental problems. Like most antidepressant medications, SSRIs take several weeks to work fully. Although SSRIs have fewer side effects than other medications, they do have some. One that causes some women to discontinue the drug is difficulty reaching orgasm. In the first few weeks, other side effects may include agitation, anxiety, or insomnia. The SSRIs should be taken in the morning so that they don't interfere with sleep. They are an excellent choice for those people with depression who do not want any sedative effects. Less common side effects include nausea, anorexia, headache, and nervousness. All of the SSRIs can cause weight loss, but the extent to which weight is lost differs among the agents. Fluoxetine (Prozac) is associated with the greatest degree of weight loss. The SSRIs can interact with a number of other drugs, such as alprazolam, cimetidine, lithium, MAOIs, and warfarin. Make sure you speak with your doctor or pharmacist before taking another drug with an SSRI.

- **Monoamine oxidase inhibitors (MAOIs).** MAOIs increase the levels of several neurotransmitters in the brain, including serotonin, norepinephrine, and dopamine. Because they affect so many neurotransmitters, they have many side effects and so are primarily used by people who have already tried several other antidepressants without success. They are also very effective in the treatment of atypical depression, which causes severe anxiety, increased appetite and weight, and severe tiredness. MAOIs tend to cause weight gain, agitation, insomnia, sexual dysfunction, increased appetite, and faintness. They can cause a severe and sudden rise in blood pressure if taken with certain drugs, including over-the-counter cold medications (such as pseudoephedrine), diet pills, and the prescription amphetamines TCAs, SSRIs, and meperidine (Demerol). While you are being treated with an MAOI, you will also need to follow a special diet that does not contain high amounts of tyramine. Foods high in tyramine are aged cheeses, fermented meats, fava or broad beans, tap beer, sauerkraut, and marmite concentrated yeast extracts. Excessive intake of tyramine with an MAOI leads to nausea, throbbing headache, rapid heartbeat, and high blood pressure.
- **Other drugs.** The development of newer antidepressants is ongoing. Bupropion (Wellbutrin) is an antidepressant that increases

dopamine. It is often preferred over the TCAs for older people because it does not cause sedation or harm the heart. Different, new antidepressants affect the neurotransmitters in the brain to varying degrees, and each has its own set of advantages and side effects. Nefazodone, the most recently approved antidepressant, does not cause weight gain, change in sexual drive, or interference

ELECTROCONVULSIVE THERAPY

Electroconvulsive therapy (ECT), sometimes referred to as "shock treatment," is a safe and effective treatment for severe depression and manic depressive disorder. This therapy is often appropriate for people who have not been helped by antidepressant medications or for older people who cannot tolerate the side effects of antidepressants or who are taking other medications that might have a dangerous interaction with antidepressants. It is not recommended if you have recently had a heart attack or have a lesion in the brain.

In electroconvulsive therapy, pulses of electrical current are carefully applied to the brain. The procedure takes only a few minutes. Why it works is unknown. When electroconvulsive therapy was first introduced in the 1930s, the dose of electrical current was much higher. The side effects were sometimes severe, and the treatment was sometimes abused. Today the technique is carefully controlled and is both safe and effective.

If you are scheduled for this therapy, you will receive general anesthesia and a muscle relaxant. The electrical current is applied through electrodes on the head, and you will not feel it. After you wake up you may feel drowsy or confused for an hour or so. You may not remember the hours or days immediately preceding the treatment, and you may have difficulty incorporating new events into your memory. The ability to incorporate memory usually returns within a few weeks but the extent of memory impairment differs based on total number of treatments and the type of electrode placement (one side of the head or both sides). For depression, the standard treatment is 6 to 12 treatments. The treatment can be done on an inpatient or outpatient basis.

ANTIDEPRESSANT DRUGS

selective serotonin reuptake
   inhibitors
  fluoxetine (Prozac)
  paroxetine (Paxil)
  sertraline (Zoloft)
tricyclic antidepressants
  amitriptyline (Elavil)
  amoxapine (Asendin)
  clomipramine (Anafranil)
  desipramine (Norpramin)
  doxepin (Sinequan)
  imipramine (Tofranil)

nortriptyline (Pamelor)
protriptyline (Vivactil)
trimipramine (Surmontil)
monoamine oxidase inhibitors
  phenelzine (Nardil)
  tranylcypromine (Parnate)
other drugs
  bupropion (Wellbutrin)
  maprotiline (Ludiomil)
  nefazodone (Serzone)
  trazodone (desyrel)
  venlafaxine (Effexor)

with blood pressure. However, it can interact with a number of drugs, including the antihistamines, terfenadine, and astemizole.

Anxiety and panic disorders

Everyone feels anxious or stressed at times. These feelings are not necessarily bad. Some stress can motivate you to accomplish things and take action in life. Feelings of anxiety can actually work in your favor by causing you to study harder before an exam or to concentrate harder on acquiring a new skill. However, anxiety can also be disabling, preventing you from participating in your usual activities and impeding you from meeting the normal challenges of life.

In a situation that normally provokes fear or extreme anxiety, chemicals called catecholamines (epinephrine, norepinephrine) stimulate the central nervous system, producing a heightened state of alertness, quickened heart rate, and tensed muscles. With an anxiety disorder, these physical symptoms are accompanied by irritability, indecision, persistent worry, feelings of inadequacy, and apprehension. The response is more intense than in a normal fearful situation. The feelings may be persistent or may appear off and on, with long periods of anticipatory anxiety. In anxiety disorders, these feelings occur in response to particular fears or when there is no identifiable external cause.

TYPES OF ANXIETY DISORDERS

Some people suffer from an overall sense of anxiety, while others experience panic attacks, phobias, or obsessive-compulsive behaviors that they cannot control. There are six specific types of anxiety disorders. These types differ in severity, types of symptoms, duration, and particularly their response to drugs and other therapies. The six types are generalized anxiety disorder, phobia (specific and social), panic disorder, obsessive-compulsive disorder, posttraumatic stress disorder, and acute stress disorder.

Generalized anxiety disorder

Generalized anxiety disorder is an overall sense of nervousness, worry, or dread, not tied to any particular situation, which persists for at least six months. Persistent anxiety is associated with at least three of the following symptoms: restlessness or feeling keyed up, tiring easily, difficulty concentrating, irritability, muscle tension, or difficulty sleeping. Unlike other anxiety disorders, this condition is chronic. It is the most common anxiety disorder and it affects about twice as many women as men.

Phobias

A phobia is an irrational fear that causes the person to avoid an object or situation. Specific phobias, in which a specific object is feared, may be triggered by an animal (dogs, snakes), natural environment (water, heights), blood (injections, medical procedures, injury), or situation (enclosed spaces, flying). Social phobia, which is twice as common in women than men, is the intense fear of suffering humiliation when under the scrutiny of others (public speaking, meeting new people, using a public restroom). In many cases the thing or situation feared may actually present a danger (fear of bee stings), but the fear is out of proportion to the potential danger. People with these phobias often admit that their fear is irrational, but they can't control the fear and so they avoid the thing that triggers it. This can disrupt daily activities. In the case of agoraphobia, a person has the fear of being alone in a situation or public place where escape may be difficult, such as in a crowd, in a check-out line, or on public transportation. If agoraphobia is severe, the person may become housebound, totally avoiding the outside community.

Panic attacks

A panic attack is an unexpected episode of intense anxiety that appears without any of the circumstances that might normally provoke panic, such as a car accident or a physical threat. You might feel as if you can't catch your breath. Your limbs may become numb. You may feel unable to speak. You may have a racing heartbeat, chest pain, dry mouth, hot and cold flashes, dizziness, or nausea. People who experience these attacks may sense immediate danger of dying or may act out of control. A typical panic attack comes on suddenly, lasts between 5 to 20 minutes, and may occur as frequently as several times a day or only once or twice a month. Panic attacks that occur while someone is sleeping are called night terrors. Someone who has at least two unexpected panic attacks followed by at least one month of persistent concern about having future attacks is said to have a panic disorder. The attacks may be triggered by a situation and they may lead to agoraphobia. Panic disorder is often associated with depression.

Obsessive-compulsive disorder

A person with obsessive-compulsive disorder is trapped in persistent anxieties and repetitive rituals that seem senseless even to her but are difficult to stop. An obsession is a thought, idea, or impulse that occurs repeatedly and is considered by the person as repugnant, such as an obsession with germs. A compulsion is an act or behavior that is repeated in an attempt to prevent the obsession, but it is senseless. A compulsive hand washer, for example, will wash her hands over and over again, sometimes 50 times a day, even though they are not dirty. The ritual, such as repeating the same sequence of hand motions or actions, can interfere with a person's ability to live a normal life because so much of her time and attention are given over to repeating the needless acts of her obsession. The compulsive act may also lead to physical ailments, such as skin disorders from repeated washing. This condition is often associated with depression.

Posttraumatic stress disorder

Posttraumatic stress disorder develops after a person has been exposed to an intensely traumatic experience such as a war, fire, or earthquake. In women, the most common cause is rape or domestic violence. The trauma overwhelms normal biological and psychological defense mechanisms, causing helplessness, vulnerability, or anger. The victim may relive the experience in dreams, flashbacks, or daydreams and may have difficulty forming relationships. Other symptoms include insomnia, difficulty in concentrating, feelings of guilt, and angry outbursts. Posttraumatic stress disorder can occur at any age. Fifty percent of people with this disorder recover completely within three months of treatment. Posttraumatic stress disorder responds poorly to drug therapy but well to behavioral and cognitive therapy. Drugs are used if there is an accompanying state of generalized anxiety. Acute stress disorder is similar to posttraumatic stress disorder but lasts only a few days or weeks instead of at least a month.

TREATMENT

See your doctor if you have anxiety that continues without relief, has no obvious cause, or is interfering with your ability to work or enjoy life. Because many anxiety disorders are caused in part by a chemical imbalance in the brain, most people cannot simply "get over it" without treatment. Anxiety disorders should be viewed like any other medical disorder. The most effective treatment is usually a combination of psychotherapy and medication. It is also important to seek medical attention because the condition may be due to a medical condition such as hypoglycemia, hyperthyroidism, or heart disease.

Psychotherapy

Psychotherapy is an important part of treating anxiety disorders. It helps the person understand the underlying motivation or trigger for the behavior and then modify the behavior. For certain types of anxiety, like phobias and obsessive-compulsive disorder, usually the most effective approach is desensitization or exposure therapy, a gradual exposure to the thing that is feared. For example, a woman who is afraid to touch a doorknob without repeatedly washing her hands afterward will be asked to touch a doorknob once without washing.

Gradually she will be asked to touch the knob more and more frequently and go for longer and longer periods without washing. When she sees that nothing bad happens, she usually will stop the hand-washing rituals. Another type of psychotherapy, known as cognitive therapy, can be effective in the treatment of generalized anxiety by helping the person identify the negative thought patterns that bring on anxiety. For panic disorder, a major part of therapy involves education and support. Relaxation training, supportive psychotherapy, and biofeedback are also used for these conditions.

Lifestyle changes

You should always seek medical help if your anxiety is persistent or is making life difficult. However, changes in your lifestyle can help support your other treatments and may reduce the need for medications. Here are some steps you can take to help yourself.

- Avoid beverages and medications that contain caffeine, including coffee, diet pills, nonprescription decongestants, and some pain relievers.
- Limit alcohol consumption. Some people turn to alcohol as a way to medicate themselves. Alcohol may temporarily mask the problem but will not cure it.
- Get regular exercise, which can boost not only your physical strength but also your well-being and self-image. It can also divert your thoughts from your anxiety.
- Learn and practice relaxation techniques, including meditation, breathing exercises, and a sequence of tensing and relaxing each muscle in your body.
- If you have concerns that keep you constantly worried, schedule a certain time in each day to think about how to deal with them. Not only will this help you manage your concerns more effectively, but when you become worried during the day, you can tell yourself to set the worries aside until your next scheduled time.

Medications

Treatment is based on your specific diagnosis (panic, phobia, obsessive-compulsive disorder). If anxiety is a symptom of depression, the depression is treated. If it is associated with a medical condition such as arrhythmia (page 189), hyperthyroidism (page 286), or chronic pain (page 210), your doctor will treat the underlying medical condition.

- **Benzodiazepines.** Often the preferred drugs for treatment of anxiety, benzodiazepines (Valium), are central nervous system depressants. This extremely large class of drugs includes long-acting, short-acting, high-potency, and low-potency medications. All benzodiazepines have four actions—antianxiety, sedation, muscle relaxation, and antiseizure—but the extent of each action differs among the drugs. For anxiety, the benzodiazepines work quickly, often within an hour, and they are an excellent choice for short-term use. Alprazolam is often considered the best drug for generalized anxiety disorder and panic attacks, while clonazepam is widely used for social phobia and panic disorder. Although very effective, the benzodiazepines have several major drawbacks. They all cause some sedation and so should be taken the first time before bedtime in a protected setting. After taking them for a while, you may need higher and higher doses to get the same effect. They cause physical and psychological dependence, especially with long-term use (more than three months) at high doses. Depending on the specific drug, its dose, and duration of use, you may experience withdrawal symptoms if you stop taking it abruptly. Instead, ask your doctor about gradually reducing the dose. Common withdrawal symptoms include anxiety, insomnia, irritability, muscle aches, nausea, depression, and fatigue. Rare symptoms include confusion, delirium, psychosis, and seizures. All benzodiazepines should not be used with alcohol. All of them cause anterograde amnesia (inability to incorporate new events into memory), difficulty concentrating, and unsteadiness (a particular problem for older people).
- **Buspirone.** A good alternative to the benzodiazepines is buspirone (BuSpar), particularly for generalized anxiety disorder. Unlike the benzodiazepines, it does not cause sedation, so people can drive while taking it. It is much less likely to cause addiction or withdrawal. However, it may take several weeks before it is effective. Buspirone also has antidepressant properties when taken in higher doses. It is a good choice if the person has both anxiety and depression.

- **Antidepressants.** Antidepressant medications are often the most effective treatment for obsessive-compulsive disorder and panic disorder. Clomipramine, fluoxetine, and fluvoxamine are the drugs of first choice for obsessive-compulsive disorder. The MAOIs, particularly phenelzine, are effective for panic attacks and social phobia. However, they are usually reserved for people who do not respond to the benzodiazepines or to other antidepressants because their use requires a special diet (see page 307). MAOIs also cause jitteriness, which may initially aggravate anxiety. Overall, the antidepressants are less addictive than the benzodiazepines, but they take longer to help relieve anxiety.
- **Beta-blockers.** Your doctor may prescribe beta-blockers because they block the chemical messengers epinephrine and norepinephrine, thereby diminishing the physical symptoms of danger, stress, or anxiety, such as racing heartbeat, sweating, and butterflies in the stomach. However, they have no effect on the psychological symptoms of anxiety. Beta-blockers, specifically propranolol, are used for mild social phobia or performance anxiety. A dose of propranolol one hour before a performance (public speaking, concert) can lessen the symptoms of anxiety. (For more about beta-blockers, see page 199.)

DRUGS FOR ANXIETY DISORDERS

antidepressants	chlordiazepoxide (Librium)
clomipramine	chlorazepate (Tranxene)
doxepin	clonazepam (Klonopin)
imipramine	diazepam (Valium)
fluoxetine	halazepam (Paxipam)
fluvoxamine	lorazepam (Ativan)
phenelzine	oxazepam (Serax)
trazodone	prazepam (Centrax)
benzodiazepines	beta-blockers (page 200)
alprazolam (Xanax)	buspirone (BuSpar)

Insomnia

Insomnia, or lack of sleep due to difficulty falling and staying asleep, is an extremely common problem. There are three basic types: difficulty falling asleep (more than 30 minutes), difficulty staying asleep, and early morning awakenings. Insomnia can be transient (lasting only a few days), short term (lasting up to three weeks), or chronic (lasting more than three weeks). It is the third most common medical complaint, following headaches and the common cold, and is particularly common among older people.

Chronic insomnia can be a symptom of a wide array of medical and psychiatric problems, including anxiety or depression; a side effect of a medication; or the result of poor sleep habits. There are also sleep disorders, such as restless leg syndrome and the breathing disorder sleep apnea, that require medical attention.

How do you know if you are getting enough sleep? The average sleep need is 8 hours, but the normal range is 5 to 10 hours a night. The best indication is how you feel during the day. If you sleep 6 hours and feel alert and well rested, then 6 hours is probably enough for you. If you feel constantly tired and lack energy or the ability to concentrate, then you probably need more sleep.

If your sleep problems are occasional or mild, try self-help techniques. If they are interfering with your life and well-being, though, talk with your doctor. Another source of help is an accredited sleep disorders clinic.

TREATMENT

When insomnia strikes, it may seem easiest to reach for a pill to help you fall asleep. But some sleeping medications are ineffective, and others addictive. The first step should be making some simple changes in your sleeping environment or schedule.

Self-help

- Probably the most important thing you can do is to go to bed and get up at the same time every day—even on weekends. This sets your body clock on a regular sleep-wake cycle.
- Don't nap during the day even if you are tired.

- Create a dark, quiet, comfortable place to sleep, and keep it the same every night.
- Exercising in the late afternoon or early evening promotes good sleep, but exercising within three hours of your bedtime can keep you awake.
- A light carbohydrate snack can help you sleep. If heartburn tends to keep you awake, skip the snack. No one should eat a heavy meal right before going to bed. A glass of warm milk or chamomile tea can be calming at bedtime. Limit yourself to one cup, though, or you may need to waken during the night to go to the bathroom.
- Limit alcohol consumption to no more than one drink a day. Don't have a nightcap—it will disturb your night's sleep. Some over-the-counter sleep aids contain alcohol. Check the label, and avoid these drugs.
- Avoid stimulants such as caffeine and tobacco in the evening. Be aware that many nonprescription remedies such as pain relievers and cold remedies contain caffeine—check the label.
- A warm bath before bedtime also helps.
- If stress and worries are contributing to your insomnia, try some stress-reduction techniques, or see your doctor or a therapist.

DRUGS THAT MAY CAUSE INSOMNIA

If you are having difficulty sleeping, the cause may be a drug or substance you are taking for another medical problem. If you are taking any of the following medications, ask your doctor if they could be interfering with your sleep.

alcohol	oral decongestants
amphetamines	levodopa
antidepressants (SSRIs only)	methylsergide
appetite suppressants	nicotine
caffeine	oral contraceptives
calcium channel blockers	theophylline
corticosteroids	thyroid replacement hormones

Medications

Nonprescription sleep aids and prescription hypnotics are among the most commonly used medications. Every year about 2 in 100 people receive a prescription for a drug to help them sleep, and 1 in 100 buys a nonprescription sleep aid. Drugs should not be the first line of treatment against sleeping problems, but when nondrug methods fail, an appropriate medication may help relieve short-term insomnia. Sleep medications are not a panacea and cannot be used over the long term. Many kinds of drugs lose their effectiveness when used every night for more than a couple of weeks, and others are habit forming. When the drug is discontinued, the insomnia may be worse than ever.

If insomnia is being caused by a breathing disorder that you may not know about, over-the-counter products can be dangerous. If you are having difficulty sleeping, see your doctor, who will want to determine whether another condition that can be treated may be causing your problem, and who can advise you on a choice of sleep medication if appropriate. The choice of treatment needs to be based on your age, type of insomnia (difficulty falling asleep, staying asleep, or early morning awakenings), other drugs you are taking for other conditions, and your lifestyle or work situation.

The drug people take most frequently to help them sleep is alcohol. While alcohol helps some people fall asleep, the sleep is often fitful. Alcohol may also cause wakefulness later in the night, often after only two or three hours of sleep. Nightly use of alcohol as a sleep aid also carries the risk of alcohol dependence. It is best not to use alcohol this way. Alcohol should never be combined with other sleep medications.

- **Antihistamines.** The two nonprescription drugs approved by the FDA as sleep aids are the antihistamines diphenhydramine (Compoz, Nytol, Sominex) and doxylamine (Unisom). Both are sedating, but they are not hypnotics. As a result, they may not cause a restful sleep. More than half of those who use these products have a residual, or "hangover," effect the next day. Although they are less effective than prescription hypnotics, they will not cause dependence. These products are most effective for people with occasional sleep problems rather than long-term insomnia. In

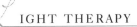

LIGHT THERAPY

Insomnia can be caused by a body clock that's out of sync with your sleep schedule. Exposure to bright daylight at midday can help keep your body clock on a normal sleep schedule. Go out for a noontime walk or sit by a bright window. If you tend to stay up too late and have trouble getting up in the morning, exposure to a couple of hours of bright light early in the morning can help set back your clock to an earlier sleep schedule. A long walk at the right time of day may be enough, but another option is light therapy using artificial lights. Ask your doctor to recommend someone trained in this treatment.

any case, they should not be used more than seven nights. They may cause a variety of side effects, including dry mouth and constipation. Antihistamines are not recommended for use by older people because they may lead to delirium and confusion. The symptoms of delirium are agitation and restlessness and sometimes hallucinations. Benzodiazepines are far safer for most older people.

- **Benzodiazepines.** These are the most common prescription drugs for insomnia. They have largely replaced barbiturates, which are more dangerous and more addictive. They can be useful for short-term or chronic sleep problems, particularly those associated with anxiety. Some benzodiazepines, such as triazolam and temazepam, induce sleep within 30 minutes to an hour, but they may not keep you asleep all night. Longer-acting drugs, such as flurazepam and quazepam, may be more effective if you suffer from difficulty staying asleep or from early morning awakening, but they may cause daytime grogginess. For many people, estazolam is the preferred drug because it induces sleep within two hours and acts through the night, but not into the following day. Although the benzodiazepines are very effective, they have several drawbacks. Long-term use may cause physical and psychological dependence. Also, you may need a progressively higher dose of the medication to get the same results. To prevent tolerance, the hypnotic benzodiazepines should be used "as needed"

MELATONIN

Melatonin, a popular alternative sleep aid, is a hormone normally manufactured by the body at night. It is sold in some drugstores as a natural supplement. Studies have suggested that small amounts of melatonin may help some people fall asleep faster. It may also shorten jet lag. However, it has not been approved by the FDA as a medication. Studies have not yet established the proper dosage, and because the manufacture is unregulated, the supplements sold in stores may not be pure. Adverse effects associated with the routine use of melatonin are not known.

rather than every night. After one good night of sleep, you should try to avoid using the hypnotic for the next one to two nights. To prevent withdrawal, these drugs should not be stopped abruptly but slowly tapered downward. Abruptly stopping a benzodiazepine hypnotic, particularly the short-acting agents, can lead to rebound insomnia. These drugs suppress the dream state during sleep, which can result in nightmares when they are discontinued. All benzodiazepines cause some degree of unsteadiness and difficulty incorporating new events into memory. In older people, short-acting or intermediate-acting agents such as temazepam and estazolam are preferred because they are rapidly removed from the body and do not cause residual effects in the morning.

- **Zolpidem.** Zolpidem (Ambien) is a newer, short-acting drug that induces sleep in one to two hours and is not likely to cause sedation during the daytime. Zolpidem can cause physical and psychological dependence. It may be less likely to cause tolerance (need for a larger dosage to get the same effect) than the benzodiazepines. Unlike the benzodiazepines, it may cause side effects of nausea and diarrhea. Zolpidem can cause confusion, which may increase the likelihood of falls, especially in older people. It should be used for no more than 7 to 10 days for short-term management of insomnia. Do not drink alcohol while taking this medication.

- **Antidepressants.** Antidepressants are sometimes prescribed in low doses as a sedative. The tricyclic antidepressants (page 306), such as amitriptyline (Elavil), trazodone, and doxepin, are among the most effective. Because they are not addictive, they can be taken over the long term. They also do not produce the rebound insomnia that many sleep medications cause when they wear off. These agents are usually the best choice if insomnia is chronic, related to depression, or resistant to the benzodiazepines or zolpidem. Antidepressants prescribed for insomnia may cause some side effects including dry mouth or morning grogginess. (For more on antidepressants, see page 305.)

DRUGS TO TREAT INSOMNIA

antihistamines
  diphenhydramine (Compoz, Nytol, Sominex)
  doxylamine (Unisom)
benzodiazepines
  estazolam (ProSom)

flurazepam (Dalmane)
quazepam (Doral)
temazepam (Restoril)
triazolam (Halcion)
zolpidem (Ambien)
antidepressants

the drug profiles

$\mathcal{A}$CE INHIBITORS (ORAL)

Including Benazepril; Captopril; Enalapril; Fosinopril; Lisinopril; Quinapril; Ramipril

ABOUT YOUR MEDICINE

ACE inhibitors are used to treat high blood pressure (hypertension). Captopril is used in some patients after a heart attack to help slow down the further weakening of the heart. Captopril is also used to treat kidney problems in some diabetic patients who use insulin to control their diabetes. In addition, some ACE inhibitors are also used to treat congestive heart failure. These medicines may also be used for other conditions as determined by your doctor.

If any of the information in this profile causes you special concern or if you want additional information about your medicine and its use, check with your doctor, nurse, or pharmacist. **Remember, keep this and all other medicines out of the reach of children and never share your medicines with others.**

BEFORE USING THIS MEDICINE

Tell your doctor, nurse, and pharmacist if you . . .
- are allergic to any medicine, either prescription or nonprescription (OTC);
- **are pregnant or intend to become pregnant while using this medicine;**
- are breast-feeding;
- are taking any other prescription or nonprescription (OTC) medicine, especially diuretics (water pills) or potassium-containing medicines or supplements;
- have any other medical problems, especially heart or blood vessel disease or kidney disease;
- are on a strict low-sodium diet or dialysis, or use low-salt milk or salt substitutes;
- have had a kidney transplant.

PROPER USE OF THIS MEDICINE

Even if you feel well and do not notice any signs of your medical problem, **take this medicine exactly as directed.**

For patients taking captopril:
- This medicine is best taken on an empty stomach 1 hour before meals, unless you are otherwise directed by your doctor.

For patients taking this medicine for high blood pressure:
- This medicine will not cure your high blood pressure, but it does help control it. You must continue to take it—even if you feel well—if you expect to keep your blood pressure down. **You may have to take high blood pressure medicine for the rest of your life.**

If you miss a dose of this medicine, take it as soon as possible. However, if it is almost time for your next dose, skip the missed dose and go back to your regular dosing schedule. Do not double doses.

Precautions While Using This Medicine

If you think that you may have become pregnant, check with your doctor immediately. Use of this medicine, especially during the second and third trimesters (after the first three months) of pregnancy, may cause serious injury or even death to the unborn child.

Check with your doctor if you become sick while taking this medicine, especially with severe or continuing vomiting or diarrhea. These conditions may cause you to lose too much water, possibly causing low blood pressure.

Dizziness, lightheadedness, or fainting may occur after the first dose, especially if you have been taking a diuretic (water pill). Make sure you know how you react to this medicine before you drive, use machines, or do other jobs that require you to be alert and clearheaded.

Avoid alcoholic beverages until you have discussed their use with your doctor. Alcohol may increase the low blood pressure effect and the possibility of dizziness and fainting.

Possible Side Effects of This Medicine

Side effects that should be reported to your doctor immediately
> RARE—Fever and chills; hoarseness; swelling of face, mouth, hands, or feet; trouble in swallowing or breathing (sudden); stomach pain, itching of skin, or yellow eyes or skin

Other side effects that should be reported to your doctor
> LESS COMMON—Dizziness, lightheadedness, or fainting; skin rash, with or without itching, fever, or joint pain
> RARE—Chest pain; fever, nausea, stomach bloating, stomach pain, or vomiting
> SIGNS OF TOO MUCH POTASSIUM IN THE BODY—Confusion; irregular heartbeat; nervousness; numbness or tingling in hands, feet, or lips; shortness of breath or difficulty breathing; weakness or heaviness of legs

Side effects that usually do not require medical attention
> These possible side effects may go away during treatment; however, if they continue or are bothersome, check with your doctor, nurse, or pharmacist.

> MORE COMMON—Cough (dry)
> LESS COMMON—Diarrhea; headache; loss of taste; nausea; unusual tiredness

> Other side effects not listed above may also occur in some patients. If you notice any other effects, check with your doctor, nurse, or pharmacist.

$\mathscr{A}$CE INHIBITORS AND HYDROCHLOROTHIAZIDE (ORAL)

Including Captopril and Hydrochlorothiazide; Enalapril and Hydrochlorothiazide; Lisinopril and Hydrochlorothiazide

ABOUT YOUR MEDICINE

ACE inhibitors and **hydrochlorothiazide** combinations are used to treat high blood pressure (hypertension). They may also be used for other conditions as determined by your doctor.

If any of the information in this profile causes you special concern or if you want additional information about your medicine and its use, check with your doctor, nurse, or pharmacist. **Remember, keep this and all other medicines out of the reach of children and never share your medicines with others.**

BEFORE USING THIS MEDICINE

Children and infants may be especially sensitive to the blood pressure–lowering effect of ACE inhibitors. **Discuss with the child's doctor the possible side effects that may be caused by this medicine.** Some of them may be serious.

Tell your doctor, nurse, and pharmacist if you . . .
- are allergic to any medicine, either prescription or nonprescription (OTC);
- are pregnant or intend to become pregnant while using this medicine;
- are breast-feeding;
- are taking any other prescription or nonprescription (OTC) medicine, especially cholestyramine, colestipol, digitalis glycosides (heart medicine), diuretics (water pills), lithium, potassium-containing medicines or supplements, or salt substitutes or low-salt milk;
- have any other medical problems, especially kidney disease;
- are on a strict low-sodium diet or dialysis;
- have had a kidney transplant.

PROPER USE OF THIS MEDICINE

Even if you feel well and do not notice any signs of your medical problem, **take this medicine exactly as directed.**

For patients taking this medicine for high blood pressure:
- This medicine will not cure your high blood pressure, but it does help control it. You must continue to take it—even if you feel well—if you expect to keep your blood pressure down. **You may have to take high blood pressure medicine for the rest of your life.**

If you miss a dose of this medicine, take it as soon as possible. However, if it is almost time for your next dose, skip the missed dose and go back to your regular dosing schedule. Do not double doses.

PRECAUTIONS WHILE USING THIS MEDICINE

If you think that you may have become pregnant, check with your doctor immediately. Use of this medicine, especially during the second and third trimesters (after the first three months) of pregnancy, may cause serious injury or even death to the unborn child.

Dizziness or lightheadedness may occur, especially after the first dose of this medicine. Make sure you know how you react to the medicine before you drive, use machines, or do other things that require you to be alert and clearheaded.

Check with your doctor if you become sick while taking this medicine, especially with severe or continuing vomiting or diarrhea. These conditions may cause you to lose too much water and lead to low blood pressure.

Dizziness, lightheadedness, or fainting may occur if you exercise or if the weather is hot. Use extra care during exercise or hot weather.

Avoid alcoholic beverages until you have discussed their use with your doctor. Alcohol may increase the low blood pressure effect and the possibility of dizziness and fainting.

POSSIBLE SIDE EFFECTS OF THIS MEDICINE

Side effects that should be reported to your doctor immediately
> RARE—Fever and chills; hoarseness; swelling of face, mouth, hands, or feet; trouble in swallowing or breathing (sudden)

Other side effects that should be reported to your doctor
> LESS COMMON—Dizziness, lightheadedness, or fainting; skin rash, with or without itching, fever, or joint pain
> RARE—Chest pain; joint pain; lower back or side pain; severe stomach pain with nausea and vomiting; unusual bleeding or bruising; yellow eyes or skin
> SIGNS OF TOO MUCH OR TOO LITTLE POTASSIUM IN THE BODY—Dryness of mouth; increased thirst; irregular heartbeats; mood or mental changes; muscle cramps or pain; numbness or tingling in hands, feet, or lips; weakness or heaviness of legs; weak pulse

Side effects that usually do not require medical attention
> These possible side effects may go away during treatment; however, if they continue or are bothersome, check with your doctor, nurse, or pharmacist.

> MORE COMMON—Cough (dry, continuing)
> LESS COMMON—Diarrhea; headache; increased sensitivity of skin to sunlight; loss of appetite; loss of taste; stomach upset; unusual tiredness

> Other side effects not listed above may also occur in some patients. If you notice any other effects, check with your doctor, nurse, or pharmacist.

$\mathscr{A}$CETAMINOPHEN (ORAL)

Including Acetaminophen; Acetaminophen and Caffeine

ABOUT YOUR MEDICINE

Acetaminophen (a-seat-a-MIN-oh-fen) is used to relieve pain and reduce fever. Unlike aspirin, it does not relieve the redness, stiffness, or swelling caused by rheumatoid arthritis. However, it may relieve pain caused by mild forms of arthritis.

If any of the information in this profile causes you special concern or if you want additional information about your medicine and its use, check with your doctor, nurse, or pharmacist. **Remember, keep this and all other medicines out of the reach of children and never share your medicines with others.**

BEFORE USING THIS MEDICINE

If you are taking this medicine without a prescription, carefully read and follow any precautions on the label. You should be especially careful if you . . .
- are allergic to any medicine, either prescription or nonprescription (OTC);
- are pregnant, intend to become pregnant, or are breast-feeding;
- are taking any other prescription or nonprescription (OTC) medicine;
- have any other medical problems, especially alcohol abuse, kidney disease, or hepatitis or other liver disease.

If you have any questions, check with your doctor, nurse, or pharmacist.

PROPER USE OF THIS MEDICINE

Unless otherwise directed by your medical doctor or dentist:
- **Do not take more of this medicine than is recommended on the package label.** If too much is taken, liver and kidney damage may occur.
- **Children up to 12 years of age should not take this medicine more than 5 times a day.**

PRECAUTIONS WHILE USING THIS MEDICINE

Check the labels of all prescription and non-prescription (over-the-counter [OTC]) medicines you now take. If any contain acetaminophen, check with your doctor or pharmacist. Taking them together with this medicine may cause an overdose.

If you will be taking more than an occasional 1 or 2 doses of acetaminophen, do not drink alcoholic beverages. To do so may increase the chance of liver damage, especially if you drink large amounts of alcoholic beverages regularly, or if you take more acetaminophen than is recommended on the package label.

Acetaminophen may interfere with the results of some medical tests. Before you have any medical tests, tell the person in charge if you have taken acetaminophen within the past 3 or 4 days. If possible, it is best to call the laboratory where the test will be done about 4 days ahead of time, to find out whether this medicine may be taken during the 3 or 4 days before the test.

For diabetic patients:

- Acetaminophen may cause false results with some blood glucose (sugar) tests. If you notice any change in your test results, or if you have any questions about this possible problem, check with your doctor, nurse, or pharmacist. This is especially important if your diabetes is not well-controlled.

For patients taking one of the products that contain caffeine in addition to acetaminophen:

- Caffeine may interfere with the results of a test that uses adenosine or dipyridamole to help find out how well your blood is flowing through certain blood vessels. Therefore, you should not have any caffeine for at least 8 to 12 hours before the test.

If you think that you or anyone else may have taken an overdose of acetaminophen, get emergency help at once, even if there are no signs of poisoning. Signs of severe poisoning may not appear for 2 to 4 days after the overdose is taken, but treatment to prevent liver damage or death must be started as soon as possible. Treatment started more than 24 hours after the overdose is taken may not be effective.

POSSIBLE SIDE EFFECTS OF THIS MEDICINE

Side effects that should be reported to your doctor immediately
   RARE—Yellow eyes or skin

Other side effects that should be reported to your doctor
   RARE—Bloody or black, tarry stools; bloody or cloudy urine; fever, chills, or sore throat (not present before being treated and not caused by the condition being treated); pain in lower back and/or side (severe and/or sharp); pinpoint red spots on skin; skin rash, hives, or itching; sores, ulcers, or white spots on lips or in mouth; sudden decrease in amount of urine; unusual bleeding or bruising; unusual tiredness or weakness

   Other side effects not listed above may also occur in some patients. If you notice any other effects, check with your doctor, nurse, or pharmacist.

*A*CYCLOVIR (ORAL)

ABOUT YOUR MEDICINE

Acyclovir (ay-SYE-kloe-veer) is used to prevent and treat the symptoms of herpes virus infections of the genitals (sex organs). It is also used to treat chickenpox and shingles. Although acyclovir will not cure herpes, it does help relieve the pain and discomfort and helps the sores (if any) heal faster. Acyclovir may also be used for other virus infections as determined by your doctor. However, it does not work in treating certain viruses, such as the common cold.

If any of the information in this profile causes you special concern or if you want additional information about your medicine and its use, check with your doctor, nurse, or pharmacist. **Remember, keep this and all other medicines out of the reach of children and never share your medicines with others.**

BEFORE USING THIS MEDICINE

Tell your doctor, nurse, and pharmacist if you . . .
* are allergic to any medicine, either prescription or nonprescription (OTC);
* are pregnant or intend to become pregnant while using this medicine;
* are breast-feeding;
* are taking any other prescription or nonprescription (OTC) medicine, especially inflammation or pain medicine, except narcotics;
* have any other medical problems.

PROPER USE OF THIS MEDICINE

Acyclovir is best used as soon as possible after the symptoms of herpes infection (for example, pain, burning, blisters) begin to appear.

Acyclovir is best taken with a full glass (8 ounces) of water.

Acyclovir capsules, tablets and oral suspension may be taken with meals.

For patients taking acyclovir for the treatment of chickenpox:
* Start using acyclovir as soon as possible after the first sign of the chickenpox rash, usually within one day.

For patients using acyclovir oral suspension:
* Use a specially marked measuring spoon or other device to measure each dose accurately. The average household teaspoon may not hold the right amount of liquid.

Do not use after the expiration date on the label. The medicine may not work as well. Check with your pharmacist if you have any questions about this.

To help clear up your herpes infection, **keep taking acyclovir for the full time of treatment,** even if your symptoms begin to clear up after a few days. **Do not miss any doses.** However, **do not use this medicine more often or for a longer time than your doctor ordered.**

If you do miss a dose of this medicine, take it as soon as possible. However, if it is almost time for your next dose, skip the missed dose and go back to your regular dosing schedule. Do not double doses.

PRECAUTIONS WHILE USING THIS MEDICINE

If your symptoms do not improve within a few days, or if they become worse, check with your doctor.

The areas affected by herpes should be kept as clean and dry as possible. Also, wear loose-fitting clothing to avoid irritating the sores (blisters).

It is important to remember that acyclovir will not keep you from spreading herpes to others.

For patients taking acyclovir for genital herpes:
- **Women with genital herpes may be more likely to get cancer of the cervix (opening to the womb).** Therefore, it is very important that Pap tests be taken at least once a year to check for cancer. Cervical cancer can be cured if found and treated early.
- Herpes infection of the genitals can be caught from or spread to your partner during any sexual activity. Even though you may get herpes if your partner has no symptoms, the infection is more likely to be spread if sores are present. This is true until the sores are completely healed and the scabs have fallen off. **Therefore, it is best to avoid any sexual activity if either you or your sexual partner has any symptoms of herpes.** The use of a latex condom ('rubber') may help prevent the spread of herpes. However, spermicidal (sperm-killing) jelly or a diaphragm will probably not help.

This medicine must not be given to other people or used for other infections unless you are otherwise directed by your doctor.

POSSIBLE SIDE EFFECTS OF THIS MEDICINE

Side effects that usually do not require medical attention

These possible side effects may go away during treatment; however, if they continue or are bothersome, check with your doctor, nurse, or pharmacist.

LESS COMMON (ESPECIALLY SEEN WITH LONG-TERM USE OR HIGH DOSES) —
Diarrhea; headache; lightheadedness; nausea or vomiting

Other side effects not listed above may also occur in some patients. If you notice any other effects, check with your doctor, nurse, or pharmacist.

$\mathcal{A}$CYCLOVIR (TOPICAL)

ABOUT YOUR MEDICINE

Topical acyclovir (ay-SYE-kloe-veer) is used to treat the symptoms of herpes virus infections of genitals (sex organs) and mucous membranes (fever blisters, oral herpes). Although topical acyclovir will not cure herpes, it may help relieve the pain and discomfort and may help the sores (if any) heal faster.

If any of the information in this profile causes you special concern or if you want additional information about your medicine and its use, check with your doctor, nurse, or pharmacist. **Remember, keep this and all other medicines out of the reach of children and never share your medicines with others.**

BEFORE USING THIS MEDICINE

Tell your doctor, nurse, and pharmacist if you . . .
- are allergic to any medicine, either prescription or nonprescription (OTC);
- are pregnant or intend to become pregnant while using this medicine;
- are breast-feeding;
- are taking any other prescription or nonprescription (OTC) medicine;
- have any other medical problems.

PROPER USE OF THIS MEDICINE

Acyclovir may come with patient information about herpes simplex infections. Read this information carefully. If you have any questions, check with your doctor, nurse, or pharmacist.

Do not use this medicine in the eyes.

Acyclovir is best used as soon as possible after the symptoms of herpes infection (for example, pain, burning, blisters) begin to appear.

Use a finger cot or rubber glove when applying this medicine. This will help keep you from spreading the infection to other areas of your body. Apply enough medicine to completely cover all the sores (blisters). A 1.25–cm (approximately 1/2-inch) strip of ointment applied to each area of the affected skin measuring 5 × 5 cm (approximately 2 × 2 inches) is usually enough, unless otherwise directed by your doctor.

To help clear up your herpes infection, **continue using acyclovir for the full time of treatment,** even if your symptoms begin to clear up after a few days. **Do not miss any doses.** However, **do not use this medicine more often or for a longer time than your doctor ordered.**

If you do miss a dose of this medicine, apply it as soon as possible. However, if it is almost time for your next dose, skip the missed dose and go back to your regular dosing schedule.

PRECAUTIONS WHILE USING THIS MEDICINE

If your symptoms do not improve within 1 week, or if they become worse, check with your doctor.

It is important to remember that acyclovir will not keep you from spreading herpes to others.

For patients using acyclovir for genital herpes:
- **Women with genital herpes may be more likely to get cancer of the cervix (opening to the womb).** Therefore, it is very important that Pap tests be taken at least once a year to check for cancer. Cervical cancer can be cured if found and treated early.
- The areas affected by herpes should be kept as clean and dry as possible. Also, wear loose-fitting clothing to avoid irritating the sores (blisters).
- Herpes infection of the genitals can be caught from or spread to your partner during any sexual activity. Even though you may get herpes if your partner has no symptoms, the infection is more likely to be spread if sores are present. This is true until the sores are completely healed and the scabs have fallen off. **Therefore, it is best to avoid any sexual activity if either you or your sexual partner has any symptoms of herpes.** The use of a latex condom ('rubber') may help prevent the spread of herpes. However, spermicidal (sperm-killing) jelly or a diaphragm will probably not help.

This medicine must not be given to other people or used for other infections unless you are otherwise directed by your doctor.

POSSIBLE SIDE EFFECTS OF THIS MEDICINE

Side effects that usually do not require medical attention
These possible side effects may go away during treatment; however, if they continue or are bothersome, check with your doctor, nurse, or pharmacist.

MORE COMMON—Mild pain, burning, or stinging
LESS COMMON OR RARE—Itching; skin rash

Other side effects not listed above may also occur in some patients. If you notice any other effects, check with your doctor, nurse, or pharmacist.

Adrenergic Bronchodilators (Inhalation)

Including Albuterol; Bitolterol;
Epinephrine; Fenoterol; Isoetharine; Isoproterenol;
Metaproterenol; Pirbuterol; Procaterol; Racepinephrine; Terbutaline

About Your Medicine

Adrenergic bronchodilators are taken by oral inhalation to treat the symptoms of bronchial asthma, chronic bronchitis, emphysema, and other lung diseases. These medicines relieve cough, wheezing, shortness of breath, and troubled breathing.

If any of the information in this profile causes you special concern or if you want additional information about your medicine and its use, check with your doctor, nurse, or pharmacist. **Remember, keep this and all other medicines out of the reach of children and never share your medicines with others.**

Before Using This Medicine

If you are using this medicine without a prescription, carefully read and follow any precautions on the label. You should be especially careful if you . . .
- are allergic to any medicine, either prescription or nonprescription (OTC);
- are pregnant, intend to become pregnant, or are breast-feeding;
- are taking **any** other prescription or nonprescription (OTC) medicine;
- have **any** other medical problems;
- are now using or have used cocaine.

If you have any questions, check with your doctor, nurse, or pharmacist.

Proper Use of This Medicine

For patients using epinephrine, isoetharine, isoproterenol, or racepinephrine:
- Do not use if the solution becomes cloudy or turns pinkish to brownish in color.

Some epinephrine preparations are available without a doctor's prescription. However, **do not use this medicine without a doctor's prescription, unless your medical problem has been diagnosed as asthma by a doctor.**

Some of these preparations may come with patient directions. Read them carefully before using this medicine.

Use this medicine only as directed. Do not use more of it and do not use it more often than recommended.

For patients using the inhalation aerosol form of this medicine:
- **Keep spray away from the eyes because it may cause irritation.**
- **Do not take more than 2 inhalations of this medicine at any one time,**

unless otherwise directed by your doctor. Allow 1 to 2 minutes after the first inhalation to make certain that a second inhalation is necessary.

- Save your applicator. Refill units may be available.
- Store away from heat and direct sunlight. Do not puncture, break, or burn container, even if it is empty.

If you are using this medicine regularly and you miss a dose, use it as soon as possible. Then use any remaining doses for that day at regularly spaced intervals. Do not double doses.

PRECAUTIONS WHILE USING THIS MEDICINE

If you still have trouble breathing after using this medicine, or if your condition becomes worse, check with your doctor at once.

If you are using the inhalation aerosol form of this medicine and you are also using a corticosteroid or ipratropium inhaler to help you breathe better, allow 5 minutes between using this medicine and the corticosteroid or ipratropium, unless otherwise directed.

POSSIBLE SIDE EFFECTS OF THIS MEDICINE

Side effects that should be reported to your doctor immediately
Bluish coloration of skin; dizziness (severe) or feeling faint; flushing or redness of face or skin (continuing); increased wheezing or difficulty in breathing; skin rash, hives, or itching; swelling of face, lips, or eyelids

Other side effects that should be reported to your doctor
RARE—Chest discomfort or pain; irregular heartbeat; numbness in hands or feet; unusual bruising
WITH HIGH DOSES—Hallucinations
POSSIBLE SIGNS OF OVERDOSE—Dizziness (severe); fast, slow, irregular, or pounding heartbeat (continuing); headache (continuing or severe); increase or decrease in blood pressure (severe); nausea or vomiting (continuing or severe); weakness (severe)

Side effects that usually do not require medical attention
These possible side effects may go away during treatment; however, if they continue or are bothersome, check with your doctor, nurse, or pharmacist.

MORE COMMON—Nervousness or restlessness; trembling
LESS COMMON—Coughing or other bronchial irritation; dizziness or lightheadedness; dryness or irritation of mouth or throat; headache; increased sweating; nausea or vomiting; trouble in sleeping; weakness

While you are using some of these medicines, you may notice an unusual or unpleasant taste. Also, pirbuterol may cause changes in smell or taste and isoproterenol may cause the saliva to turn pinkish to red. These effects may be expected and will go away when you stop using the medicine.

Other side effects not listed above may also occur in some patients. If you notice any other effects, check with your doctor, nurse, or pharmacist.

ALENDRONATE (ORAL)*

ABOUT YOUR MEDICINE

Alendronate (a-LEN-dro-nate) is used to treat osteoporosis (thinning of the bone) in women after menopause. It may also be used to treat Paget's disease of bone.

If any of the information in this profile causes you special concern or if you want additional information about your medicine and its use, check with your doctor, nurse, or pharmacist. **Remember, keep this and all other medicines out of the reach of children and never share your medicines with others.**

BEFORE USING THIS MEDICINE

Tell your doctor, nurse, and pharmacist if you . . .
- are allergic to any medicine, either prescription or nonprescription (OTC);
- are pregnant or intend to become pregnant while using this medicine;
- are breast feeding;
- are taking any other prescription or nonprescription (OTC) medicine;
- have any other medical problems, especially hypocalcemia (low blood levels of calcium) or kidney problems.

PROPER USE OF THIS MEDICINE

Take alendronate with a full glass (6 to 8 ounces) of plain water on an empty stomach. It should be taken in the morning at least 30 minutes before any food, beverage, or other medicines. Food and beverages such as mineral water, coffee, tea, or juice will decrease the amount of alendronate absorbed by the body. Medicines such as antacids or calcium or vitamin supplements will also decrease the absorption of alendronate.

Do not lie down for 30 minutes after taking alendronate. This will help prevent irritation to your esophagus.

Your doctor may recommend that you eat a balanced diet with an adequate amount of calcium and vitamin D (found in milk or other dairy products). However, do not

*This profile has been developed by the USP based primarily on labeling provided by the manufacturer at the time of its approval. This information is intended for use as a temporary educational aid until the drug has been assessed by USP advisory panels. The information does not cover all possible uses, actions, precautions, side effects, or interactions of this medicine. It is not intended as medical advice for individual problems.

take any food, beverages, or calcium or vitamin supplements within 30 minutes of taking alendronate. To do so may keep this medicine from working properly.

If you miss a dose of this medicine, do not take the missed dose at all and do not double the next one. Instead, go back to your regular dosing schedule.

POSSIBLE SIDE EFFECTS OF THIS MEDICINE

Side effects that should be reported to your doctor
> MORE COMMON—Abdominal pain
> LESS COMMON—Bone or muscle pain; nausea; vomiting
> RARE—Skin rash

Side effects that usually do not require medical attention
> These possible side effects may go away during treatment; however, if they continue or are bothersome, check with your doctor, nurse, or pharmacist.
>
> LESS COMMON—Altered sense of taste; constipation; diarrhea; difficulty swallowing; full or bloated feeling in the stomach; gas; headache; heartburn; irritation or pain of the esophagus

Other side effects not listed above may also occur in some patients. If you notice any other effects, check with your doctor, nurse, or pharmacist.

$\mathcal{A}$LLOPURINOL (ORAL)

ABOUT YOUR MEDICINE

Allopurinol (al-oh-PURE-i-nole) is used to treat chronic gout. It helps to prevent gout attacks, but will not relieve an attack that has already started. Allopurinol is also used to prevent or treat medical problems caused by too much uric acid in the body, including certain kinds of kidney stones or other kidney problems.

If any of the information in this profile causes you special concern or if you want additional information about your medicine and its use, check with your doctor, nurse, or pharmacist. **Remember, keep this and all other medicines out of the reach of children and never share your medicines with others.**

BEFORE USING THIS MEDICINE

Tell your doctor, nurse, and pharmacist if you . . .
- are allergic to any medicine, either prescription or nonprescription (OTC);
- are pregnant or intend to become pregnant while using this medicine;
- are breast-feeding;

- are taking any other prescription or nonprescription (OTC) medicine, especially anticoagulants, azathioprine, or mercaptopurine;
- have any other medical problems, especially diabetes mellitus (sugar diabetes), high blood pressure, or kidney disease.

PROPER USE OF THIS MEDICINE

If this medicine upsets your stomach, take it after meals. If stomach upset (nausea, vomiting, diarrhea, or stomach pain) continues, check with your doctor.

In order for this medicine to help you, it must be taken regularly as ordered.

If you are taking allopurinol to prevent gout attacks and they continue, **keep taking this medicine, even if you are taking another medicine for the attacks.**

To help prevent kidney stones while taking allopurinol, adults should drink at least 10 to 12 full glasses (8 ounces each) of fluids each day unless otherwise directed by their doctor. Check with your doctor about the amount of fluids to be taken each day by children being treated with this medicine. Also, your doctor may want you to take another medicine to make your urine less acid.

If you miss a dose of this medicine, take it as soon as possible. However, if it is almost time for your next dose, skip the missed dose and go back to your regular dosing schedule. Do not double doses.

PRECAUTIONS WHILE USING THIS MEDICINE

Drinking too much alcohol may increase the amount of uric acid in the blood and lessen the effects of allopurinol. Therefore, people with gout and other people with too much uric acid in the body should be careful to limit the amount of alcohol they drink.

Check with your doctor immediately if you notice a skin rash, hives, or itching while taking allopurinol or if chills, fever, joint pain, muscle aches or pains, sore throat, or nausea or vomiting occur, especially if they occur together with or shortly after a skin rash. Very rarely, these effects may be the first signs of a serious reaction to the medicine.

This medicine may cause some people to become drowsy or less alert than they are normally. **Make sure you know how you react to this medicine before you drive, use machines, or do other jobs that require you to be alert.**

POSSIBLE SIDE EFFECTS OF THIS MEDICINE

Side effects that should be reported to your doctor immediately

Stop taking this medicine and check with your doctor immediately if you notice:

MORE COMMON—Skin rash or sores, hives, or itching

RARE—Black, tarry stools; bleeding sores on lips; blood in urine or stools; chills, fever, muscle aches or pains, nausea, or vomiting, especially if occurring with or shortly after a skin rash; difficult or painful urination; pinpoint red spots on skin; red and/or irritated eyes; redness, tenderness, burning, or peeling of skin; red, thickened, or scaly skin; shortness of breath, troubled breathing, tightness in chest, or wheezing; sores, ulcers, or white spots in mouth or on lips; sore throat and fever; sudden decrease in urine; swelling in upper abdominal (stomach) area; swelling of face, feet, fingers, or lower legs; swollen and/or painful glands; unusual bleeding or bruising; unusual tiredness or weakness; weight gain (rapid); yellow eyes or skin

Other side effects that should be reported to your doctor

RARE—Loosening of fingernails; numbness, tingling, pain, or weakness in hands or feet; pain in lower back or side; unexplained nosebleeds

Other side effects not listed above may also occur in some patients. If you notice any other effects, check with your doctor, nurse, or pharmacist.

ALPHA₁-BLOCKERS (ORAL)

Including Doxazosin; Prazosin; Terazosin

ABOUT YOUR MEDICINE

Alpha₁-blockers are used to treat high blood pressure (hypertension). Doxazosin and terazosin are also used to treat benign enlargement of the prostate (benign prostatic hyperplasia [BPH]). These medicines may also be used for other conditions as determined by your doctor.

If any of the information in this profile causes you special concern or if you want additional information about your medicine and its use, check with your doctor, nurse, or pharmacist. **Remember, keep this and all other medicines out of the reach of children and never share your medicines with others.**

BEFORE USING THIS MEDICINE

Tell your doctor, nurse, and pharmacist if you . . .
- are allergic to any medicine, either prescription or nonprescription (OTC);
- are pregnant or intend to become pregnant while using this medicine;
- are breast-feeding;
- are taking any other prescription or nonprescription (OTC) medicine, especially medicines for appetite control, asthma, colds, cough, hay fever, or sinus;
- have any other medical problems, especially heart disease.

PROPER USE OF THIS MEDICINE

For patients taking this medicine for high blood pressure:
- This medicine will not cure your high blood pressure but it does help control it. You must continue to take it—even if you feel well—if you expect to keep your blood pressure down. **You may have to take high blood pressure medicine for the rest of your life.**

For patients taking doxazosin or terazosin for benign enlargement of the prostate:
- Remember that this medicine will not shrink the size of your prostate, but it does help to relieve the symptoms.
- It may take up to 6 weeks before your symptoms get better.

If you miss a dose of this medicine, take it as soon as possible. However, if it is almost time for your next dose, skip the missed dose and go back to your regular dosing schedule. Do not double doses.

PRECAUTIONS WHILE USING THIS MEDICINE

Dizziness, lightheadedness, or sudden fainting may occur after you take this medicine, especially when you get up from a sitting or lying position. These effects are more likely to occur when you take the first dose of this medicine. Taking the first dose at bedtime may prevent problems. However, **be especially careful if you need to get up during the night.** These effects may also occur with any doses you take after the first dose. Getting up slowly may help lessen this problem. **If you feel dizzy, lie down so that you do not faint.** Then sit for a few minutes before standing to prevent the dizziness from returning.

The dizziness, lightheadedness, or fainting is more likely to occur if you drink alcohol, stand for long periods of time, exercise, or if the weather is hot. **While you are taking this medicine, be careful to limit the amount of alcohol you drink. Also, use extra care during exercise or hot weather or if you must stand for long periods of time.**

This medicine may cause some people to become drowsy or less alert than they are normally. **Make sure you know how you react to this medicine before you drive, use machines, or do other jobs that could be dangerous if you are dizzy, drowsy, or are not alert.** After you have taken several doses of this medicine, these effects should lessen.

POSSIBLE SIDE EFFECTS OF THIS MEDICINE

The following side effects may occur more or less often than listed, depending on which medicine you are taking.

Side effects that should be reported to your doctor
LESS COMMON—Dizziness; dizziness or lightheadedness when standing up; fainting (sudden); fast, irregular, or pounding heartbeat; loss of bladder control (prazosin only); shortness of breath; swelling of feet or lower legs

RARE—Chest pain; continuing, painful, inappropriate erection of the penis (prazosin only); shortness of breath (prazosin only)

Side effects that usually do not require medical attention

These possible side effects may go away during treatment; however, if they continue or are bothersome, check with your doctor, nurse, or pharmacist.

MORE COMMON—Drowsiness; headache; unusual tiredness or weakness

LESS COMMON—Dryness of mouth (prazosin only); nausea; nervousness (doxazosin and prazosin only)

FOR DOXAZOSIN ONLY (IN ADDITION TO THOSE LISTED ABOVE)—Restlessness; runny nose; unusual irritability

FOR PRAZOSIN ONLY—RARE (IN ADDITION TO THOSE LISTED ABOVE)— Frequent urge to urinate

FOR TERAZOSIN ONLY (IN ADDITION TO THOSE LISTED ABOVE)—Back or joint pain; blurred vision; stuffy nose

Other side effects not listed above may also occur in some patients. If you notice any other effects, check with your doctor, nurse, or pharmacist.

ᴀMIODARONE (ORAL)

ABOUT YOUR MEDICINE

Amiodarone (am-ee-OH-da-rone) is an antiarrhythmic. It is used to correct irregular heartbeats to a normal rhythm.

If any of the information in this profile causes you special concern or if you want additional information about your medicine and its use, check with your doctor, nurse, or pharmacist. **Remember, keep this and all other medicines out of the reach of children and never share your medicines with others.**

BEFORE USING THIS MEDICINE

Tell your doctor, nurse, and pharmacist if you . . .
- are allergic to any medicine, either prescription or nonprescription (OTC);
- are pregnant or intend to become pregnant while using this medicine;
- are breast-feeding;
- are taking any other prescription or nonprescription (OTC) medicine, especially anticoagulants, other heart medicine, or phenytoin;
- have any other medical problems.

PROPER USE OF THIS MEDICINE

Take amiodarone exactly as directed by your doctor even though you may feel well. Do not take more medicine than ordered and do not miss any doses.

If you do miss a dose of this medicine, do not take the missed dose at all and do not double the next one. Instead, go back to your regular dosing schedule. If you miss two or more doses in a row, check with your doctor.

PRECAUTIONS WHILE USING THIS MEDICINE

It is important that your doctor check your progress at regular visits to make sure the medicine is working properly.

Your doctor may want you to carry a medical identification card or bracelet stating that you are taking this medicine.

Before having any kind of surgery or dental or emergency treatment, tell the physician or dentist in charge that you are taking this medicine.

Amiodarone increases the sensitivity of your skin to sunlight; too much exposure could cause a serious burn. Your skin may continue to be sensitive to sunlight for several months after treatment with this medicine is stopped. A burn can occur even through window glass or thin cotton clothing. If you must go out in the sunlight, **cover your skin and wear a wide-brimmed hat. A special sun-blocking cream should also be used**; it must contain zinc or titanium oxide because other sunscreens will not work. **In case of a severe burn, check with your doctor.**

After you have taken this medicine for a long time, it may cause a blue-gray color to appear on your skin, especially in areas exposed to the sun, such as your face, neck, and arms. This color will usually fade after treatment with amiodarone has ended, although it may take several months. However, check with your doctor if this effect occurs.

POSSIBLE SIDE EFFECTS OF THIS MEDICINE

Side effects that should be reported to your doctor immediately
    MORE COMMON—Cough; painful breathing; shortness of breath

Other side effects that should be reported to your doctor
    MORE COMMON—Fever (slight); numbness or tingling in fingers or toes; sensitivity of skin to sunlight; trembling or shaking of hands; trouble in walking; unusual and uncontrolled movements of the body; weakness of arms or legs
    LESS COMMON—Blue-gray coloring of skin on face, neck, and arms; blurred vision or blue-green halos seen around objects; coldness; dry eyes; dry, puffy skin; fast or irregular heartbeat; nervousness; pain and swelling in scrotum; sensitivity of eyes to light; sensitivity to heat; slow heartbeat; sweating; swelling of feet or lower legs; trouble in sleeping; unusual tiredness; weight gain or loss
    RARE—Skin rash; yellow eyes or skin

Side effects that usually do not require medical attention

These possible side effects may go away during treatment; however, if they continue or are bothersome, check with your doctor, nurse, or pharmacist.

MORE COMMON—Constipation; headache; loss of appetite; nausea and vomiting

Other side effects not listed above may also occur in some patients. If you notice any other effects, check with your doctor, nurse, or pharmacist.

After you stop using this medicine, your body may need time to adjust. The length of time this takes depends on the amount of medicine you were using and how long you used it. **During this time check with your doctor** if you notice cough, fever (slight), painful breathing, or shortness of breath.

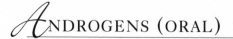NDROGENS (ORAL)

Including Fluoxymesterone; Methyltestosterone

ABOUT YOUR MEDICINE

Androgens (AN-droe-jens) are male hormones which are necessary for the normal sexual development of males. Androgens are used for several reasons: to replace the hormone when the body is unable to produce enough; to stimulate the beginning of puberty in certain boys who are late starting puberty naturally; to treat certain types of breast cancer in females. Some of these medicines may also be used for other conditions as determined by your doctor.

There is no good medical evidence to support the belief that use of androgens in athletes will increase muscle strength. When used for this purpose, they may even be dangerous because of their side effects. Also, use of androgens can lead to disqualification of athletes in most athletic events.

If any of the information in this profile causes you special concern or if you want additional information about your medicine and its use, check with your doctor, nurse, or pharmacist. **Remember, keep this and all other medicines out of the reach of children and never share your medicines with others.**

BEFORE USING THIS MEDICINE

Tell your doctor, nurse, and pharmacist if you . . .
- are allergic to any medicine, either prescription or nonprescription (OTC);
- are pregnant or intend to become pregnant while using this medicine;
- are breast-feeding;

- are taking **any** other prescription or nonprescription (OTC) medicine;
- have **any** other medical problems.

PROPER USE OF THIS MEDICINE

Take this medicine only as directed. Do not take more of it and do not take it more often than ordered. To do so may increase side effects.

For patients taking the capsule or regular tablet form of this medicine:
- Take this medicine with food to lessen possible stomach upset.

For patients taking the buccal tablet form of methyltestosterone:
- **This medicine should not be swallowed whole.** Place the tablet in the upper or lower pouch between your gum and the side of your cheek. Let the tablet slowly dissolve there. Do not eat, drink, chew, or smoke while the tablet is dissolving.

If you miss a dose of this medicine and your dosing schedule is:
- One dose a day—Take the missed dose as soon as possible. However, if you do not remember it until the next day, skip the missed dose. Do not double doses.
- More than one dose a day—Take the missed dose as soon as possible. However, if almost time for your next dose, skip the missed dose. Do not double doses.

If you have any questions about this, check with your doctor.

PRECAUTIONS WHILE USING THIS MEDICINE

Your doctor should check your progress at regular visits to make sure this medicine does not cause unwanted effects.

Androgens can decrease the amount of sperm made. Also, androgens may cause children to stop growing early or to develop too fast sexually.

POSSIBLE SIDE EFFECTS OF THIS MEDICINE

Tumors of the liver or liver disease have occurred with long-term, high-dose therapy with androgens. These effects are rare but can be very serious.

Side effects that should be reported to your doctor immediately
For both females and males

LESS COMMON—Yellow eyes or skin
RARE—(with long-term use and/or high doses)—Black, tarry, or light-colored stools; dark-colored urine; purple or red spots on body or inside the mouth or nose; sore throat or fever; vomiting of blood

Other side effects that should be reported to your doctor
For both females and males

LESS COMMON—Changes in skin color; confusion; dizziness; flushing of skin; headache (frequent or continuing); mental depression; nausea or vomiting;

shortness of breath; skin rash or itching; swelling of feet or lower legs; unusual bleeding; unusual tiredness; weight gain (rapid)

RARE—(with long-term use and/or high doses)—Hives; loss of appetite (continuing); pain, tenderness, or swelling in the abdominal or stomach area; unpleasant breath odor (continuing)

For females only

MORE COMMON—Acne or oily skin; enlarged clitoris; hair loss; hoarseness or deepening of voice; irregular periods; unnatural hair growth

For sexually mature males only

MORE COMMON—Acne; breast soreness; frequent or continuing erections; frequent urge to urinate; increased breast size

LESS COMMON—Chills; pain in scrotum or groin

For elderly patients only

LESS COMMON—Difficult or frequent urination (in males); increase in sexual desire

Other side effects not listed above may also occur in some patients. If you notice any other effects, check with your doctor, nurse, or pharmacist.

ANESTHETICS (TOPICAL)

Including Benzocaine; Benzocaine and
Menthol; Butamben; Dibucaine; Lidocaine; Pramoxine;
Pramoxine and Menthol; Tetracaine; Tetracaine and Menthol

ABOUT YOUR MEDICINE

Topical anesthetics (an-ess-THET-iks) are used to relieve pain and itching caused by conditions such as sunburn or other minor burns, insect bites or stings, poison ivy, poison oak, poison sumac, and minor cuts and scratches.

If any of the information in this profile causes you special concern or if you want additional information about your medicine and its use, check with your doctor, nurse, or pharmacist. **Remember, keep this and all other medicines out of the reach of children and never share your medicines with others.**

BEFORE USING THIS MEDICINE

If you are using this medicine without a prescription, carefully read and follow any precautions on the label. You should be especially careful if you . . .

- are allergic to any medicine, either prescription or nonprescription (OTC);
- are pregnant, intend to become pregnant, or are breast-feeding;
- are taking any other prescription or nonprescription (OTC) medicine;
- have any other medical problems.

If you have any questions, check with your doctor, nurse, or pharmacist.

PROPER USE OF THIS MEDICINE

Unless otherwise directed by your doctor, **do not use this medicine on large areas, especially if the skin is broken or scraped. Also, do not use it more often than directed on the package label, or for more than a few days at a time.** To do so may increase the chance of unwanted effects. This is especially important when benzocaine is used for children younger than 2 years of age.

This medicine should be used only for problems being treated by your doctor or conditions listed in the package directions. **Check with your doctor before using it for other problems, especially if you think that an infection may be present.** This medicine should not be used to treat certain kinds of skin infections or serious problems, such as severe burns.

Do not use any product containing alcohol near a fire or open flame, or while smoking. Also, do not smoke after applying one of these products until it has completely dried.

If you are using this medicine on your face, **be very careful not to get it in your eyes, mouth, or nose.** If you are using an aerosol or spray form of this medicine, do not spray it directly on your face. Instead, use your hand or an applicator (for example, a sterile gauze pad or cotton swab) to apply the medicine.

For patients using butamben: Butamben may stain clothing and discolor hair. It may not be possible to remove the stains. To avoid this, do not touch your clothing or your hair while applying the medicine. Also, cover the treated area with a loose bandage after applying butamben, to protect your clothes.

To use lidocaine film-forming gel:
- First dry the area with a clean cloth or a piece of gauze. Then apply the medicine. The medicine should dry, forming a clear film, after about 1 minute.

If your doctor has ordered you to use this medicine according to a regular schedule and you miss a dose, use it as soon as possible. However, if it is almost time for your next dose, skip the missed dose and use your next dose at the regularly scheduled time.

PRECAUTIONS WHILE USING THIS MEDICINE

After applying this medicine to the skin of a child, **watch the child carefully to make sure that he or she does not get any of the medicine into his or her mouth.** Topical anesthetics can cause serious side effects, especially in children, if any of the medicine gets into the mouth or is swallowed.

Stop using this medicine and check with your doctor:
- If your condition does not improve within 7 days, or if it gets worse.
- If the area you are treating becomes infected.
- If you notice a skin rash, burning, stinging, swelling, or any other sign of irritation that was not present when you began using this medicine.
- If you swallow any of the medicine.

POSSIBLE SIDE EFFECTS OF THIS MEDICINE

Side effects that should be reported to your doctor immediately

LESS COMMON—Large swellings that look like hives on the skin or in the mouth or throat

SIGNS OF TOO MUCH MEDICINE BEING ABSORBED BY THE BODY—VERY RARE— Blurred or double vision; confusion; convulsions (seizures); dizziness or lightheadedness; drowsiness; feeling hot, cold, or numb; headache; increased sweating; ringing or buzzing in the ears; shivering or trembling; slow or irregular heartbeat; trouble breathing; unusual anxiety, excitement, nervousness, or restlessness; unusual paleness; unusual tiredness or weakness

Other side effects that should be reported to your doctor

Burning, stinging, or tenderness not present before treatment; skin rash, redness, itching, or hives

Other side effects not listed above may also occur in some patients. If you notice any other effects, check with your doctor, nurse, or pharmacist.

ANESTHETICS, LOCAL (INJECTION)

Including Bupivacaine; Chloroprocaine; Etidocaine; Etidocaine and Epinephrine; Lidocaine; Mepivacaine; Mepivacaine and Levonordefrin; Prilocaine; Prilocaine and Epinephrine; Procaine; Propoxycaine and Procaine; Tetracaine

ABOUT YOUR MEDICINE

Local anesthetics (an-ess-THET-iks) are given by injection to cause loss of feeling before and during surgery, dental procedures (including dental surgery), or labor and delivery. These medicines do not cause loss of consciousness.

These medicines are given only by or under the immediate supervision of a physician or dentist, or by a specially trained nurse, in the doctor's office or in a hospital.

If any of the information in this profile causes you special concern or if you want additional information about your medicine and its use, check with your physician, dentist, nurse, or pharmacist.

BEFORE RECEIVING THIS MEDICINE

Tell your physician, dentist, or nurse if you . . .
- are allergic to any medicine, either prescription or nonprescription (OTC);
- are pregnant or intend to become pregnant while using this medicine;
- are breast-feeding;
- are taking any other prescription or nonprescription (OTC) medicine;
- have any other medical problems;
- use cocaine or other drugs.

PRECAUTIONS AFTER RECEIVING THIS MEDICINE

For patients going home before the numbness or loss of feeling caused by the anesthetic wears off:
- During the time that the injected area feels numb, serious injury can occur without your knowing about it. Be especially careful to avoid injury until the anesthetic wears off or feeling returns to the area.
- If you have received the local anesthetic injection in your mouth, do not chew gum or food while your mouth feels numb. You may injure yourself by biting your tongue or the inside of your cheeks.

POSSIBLE SIDE EFFECTS OF THIS MEDICINE

Side effects that should be reported to your doctor immediately
LESS COMMON OR RARE—Skin rash, hives, or itching

Also, check with your dentist if you have received the anesthetic for dental work, and the feeling of numbness or tingling in your lips and mouth does not go away within a few hours, or if you have difficulty in opening your mouth.

Other side effects not listed above may also occur in some patients. If you notice any other effects, check with your physician or dentist.

*A*NTACIDS, ALUMINUM-CONTAINING (ORAL)

Including Aluminum Carbonate, Basic;
Aluminum Hydroxide; Dihydroxyaluminum
Aminoacetate; Dihydroxyaluminum Sodium Carbonate

ABOUT YOUR MEDICINE

Antacids are taken by mouth to relieve heartburn, sour stomach, or acid indigestion. Antacids may also be used to treat the symptoms of stomach or duodenal ulcers.

Some antacids, such as aluminum carbonate and aluminum hydroxide, may be prescribed with a low-phosphate diet to treat hyperphosphatemia (too much phosphate in the blood) or to prevent the formation of some kinds of kidney stones. Aluminum hydroxide may also be used for other conditions as determined by your doctor.

If any of the information in this profile causes you special concern or if you want additional information about your medicine and its use, check with your doctor, nurse, or pharmacist. **Remember, keep this and all other medicines out of the reach of children and never share your medicines with others.**

BEFORE USING THIS MEDICINE

If you are taking this medicine without a prescription, carefully read and follow any precautions on the label. You should be especially careful if you . . .
- are allergic to any medicine, either prescription or nonprescription (OTC);
- are pregnant, intend to become pregnant, or are breast-feeding;
- are taking any other prescription or nonprescription (OTC) medicine, especially fluoroquinolones (medicine for infection), isoniazid, ketoconazole, mecamylamine, methenamine, or tetracyclines (medicine for infection);
- have any other medical problems, especially Alzheimer's disease, appendicitis (or signs of), constipation (severe and continuing), edema (swelling of feet or lower legs), heart disease, hemorrhoids, intestinal blockage, kidney disease, liver disease, or toxemia of pregnancy.

If you have any questions, check with your doctor, nurse, or pharmacist.

PROPER USE OF THIS MEDICINE

For safe and effective use of this medicine:
- Follow your doctor's instructions if this medicine was prescribed.
- Follow the manufacturer's package directions if you are treating yourself.

For patients taking this medicine for a stomach or duodenal ulcer:
- **Take it exactly as directed and for the full time of treatment as ordered by your doctor** to obtain maximum relief of your symptoms.

- Take it 1 and 3 hours after meals and at bedtime for best results, unless otherwise directed by your doctor.

For patients taking aluminum carbonate or aluminum hydroxide to prevent kidney stones: Drink plenty of fluids unless otherwise directed by your doctor.

For patients taking aluminum carbonate or aluminum hydroxide for hyperphosphatemia (too much phosphate in the blood): Your doctor may want you to follow a low-phosphate diet. If you have any questions about this, check with your doctor.

If your doctor has told you to take this medicine on a regular schedule and you miss a dose, take it as soon as possible. However, if it is almost time for your next dose, skip the missed dose and go back to your regular dosing schedule. Do not double doses.

PRECAUTIONS WHILE USING THIS MEDICINE

If this medicine has been ordered by your doctor and you will be taking it in large doses, or for a long time, your doctor should check your progress at regular visits.

Do not take this medicine:
- **—if you have any signs of appendicitis or inflamed bowel** (such as stomach or lower abdominal pain, cramping, bloating, soreness, nausea, or vomiting). Instead, check with your doctor as soon as possible.
- **—within 1 to 2 hours or more of taking other medicine by mouth.** To do so may keep the other medicine from working properly.
- **—for more than 2 weeks unless otherwise directed by your doctor.** Antacids should be used only for occasional relief.

Some antacids contain a large amount of sodium. If you have any questions about this, check with your doctor or pharmacist.

If your stomach problem is not helped by the antacid or if it keeps coming back, check with your doctor.

POSSIBLE SIDE EFFECTS OF THIS MEDICINE

Along with its needed effects, a medicine may cause some unwanted effects. When antacids are used at recommended doses, side effects that require medical attention usually do not occur.

Side effects that usually do not require medical attention
These possible side effects may go away during treatment; however, if they continue or are bothersome, check with your doctor, nurse, or pharmacist.

MORE COMMON—CHALKY taste

Other side effects not listed above may also occur in some patients. If you notice any other effects, check with your doctor, nurse, or pharmacist.

Antacids, Aluminum-, Calcium-, and Magnesium-Containing (Oral)

Including Simethicone, Alumina,
Calcium Carbonate, and Magnesia

About Your Medicine

Antacids are taken by mouth to relieve heartburn, sour stomach, or acid indigestion. Some antacid combinations also contain simethicone, which may relieve the symptoms of excess gas. Antacids alone or in combination with simethicone may also be used to treat the symptoms of stomach or duodenal ulcers.

If any of the information in this profile causes you special concern or if you want additional information about your medicine and its use, check with your doctor, nurse, or pharmacist. **Remember, keep this and all other medicines out of the reach of children and never share your medicines with others.**

Before Using This Medicine

If you are taking this medicine without a prescription, carefully read and follow any precautions on the label. You should be especially careful if you . . .
- are allergic to any medicine, either prescription or nonprescription (OTC);
- are pregnant, intend to become pregnant, or are breast-feeding;
- are taking any other prescription or nonprescription (OTC) medicine, especially cellulose sodium phosphate, fluoroquinolones (medicine for infection), isoniazid, ketoconazole, mecamylamine, methenamine, sodium polystyrene sulfonate, or tetracyclines (medicine for infection);
- have any other medical problems, especially Alzheimer's disease, appendicitis (or signs of), constipation (severe and continuing), edema (swelling of feet or lower legs), heart disease, hemorrhoids, ileostomy, intestinal blockage, kidney disease, liver disease, sarcoidosis, toxemia of pregnancy, or underactive parathyroid glands.

If you have any questions, check with your doctor, nurse, or pharmacist.

Proper Use of This Medicine

For safe and effective use of this medicine:
- Follow your doctor's instructions if this medicine was prescribed.
- Follow the manufacturer's package directions if you are treating yourself.

For patients taking this medicine for a stomach or duodenal ulcer:
- **Take it exactly as directed and for the full time of treatment as ordered by your doctor** to obtain maximum relief of your symptoms.
- Take it 1 and 3 hours after meals and at bedtime for best results, unless otherwise directed by your doctor.

If your doctor has told you to take this medicine on a regular schedule and you miss a dose, take it as soon as possible. However, if it is almost time for your next dose, skip the missed dose and go back to your regular dosing schedule. Do not double doses.

PRECAUTIONS WHILE USING THIS MEDICINE

If this medicine has been ordered by your doctor and you will be taking it in large doses, or for a long time, your doctor should check your progress at regular visits.

Do not take this medicine:
> —**if you have any signs of appendicitis or inflamed bowel** (such as stomach or lower abdominal pain, cramping, bloating, soreness, nausea, or vomiting). Instead, check with your doctor as soon as possible.
> —**within 1 to 2 hours or more of taking other medicine by mouth.** To do so may keep the other medicine from working properly.
> —**for more than 2 weeks unless otherwise directed by your doctor.** Antacids should be used only for occasional relief.

Some antacids contain a large amount of sodium. If you have any questions about this, check with your doctor or pharmacist.

If your stomach problem is not helped by the antacid or if it keeps coming back, check with your doctor.

Do not take the antacid with large amounts of milk or milk products. To do so may increase the chance of side effects.

POSSIBLE SIDE EFFECTS OF THIS MEDICINE

Along with its needed effects, a medicine may cause some unwanted effects. When antacids are used at recommended doses, side effects that require medical attention usually do not occur.

Side effects that usually do not require medical attention
> These possible side effects may go away during treatment; however, if they continue or are bothersome, check with your doctor, nurse, or pharmacist.
>
> MORE COMMON—Chalky taste
> LESS COMMON—Constipation (mild); diarrhea; increased thirst; speckling or whitish discoloration of stools; stomach cramps
>
> Other side effects not listed above may also occur in some patients. If you notice any other effects, check with your doctor, nurse, or pharmacist.

ANTACIDS, ALUMINUM- AND MAGNESIUM-CONTAINING (ORAL)

Including Alumina and Magnesia;
Alumina,Magnesia, and Simethicone; Alumina
and Magnesium Carbonate; Alumina and Magnesium
Trisilicate; Magnesium Trisilicate, Alumina, and Magnesia;
Simethicone, Alumina, Magnesium Carbonate, and Magnesia

ABOUT YOUR MEDICINE

Antacids are taken by mouth to relieve heartburn, sour stomach, or acid indigestion. Some antacid combinations also contain simethicone, which may relieve the symptoms of excess gas. Antacids alone or in combination with simethicone may also be used to treat the symptoms of stomach or duodenal ulcers.

If any of the information in this profile causes you special concern or if you want additional information about your medicine and its use, check with your doctor, nurse, or pharmacist. **Remember, keep this and all other medicines out of the reach of children and never share your medicines with others.**

USING THIS MEDICINE

If you are taking this medicine without a prescription, carefully read and follow any precautions on the label. You should be especially careful if you . . .
- are allergic to any medicine, either prescription or nonprescription (OTC);
- are pregnant, intend to become pregnant, or are breast-feeding;
- are taking any other prescription or nonprescription (OTC) medicine, especially cellulose sodium phosphate, fluoroquinolones (medicine for infection), isoniazid, ketoconazole, mecamylamine, methenamine, sodium polystyrene sulfonate resin (SPSR), or tetracyclines (medicine for infection);
- have any other medical problems, especially Alzheimer's disease, appendicitis (or signs of), constipation (severe and continuing), edema (swelling of feet or lower legs), heart disease, hemorrhoids, ileostomy, intestinal blockage, kidney disease, liver disease, or toxemia of pregnancy.

If you have any questions, check with your doctor, nurse, or pharmacist.

PROPER USE OF THIS MEDICINE

For safe and effective use of this medicine:
- Follow your doctor's instructions if this medicine was prescribed.
- Follow the manufacturer's package directions if you are treating yourself.

For patients taking this medicine for a stomach or duodenal ulcer:
- **Take it exactly as directed and for the full time of treatment as ordered by your doctor** to obtain maximum relief of your symptoms.

- Take it 1 and 3 hours after meals and at bedtime for best results, unless otherwise directed by your doctor.

If your doctor has told you to take this medicine on a regular schedule and you miss a dose, take it as soon as possible. However, if it is almost time for your next dose, skip the missed dose and go back to your regular dosing schedule. Do not double doses.

PRECAUTIONS WHILE USING THIS MEDICINE

If this medicine has been ordered by your doctor and if you will be taking it in large doses, or for a long time, your doctor should check your progress at regular visits.

Do not take this medicine:
   —**if you have any signs of appendicitis or inflamed bowel** (such as stomach or lower abdominal pain, cramping, bloating, soreness, nausea, or vomiting). Instead, check with your doctor as soon as possible.
   —**within 1 to 2 hours or more of taking other medicine by mouth.** To do so may keep the other medicine from working as well.
   —**for more than 2 weeks unless otherwise directed by your doctor.** Antacids should be used only for occasional relief.

Some antacids contain a large amount of sodium. If you have any questions about this, check with your doctor or pharmacist.

If your stomach problem is not helped by the antacid or if it keeps coming back, check with your doctor.

POSSIBLE SIDE EFFECTS OF THIS MEDICINE

Along with its needed effects, a medicine may cause some unwanted effects. When antacids are used at recommended doses, side effects that require medical attention usually do not occur.

Side effects that usually do not require medical attention
   These possible side effects may go away during treatment; however, if they continue or are bothersome, check with your doctor, nurse, or pharmacist.

   MORE COMMON—Chalky taste
   LESS COMMON—Constipation (mild); diarrhea or laxative effect; increase in thirst; speckling or whitish discoloration of stools; stomach cramps

   Other side effects not listed above may also occur in some patients. If you notice any other effects, check with your doctor, nurse, or pharmacist.

ANTACIDS, CALCIUM CARBONATE–CONTAINING (ORAL)

Including Calcium Carbonate; Calcium Carbonate and Simethicone

ABOUT YOUR MEDICINE

Antacids are taken by mouth to relieve heartburn, sour stomach, or acid indigestion. Some antacid combinations also contain simethicone, which may relieve the symptoms of excess gas. Antacids alone or in combination with simethicone may also be used to treat the symptoms of stomach or duodenal ulcers.

If any of the information in this profile causes you special concern or if you want additional information about your medicine and its use, check with your doctor, nurse, or pharmacist. **Remember, keep this and all other medicines out of the reach of children and never share your medicines with others.**

BEFORE USING THIS MEDICINE

If you are taking this medicine without a prescription, carefully read and follow any precautions on the label. You should be especially careful if you . . .
- are allergic to any medicine, either prescription or nonprescription (OTC);
- are pregnant, intend to become pregnant, or are breast-feeding;
- are taking any other prescription or nonprescription (OTC) medicine, especially cellulose sodium phosphate, fluoroquinolones (medicine for infection), ketoconazole, mecamylamine, methenamine, sodium polystyrene sulfonate, or tetracyclines (medicine for infection);
- have any other medical problems, especially appendicitis (or signs of), constipation (severe and continuing), edema (swelling of feet or lower legs), heart disease, hemorrhoids, ileostomy, intestinal blockage, kidney disease, liver disease, sarcoidosis, toxemia of pregnancy, or underactive parathyroid glands.

If you have any questions, check with your doctor, nurse, or pharmacist.

PROPER USE OF THIS MEDICINE

For safe and effective use of this medicine:
- Follow your doctor's instructions if this medicine was prescribed.
- Follow the manufacturer's package directions if you are treating yourself.

For patients taking this medicine for a stomach or duodenal ulcer:
- **Take it exactly as directed and for the full time of treatment as ordered by your doctor** to obtain maximum relief of your symptoms.
- Take it 1 and 3 hours after meals and at bedtime for best results, unless otherwise directed by your doctor.

If your doctor has told you to take this medicine on a regular schedule and you miss a dose, take it as soon as possible. However, if it is almost time for your next dose, skip the missed dose and go back to your regular dosing schedule. Do not double doses.

PRECAUTIONS WHILE USING THIS MEDICINE

If this medicine has been ordered by your doctor and you will be taking it in large doses, or for a long time, your doctor should check your progress at regular visits.

Do not take this medicine:
—**if you have any signs of appendicitis or inflamed bowel** (such as stomach or lower abdominal pain, cramping, bloating, soreness, nausea, or vomiting). Instead, check with your doctor as soon as possible.
—**within 1 to 2 hours or more of taking other medicine by mouth.** To do so may keep the other medicine from working properly.
—**for more than 2 weeks unless otherwise directed by your doctor.** Antacids should be used only for occasional relief.

Some antacids contain a large amount of sodium. If you have any questions about this, check with your doctor or pharmacist.

If your stomach problem is not helped by the antacid or if it keeps coming back, check with your doctor.

Do not take the antacid with large amounts of milk or milk products. To do so may increase the chance of side effects.

POSSIBLE SIDE EFFECTS OF THIS MEDICINE

Along with its needed effects, a medicine may cause some unwanted effects. When antacids are used at recommended doses, side effects that require medical attention usually do not occur.

Side effects that usually do not require medical attention
These possible side effects may go away during treatment; however, if they continue or are bothersome, check with your doctor, nurse, or pharmacist.

MORE COMMON—Chalky taste
LESS COMMON—Constipation (mild)

Other side effects not listed above may also occur in some patients. If you notice any other effects, check with your doctor, nurse, or pharmacist.

ANTIARRHYTHMICS, TYPE I (ORAL)

Including Disopyramide; Encainide; Flecainide; Mexiletine;
Moricizine; Procainamide; Propafenone; Quinidine; Tocainide

ABOUT YOUR MEDICINE

Type I antiarrhythmics are used to correct irregular heartbeats to a normal rhythm and to slow an overactive heart.

There is a chance that these medicines may cause new heart rhythm problems when they are used. Usually this effect is rare and mild. However, some of these medicines are more likely than others to cause this effect. For example, encainide and flecainide have been shown to cause severe problems in some patients, and so they are only used to treat serious heart rhythm problems. Discuss this possible effect with your doctor.

If any of the information in this profile causes you special concern or if you want additional information about your medicine and its use, check with your doctor, nurse, or pharmacist. **Remember, keep this and all other medicines out of the reach of children and never share your medicines with others.**

BEFORE USING THIS MEDICINE

Tell your doctor, nurse, and pharmacist if you . . .
- are allergic to any medicine, either prescription or nonprescription (OTC);
- are pregnant or intend to become pregnant while using this medicine;
- are breast-feeding;
- are taking **any** other prescription or nonprescription (OTC) medicine;
- have **any** other medical problems.

PROPER USE OF THIS MEDICINE

Take this medicine exactly as directed by your doctor, even though you may feel well. Do not take more medicine than ordered.

For patients taking the extended-release capsules or tablets:
- Swallow whole without breaking, crushing, or chewing.

It is best to take each dose at evenly spaced times day and night.

For patients taking mexiletine:
- To lessen the possibility of stomach upset, this medicine should be taken with food or immediately after meals or with milk or an antacid.

If you miss a dose of this medicine, take it as soon as possible. However, if you do not remember until it is almost time for the next dose, skip the missed dose and go back to your regular dosing schedule. Do not double doses.

PRECAUTIONS WHILE USING THIS MEDICINE

It is important that your doctor check your progress at regular visits to make sure the medicine is working properly to help your heart.

Do not suddenly stop taking this medicine without first checking with your doctor. Stopping it suddenly may cause a serious change in heart activity.

Dizziness or lightheadedness or blurred vision may occur. **Make sure you know how you react to this medicine before you drive, use machines, or do other jobs that require you to be alert and able to see well.**

For patients taking disopyramide:
- If signs of hypoglycemia (low blood sugar) such as chills, hunger, nausea, nervousness, or sweating appear, eat or drink a food containing sugar and call your doctor right away.
- **Use extra care not to become overheated during exercise or hot weather,** since this medicine will often make you sweat less and could possibly result in heat stroke.

POSSIBLE SIDE EFFECTS OF THIS MEDICINE

Side effects that should be reported to your doctor immediately
FOR QUINIDINE ONLY, ESPECIALLY AFTER THE FIRST DOSE OR FIRST FEW DOSES—Breathing difficulty; changes in vision; dizziness, lightheadedness, or fainting; fever; severe headache; ringing in ears; skin rash

Other side effects that should be reported to your doctor
FOR ALL ANTIARRHYTHMICS—Chest pain; fast or irregular heartbeat; fever or chills; shortness of breath or painful breathing; skin rash or itching; unusual bleeding or bruising

FOR DISOPYRAMIDE (IN ADDITION TO ABOVE)—Difficult urination; swelling of feet or lower legs

FOR ENCAINIDE, FLECAINIDE, MORICIZINE, AND PROPAFENONE (IN ADDITION TO ABOVE)—Swelling of feet or lower legs; trembling or shaking

Side effects that usually do not require medical attention
These possible side effects may go away during treatment; however, if they continue or are bothersome, check with your doctor, nurse, or pharmacist.

FOR ALL ANTIARRHYTHMICS—Blurred or double vision; dizziness or lightheadedness

FOR DISOPYRAMIDE (IN ADDITION TO ABOVE)—Dry mouth and throat

FOR FLECAINIDE (IN ADDITION TO ABOVE)—Seeing spots

FOR MEXILETINE (IN ADDITION TO ABOVE)—Heartburn; nausea and vomiting; nervousness; trembling or shaking of hands; unsteadiness or trouble walking

FOR PROCAINAMIDE (IN ADDITION TO ABOVE)—Diarrhea; loss of appetite

FOR PROPAFENONE (IN ADDITION TO ABOVE)—Change in taste

FOR QUINIDINE (IN ADDITION TO ABOVE)—Bitter taste; diarrhea; flushing of skin with itching; loss of appetite; nausea or vomiting; stomach pain or cramps

FOR TOCAINIDE (IN ADDITION TO ABOVE)—Loss of appetite; nausea

Other side effects not listed above may also occur in some patients. If you notice any other effects, check with your doctor, nurse, or pharmacist.

ANTICHOLINERGICS/ANTISPASMODICS (ORAL)

Including Anisotropine; Atropine; Belladonna; Clidinium; Dicyclomine; Glycopyrrolate; Homatropine; Hyoscyamine; Mepenzolate; Methantheline; Methscopolamine; Pirenzepine; Propantheline; Scopolamine

ABOUT YOUR MEDICINE

The **anticholinergics/antispasmodics** are used to relieve cramps or spasms of the stomach, intestines, and bladder. Some are used together with antacids or other medicine in the treatment of peptic ulcer. Others are used to prevent nausea, vomiting, and motion sickness. Some anticholinergics are also used to treat poisoning caused by medicines such as neostigmine and physostigmine, certain types of mushrooms, and poisoning by "nerve" gases or organic phosphorous pesticides. Also, anticholinergics can be used for painful menstruation, runny nose, and to prevent urination during sleep. These medicines may also be used for other conditions as determined by your doctor.

If any of the information in this profile causes you special concern or if you want additional information about your medicine and its use, check with your doctor, nurse, or pharmacist. **Remember, keep this and all other medicines out of the reach of children and never share your medicines with others.**

BEFORE USING THIS MEDICINE

Tell your doctor, nurse, and pharmacist if you . . .
- are allergic to any medicine, either prescription or nonprescription (OTC);
- are pregnant or intend to become pregnant while using this medicine;
- are breast-feeding;
- are taking **any** other prescription or nonprescription (OTC) medicine;
- have **any** other medical problems.

PROPER USE OF THIS MEDICINE

Take this medicine only as directed. Do not take more of it, do not take it more often, and do not take it for a longer period of time than ordered.

Take this medicine 30 minutes to 1 hour before meals unless otherwise directed.

If you miss a dose of this medicine, take it as soon as possible. However, if it is almost time for your next dose, skip the missed dose and go back to your regular dosing schedule. Do not double doses.

PRECAUTIONS WHILE USING THIS MEDICINE

If you think you or someone else may have taken an overdose, get emergency help at once. Taking an overdose of any of these medicines or taking scopolamine with alcohol or other CNS depressants may lead to unconsciousness and possibly death. Some signs of overdose are clumsiness or unsteadiness; confusion; dizziness; fever; hallucinations (seeing, hearing, or feeling things that are not there); severe drowsiness; slurred speech; unusual excitement, nervousness, restlessness, or irritability; unusually fast heartbeat; and unusual warmth, dryness, and flushing of skin.

These medicines may make you sweat less, causing your body temperature to rise. **Use care not to become overheated during exercise or hot weather** since overheating may result in heat stroke. Also, hot baths or saunas may make you dizzy or faint while you are taking this medicine.

Check with your doctor before you stop using this medicine. Your doctor may want you to reduce gradually the amount you are using before stopping completely.

Anticholinergics may cause some people to have blurred vision. **Make sure your vision is clear before you drive or do other jobs that require you to see well.** These medicines may also cause your eyes to become more sensitive to light. Wearing sunglasses may help lessen the discomfort from bright light.

These medicines, especially in high doses, may cause some people to become dizzy or drowsy. **Make sure you know how you react to this medicine before you drive, use machines, or do other jobs that require you to be alert.**

For patients taking scopolamine: This medicine will add to the effects of alcohol and other CNS depressants (medicines that may make you drowsy or less alert). **Check with your doctor before taking any such depressants while you are taking this medicine.**

POSSIBLE SIDE EFFECTS OF THIS MEDICINE

Side effects that should be reported to your doctor
> RARE—Confusion (especially in the elderly); dizziness, lightheadedness (continuing), or fainting; eye pain; skin rash or hives

Side effects that usually do not require medical attention
> These possible side effects may go away during treatment; however, if they continue or are bothersome, check with your doctor, nurse, or pharmacist.

MORE COMMON—Constipation; decreased sweating; dryness of mouth, nose, throat, or skin

Other side effects not listed above may also occur in some patients. If you notice any other effects, check with your doctor, nurse, or pharmacist.

For patients using scopolamine: After you stop using scopolamine, your body may need time to adjust. The length of time this takes depends on the amount of scopolamine you were using and how long you used it. During this time check with your doctor if you notice anxiety, irritability, nightmares, or trouble in sleeping.

ANTICOAGULANTS (ORAL)

Including Anisindione; Dicumarol; Warfarin

ABOUT YOUR MEDICINE

Oral anticoagulants decrease the clotting ability of the blood and therefore help prevent harmful clots from forming in the blood vessels. These medicines are sometimes called "blood thinners," although they do not actually thin the blood. They will not dissolve clots that already have formed. However, they may prevent clots from becoming larger and causing more serious problems.

If any of the information in this profile causes you special concern or if you want additional information about your medicine and its use, check with your doctor, nurse, or pharmacist. **Remember, keep this and all other medicines out of the reach of children and never share your medicines with others.**

BEFORE USING THIS MEDICINE

In order for an anticoagulant to help you without causing serious bleeding, it must be used properly and all of the precautions concerning its use must be followed exactly. Be sure that you have discussed the use of this medicine with the doctor or pharmacist who is following your treatment. It is very important that you understand all directions and that you are willing and able to follow them exactly.

Tell your doctor, nurse, and pharmacist if you . . .
- are allergic to any medicine, either prescription or nonprescription (OTC);
- are pregnant or intend to become pregnant while using this medicine;
- are breast-feeding;
- are taking **any** other prescription or nonprescription (OTC) medicine;
- have **any** other medical problems.

Proper Use of This Medicine

Take this medicine exactly as directed. Do not take more or less of it, do not take it more often, and do not take it for a longer time than ordered. This is especially important for elderly patients, who are especially sensitive to the effects of anticoagulants. **Your blood must be checked regularly.**

If you miss a dose of this medicine, take it as soon as possible if you remember the same day. However, if you do not remember until the next day, do not take the missed dose at all and do not double the next one. **Doubling the dose may cause bleeding.** Be sure to give the doctor or pharmacist who is following your treatment a record of any doses you miss.

Precautions While Using This Medicine

Tell all physicians, dentists, and pharmacists you go to that you are taking this medicine. You should also carry identification stating that you are taking it.

Always check with your doctor or pharmacist before you start or stop taking any other medicine. This includes any nonprescription medicine, even aspirin and acetaminophen. Many medicines change the way this medicine affects your body. In addition, drinking too much alcohol may change the way this medicine works.

Anticoagulants are also affected by vitamin K (found in meats, dairy products, green leafy vegetables, and some vitamin and nutrition products). Check with your doctor before changing your eating habits, if you are unable to eat for a few days, or have stomach upset, diarrhea, or fever.

Possible Side Effects of This Medicine

Side effects that should be reported immediately

LESS COMMON OR RARE—Blue or purple color and pain in toes; cloudy or dark urine; difficult or painful urination; sores, ulcers, or white spots in mouth or throat; sore throat, fever, chills, or unusual tiredness or weakness; sudden decrease in amount of urine; swelling of face, feet, or lower legs; unusual weight gain; yellow eyes or skin

SIGNS OF BLEEDING INSIDE THE BODY—Abdominal pain or swelling; back pain; bloody or black, tarry stools; bloody urine; constipation; coughing up blood; dizziness; headache (severe or continuing); joint pain, stiffness, or swelling; vomiting blood or material that looks like coffee grounds

SIGNS OF OVERDOSE—Bleeding from gums when brushing teeth; unexplained bruising, nosebleeds, or purplish areas on skin; unusually heavy bleeding from cuts; unusually heavy or unexpected menstrual bleeding

Other side effects that should be reported

LESS COMMON OR RARE—Diarrhea; itching, skin rash, or hives; nausea or vomiting; stomach cramps or pain

Side effects that usually do not require medical attention

These possible side effects may go away during treatment; however, if they continue or are bothersome, check with your doctor, nurse, or pharmacist.

MORE COMMON—Bloated stomach or gas

Anisindione may cause your urine to turn orange. Since it may be hard to tell the difference between blood in the urine and this color change, check with your doctor if you notice any color change in your urine.

Other side effects not listed above may also occur in some patients. If you notice any other effects, check with your doctor, nurse, or pharmacist.

Antidiabetics (Oral)

Including Acetohexamide; Chlorpropamide; Glipizide; Glyburide; Tolazamide; Tolbutamide

ABOUT YOUR MEDICINE

Oral antidiabetics (diabetes medicine you take by mouth) are used to treat certain types of diabetes mellitus (sugar diabetes). Chlorpropamide may also be used for other conditions as determined by your doctor.

If any of the information in this profile causes you special concern or if you want additional information about your medicine and its use, check with your doctor, nurse, or pharmacist. **Remember, keep this and all other medicines out of the reach of children and never share your medicines with others.**

BEFORE USING THIS MEDICINE

Tell your doctor, nurse, and pharmacist if you . . .

- are allergic to any medicine, either prescription or nonprescription (OTC);
- are pregnant or intend to become pregnant while using this medicine;
- are breast-feeding;
- are taking any other prescription or nonprescription (OTC) medicine, especially anticoagulants (blood thinners); aspirin or other salicylates; beta-blockers; chloramphenicol; guanethidine; MAO inhibitors; medicines for coughs, colds, asthma, hay fever, or appetite control; or sulfonamides (sulfa drugs);
- have any other medical problems, especially kidney, liver, or thyroid disease; severe infection; or underactive adrenal or pituitary glands;
- are taking chlorpropamide and have heart disease.

PROPER USE OF THIS MEDICINE

Follow carefully the special meal plan your doctor gave you. This is the most important part of controlling your condition, and is necessary if the medicine is to work properly. Also, test for sugar in your blood or urine as directed.

Take this medicine only as directed. Do not take more or less of it than your doctor ordered, and take it at the same time each day.

If you miss a dose of this medicine, take it as soon as possible. However, if it is almost time for your next dose, skip the missed dose and go back to your regular dosing schedule. Do not double doses.

PRECAUTIONS WHILE USING THIS MEDICINE

Avoid drinking alcoholic beverages until you have discussed their use with your doctor. They may affect diet, produce low blood sugar, and cause other side effects.

Eat or drink something containing sugar and check with your doctor right away if mild symptoms of low blood sugar (hypoglycemia) appear. Good sources of sugar are glucose tablets or gel, fruit juice, corn syrup, honey, regular (non-diet) soft drinks, or sugar dissolved in water. It is a good idea to check your blood sugar to confirm that it is low.

If severe symptoms such as convulsions (seizures) or unconsciousness occur, diabetics should not eat or drink anything. There is a chance that they could choke from not swallowing correctly. Emergency medical help should be obtained immediately.

Symptoms of low blood sugar include abdominal or stomach pain (mild); anxious feeling; chills (continuing); cold sweats; confusion; convulsions (seizures); cool pale skin; difficulty in thinking; drowsiness; excessive hunger; headache (continuing); nausea or vomiting (continuing); nervousness; rapid heartbeat; shakiness; unconsciousness; unsteady walk; unusual tiredness or weakness; or vision changes. **These symptoms may occur if you** delay or miss a meal or snack, exercise much more than usual, cannot eat because of nausea and vomiting, or drink a significant amount of alcohol. **Tell someone to take you to your doctor or to a hospital right away if the symptoms do not improve after eating or drinking a sweet food.**

POSSIBLE SIDE EFFECTS OF THIS MEDICINE

Side effects that should be reported to your doctor

> RARE—Chest pain; chills; coughing up blood; dark urine; fever; general feeling of illness; increased amounts of sputum (phlegm); increased sweating; itching of the skin; light-colored stools; sore throat; troubled breathing; unusual bleeding or bruising; unusual tiredness or weakness (continuing and unexplained); yellow eyes or skin

Side effects that usually do not require medical attention

These possible side effects may go away during treatment; however, if they continue or are bothersome, check with your doctor, nurse, or pharmacist.

MORE COMMON—Changes in taste (for tolbutamide); constipation; diarrhea; dizziness; drowsiness (mild); headache; heartburn; increased or decreased appetite; nausea; stomach pain, fullness, or discomfort; vomiting

LESS COMMON—Hives; increased sensitivity of skin to sun; skin redness, itching, or rash

Other side effects not listed above may also occur in some patients. If you notice any other effects, check with your doctor, nurse, or pharmacist.

$\mathcal{A}$NTIDYSKINETICS (ORAL)

Including Benztropine; Biperiden;
Ethopropazine; Procyclidine; Trihexyphenidyl

ABOUT YOUR MEDICINE

Antidyskinetics (an-tye-dis-kin-ET-iks) are used to treat Parkinson's disease, sometimes referred to as "shaking palsy." Antidyskinetics are also used to control certain side effects of other medicines. Antidyskinetics may also be used for other conditions as determined by your doctor.

If any of the information in this profile causes you special concern or if you want additional information about your medicine and its use, check with your doctor, nurse, or pharmacist. **Remember, keep this and all other medicines out of the reach of children and never share your medicines with others.**

BEFORE USING THIS MEDICINE

Tell your doctor, nurse, and pharmacist if you . . .
- are allergic to any medicine, either prescription or nonprescription (OTC);
- are pregnant or intend to become pregnant while using this medicine;
- are breast-feeding;
- are taking any other prescription or nonprescription (OTC) medicine, especially antacids, anticholinergics (medicine for abdominal or stomach spasms or cramps), CNS depressants, or tricyclic antidepressants;
- have any other medical problems, especially difficult urination; glaucoma; heart or blood vessel disease; intestinal blockage; myasthenia gravis; or uncontrolled movements of hands, mouth, or tongue.

Proper Use of This Medicine

Take this medicine only as directed. Do not take more of it, do not take it more often, and do not take it for a longer period of time than your doctor ordered. To lessen stomach upset, take this medicine with meals or right after meals.

If you miss a dose of this medicine, take it as soon as possible. However, if it is within 2 hours of your next dose, skip the missed dose and go back to your regular dosing schedule. Do not double doses.

Precautions While Using This Medicine

Your doctor should check your progress at regular visits, especially for the first few months you take this medicine. Your doctor may also want you to have your eyes examined before and also sometime later during treatment.

Do not stop taking this medicine without first checking with your doctor. Your doctor may want you to reduce your dose gradually.

This medicine will add to the effects of alcohol and other CNS depressants (medicines that slow down your nervous system). **Check with your doctor before taking any such depressants while you are using this medicine.**

Antidyskinetics may cause some people to have blurred vision or to become drowsy, dizzy, or less alert than they are normally. **Make sure you know how you react to this medicine before you drive, use machines, or do other jobs that require you to be alert or able to see well.**

Antidyskinetics will often reduce your tolerance to heat, since they make you sweat less, causing your body temperature to increase. **Use extra care not to become overheated during exercise or hot weather while you are taking this medicine as this could possibly result in heat stroke.** Also, hot baths or saunas may make you feel dizzy or faint while you are taking this medicine.

If you think you or anyone else has taken an overdose of this medicine, get emergency help at once. Overdose may lead to unconsciousness. Some signs of an overdose are clumsiness; hallucinations; seizures; severe drowsiness; severe dryness of mouth, nose, and throat; troubled breathing; unusually fast heartbeat; or unusual warmth, dryness, and flushing of the skin.

Possible Side Effects of This Medicine

Side effects that should be reported to your doctor
> RARE—Confusion; eye pain; skin rash

Side effects that usually do not require medical attention
> These possible side effects may go away during treatment; however, if they continue or are bothersome, check with your doctor, nurse, or pharmacist.
>
> MORE COMMON—Blurred vision; constipation; decreased sweating; difficult or painful urination; drowsiness; dryness of mouth, nose, or throat; increased sensitivity of eyes to light; nausea or vomiting

Other side effects not listed above may also occur in some patients. If you notice any other effects, check with your doctor, nurse, or pharmacist.

After you stop using this medicine, your body may need time to adjust. The length of time this takes depends on how long you used this medicine. **During this period of time, check with your doctor** if you have anxiety; difficulty in speaking or swallowing; loss of balance control; muscle spasms, especially of face, neck, and back; restlessness; shuffling walk; trembling and shaking of hands and fingers; or unusually fast heartbeat.

ANTIHISTAMINES (ORAL)

Including Astemizole; Azatadine; Bromodiphenhydramine; Brompheniramine; Cetirizine; Chlorpheniramine; Clemastine; Cyproheptadine; Dexchlorpheniramine; Dimenhydrinate; Diphenhydramine; Doxylamine; Hydroxyzine; Loratadine; Phenindamine; Pyrilamine; Terfenadine; Tripelennamine; Triprolidine

ABOUT YOUR MEDICINE

Antihistamines (an-tye-HIST-a-meens) are used to relieve or prevent the symptoms of hay fever and other types of allergy. Some of the antihistamines are also used to prevent motion sickness, nausea, vomiting, and dizziness. In patients with Parkinson's disease, diphenhydramine may be used to decrease stiffness and tremors. In addition, since antihistamines may cause drowsiness as a side effect, some of them may be used to help people go to sleep. Hydroxyzine is used in the treatment of nervous and emotional conditions to help control anxiety. It can also be used to help control anxiety and produce sleep before surgery. Antihistamines may also be used for other conditions as determined by your doctor.

If this medicine was prescribed for you and any of the information in this profile causes you special concern or if you want additional information about your medicine and its use, check with your doctor, nurse, or pharmacist. **Remember, keep this and all other medicines out of the reach of children and never share your medicines with others.**

BEFORE USING THIS MEDICINE

If you are taking this medicine without a prescription, carefully read and follow any precautions on the label. You should be especially careful if you . . .

- are allergic to any medicine, either prescription or nonprescription (OTC);

- are pregnant, intend to become pregnant, or are breast-feeding;
- are taking any other prescription or nonprescription (OTC) medicine, especially CNS depressants, MAO inhibitors, or anticholinergics (medicine for abdominal or stomach spasms or cramps);
- are taking astemizole or terfenadine and are also taking bepridil, clarithromycin, disopyramide, erythromycin, itraconazole, ketoconazole, maprotiline, phenothiazines, pimozide, procainamide, quinidine, or tricyclic antidepressants;
- have any other medical problems, especially difficult urination, enlarged prostate, glaucoma, or urinary tract blockage;
- are taking astemizole or terfenadine and have heart rhythm problems (history of), low potassium blood levels, or liver disease.

If you have any questions, check with your doctor, nurse, or pharmacist.

PROPER USE OF THIS MEDICINE

Antihistamines are used to relieve or prevent the symptoms of your medical problem. Take them only as directed. Do not take more of them and do not take them more often than your doctor ordered. To do so may increase the chance of side effects.

Antihistamines can be taken with food or a glass of water or milk to lessen stomach irritation if necessary. However, astemizole and loratadine should be taken on an empty stomach.

If you are taking the extended-release tablet form of this medicine, swallow the tablets whole. Do not break, crush, or chew before swallowing.

If you must take this medicine regularly and you miss a dose, take it as soon as possible. However, if it is almost time for your next dose, skip the missed dose and go back to your regular dosing schedule. Do not double doses.

PRECAUTIONS WHILE USING THIS MEDICINE

Antihistamines will add to the effects of alcohol and other CNS depressants (medicines that slow down the nervous system). **Check with your doctor before taking any such depressants while you are using this medicine.**

This medicine may cause some people to become drowsy or less alert than they are normally. Even if taken at bedtime, it may cause some people to feel drowsy or less alert on arising. Drowsiness is less likely with cetirizine, and rare with astemizole, loratadine, and terfenadine; however, **make sure you know how you react to any antihistamine before you drive, use machines, or do other jobs that require you to be alert.**

POSSIBLE SIDE EFFECTS OF THIS MEDICINE

Side effects that should be reported to your doctor immediately
LESS COMMON OR RARE (WITH HIGH DOSES OF ASTEMIZOLE AND TERFENADINE ONLY)—Fast or irregular heartbeat

Other side effects that should be reported to your doctor

LESS COMMON OR RARE—Sore throat and fever; unusual bleeding or bruising; unusual tiredness or weakness

Side effects that usually do not require medical attention

These possible side effects may go away during treatment; however, if they continue or are bothersome, check with your doctor, nurse, or pharmacist.

MORE COMMON (LESS COMMON WITH CETIRIZINE; RARE WITH ASTEMIZOLE, LORATADINE, AND TERFENADINE)—Drowsiness; thickening of mucus

Other side effects not listed above may also occur in some patients. If you notice any other effects, check with your doctor, nurse, or pharmacist.

$\mathcal{A}$NTIHISTAMINES AND DECONGESTANTS (ORAL)

ABOUT YOUR MEDICINE

Antihistamine (an-tye-HIST-a-meen) and **decongestant** (dee-kon-JES-tant) combinations are used to treat the nasal congestion (stuffy nose), sneezing, and runny nose caused by colds and hay fever.

If this medicine was prescribed for you and any of the information in this profile causes you special concern or if you want additional information about your medicine and its use, check with your doctor, nurse, or pharmacist. **Remember, keep this and all other medicines out of the reach of children and never share your medicines with others.**

BEFORE USING THIS MEDICINE

If you are taking this medicine without a prescription, carefully read and follow any precautions on the label. You should be especially careful if you . . .

- are allergic to any medicine, either prescription or nonprescription (OTC);
- are pregnant, intend to become pregnant, or are breast-feeding;
- are taking any other prescription or nonprescription (OTC) medicine, especially beta-blockers, CNS depressants and stimulants, MAO inhibitors, maprotiline, medicine for abdominal or stomach spasms or cramps, phenothiazines, rauwolfia alkaloids, or tricyclic antidepressants (medicine for depression);
- are taking clarithromycin, erythromycin, itraconazole, or ketoconazole and are also taking the combination that contains terfenadine;
- have any other medical problems, especially high blood pressure, liver

disease (for terfenadine-containing combination only), or urinary tract blockage.

If you have any questions, check with your doctor, nurse, or pharmacist.

PROPER USE OF THIS MEDICINE

Take this medicine only as directed. Do not take more of it and do not take it more often than recommended on the label, unless otherwise directed by your doctor. To do so may increase the chance of side effects.

Antihistamine and decongestant combinations may be taken with food or a glass of water or milk to lessen stomach irritation, if necessary.

For patients taking the extended-release capsule or tablet form of this medicine:
- Swallow it whole.
- Do not crush, break, or chew before swallowing.
- If the capsule is too large to swallow, you may mix the contents of the capsule with applesauce, jelly, honey, or syrup and swallow without chewing.

If you must take this medicine regularly and you miss a dose, take it as soon as possible. However, if it is almost time for your next dose, skip the missed dose and go back to your regular dosing schedule. Do not double doses.

PRECAUTIONS WHILE USING THIS MEDICINE

The antihistamine in this medicine will add to the effects of alcohol and other CNS depressants (medicines that slow down the nervous system). **Check with your doctor before taking any such depressants while you are taking this medicine.**

The antihistamine may also cause some people to become drowsy, dizzy, or less alert than they are normally. This side effect is less likely to occur with the loratadine or terfenadine-containing combinations; however, **make sure you know how you react to this medicine before you drive, use machines, or do other jobs that require you to be alert.**

The decongestant in this medicine may add to the effects of phenylpropanolamine-containing diet aids. **Do not use medicines for diet or appetite control while taking this medicine unless you have first checked with your doctor.**

The decongestant may also cause some people to be nervous or restless or to have trouble in sleeping. If you have trouble in sleeping, **take the last dose of this medicine for each day a few hours before bedtime.**

POSSIBLE SIDE EFFECTS OF THIS MEDICINE

Although serious side effects occur rarely when this medicine is taken as recommended, they may be more likely to occur if too much medicine is taken or if it is taken in large doses, or for a long period of time.

Side effects that should be reported to your doctor immediately
> RARE—Fast or irregular heartbeat

Other side effects that should be reported to your doctor
> RARE—Mood or mental changes; sore throat and fever; tightness in chest; unusual bleeding or bruising; unusual tiredness or weakness

Side effects that usually do not require medical attention
> These possible side effects may go away during treatment; however, if they continue or are bothersome, check with your doctor, nurse, or pharmacist.
>
> MORE COMMON (RARE WITH TERFENADINE-CONTAINING COMBINATION)— Drowsiness; thickening of the bronchial secretions
>
> Other side effects not listed above may also occur in some patients. If you notice any other effects, check with your doctor, nurse, or pharmacist.

ANTIHISTAMINES, DECONGESTANTS, AND ANALGESICS (ORAL)

ABOUT YOUR MEDICINE

Antihistamine, decongestant, and **analgesic** combinations are taken by mouth to relieve the sneezing, runny nose, sinus and nasal congestion (stuffy nose), fever, headache, and aches and pain, of colds, influenza, and hay fever. These combinations do not contain any ingredient to relieve coughs.

Some of these medicines are available without a prescription. However, your doctor may have special instructions for your medical condition.

If any of the information in this profile causes you special concern or if you want additional information about your medicine and its use, check with your doctor, nurse, or pharmacist. **Remember, keep this and all other medicines out of the reach of children and never share your medicines with others.**

BEFORE USING THIS MEDICINE

Do not give a medicine containing aspirin or other salicylates to a child or a teenager with a fever or other symptoms of a virus infection, especially flu or chickenpox, without first discussing this with your child's doctor.

If you are taking this medicine without a prescription, carefully read and follow any precautions on the label. You should be especially careful if you . . .
- are allergic to any medicine, either prescription or nonprescription (OTC);
- are pregnant, intend to become pregnant, or are breast-feeding;

- are taking **any** other prescription or nonprescription (OTC) medicine;
- have **any** other medical problems.

If you have any questions, check with your doctor, nurse, or pharmacist.

PROPER USE OF THIS MEDICINE

Take this medicine only as directed. Do not take more of it and do not take it more often than recommended on the label, unless otherwise directed by your doctor. To do so may increase the chance of side effects.

If this medicine irritates your stomach, you may take it with food or a glass of water or milk to lessen the irritation.

If you must take this medicine regularly and you miss a dose, take it as soon as possible. However, if it is almost time for your next dose, skip the missed dose and go back to your regular dosing schedule. Do not double doses.

PRECAUTIONS WHILE USING THIS MEDICINE

Check with your doctor if your symptoms do not improve or become worse, or if you have a high fever.

This medicine will add to the effects of alcohol and other CNS depressants (medicines that slow down the nervous system). **Check with your doctor before taking any such depressants while you are taking this medicine.**

Do not drink alcoholic beverages while taking this medicine. To do so may increase the chance of serious side effects.

The antihistamine in this medicine may cause some people to become drowsy, dizzy, or less alert than they are normally. **Make sure you know how you react before you drive, use machines, or do other jobs that require you to be alert.**

The decongestant in this medicine may cause some people to become nervous or restless or to have trouble in sleeping. If you have trouble in sleeping, **take the last dose of this medicine for each day a few hours before bedtime.** If you have any questions about this, check with your doctor.

POSSIBLE SIDE EFFECTS OF THIS MEDICINE

Side effects that should be reported to your doctor

MORE COMMON—Nausea or vomiting; stomach pain (mild)

LESS COMMON OR RARE—Bloody or black tarry stools; changes in urine or problems with urination; skin rash, hives, or itching; sore throat and fever; swelling of face, feet, or lower legs; tightness in chest; unusual bleeding or bruising; unusual tiredness or weakness; vomiting of blood or material that looks like coffee grounds; weight gain (unusual); yellow eyes or skin

Side effects that usually do not require medical attention

These possible side effects may go away during treatment; however, if they continue or are bothersome, check with your doctor, nurse, or pharmacist.

MORE COMMON—Drowsiness; heartburn or indigestion (for salicylate-containing medicines); thickening of mucus

Other side effects not listed above may also occur in some patients. If you notice any other effects, check with your doctor, nurse, or pharmacist.

ANTI-INFLAMMATORY DRUGS (NSAIDS) (ORAL)

Including Buffered Phenylbutazone; Diclofenac; Diflunisal; Etodolac; Fenoprofen; Floctafenine; Flurbiprofen; Ibuprofen; Indomethacin; Ketoprofen; Meclofenamate; Mefenamic Acid; Nabumetone; Naproxen; Oxaprozin; Phenylbutazone; Piroxicam; Sulindac; Tiaprofenic Acid; Tolmetin

ABOUT YOUR MEDICINE

Nonsteroidal anti-inflammatory drugs (NSAIDs) are used for inflammation, swelling, stiffness, and joint pain. Some are also used to relieve gout, menstrual cramps, or other kinds of pain. Ibuprofen and naproxen are also used to reduce fever. Meclofenamate is also used to lessen heavy menstrual bleeding. They may also be used for other conditions as determined by your doctor.

If any of the information in this profile causes you special concern or if you want additional information about your medicine and its use, check with your doctor, nurse, or pharmacist. **Remember, keep this and all other medicines out of the reach of children and never share your medicines with others.**

BEFORE USING THIS MEDICINE

If you are taking this medicine without a prescription, carefully read and follow any precautions on the label. You should be especially careful if you . . .
- are allergic to any medicine, either prescription or nonprescription (OTC);
- are pregnant, intend to become pregnant, or are breast-feeding;
- are taking **any** other prescription or nonprescription (OTC) medicine;
- have **any** other medical problems.

If you have any questions, check with your doctor, nurse, or pharmacist.

PROPER USE OF THIS MEDICINE

Always take NSAIDs with food or antacids and an 8-ounce glass of water. Do not take more of this medicine, do not take it more often, and do not take it for a longer time than directed.

When used for arthritis, this medicine must be taken regularly as ordered.

If you are taking this medicine regularly and you miss a dose, take it as soon as possible. However, if it is almost time for your next dose, skip the missed dose and go back to your regular schedule. Do not double doses.

PRECAUTIONS WHILE USING THIS MEDICINE

It is important to have regular check-ups if you are taking this medicine regularly. Serious side effects, such as ulcers or bleeding, can occur.

Do not take other anti-inflammatories, including aspirin, regularly or drink alcohol while taking this medicine, unless otherwise directed by your doctor.

This medicine may cause some people to become drowsy, dizzy, or less alert than they are normally. Make sure you know how you react before you drive, use machines, or do other jobs that require you to be alert.

POSSIBLE SIDE EFFECTS OF THIS MEDICINE

Stop taking this medicine and get emergency help right away if you notice: fainting; irregular breathing, heartbeat, or pulse; hive-like swellings (large) on face or tongue; puffiness or swelling of the eyelids or around the eyes; or shortness of breath, troubled breathing, wheezing, or tightness in chest.

Stop taking this medicine and check with your doctor immediately if you notice severe abdominal or stomach pain, cramping, or burning; bloody or black, tarry stools; chest pain; convulsions (seizures); diarrhea (mefenamic acid only); fever; pinpoint red spots on skin; severe and continuing nausea, heartburn, or indigestion; sores, ulcers, or white spots on lips or in mouth; swelling of face, hands, feet, or lower legs (phenylbutazone only); spitting up blood; unusual bleeding or bruising; vomiting blood or material that looks like coffee grounds; or weight gain (rapid—phenylbutazone only).

Other side effects that should be reported to your doctor

MORE COMMON—Headache (for indomethacin); skin rash

LESS COMMON OR RARE—Bladder pain; bleeding from cuts that lasts longer than usual; bleeding or crusting sores on lips; bloody or cloudy urine or problems with urination; burning feeling in throat, chest, or stomach; change in urine color or odor; changes in hearing; confusion or forgetfulness; cough or hoarseness; diarrhea (severe); difficulty speaking or swallowing; fast or pounding heartbeat; hallucinations; headache (severe) with stiff neck or back; hives, itching, or other skin problems; increased blood pressure; irritated tongue; light-colored stools; loose or splitting fingernails; mood changes; muscle cramps, pain, or weakness, or uncontrollable muscle movements; numbness, tingling, pain, or weakness in hands or feet; lower back or side pain (severe); painful or swollen glands; pain or redness in eyes; ringing or buzzing in ears; runny nose or sneezing; sore throat or fever; swelling of face, lips, tongue, hands, feet, or lower legs; swelling or tenderness in upper stomach; unusual thirst; unusual tiredness or weakness; weight gain (rapid); vision problems; yellow eyes or skin

Side effects that usually do not require medical attention

These possible side effects may go away during treatment; however, if they continue or are bothersome, check with your doctor, nurse, or pharmacist.

MORE COMMON—Bloated feeling or gas; diarrhea, mild nausea, or vomiting; dizziness, lightheadedness, or drowsiness; headache; mild heartburn, indigestion, or stomach pain or cramps

Other side effects not listed above may also occur in some patients. If you notice any other effects, check with your doctor, nurse, or pharmacist.

Antithyroid Agents (Oral)

Including Methimazole; Propylthiouracil

About Your Medicine

Methimazole (meth-IM-a-zole) and **propylthiouracil** (proe-pill-thye-oh-YOOR-a-sill) are used to treat conditions in which the thyroid gland produces too much thyroid hormone.

If any of the information in this profile causes you special concern or if you want additional information about your medicine and its use, check with your doctor, nurse, or pharmacist. **Remember, keep this and all other medicines out of the reach of children and never share your medicines with others.**

Before Using This Medicine

Tell your doctor, nurse, and pharmacist if you . . .
- are allergic to any medicine, either prescription or nonprescription (OTC);
- are pregnant or intend to become pregnant while using this medicine;
- are breast-feeding;
- are taking any other prescription or nonprescription (OTC) medicine,

especially amiodarone, anticoagulants (blood thinners), digitalis medicines, iodinated glycerol, or potassium iodide;
- have any other medical problems, especially liver disease.

PROPER USE OF THIS MEDICINE

Use this medicine only as directed by your doctor. Do not use more or less of it and do not use it more often or for a longer time than your doctor ordered.

In order for it to work properly, **this medicine must be taken every day in regularly spaced doses, as ordered by your doctor.**

Food in your stomach may change the amount of methimazole that is able to enter the bloodstream. To make sure that you always get the same effects, try to take methimazole at the same time in relation to meals every day. That is, always take it with meals or always take it on an empty stomach.

If you miss a dose of this medicine, take it as soon as possible. If it is almost time for your next dose, take both doses together. Then go back to your regular dosing schedule. If you miss more than one dose or if you have any questions about this, check with your doctor.

PRECAUTIONS WHILE USING THIS MEDICINE

It is very important that your doctor check your progress at regular intervals in order to make sure that this medicine is working properly and to check for unwanted effects.

It may take several days or weeks for this medicine to work. However, **do not stop taking this medicine without first checking with your doctor.** Some medical problems may require several years of continuous treatment.

Before having any kind of surgery or dental or emergency treatment, **tell the physician or dentist in charge that you are taking this medicine.**

Check with your doctor right away if you get an injury, infection, or illness of any kind. Your doctor may want you to stop taking this medicine or change the amount you are taking.

POSSIBLE SIDE EFFECTS OF THIS MEDICINE

Side effects that should be reported to your doctor immediately
    LESS COMMON—Cough; fever or chills (continuing or severe); general feeling of discomfort, illness, or weakness; hoarseness; mouth sores; pain, swelling, or redness of joints; throat infection
    RARE—Yellow eyes or skin

Other side effects that should be reported to your doctor
    MORE COMMON—Fever (mild and temporary); skin rash or itching
    RARE—Backache; black, tarry stools; blood in urine or stools; changes in menstrual periods; coldness; constipation; diarrhea; dry, puffy skin; fast or

irregular heartbeat; headache; increase in bleeding or bruising; increase or decrease in urination; listlessness or sleepiness; muscle aches; numbness or tingling of fingers, toes, or face; pinpoint red spots on skin; shortness of breath; swelling of feet or lower legs; swollen lymph nodes; swollen salivary glands; unusual tiredness or weakness; weight gain (unusual)

Side effects that usually do not require medical attention

These possible side effects may go away during treatment; however, if they continue or are bothersome, check with your doctor, nurse, or pharmacist.

LESS COMMON—Dizziness; loss of taste (for methimazole); nausea; stomach pain; vomiting

Other side effects not listed above may also occur in some patients. If you notice any other effects, check with your doctor, nurse, or pharmacist.

$\mathcal{A}$PPETITE SUPPRESSANTS (ORAL)

Including Benzphetamine;
Diethylpropion; Mazindol; Phendimetrazine; Phentermine

ABOUT YOUR MEDICINE

Appetite suppressants are used in the short-term treatment of obesity. For a few weeks these medicines in combination with dieting and exercise can help obese patients lose weight. However, since their appetite-reducing effect is only temporary, they are useful only for the first few weeks of dieting until new eating habits are established.

If any of the information in this profile causes you special concern or if you want additional information about your medicine and its use, check with your doctor, nurse, or pharmacist. **Remember, keep this and all other medicines out of the reach of children and never share your medicines with others.**

BEFORE USING THIS MEDICINE

Tell your doctor, nurse, and pharmacist if you . . .
- are allergic to any medicine, either prescription or nonprescription (OTC);
- are pregnant or intend to become pregnant while using this medicine;
- are breast-feeding;
- are taking any other prescription or nonprescription (OTC) medicine, especially MAO inhibitors;
- have any other medical problems, especially alcoholism, drug abuse or

dependence (or history of), glaucoma, heart or blood vessel disease, high blood pressure, kidney disease, mental illness (severe), or overactive thyroid.

PROPER USE OF THIS MEDICINE

Take this medicine only as directed by your doctor. Do not take more of it, do not take it more often, and do not take it for a longer period of time than your doctor ordered. If too much is taken, it may become habit-forming.

If you think this medicine is not working properly after you have taken it for a few weeks, do not increase the dose. Instead, check with your doctor.

For patients taking the short-acting form of this medicine (effects last only a few hours):
- Take the last dose for each day about 4 to 6 hours before bedtime to help prevent trouble in sleeping.

For patients taking the long-acting form of this medicine (effects last 8 hours or more):
- Take the daily dose about 10 to 14 hours before bedtime to help prevent trouble in sleeping.
- The capsules or tablets are to be swallowed whole. Do not break, crush, or chew before swallowing.

PRECAUTIONS WHILE USING THIS MEDICINE

If you have taken this medicine for a while, do not stop taking it without first checking with your doctor. Your doctor may want you to reduce gradually the amount you are taking before stopping completely.

This medicine may cause some people to become dizzy, lightheaded, drowsy, or less alert than they are normally. **Make sure you know how you react to this medicine before you drive, use machines, or do other jobs that require you to be alert.**

Before having any kind of surgery or dental or emergency treatment, tell the physician or dentist in charge that you are using this medicine. Taking appetite suppressants together with medicines that are used during surgery or dental or emergency treatments may cause serious side effects.

If you have been taking this medicine for a long time or in large doses and **you think you may have become mentally or physically dependent on it, check with your doctor.**

POSSIBLE SIDE EFFECTS OF THIS MEDICINE

Side effects that should be reported to your doctor
MORE COMMON—Increased blood pressure
LESS COMMON OR RARE—Confusion; mental depression; skin rash or hives; sore throat and fever; unusual bleeding or bruising

Side effects that usually do not require medical attention

These possible side effects may go away during treatment; however, if they continue or are bothersome, check with your doctor, nurse, or pharmacist.

False sense of well-being; irritability; nervousness; restlessness; trouble in sleeping

After the stimulant side effects have worn off, drowsiness, trembling, unusual tiredness or weakness, or mental depression may occur.

Other side effects not listed above may also occur in some patients. If you notice any other effects, check with your doctor, nurse, or pharmacist.

After you stop using this medicine, your body may need time to adjust. This may take several days or more. **Check with your doctor if you experience** mental depression, nausea or vomiting, stomach cramps or pain, trembling, or unusual tiredness or weakness.

ASTEMIZOLE (ORAL)

ABOUT YOUR MEDICINE

Astemizole (a-STEM-mi-zole) is used to relieve or prevent the symptoms of hay fever and other types of allergy. Astemizole may also be used for other conditions as determined by your doctor.

If any of the information in this profile causes you special concern or if you want additional information about your medicine and its use, check with your doctor, nurse, or pharmacist. **Remember, keep this and all other medicines out of the reach of children and never share your medicines with others.**

BEFORE USING THIS MEDICINE

Tell your doctor, nurse, and pharmacist if you . . .
- are allergic to any medicine, either prescription or nonprescription (OTC);
- are pregnant or intend to become pregnant;
- are breast-feeding;
- are taking any other prescription or nonprescription (OTC) medicine, especially bepridil, clarithromycin, disopyramide, erythromycin, itraconazole, ketoconazole, maprotiline, phenothiazines, pimozide, procainamide, quinidine, or tricyclic antidepressants;
- have any other medical problems, especially difficult urination, enlarged prostate, glaucoma, heart rhythm problems (history of), liver disease, low potassium blood levels, or urinary tract blockage.

PROPER USE OF THIS MEDICINE

Astemizole is used to relieve or prevent the symptoms of your medical problem. Take it only as directed. Do not take more of it and do not take it more often than your doctor ordered. To do so may increase the chance of side effects.

Astemizole should be taken on an empty stomach.

If you must take this medicine regularly and you miss a dose, take it as soon as possible. However, if it is almost time for your next dose, skip the missed dose and go back to your regular dosing schedule. Do not double doses.

POSSIBLE SIDE EFFECTS OF THIS MEDICINE

Side effects that should be reported to your doctor immediately
> LESS COMMON OR RARE (WITH HIGH DOSES)—Fast or irregular heartbeat

Other side effects that should be reported to your doctor
> LESS COMMON OR RARE—Sore throat and fever; unusual bleeding or bruising; unusual tiredness or weakness

Side effects that usually do not require medical attention
> These possible side effects may go away during treatment; however, if they continue or are bothersome, check with your doctor, nurse, or pharmacist.
>
> RARE—Drowsiness; thickening of mucus
>
> Other side effects not listed above may also occur in some patients. If you notice any other effects, check with your doctor, nurse, or pharmacist.

AZITHROMYCIN (ORAL)

ABOUT YOUR MEDICINE

Azithromycin (az-ith-roe-MYE-sin) is used to treat bacterial infections in many different parts of the body. However, this medicine will not work for colds, flu, or other virus infections. Azithromycin may be used for other problems as determined by your doctor.

If any of the information in this profile causes you special concern or if you want additional information about your medicine and its use, check with your doctor, nurse, or pharmacist. **Remember, keep this and all other medicines out of the reach of children and never share your medicines with others.**

Before Using This Medicine

Tell your doctor, nurse, and pharmacist if you . . .
- are allergic to any medicine, either prescription or nonprescription (OTC);
- are pregnant or intend to become pregnant while using this medicine;
- are breast-feeding;
- are taking any other prescription or nonprescription (OTC) medicine, especially aluminum- and magnesium-containing antacids;
- have any other medical problems.

Proper Use of This Medicine

Azithromycin should be taken at least one hour before or at least 2 hours after meals. Taking azithromycin with food may decrease the amount of medicine that gets into your blood and may keep the medicine from working properly.

To help clear up your infection completely, **keep taking azithromycin for the full time of treatment,** even if you begin to feel better after a few days. If you stop taking this medicine too soon, your symptoms may return.

If you miss a dose of this medicine, take it as soon as possible. However, if it is almost time for your next dose, skip the missed dose and go back to your regular dosing schedule. Do not double doses.

Precautions While Using This Medicine

If your symptoms do not improve within a few days, or if they become worse, check with your doctor.

Possible Side Effects of This Medicine

Side effects that should be reported to your doctor immediately
> **Stop taking this medicine and get emergency help immediately if any of the following side effects occur:**
>
> RARE—Difficulty in breathing; fever; joint pain; skin rash; swelling of face, mouth, neck, hands, and feet

Side effects that usually do not require medical attention
> These possible side effects may go away during treatment; however, if they continue or are bothersome, check with your doctor, nurse, or pharmacist.
>
> LESS COMMON—Diarrhea; nausea; stomach pain or discomfort; vomiting
> RARE—Dizziness; headache
>
> Other side effects not listed above may also occur in some patients. If you notice any other effects, check with your doctor, nurse, or pharmacist.

$\mathcal{A}$ZOLE ANTIFUNGALS (ORAL)

Including Fluconazole; Itraconazole; Ketoconazole

ABOUT YOUR MEDICINE

Azole (AY-zole) **antifungals** are used to treat serious fungus infections that may occur in different parts of the body. These medicines may also be used for other problems as determined by your doctor.

If any of the information in this profile causes you special concern or if you want additional information about your medicine and its use, check with your doctor, nurse, or pharmacist. **Remember, keep this and all other medicines out of the reach of children and never share your medicines with others.**

BEFORE USING THIS MEDICINE

Tell your doctor, nurse, and pharmacist if you . . .
- are allergic to any medicine, either prescription or nonprescription (OTC);
- are pregnant or intend to become pregnant while using this medicine;
- are breast-feeding;
- are taking **any** other prescription or nonprescription (OTC) medicine;
- have any other medical problems, especially achlorhydria (absence of stomach acid), alcohol abuse (or history of), hypochlorhydria (decreased amount of stomach acid), or kidney or liver disease.

PROPER USE OF THIS MEDICINE

Itraconazole and ketoconazole should be taken with a meal or snack.

For patients taking the oral liquid form of ketoconazole:
- Use a specially marked measuring spoon or other device to measure each dose. The average household teaspoon may not hold the right amount.

If you have achlorhydria or hypochlorhydria and you are taking itraconazole or ketoconazole, your doctor may have special instructions for you. Your doctor may want you to take your medicine with an acidic drink, such as cola or seltzer water, or mixed into a special solution of weak hydrochloric acid. Be sure to follow your doctor's instructions carefully.

To help clear up your infection completely, **it is very important that you keep taking this medicine for the full time of treatment.**

This medicine works best when there is a constant amount in the blood. **To help keep this amount constant, do not miss any doses. Also, it is best to take each dose at the same time every day.** If you need help in planning the best time to take your medicine, check with your doctor, nurse, or pharmacist.

If you do miss a dose of this medicine, take it as soon as possible. However, if it is almost time for your next dose, skip the missed dose and go back to your regular dosing schedule. Do not double doses.

PRECAUTIONS WHILE USING THIS MEDICINE

It is important that your doctor check your progress at regular visits.

If your symptoms do not improve within a few weeks (or months for some infections), or if they become worse, check with your doctor.

Itraconazole and ketoconazole should not be taken with astemizole (e.g., Hismanal), cisapride (e.g., Propulsid), or terfenadine (e.g., Seldane). Doing so may increase the risk of serious side effects affecting the heart.

Liver problems may be more likely to occur if you drink alcoholic beverages while you are taking ketoconazole. Alcoholic beverages may also cause stomach pain, nausea, vomiting, headache, or flushing or redness of the face. Other alcohol-containing preparations (for example, elixirs, cough syrups, tonics) may also cause problems. These problems may occur for at least a day after you stop taking ketoconazole. Therefore, **you should not drink alcoholic beverages while you are taking ketoconazole and for at least a day after you stop taking it.**

If you are taking antacids, cimetidine, famotidine, nizatidine, ranitidine, or omeprazole while you are taking itraconazole or ketoconazole, take them at least 2 hours after you take itraconazole or ketoconazole.

Ketoconazole may cause your eyes to become more sensitive to light than they are normally. Wearing sunglasses and avoiding too much exposure to bright light may help lessen the discomfort.

POSSIBLE SIDE EFFECTS OF THIS MEDICINE

Side effects that should be reported to your doctor immediately
> LESS COMMON OR RARE—Dark or amber urine; fever, chills, or sore throat; loss of appetite; pale stools; reddening, blistering, peeling, or loosening of skin and mucous membranes; skin rash or itching; stomach pain; unusual bleeding or bruising; unusual tiredness or weakness; yellow eyes or skin

Side effects that usually do not require medical attention
> These possible side effects may go away during treatment; however, if they continue or are bothersome, check with your doctor, nurse, or pharmacist.

> LESS COMMON—Constipation; diarrhea; dizziness; drowsiness; flushing or redness of the face or skin; headache; nausea; vomiting
> RARE (FOR KETOCONAZOLE ONLY)—Decreased sexual ability or enlarged breasts in males; increased sensitivity of eyes to light; menstrual irregularities

> Other side effects not listed above may also occur in some patients. If you notice any other effects, check with your doctor, nurse, or pharmacist.

Azole Antifungals (Vaginal)

Including Butoconazole; Clotrimazole;
Econazole; Miconazole; Terconazole; Tioconazole

About Your Medicine

Vaginal azole (AZ-ole) **antifungals** are used to treat fungus (yeast) infections of
the vagina.

If any of the information in this profile causes you special concern or if you want
additional information about your medicine and its use, check with your doctor,
nurse, or pharmacist. **Remember, keep this and all other medicines out of the
reach of children and never share your medicines with others.**

Before Using This Medicine

Tell your doctor, nurse, and pharmacist if you . . .
- are allergic to any medicine, either prescription or nonprescription (OTC);
- are pregnant or intend to become pregnant while using this medicine;
- are breast-feeding;
- are taking any other prescription or nonprescription (OTC) medicine;
- use condoms, a cervical cap, or a diaphragm for birth control;
- have any other medical problems.

Proper Use of This Medicine

Vaginal azole antifungals usually come with patient directions. Read them carefully
before using this medicine.

Use this medicine at bedtime, unless otherwise directed by your doctor. The vaginal
tampon form of miconazole should be left in the vagina overnight and removed the
next morning.

To help clear up your infection completely, **it is very important that you keep
using this medicine for the full time of treatment,** even if your symptoms begin
to clear up after a few days. If you stop using this medicine too soon, your symptoms
may return. **Do not miss any doses.** Also, **do not stop using this medicine if your
menstrual period starts during the time of treatment.**

If you do miss a dose of this medicine, insert it as soon as possible. However, if it
is almost time for your next dose, skip the missed dose and go back to your regular
dosing schedule.

Precautions While Using This Medicine

If your symptoms do not improve within a few days, or if they become worse, check
with your doctor.

Vaginal medicines usually will come out of the vagina during treatment. To keep
the medicine from getting on your clothing, wear a minipad or sanitary napkin. The

use of nonmedicated tampons (like those used for menstrual periods) is not recommended since they may soak up the medicine.

To help clear up your infection completely and to help make sure it does not return, good health habits are also required.

- Wear cotton panties (or panties or pantyhose with cotton crotches) instead of synthetic (for example, nylon or rayon) panties.
- Wear only clean panties.

Many vaginal infections are spread by having sex. A male sexual partner may carry the fungus on or in his penis. While you are using this medicine, it may be a good idea for your partner to wear a condom during sex to avoid reinfection. Also, it may be necessary for your partner to be treated. **Do not stop using this medicine if you have sex during treatment.**

Some women may want to use a douche before the next dose. Some doctors will allow the use of a vinegar and water douche or other douche. However, others do not allow any douching. If you do use a douche, **do not overfill the vagina.** To do so may push the douche up into the uterus and possibly cause inflammation or infection. Also, **do not douche if you are pregnant since this may harm the fetus.** If you have any questions about this, check with your doctor, nurse, or pharmacist.

This medicine must not be given to other people or used for other infections unless otherwise directed by your doctor.

POSSIBLE SIDE EFFECTS OF THIS MEDICINE

Side effects that should be reported to your doctor

LESS COMMON—Vaginal burning, itching, discharge, or other irritation not present before use of this medicine

RARE—Skin rash or hives

Side effects that usually do not require medical attention

These possible side effects may go away during treatment; however, if they continue or are bothersome, check with your doctor, nurse, or pharmacist.

LESS COMMON OR RARE—Abdominal or stomach cramps or pain; burning or irritation of penis of sexual partner; headache

Other side effects not listed above may also occur in some patients. If you notice any other effects, check with your doctor, nurse, or pharmacist.

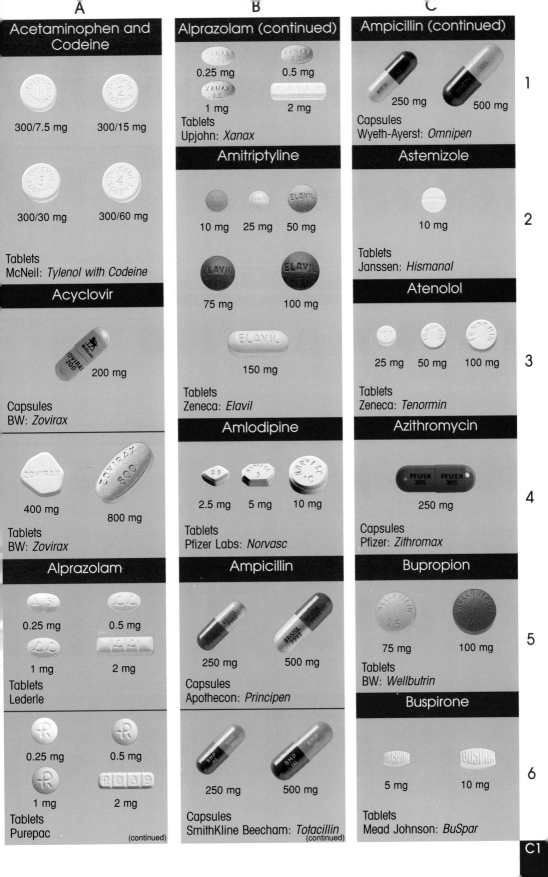

A

Acetaminophen and Codeine

300/7.5 mg 300/15 mg

300/30 mg 300/60 mg

Tablets
McNeil: *Tylenol with Codeine*

Acyclovir

200 mg

Capsules
BW: *Zovirax*

400 mg 800 mg

Tablets
BW: *Zovirax*

Alprazolam

0.25 mg 0.5 mg

1 mg 2 mg

Tablets
Lederle

0.25 mg 0.5 mg

1 mg 2 mg

Tablets
Purepac

(continued)

B

Alprazolam (continued)

0.25 mg 0.5 mg

1 mg 2 mg

Tablets
Upjohn: *Xanax*

Amitriptyline

10 mg 25 mg 50 mg

75 mg 100 mg

150 mg

Tablets
Zeneca: *Elavil*

Amlodipine

2.5 mg 5 mg 10 mg

Tablets
Pfizer Labs: *Norvasc*

Ampicillin

250 mg 500 mg

Capsules
Apothecon: *Principen*

250 mg 500 mg

Capsules
SmithKline Beecham: *Totacillin*
(continued)

C

Ampicillin (continued)

250 mg 500 mg

Capsules
Wyeth-Ayerst: *Omnipen*

Astemizole

10 mg

Tablets
Janssen: *Hismanal*

Atenolol

25 mg 50 mg 100 mg

Tablets
Zeneca: *Tenormin*

Azithromycin

250 mg

Capsules
Pfizer: *Zithromax*

Bupropion

75 mg 100 mg

Tablets
BW: *Wellbutrin*

Buspirone

5 mg 10 mg

Tablets
Mead Johnson: *BuSpar*

1

2

3

4

5

6

C1

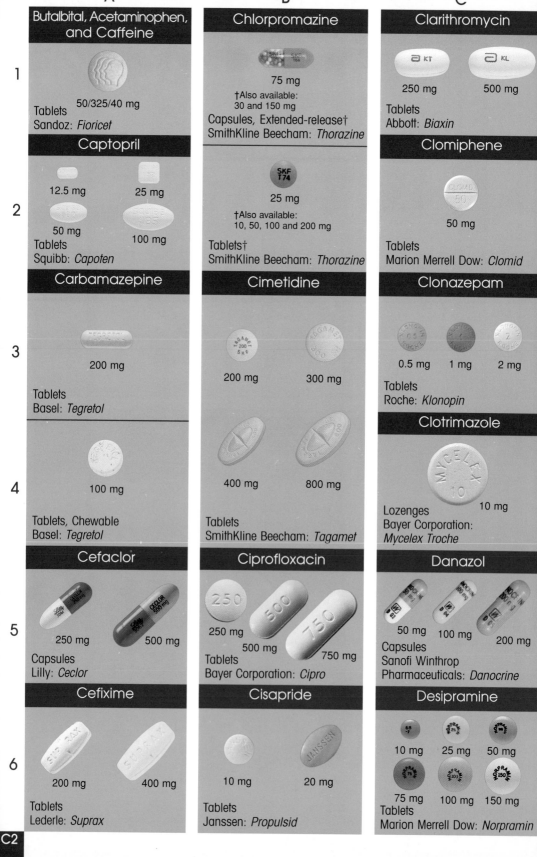

A

Butalbital, Acetaminophen, and Caffeine

1. 50/325/40 mg
    Tablets
    Sandoz: *Fioricet*

Captopril

2. 12.5 mg
    25 mg
    50 mg
    100 mg
    Tablets
    Squibb: *Capoten*

Carbamazepine

3. 200 mg
    Tablets
    Basel: *Tegretol*

4. 100 mg
    Tablets, Chewable
    Basel: *Tegretol*

Cefaclor

5. 250 mg
    500 mg
    Capsules
    Lilly: *Ceclor*

Cefixime

6. 200 mg
    400 mg
    Tablets
    Lederle: *Suprax*

B

Chlorpromazine

1. 75 mg
    †Also available:
    30 and 150 mg
    Capsules, Extended-release†
    SmithKline Beecham: *Thorazine*

2. SKF
    T74
    25 mg
    †Also available:
    10, 50, 100 and 200 mg
    Tablets†
    SmithKline Beecham: *Thorazine*

Cimetidine

3. 200 mg
    300 mg

4. 400 mg
    800 mg
    Tablets
    SmithKline Beecham: *Tagamet*

Ciprofloxacin

5. 250 mg
    500 mg
    750 mg
    Tablets
    Bayer Corporation: *Cipro*

Cisapride

6. 10 mg
    20 mg
    Tablets
    Janssen: *Propulsid*

C

Clarithromycin

1. 250 mg
    500 mg
    Tablets
    Abbott: *Biaxin*

Clomiphene

2. 50 mg
    Tablets
    Marion Merrell Dow: *Clomid*

Clonazepam

3. 0.5 mg
    1 mg
    2 mg
    Tablets
    Roche: *Klonopin*

Clotrimazole

4. MYCELEX
    10
    10 mg
    Lozenges
    Bayer Corporation:
    Mycelex Troche

Danazol

5. 50 mg
    100 mg
    200 mg
    Capsules
    Sanofi Winthrop
    Pharmaceuticals: *Danocrine*

Desipramine

6. 10 mg
    25 mg
    50 mg
    75 mg
    100 mg
    150 mg
    Tablets
    Marion Merrell Dow: *Norpramin*

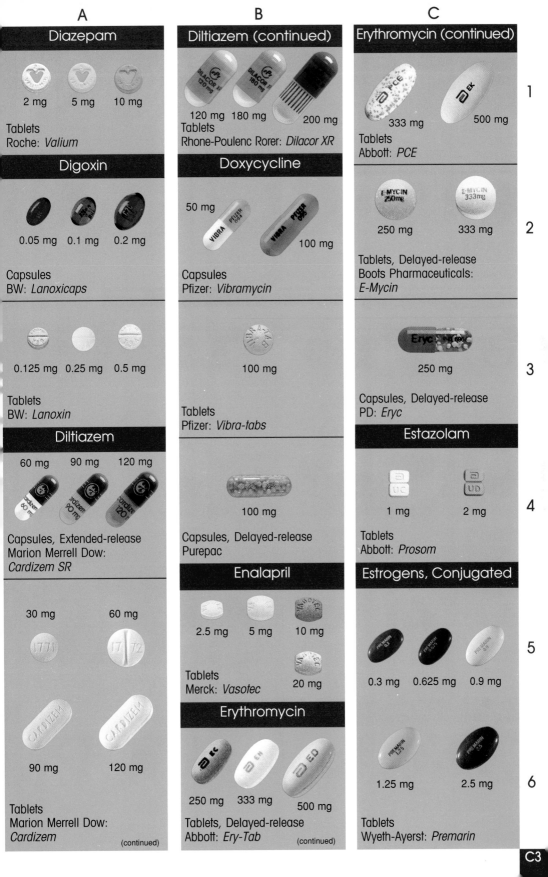

A

Diazepam

2 mg 5 mg 10 mg

Tablets
Roche: *Valium*

Digoxin

0.05 mg 0.1 mg 0.2 mg

Capsules
BW: *Lanoxicaps*

0.125 mg 0.25 mg 0.5 mg

Tablets
BW: *Lanoxin*

Diltiazem

60 mg 90 mg 120 mg

Capsules, Extended-release
Marion Merrell Dow:
Cardizem SR

30 mg 60 mg

90 mg 120 mg

Tablets
Marion Merrell Dow:
Cardizem

(continued)

B

Diltiazem (continued)

120 mg 180 mg 200 mg

Tablets
Rhone-Poulenc Rorer: *Dilacor XR*

Doxycycline

50 mg 100 mg

Capsules
Pfizer: *Vibramycin*

100 mg

Tablets
Pfizer: *Vibra-tabs*

100 mg

Capsules, Delayed-release
Purepac

Enalapril

2.5 mg 5 mg 10 mg

20 mg

Tablets
Merck: *Vasotec*

Erythromycin

250 mg 333 mg 500 mg

Tablets, Delayed-release
Abbott: *Ery-Tab*

(continued)

C

Erythromycin (continued)

333 mg 500 mg

1

Tablets
Abbott: *PCE*

250 mg 333 mg

2

Tablets, Delayed-release
Boots Pharmaceuticals:
E-Mycin

250 mg

3

Capsules, Delayed-release
PD: *Eryc*

Estazolam

1 mg 2 mg

4

Tablets
Abbott: *Prosom*

Estrogens, Conjugated

0.3 mg 0.625 mg 0.9 mg

5

1.25 mg 2.5 mg

6

Tablets
Wyeth-Ayerst: *Premarin*

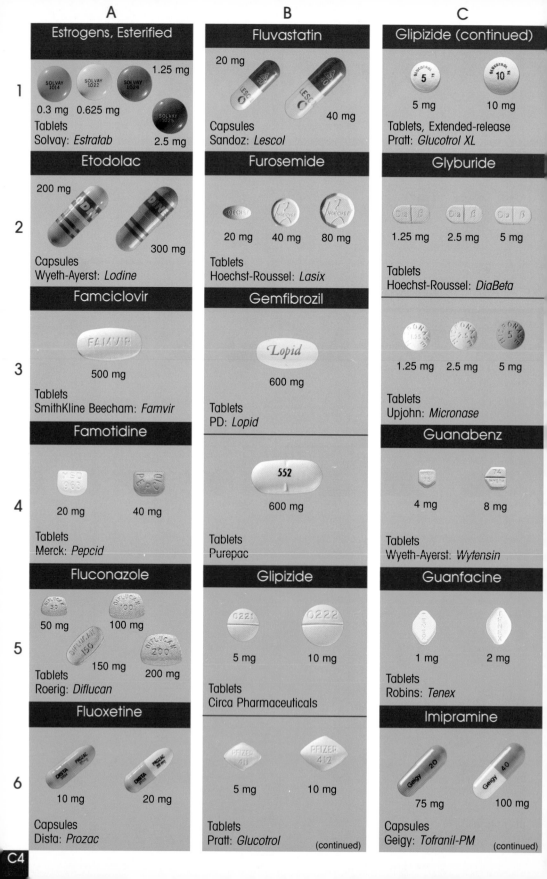

A

Estrogens, Esterified

1
SOLVAY 1014 — 0.3 mg
SOLVAY 1022 — 0.625 mg
SOLVAY 1024 — 1.25 mg
SOLVAY 1025 — 2.5 mg
Tablets
Solvay: *Estratab*

Etodolac

2
200 mg
300 mg
Capsules
Wyeth-Ayerst: *Lodine*

Famciclovir

3
FAMVIR
500 mg
Tablets
SmithKline Beecham: *Famvir*

Famotidine

4
MSD 963 — 20 mg
PEPCID — 40 mg
Tablets
Merck: *Pepcid*

Fluconazole

5
50 mg
100 mg
150 mg
200 mg
Tablets
Roerig: *Diflucan*

Fluoxetine

6
DISTA PROZAC — 10 mg
DISTA PROZAC 20 mg — 20 mg
Capsules
Dista: *Prozac*

B

Fluvastatin

1
20 mg
40 mg
Capsules
Sandoz: *Lescol*

Furosemide

2
20 mg
40 mg
80 mg
Tablets
Hoechst-Roussel: *Lasix*

Gemfibrozil

3
Lopid
600 mg
Tablets
PD: *Lopid*

4
552
600 mg
Tablets
Purepac

Glipizide

5
0221 — 5 mg
0222 — 10 mg
Tablets
Circa Pharmaceuticals

6
PFIZER 411 — 5 mg
PFIZER 412 — 10 mg
Tablets
Pratt: *Glucotrol*

(continued)

C

Glipizide (continued)

1
GLUCOTROL XL 5 — 5 mg
GLUCOTROL XL 10 — 10 mg
Tablets, Extended-release
Pratt: *Glucotrol XL*

Glyburide

2
Dia ß — 1.25 mg
Dia ß — 2.5 mg
Dia ß — 5 mg
Tablets
Hoechst-Roussel: *DiaBeta*

MICRONASE 1.25 — 1.25 mg
MICRONASE 2.5 — 2.5 mg
MICRONASE 5 — 5 mg
Tablets
Upjohn: *Micronase*

Guanabenz

3
4 mg
74 WYETH — 8 mg
Tablets
Wyeth-Ayerst: *Wytensin*

Guanfacine

5
1 mg
2 mg
Tablets
Robins: *Tenex*

Imipramine

6
Geigy 20 — 75 mg
Geigy 40 — 100 mg
Capsules
Geigy: *Tofranil-PM*

(continued)

A

Imipramine (continued)

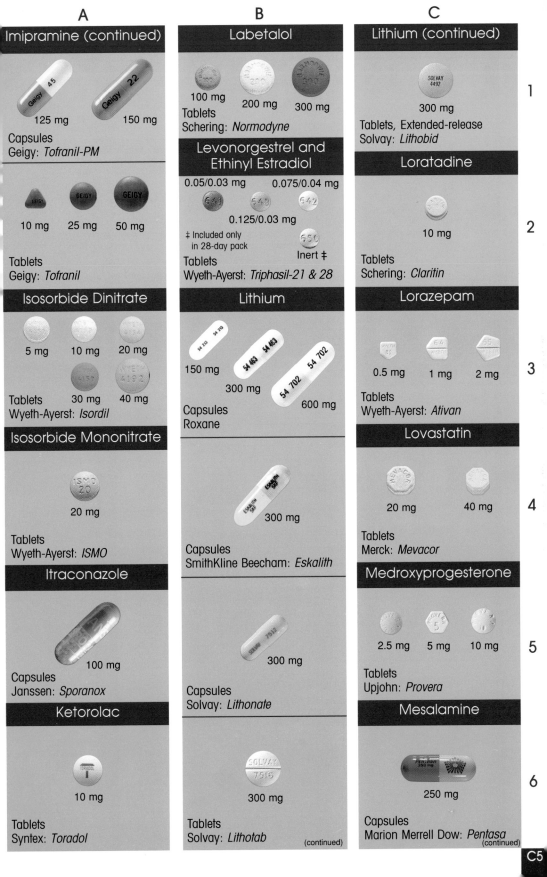

125 mg   150 mg

Capsules
Geigy: *Tofranil-PM*

10 mg   25 mg   50 mg

Tablets
Geigy: *Tofranil*

Isosorbide Dinitrate

5 mg   10 mg   20 mg

30 mg   40 mg

Tablets
Wyeth-Ayerst: *Isordil*

Isosorbide Mononitrate

20 mg

Tablets
Wyeth-Ayerst: *ISMO*

Itraconazole

100 mg

Capsules
Janssen: *Sporanox*

Ketorolac

10 mg

Tablets
Syntex: *Toradol*

B

Labetalol

100 mg   200 mg   300 mg

Tablets
Schering: *Normodyne*

Levonorgestrel and Ethinyl Estradiol

0.05/0.03 mg   0.075/0.04 mg

0.125/0.03 mg

‡ Included only
in 28-day pack   Inert ‡

Tablets
Wyeth-Ayerst: *Triphasil-21 & 28*

Lithium

150 mg

300 mg

600 mg

Capsules
Roxane

300 mg

Capsules
SmithKline Beecham: *Eskalith*

300 mg

Capsules
Solvay: *Lithonate*

300 mg

Tablets
Solvay: *Lithotab*

(continued)

C

Lithium (continued)

300 mg

Tablets, Extended-release
Solvay: *Lithobid*

Loratadine

10 mg

Tablets
Schering: *Claritin*

Lorazepam

0.5 mg   1 mg   2 mg

Tablets
Wyeth-Ayerst: *Ativan*

Lovastatin

20 mg   40 mg

Tablets
Merck: *Mevacor*

Medroxyprogesterone

2.5 mg   5 mg   10 mg

Tablets
Upjohn: *Provera*

Mesalamine

250 mg

Capsules
Marion Merrell Dow: *Pentasa*

(continued)

1

2

3

4

5

6

A

Mesalamine (continued)

1

400 mg

Tablets, Delayed -release
P & GP: *Asacol*

Methotrexate

2

2.5 mg

Tablets
Barr

Methyldopa

3

125 mg   250 mg   500 mg

Tablets
Geneva

4

125 mg   250 mg

500 mg

Tablets
Merck: *Aldomet*

5

250 mg   500 mg

Tablets
Rugby

6

250 mg   500 mg

Tablets
Schein/Danbury

B

Misoprostol

1

0.1 mg   0.2 mg

Tablets
Searle: *Cytotec*

Nabumetone

2

500 mg   750 mg

Tablets
SmithKline Beecham: *Relafen*

Naproxen

3

521
250 mg

522
375 mg

523
500 mg

Tablets
Purepac

4

250 mg

375 mg

500 mg

Tablets
Syntex: *Naprosyn*

5

375 mg   500 mg

Tablets, Delayed-release
Syntex: *E-C Naprosyn*

Niacin

6

125 mg   250 mg   500 mg

Capsules, Extended-release
Rhone-Poulenc Rorer: *Nicobid*
(conitnued)

C

Niacin (continued)

1

500 mg

Tablets
Rhone-Poulenc Rorer: *Nicolar*

2

250 mg   500 mg   750 mg

Tablets, Extended-release
Upsher-Smith: *Slo-Niacin*

Nifedipine

3

10 mg   20 mg

Capsules
Pratt: *Procardia*

4

30 mg   60 mg   90 mg

Tablets, Extended-release
Pratt: *Procardia XL*

Norethindrone and Ethinyl Estradiol

5

1/0.035 mg   Inert ‡

‡ Included only in 28-day pack

Tablets
Ortho: *Ortho-Novum 1/35-21and -28*

6

0.5/0.035 mg   0.75/0.035 mg

1/0.035 mg   Inert ‡

‡ Included only in
28-day pack

Tablets
Ortho: *Ortho-Novum 7/7/7-21and -28*

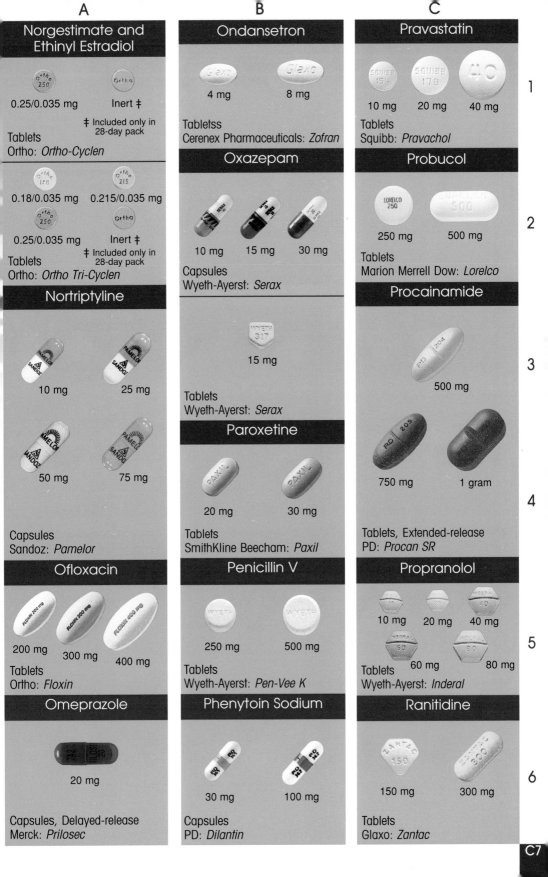

A

Norgestimate and Ethinyl Estradiol

0.25/0.035 mg   Inert ‡

‡ Included only in 28-day pack

Tablets
Ortho: *Ortho-Cyclen*

0.18/0.035 mg   0.215/0.035 mg

0.25/0.035 mg   Inert ‡

‡ Included only in 28-day pack

Tablets
Ortho: *Ortho Tri-Cyclen*

Nortriptyline

10 mg   25 mg

50 mg   75 mg

Capsules
Sandoz: *Pamelor*

Ofloxacin

200 mg   300 mg   400 mg

Tablets
Ortho: *Floxin*

Omeprazole

20 mg

Capsules, Delayed-release
Merck: *Prilosec*

B

Ondansetron

4 mg   8 mg

Tabletss
Cerenex Pharmaceuticals: *Zofran*

Oxazepam

10 mg   15 mg   30 mg

Capsules
Wyeth-Ayerst: *Serax*

15 mg

Tablets
Wyeth-Ayerst: *Serax*

Paroxetine

20 mg   30 mg

Tablets
SmithKline Beecham: *Paxil*

Penicillin V

250 mg   500 mg

Tablets
Wyeth-Ayerst: *Pen-Vee K*

Phenytoin Sodium

30 mg   100 mg

Capsules
PD: *Dilantin*

C

Pravastatin

10 mg   20 mg   40 mg

Tablets
Squibb: *Pravachol*

Probucol

250 mg   500 mg

Tablets
Marion Merrell Dow: *Lorelco*

Procainamide

500 mg

750 mg   1 gram

Tablets, Extended-release
PD: *Procan SR*

Propranolol

10 mg   20 mg   40 mg

60 mg   80 mg

Tablets
Wyeth-Ayerst: *Inderal*

Ranitidine

150 mg   300 mg

Tablets
Glaxo: *Zantac*

1

2

3

4

5

6

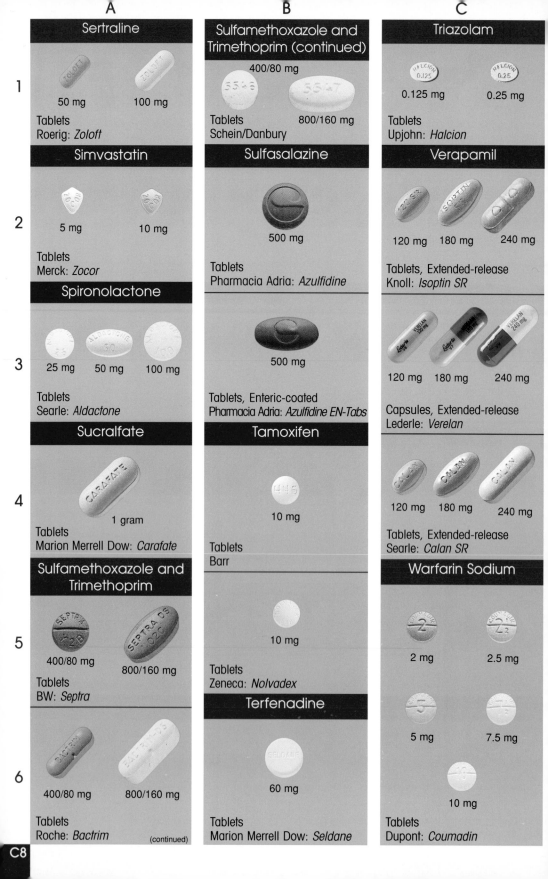

A

Sertraline

1 — 50 mg   100 mg

Tablets
Roerig: *Zoloft*

Simvastatin

2 — 5 mg   10 mg

Tablets
Merck: *Zocor*

Spironolactone

3 — 25 mg   50 mg   100 mg

Tablets
Searle: *Aldactone*

Sucralfate

4 — 1 gram

Tablets
Marion Merrell Dow: *Carafate*

Sulfamethoxazole and Trimethoprim

5 — 400/80 mg   800/160 mg

Tablets
BW: *Septra*

6 — 400/80 mg   800/160 mg

Tablets
Roche: *Bactrim*   (continued)

B

Sulfamethoxazole and Trimethoprim (continued)

1 — 400/80 mg   800/160 mg

Tablets
Schein/Danbury

Sulfasalazine

2 — 500 mg

Tablets
Pharmacia Adria: *Azulfidine*

3 — 500 mg

Tablets, Enteric-coated
Pharmacia Adria: *Azulfidine EN-Tabs*

Tamoxifen

4 — 10 mg

Tablets
Barr

5 — 10 mg

Tablets
Zeneca: *Nolvadex*

Terfenadine

6 — 60 mg

Tablets
Marion Merrell Dow: *Seldane*

C

Triazolam

1 — 0.125 mg   0.25 mg

Tablets
Upjohn: *Halcion*

Verapamil

2 — 120 mg   180 mg   240 mg

Tablets, Extended-release
Knoll: *Isoptin SR*

3 — 120 mg   180 mg   240 mg

Capsules, Extended-release
Lederle: *Verelan*

4 — 120 mg   180 mg   240 mg

Tablets, Extended-release
Searle: *Calan SR*

Warfarin Sodium

5 — 2 mg   2.5 mg

5 mg   7.5 mg

6 — 10 mg

Tablets
Dupont: *Coumadin*

$\mathscr{B}$ARBITURATES (ORAL)

Including Amobarbital; Aprobarbital;
Butabarbital; Mephobarbital; Metharbital; Pentobarbital;
Phenobarbital; Secobarbital; Secobarbital and Amobarbital

ABOUT YOUR MEDICINE

Barbiturates belong to the group of medicines called central nervous system (CNS) depressants. Some barbiturates may be used before surgery to relieve anxiety. In addition, some are also used to help control seizures in certain disorders, such as epilepsy. Barbiturates may also be used for other conditions as determined by your doctor.

If any of the information in this profile causes you special concern or if you want additional information about your medicine and its use, check with your doctor, nurse, or pharmacist. **Remember, keep this and all other medicines out of the reach of children and never share your medicines with others.**

BEFORE USING THIS MEDICINE

Tell your doctor, nurse, and pharmacist if you . . .
- are allergic to any medicine, either prescription or nonprescription (OTC);
- are pregnant or intend to become pregnant while using this medicine;
- are breast-feeding;
- are taking **any** other prescription or nonprescription (OTC) medicine;
- have **any** other medical problems.

PROPER USE OF THIS MEDICINE

Use this medicine only as directed. If too much is used, it may become habit-forming. Even if you think this medicine is not working, **do not increase the dose.** Instead, check with your doctor.

If you are taking this medicine for epilepsy, it must be taken every day in regularly spaced doses in order for it to control your seizures.

If you are taking this medicine regularly and you miss a dose, take it as soon as possible. However, if it is almost time for your next dose, skip the missed dose and go back to your regular dosing schedule. Do not double doses.

PRECAUTIONS WHILE USING THIS MEDICINE

If you will be taking this medicine regularly for a long time, do not stop taking it without first checking with your doctor.

Barbiturates will add to the effects of alcohol and other CNS depressants. **Check with your doctor before taking any such depressants while taking this medicine.**

This medicine may cause some people to become dizzy, lightheaded, drowsy, or less alert than they are normally. Even if taken at bedtime, it may cause these effects on arising. **Make sure you know how you react before you drive, use machines, or do other jobs that require you to be alert.**

Birth control pills containing estrogen may not work properly if you take them while taking barbiturates. Unplanned pregnancies may occur. Use a different or additional means of birth control while you are taking barbiturates. If you have any questions about this, check with your doctor or pharmacist.

If you have been using this medicine for a long time and you think that you may have become mentally or physically dependent on it, check with your doctor. Some signs of mental or physical dependence are:
 —a strong desire or need to continue taking the medicine.
 —a need to increase the dose to receive the effects of the medicine.
 —withdrawal side effects after the medicine is stopped.

If you think you or someone else may have taken an overdose, get emergency help at once. Taking an overdose of a barbiturate or taking alcohol or other CNS depressants with it may lead to death. Some signs of overdose are decrease in reflexes; severe drowsiness, confusion, or weakness; shortness of breath or slow or troubled breathing; slurred speech; staggering; and slow heartbeat.

POSSIBLE SIDE EFFECTS OF THIS MEDICINE

Side effects that should be reported to your doctor immediately
 RARE—Bleeding sores on lips; chest pain; fever; muscle or joint pain; red, thickened, or scaly skin; skin rash or hives; sores or white spots in mouth (painful); sore throat; swelling of eyelids, face, or lips; wheezing or tightness in chest

Other side effects that should be reported to your doctor
 LESS COMMON—Confusion; mental depression; unusual excitement
 RARE—Hallucinations; unusual bleeding, bruising, tiredness, or weakness
 WITH LONG-TERM OR CHRONIC USE—Bone pain or aching; loss of appetite; muscle weakness; weight loss (unusual); yellow eyes or skin

Side effects that usually do not require medical attention
 These possible side effects may go away during treatment; however, if they continue or are bothersome, check with your doctor, nurse, or pharmacist.

 MORE COMMON—Clumsiness or unsteadiness, dizziness or lightheadedness, drowsiness, "hangover" effect

 Other side effects not listed above may also occur in some patients. If you notice any other effects, check with your doctor, nurse, or pharmacist.

After you stop using this medicine, your body may need time to adjust. If you took this medicine in high doses or for a long time, this may take up to about 15 days. Check with your doctor **if you experience anxiety; convulsions (seizures);**

dizziness or lightheadedness; faint feeling; hallucinations; muscle twitching; nausea or vomiting; trembling of hands; trouble in sleeping, increased dreaming, or nightmares; vision problems; or weakness.

BENZODIAZEPINES (ORAL)

Including Alprazolam; Bromazepam; Chlordiazepoxide; Clonazepam; Clorazepate; Diazepam; Estazolam; Flurazepam; Halazepam; Ketazolam; Lorazepam; Nitrazepam; Oxazepam; Prazepam; Quazepam; Temazepam; Triazolam

ABOUT YOUR MEDICINE

Benzodiazepines (ben-zoe-dye-AZ-e-peens) are used to relieve nervousness or tension, and to treat insomnia (trouble in sleeping). For these conditions, benzodiazepines are used only for a short time. Some benzodiazepines may also be used to relax muscles or relieve muscle spasm, and to treat panic disorders and certain convulsive disorders, such as epilepsy. Benzodiazepines may also be used for other conditions as determined by your doctor. Benzodiazepines should not be used for nervousness or tension caused by the stress of everyday life.

If any of the information in this profile causes you special concern or if you want additional information about your medicine and its use, check with your doctor, nurse, or pharmacist. **Remember, keep this and all other medicines out of the reach of children and never share your medicines with others.**

BEFORE USING THIS MEDICINE

Tell your doctor, nurse, and pharmacist if you . . .
- are allergic to any medicine, either prescription or nonprescription (OTC);
- are pregnant or intend to become pregnant while using this medicine;
- are breast-feeding;
- are taking any other prescription or nonprescription (OTC) medicine, especially other CNS depressants;
- have any other medical problems, especially asthma, bronchitis, emphysema, or other chronic lung disease; glaucoma; or myasthenia gravis.

PROPER USE OF THIS MEDICINE

Take this medicine only as directed by your doctor. Do not take more of it, do not take it more often, and do not take it for a longer time than your doctor ordered. If too much is taken, it may become habit-forming.

If you think this medicine is not working properly after you have taken it for a few weeks, **do not increase the dose.** Instead, check with your doctor.

If you are taking this medicine for epilepsy, it must be taken every day in regularly spaced doses in order for it to control your seizures.

If you are taking this medicine for insomnia, do not take it if you cannot get a full night's sleep (7 to 8 hours). Otherwise, you may feel drowsy and have memory problems because the effects of the medicine have not worn off.

If you are taking this medicine regularly (for example, every day) and you miss a dose, take it right away if you remember within an hour or so of the missed dose. However, if you do not remember until later, skip the missed dose and go back to your regular dosing schedule. Do not double doses.

PRECAUTIONS WHILE USING THIS MEDICINE

This medicine will add to the effects of alcohol and other CNS depressants (medicines that may make you drowsy or less alert). **Check with your doctor before taking any such depressants while you are taking this medicine.**

Benzodiazepines may cause some people to become drowsy. **Make sure you know how you react to this medicine before you drive, use machines, or do other jobs that require you to be alert.**

If you think you or someone else may have taken an overdose, get emergency help at once. Some signs of an overdose are continuing slurred speech or confusion, severe drowsiness, severe weakness, and staggering.

POSSIBLE SIDE EFFECTS OF THIS MEDICINE

Side effects that should be reported to your doctor

> LESS COMMON OR RARE—Behavior problems, including difficulty in concentrating and outbursts of anger; confusion or mental depression; convulsions (seizures); hallucinations; memory problems; muscle weakness; skin rash or itching; sore throat, fever, and chills; ulcers or sores in mouth or throat (continuing); uncontrolled movements of body, including the eyes; unusual bleeding or bruising; unusual excitement, nervousness, or irritability; unusual tiredness or weakness; yellow eyes or skin
>
> SIGNS OF OVERDOSE—Confusion (continuing); drowsiness (severe); shakiness; shortness of breath or troubled breathing; slow heartbeat; slow reflexes; slurred speech (continuing); staggering; weakness (severe)

Side effects that usually do not require medical attention

> These possible side effects may go away during treatment; however, if they continue or are bothersome, check with your doctor, nurse, or pharmacist.
>
> MORE COMMON—Clumsiness or unsteadiness; dizziness or lightheadedness; drowsiness; slurred speech
>
> Other side effects not listed above may also occur in some patients. If you notice any other effects, check with your doctor, nurse, or pharmacist.

After you stop using this medicine, your body may need time to adjust. If you took this medicine in high doses or for a long time, this may take up to 3 weeks. **During this time, check with your doctor if you experience** fast or pounding heartbeat; increased sense of hearing; increased sensitivity to touch and pain; increased sweating; mental depression; muscle or stomach cramps; nausea or vomiting; sensitivity of eyes to light; tingling, burning, or prickly sensations; trembling; trouble in sleeping; or if you are unusually irritable, nervous, or confused.

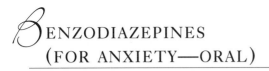

$\mathcal{B}$ENZODIAZEPINES (FOR ANXIETY—ORAL)

Including Alprazolam; Bromazepam;
Chlordiazepoxide; Clorazepate; Diazepam;
Halazepam; Ketazolam; Lorazepam; Oxazepam; Prazepam

About Your Medicine

Benzodiazepines (ben-zoe-dye-AZ-e-peens) are used to relieve anxiety, nervousness, or tension. Benzodiazepines should not be used for anxiety, nervousness, or tension caused by the stress of everyday life. Alprazolam, lorazepam, and oxazepam are also used to help control anxiety that sometimes occurs with mental depression. Benzodiazepines may also be used for other conditions as determined by your doctor.

If any of the information in this profile causes you special concern or if you want additional information about your medicine and its use, check with your doctor, nurse, or pharmacist. **Remember, keep this and all other medicines out of the reach of children and never share your medicines with others.**

Before Using This Medicine

Tell your doctor, nurse, and pharmacist if you . . .
- are allergic to any medicine, either prescription or nonprescription (OTC);
- are pregnant or intend to become pregnant while using this medicine;
- are breast-feeding;
- are taking any other prescription or nonprescription (OTC) medicine, especially other CNS depressants;
- have any other medical problems, especially asthma, bronchitis, emphysema, or other chronic lung disease; glaucoma; or myasthenia gravis.

PROPER USE OF THIS MEDICINE

Take this medicine only as directed by your doctor. Do not take more of it, do not take it more often, and do not take it for a longer time than your doctor ordered. If too much is taken, it may become habit-forming.

If you think this medicine is not working properly after you have taken it for a few weeks, **do not increase the dose.** Instead, check with your doctor.

If you are taking this medicine regularly (for example, every day) and you miss a dose, take it right away if you remember within an hour or so of the missed dose. However, if you do not remember until later, skip the missed dose and go back to your regular dosing schedule. Do not double doses.

PRECAUTIONS WHILE USING THIS MEDICINE

This medicine will add to the effects of alcohol and other CNS depressants (medicines that may make you drowsy or less alert). **Check with your doctor before taking any such depressants while you are taking this medicine.**

Benzodiazepines may cause some people to become drowsy. **Make sure you know how you react to this medicine before you drive, use machines, or do other jobs that require you to be alert.**

POSSIBLE SIDE EFFECTS OF THIS MEDICINE

Side effects that should be reported to your doctor

LESS COMMON OR RARE—Behavior problems, including difficulty in concentrating and outbursts of anger; confusion or mental depression; convulsions (seizures); hallucinations; impaired memory; muscle weakness; skin rash or itching; sore throat, fever, and chills; ulcers or sores in mouth or throat (continuing); uncontrolled movements of body, including the eyes; unusual bleeding or bruising; unusual excitement, nervousness, or irritability; unusual tiredness or weakness; yellow eyes or skin

SIGNS OF OVERDOSE—Confusion (continuing); drowsiness (severe); shakiness; shortness of breath or troubled breathing; slow heartbeat; slow reflexes; slurred speech (continuing); staggering; weakness (severe)

Side effects that usually do not require medical attention

These possible side effects may go away during treatment; however, if they continue or are bothersome, check with your doctor, nurse, or pharmacist.

MORE COMMON—Clumsiness or unsteadiness; dizziness or lightheadedness; drowsiness; slurred speech

Other side effects not listed above may also occur in some patients. If you notice any other effects, check with your doctor, nurse, or pharmacist.

After you stop using this medicine, your body may need time to adjust. If you took this medicine in high doses or for a long time, this may take up to 3 weeks. **During this time check with your doctor if you experience** fast or pounding heartbeat; increased sense of hearing; increased sensitivity to touch and pain; increased sweating; mental depression; muscle or stomach cramps; nausea or vomiting; sensitivity of eyes to light; tingling, burning, or prickly sensations; trembling; trouble in sleeping; or if you are unusually irritable, nervous, or confused.

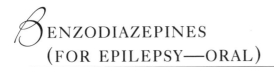

BENZODIAZEPINES (FOR EPILEPSY—ORAL)

Including Clonazepam; Clorazepate; Diazepam; Nitrazepam

ABOUT YOUR MEDICINE

Benzodiazepines (ben-zoe-dye-AZ-e-peens) are used to treat certain convulsive disorders, such as epilepsy. Benzodiazepines may also be used for other conditions as determined by your doctor.

If any of the information in this profile causes you special concern or if you want additional information about your medicine and its use, check with your doctor, nurse, or pharmacist. **Remember, keep this and all other medicines out of the reach of children and never share your medicines with others.**

BEFORE USING THIS MEDICINE

Tell your doctor, nurse, and pharmacist if you . . .
- are allergic to any medicine, either prescription or nonprescription (OTC);
- are pregnant or intend to become pregnant while using this medicine;
- are breast-feeding;
- are taking any other prescription or nonprescription (OTC) medicine, especially other CNS depressants;
- have any other medical problems, especially asthma, bronchitis, emphysema, or other chronic lung disease; glaucoma; or myasthenia gravis.

PROPER USE OF THIS MEDICINE

Take this medicine only as directed by your doctor. Do not take more of it, do not take it more often, and do not take it for a longer time than your doctor ordered. If too much is taken, it may become habit-forming.

If you think this medicine is not working properly after you have taken it for a few weeks, **do not increase the dose.** Instead, check with your doctor.

This medicine must be taken every day in regularly spaced doses in order for it to control your seizures.

If you are taking this medicine regularly (for example, every day) and you miss a dose, take it right away if you remember within an hour or so of the missed dose. However, if you do not remember until later, skip the missed dose and go back to your regular dosing schedule. Do not double doses.

Precautions While Using This Medicine

This medicine will add to the effects of alcohol and other CNS depressants (medicines that may make you drowsy or less alert). **Check with your doctor before taking any such depressants while you are taking this medicine.**

Benzodiazepines may cause some people to become drowsy. **Make sure you know how you react to this medicine before you drive, use machines, or do other jobs that require you to be alert.**

If you think you or someone else may have taken an overdose, get emergency help at once. Some signs of an overdose are continuing slurred speech or confusion, severe drowsiness, severe weakness, and staggering.

Possible Side Effects of This Medicine

Side effects that should be reported to your doctor
> Less Common or Rare—Behavior problems, including difficulty in concentrating and outbursts of anger; confusion or mental depression; convulsions (seizures); hallucinations; impaired memory; muscle weakness; skin rash or itching; sore throat, fever, and chills; ulcers or sores in mouth or throat (continuing); uncontrolled movements of body, including the eyes; unusual bleeding or bruising; unusual excitement, nervousness, or irritability; unusual tiredness or weakness; yellow eyes or skin
> Signs of Overdose—Confusion (continuing); drowsiness (severe); shakiness; shortness of breath or troubled breathing; slow heartbeat; slow reflexes; slurred speech (continuing); staggering; weakness (severe)

Side effects that usually do not require medical attention
> These possible side effects may go away during treatment; however, if they continue or are bothersome, check with your doctor, nurse, or pharmacist.

> More Common—Clumsiness or unsteadiness; dizziness or lightheadedness; drowsiness; slurred speech

> Other side effects not listed above may also occur in some patients. If you notice any other effects, check with your doctor, nurse, or pharmacist.

After you stop using this medicine, your body may need time to adjust. If you took this medicine in high doses or for a long time, this may take up to 3 weeks. **During this time check with your doctor if you experience** fast or pounding heartbeat; increased sense of hearing; increased sensitivity to touch and pain;

increased sweating; mental depression; muscle or stomach cramps; nausea or vomiting; sensitivity of eyes to light; tingling, burning, or prickly sensations; trembling; trouble in sleeping; or if you are unusually irritable, nervous, or confused.

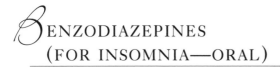

BENZODIAZEPINES (FOR INSOMNIA—ORAL)

Including Alprazolam; Bromazepam; Chlordiazepoxide; Clorazepate; Diazepam; Estazolam; Flurazepam; Halazepam; Ketazolam; Lorazepam; Nitrazepam; Oxazepam; Prazepam; Quazepam; Temazepam; Triazolam

ABOUT YOUR MEDICINE

Benzodiazepines (ben-zoe-dye-AZ-e-peens) are used to treat insomnia (trouble in sleeping). Benzodiazepines may also be used for other conditions as determined by your doctor.

If any of the information in this profile causes you special concern or if you want additional information about your medicine and its use, check with your doctor, nurse, or pharmacist. **Remember, keep this and all other medicines out of the reach of children and never share your medicines with others.**

BEFORE USING THIS MEDICINE

Tell your doctor, nurse, and pharmacist if you . . .
- are allergic to any medicine, either prescription or nonprescription (OTC);
- are pregnant or intend to become pregnant while using this medicine;
- are breast-feeding;
- are taking any other prescription or nonprescription (OTC) medicine, especially other CNS depressants;
- have any other medical problems, especially asthma, bronchitis, emphysema, or other chronic lung disease; glaucoma; or myasthenia gravis.

PROPER USE OF THIS MEDICINE

Take this medicine only as directed by your doctor. Do not take more of it, do not take it more often, and do not take it for a longer time than your doctor ordered. If too much is taken, it may become habit-forming.

If you think this medicine is not working properly after you have taken it for a few weeks, **do not increase the dose.** Instead, check with your doctor.

Do not take this medicine if you cannot get a full night's sleep (7 or 8 hours). Otherwise, you may feel drowsy and have memory problems because the effects of the medicine have not worn off.

PRECAUTIONS WHILE USING THIS MEDICINE

This medicine will add to the effects of alcohol and other CNS depressants (medicines that may make you drowsy or less alert). **Check with your doctor before taking any such depressants while you are taking this medicine.**

Benzodiazepines may cause some people to become drowsy. **Make sure you know how you react to this medicine before you drive, use machines, or do other jobs that require you to be alert.**

POSSIBLE SIDE EFFECTS OF THIS MEDICINE

Side effects that should be reported to your doctor
> LESS COMMON OR RARE—Behavior problems, including difficulty in concentrating and outbursts of anger; confusion or mental depression; convulsions (seizures); hallucinations; impaired memory; muscle weakness; skin rash or itching; sore throat, fever, and chills; ulcers or sores in mouth or throat (continuing); uncontrolled movements of body, including the eyes; unusual bleeding or bruising; unusual excitement, nervousness, or irritability; unusual tiredness or weakness; yellow eyes or skin
> SIGNS OF OVERDOSE—Confusion (continuing); drowsiness (severe); shakiness; shortness of breath or troubled breathing; slow heartbeat; slow reflexes; slurred speech (continuing); staggering; weakness (severe)

Side effects that usually do not require medical attention
> These possible side effects may go away during treatment; however, if they continue or are bothersome, check with your doctor, nurse, or pharmacist.
>
> MORE COMMON—Clumsiness or unsteadiness; dizziness or lightheadedness; drowsiness; slurred speech
>
> Other side effects not listed above may also occur in some patients. If you notice any other effects, check with your doctor, nurse, or pharmacist.

After you stop using this medicine, your body may need time to adjust. If you took this medicine in high doses or for a long time, this may take up to 3 weeks. **During this time check with your doctor if you experience** fast or pounding heartbeat; increased sense of hearing; increased sensitivity to touch and pain; increased sweating; mental depression; muscle or stomach cramps; nausea or vomiting; sensitivity of eyes to light; tingling, burning, or prickly sensations; trembling; trouble in sleeping; or if you are unusually irritable, nervous, or confused.

ℬETA-BLOCKERS (ORAL)

Including Acebutolol; Atenolol; Betaxolol;
Bisoprolol; Carteolol; Labetalol; Metoprolol; Nadolol;
Oxprenolol; Penbutolol; Pindolol; Propranolol; Sotalol; Timolol

ABOUT YOUR MEDICINE

Beta-blockers are used to treat high blood pressure. Some are also used in the relief of angina (chest pain) and in heart attack patients to help prevent additional heart attacks. Some beta-blockers are also used to correct irregular heartbeats, prevent migraine headaches, and treat tremors. Beta-blockers may also be used for other conditions as determined by your doctor.

If any of the information in this profile causes you special concern or if you want additional information about your medicine and its use, check with your doctor, nurse, or pharmacist. **Remember, keep this and all other medicines out of the reach of children and never share your medicines with others.**

BEFORE USING THIS MEDICINE

Tell your doctor, nurse, and pharmacist if you . . .
- are allergic to any medicine, either prescription or nonprescription (OTC);
- are pregnant or intend to become pregnant while using this medicine;
- are breast-feeding;
- are taking any other prescription or nonprescription (OTC) medicine, especially allergy shots or allergy skin testing; aminophylline; caffeine; calcium channel blockers; clonidine; diabetes medicine; dyphylline; guanabenz; insulin; MAO inhibitors; oxtriphylline; theophylline; or medicines for appetite control, asthma, colds, cough, hay fever, or sinus;
- have any other medical problems, especially allergy, asthma or other lung disease, diabetes, heart or blood vessel disease, mental depression, or overactive thyroid;
- use cocaine.

PROPER USE OF THIS MEDICINE

Even if you feel well, **take this medicine exactly as directed.**

Ask your doctor about your pulse rate before and after taking beta-blockers. Then, while you are taking this medicine, check your pulse regularly. If it is much slower than your usual rate (or less than 50 beats per minute), check with your doctor. A pulse rate that is too slow may cause circulation problems.

If you are taking this medicine for high blood pressure, remember that it will not cure your high blood pressure, but it does help control it. You must continue to take it—even if you feel well—if you expect to keep your blood pressure down. **You may have to take medicine for the rest of your life.**

Do not miss any doses, especially if you are taking only one dose a day. Some conditions may become worse when this medicine is not taken regularly.

If you do miss a dose of this medicine, take it as soon as possible. However, if it is within 4 hours of your next dose (8 hours when taking atenolol, betaxolol, carteolol, labetalol, nadolol, penbutolol, sotalol, or extended-release oxprenolol or propranolol), skip the missed dose and go back to your regular dosing schedule. Do not double doses.

PRECAUTIONS WHILE USING THIS MEDICINE

Do not stop taking this medicine without first checking with your doctor.
For diabetic patients:
- **This medicine may cause your blood sugar levels to fall. Also, this medicine may cover up signs of hypoglycemia (low blood sugar).**

This medicine may cause some people to become dizzy, drowsy, or lightheaded. **Make sure you know how you react before you drive, use machines, or do other jobs that require you to be alert.**

Chest pain resulting from exercise or physical exertion is usually reduced or prevented by this medicine. This may tempt a patient to be overly active. **Make sure you discuss with your doctor a safe amount of exercise for you.**

POSSIBLE SIDE EFFECTS OF THIS MEDICINE

Side effects that should be reported to your doctor
> LESS COMMON—Breathing difficulty; cold hands and feet; mental depression; shortness of breath; slow heartbeat (especially less than 50 beats per minute); swelling of ankles, feet, and/or lower legs
>
> RARE—Back pain or joint pain; chest pain; confusion (especially in elderly); dark urine (for acebutolol, bisoprolol, or labetalol); dizziness or lightheadedness when getting up from a lying or sitting position; fever and sore throat; hallucinations; irregular heartbeat; red, scaling, or crusted skin; skin rash; unusual bleeding and bruising; yellow eyes or skin (for acebutolol, bisoprolol, or labetalol)

Side effects that usually do not require medical attention
> These possible side effects may go away during treatment; however, if they continue or are bothersome, check with your doctor, nurse, or pharmacist.
>
> MORE COMMON—Decreased sexual ability; dizziness or lightheadedness; drowsiness (slight); trouble in sleeping; unusual tiredness or weakness
>
> After you have been taking a beta-blocker for a while, it may cause unpleasant or even harmful effects if you stop taking it too suddenly. Check with your doctor right away if you notice chest pain, fast or irregular heartbeat, general feeling of body discomfort or weakness, shortness of breath (sudden), sweating, or trembling.

Other side effects not listed above may also occur in some patients. If you notice any other effects, check with your doctor, nurse, or pharmacist.

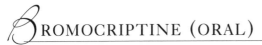ROMOCRIPTINE (ORAL)

ABOUT YOUR MEDICINE

Bromocriptine (broe-moe-KRIP-teen) is used to treat certain menstrual problems or to stop milk production in some women or men who have abnormal milk leakage. It is also used to treat infertility in men and women. Bromocriptine is also used to treat Parkinson's disease, acromegaly (over-production of growth hormone), and pituitary prolactinomas (tumors of the pituitary gland). It may also be used for other conditions as determined by your doctor.

If any of the information in this profile causes you special concern or if you want additional information about your medicine and its use, check with your doctor, nurse, or pharmacist. **Remember, keep this and all other medicines out of the reach of children and never share your medicines with others.**

BEFORE USING THIS MEDICINE

Tell your doctor, nurse, and pharmacist if you . . .
- are allergic to any medicine, either prescription or nonprescription (OTC);
- are pregnant or intend to become pregnant while using this medicine;
- are breast-feeding;
- are taking any other prescription or nonprescription (OTC) medicine, especially ergot alkaloids;
- have any other medical problems, especially high blood pressure (history of or pregnancy-induced).

PROPER USE OF THIS MEDICINE

If bromocriptine upsets your stomach, it may be taken with meals or milk or at bedtime. If stomach upset continues, check with your doctor.

If you miss a dose of this medicine, take the missed dose if you remember it within 4 hours. However, if a longer time has passed, skip the missed dose and go back to your regular schedule. Do not double doses.

PRECAUTIONS WHILE USING THIS MEDICINE

This medicine may cause some people to become drowsy, dizzy, or less alert than they are normally. **Make sure you know how you react before you drive, use machines, or do other jobs that require you to be alert.**

Dizziness is more likely to occur after the first dose of bromocriptine. Taking the first dose vaginally or at bedtime or when you are able to lie down may lessen problems. It may also be helpful if you get up slowly from a lying or sitting position.

It may take several weeks for bromocriptine to work. Do not stop taking it or reduce the amount you are taking without first checking with your doctor.

For females who are able to bear children:
- It is best to use some type of birth control while you are taking bromocriptine. However, do not use oral contraceptives (the "Pill") since they may prevent bromocriptine from working. For women using bromocriptine for infertility, tell your doctor when your normal menstrual cycle returns. If you wish to become pregnant, you and your doctor should decide on the best time for you to stop using birth control.
- Tell your doctor right away if you think you have become pregnant. You and your doctor should discuss whether you should continue to take bromocriptine during pregnancy. **Check with your doctor right away** if you develop blurred vision, a sudden headache, or severe nausea and vomiting.

Drinking alcohol while you are taking bromocriptine may cause you to have a certain reaction. **Avoid alcohol until you have discussed this with your doctor.**

POSSIBLE SIDE EFFECTS OF THIS MEDICINE

Some serious side effects have occurred during the use of bromocriptine to stop milk flow after pregnancy or abortion. These side effects have included strokes, seizures (convulsions), and heart attacks. Some deaths have also occurred. You should discuss with your doctor the good that this medicine will do as well as the risks of using it.

Side effects that should be reported to your doctor immediately
> RARE—Black, tarry stools; bloody vomit; chest pain (severe); convulsions (seizures); fainting; fast heartbeat; headache (unusual); increased sweating; nausea and vomiting (severe); nervousness; shortness of breath (unexplained); vision changes (such as blurred vision or temporary blindness); weakness (sudden)

Other side effects that should be reported to your doctor
> LESS COMMON (REPORTED MORE OFTEN IN PATIENTS WITH PARKINSON'S DISEASE)—Confusion; hallucinations; uncontrolled movements of the body
> RARE—Abdominal or stomach pain (continuing or severe); increased frequency of urination; loss of appetite (continuing); lower back pain; runny nose (continuing); weakness

Side effects that usually do not require medical attention
> These possible side effects may go away during treatment; however, if they continue or are bothersome, check with your doctor, nurse, or pharmacist.

> MORE COMMON—Dizziness or lightheadedness; nausea

Other side effects not listed above may also occur in some patients. If you notice any other effects, check with your doctor, nurse, or pharmacist.

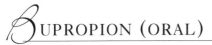

BUPROPION (ORAL)

ABOUT YOUR MEDICINE

Bupropion (byoo-PROE-pee-on) is used to relieve mental depression.

If any of the information in this profile causes you special concern or if you want additional information about your medicine and its use, check with your doctor, nurse, or pharmacist. **Remember, keep this and all other medicines out of the reach of children and never share your medicines with others.**

BEFORE USING THIS MEDICINE

Tell your doctor, nurse, and pharmacist if you . . .
- are allergic to any medicine, either prescription or nonprescription (OTC);
- are pregnant or intend to become pregnant while using this medicine;
- are breast-feeding;
- are taking any other prescription or nonprescription (OTC) medicine, especially antipsychotics (medicine for mental illness), fluoxetine, lithium, MAO inhibitors, maprotiline, trazodone, or tricyclic antidepressants;
- have any other medical problems, especially anorexia nervosa; brain tumor; bulimia; head injury (history of); heart attack (recent); kidney disease; liver disease; other nervous, mental, or emotional conditions; or seizure disorder.

PROPER USE OF THIS MEDICINE

Use bupropion only as directed by your doctor. Do not use more of it, do not use it more often, and do not use it for a longer time than your doctor ordered. To do so may increase the chance of side effects.

To lessen stomach upset, this medicine may be taken with food, unless your doctor has told you to take it on an empty stomach.

Usually this medicine must be taken for several weeks before you feel better. Your doctor should check your progress at regular visits.

If you miss a dose of this medicine, take it as soon as possible. However, if it is within 4 hours of your next dose, skip the missed dose and go back to your regular dosing schedule. Do not double doses.

PRECAUTIONS WHILE USING THIS MEDICINE

Your doctor should check your progress at regular visits, especially during the first few months of treatment with this medicine. The amount of bupropion you take may have to be changed often to meet the needs of your condition and to help avoid unwanted effects.

If you have been taking this medicine regularly, do not stop taking it without first checking with your doctor. Your doctor may want you to reduce gradually the amount you are taking before stopping completely. This will help reduce the chance of side effects.

Drinking of alcoholic beverages should be limited or avoided, if possible, while taking bupropion. This will help prevent unwanted effects.

This medicine may cause some people to feel a false sense of well-being, or to become drowsy, dizzy, or less alert than they are normally. **Make sure you know how you react to this medicine before you drive, use machines, or do other jobs that require you to be alert and clearheaded.**

POSSIBLE SIDE EFFECTS OF THIS MEDICINE

Side effects that should be reported to your doctor

MORE COMMON—Agitation or excitement; anxiety; confusion; fast or irregular heartbeat; headache (severe); restlessness; trouble in sleeping
LESS COMMON—Hallucinations; skin rash
RARE—Fainting; seizures (convulsions), especially with higher doses

Side effects that usually do not require medical attention

These possible side effects may go away during treatment; however, if they continue or are bothersome, check with your doctor, nurse, or pharmacist.

MORE COMMON—Constipation; decrease in appetite; dizziness; dryness of mouth; increased sweating; nausea or vomiting; tremor; weight loss (unusual)
LESS COMMON—Blurred vision; difficulty in concentration; drowsiness; fever or chills; hostility or anger; sleep problems; tiredness; unusual feeling of well-being

Other side effects not listed above may also occur in some patients. If you notice any other effects, check with your doctor, nurse, or pharmacist.

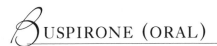USPIRONE (ORAL)

ABOUT YOUR MEDICINE

Buspirone (byoo-SPYE-rone) is used to treat certain anxiety disorders or to relieve the symptoms of anxiety. However, buspirone is usually not used for anxiety or tension caused by the stress of everyday life.

If any of the information in this profile causes you special concern or if you want additional information about your medicine and its use, check with your doctor, nurse, or pharmacist. **Remember, keep this and all other medicines out of the reach of children and never share your medicines with others.**

BEFORE USING THIS MEDICINE

Tell your doctor, nurse, and pharmacist if you . . .
- are allergic to any medicine, either prescription or nonprescription (OTC);
- are pregnant or intend to become pregnant while using this medicine;
- are breast-feeding;
- are taking any other prescription or nonprescription (OTC) medicine, especially MAO inhibitors;
- have any other medical problems.

PROPER USE OF THIS MEDICINE

Take buspirone only as directed by your doctor. Do not take more of it, do not take it more often, and do not take it for a longer time than your doctor ordered. To do so may increase the chance of unwanted effects.

After you begin taking buspirone, 1 to 2 weeks may pass before you feel the full effects of the medicine.

If you are taking this medicine regularly and you miss a dose, take it as soon as possible. However, if it is almost time for your next dose, skip the missed dose and go back to your regular dosing schedule. Do not double doses.

PRECAUTIONS WHILE USING THIS MEDICINE

If you will be using buspirone regularly for a long time, your doctor should check your progress at regular visits to make sure the medicine does not cause unwanted effects.

Buspirone when taken with alcohol or other CNS depressants (medicines that slow down the nervous system) may increase the chance of drowsiness. Check with your doctor before taking any such depressants while you are taking this medicine.

Buspirone may cause some people to become dizzy, lightheaded, drowsy, or less alert than they are normally. **Make sure you know how you react to this medicine before you drive, use machines, or do other jobs that require you to be alert.**

If you think you or someone else may have taken an overdose of buspirone, get emergency help at once. Some signs of an overdose are severe dizziness or drowsiness; severe stomach upset, including nausea or vomiting; or unusually small pupils.

POSSIBLE SIDE EFFECTS OF THIS MEDICINE

Side effects that should be reported to your doctor

RARE—Chest pain; confusion or mental depression; fast or pounding heartbeat; muscle weakness; numbness, tingling, pain, or weakness in hands or feet; sore throat or fever; uncontrolled movements of the body

Side effects that usually do not require medical attention

These possible side effects may go away during treatment; however, if they continue or are bothersome, check with your doctor, nurse, or pharmacist.

MORE COMMON—Dizziness or lightheadedness; headache; nausea; restlessness, nervousness, or unusual excitement

LESS COMMON OR RARE—Blurred vision; decreased concentration; drowsiness; dryness of mouth; muscle pain, spasms, cramps, or stiffness; ringing in the ears; stomach upset; trouble in sleeping, nightmares, or vivid dreams; unusual tiredness or weakness

Other side effects not listed above may also occur in some patients. If you notice any other effects, check with your doctor, nurse, or pharmacist.

ℬUTALBITAL AND ACETAMINOPHEN (ORAL)

Including Butalbital and Acetaminophen; Butalbital, Acetaminophen, and Caffeine

ABOUT YOUR MEDICINE

Butalbital (byoo-TAL-bi-tal) and **acetaminophen** (a-seat-a-MIN-oh-fen) combination is a pain reliever and relaxant. It is used to treat tension headaches.

If any of the information in this profile causes you special concern or if you want additional information about your medicine and its use, check with your doctor, nurse, or pharmacist. **Remember, keep this and all other medicines out of the reach of children and never share your medicines with others.**

Before Using This Medicine

Tell your doctor, nurse, and pharmacist if you . . .
- are allergic to any medicine, either prescription or nonprescription (OTC);
- are pregnant or intend to become pregnant while using this medicine;
- are breast-feeding;
- are taking **any** other prescription or nonprescription (OTC) medicine;
- have **any** other medical problems.

Proper Use of This Medicine

Take this medicine only as directed by your doctor. Too much of this medicine may cause mental or physical dependence.

This medicine will relieve a headache best if you **take it as soon as the headache begins.** If you get warning signs of a migraine, take this medicine as soon as you are sure that the migraine is coming. **Lying down in a quiet, dark room for a while after taking the medicine also helps to relieve headaches.**

People who get a lot of headaches may need to take a different medicine to help prevent headaches. **It is important that you follow your doctor's directions about taking the other medicine, even if your headaches continue.**

If you must take this medicine regularly and you miss a dose, take it as soon as you remember. However, if it is almost time for your next dose, skip the missed dose and go back to your regular dosing schedule. **Do not double doses.**

Precautions While Using This Medicine

Check with your doctor if this medicine stops working as well as it did when you first started using it, or if your headaches are coming more often. Do not try to get better relief by increasing the amount of medicine you take. **Continuing to take this medicine will cause even more headaches later on. Check the labels of all prescription and nonprescription medicines you now take.** If any contain a barbiturate or acetaminophen, be especially careful, since taking them while taking this medicine may lead to overdose.

The butalbital in this medicine will add to the effects of alcohol and other CNS depressants. Also, drinking large amounts of alcoholic beverages regularly may increase the chance of liver damage. **Check with your doctor before taking any such depressants while you are taking this medicine.**

This medicine may cause some people to become drowsy, dizzy, or lightheaded. **Make sure you know how you react to this medicine before you drive, use machines, or do other jobs that require you to be alert and clearheaded.**

If you have been taking large amounts of this medicine, or if you have been taking it regularly for several weeks or more, **do not suddenly stop taking it without first checking with your doctor.**

If you think you or someone else in your home may have taken an overdose of this medicine, get emergency help at once. Taking an overdose of this medicine or taking alcohol or CNS depressants with this medicine may lead to unconsciousness or possibly death. Signs of butalbital overdose include severe drowsiness, confusion, or weakness; shortness of breath or unusually slow or troubled breathing; slurred speech; staggering; and unusually slow heartbeat.

POSSIBLE SIDE EFFECTS OF THIS MEDICINE

Side effects that should be reported to your doctor immediately

RARE—Bleeding or crusting sores on lips; chest pain; fever with or without chills; hive-like swellings (large) on eyelids, face, lips, or tongue; muscle cramps or pain; red, thickened, or scaly skin; shortness of breath, troubled breathing, tightness in chest, or wheezing; skin rash, itching, or hives; sores, ulcers, or white spots in mouth (painful); sore throat

Other side effects that should be reported to your doctor

LESS COMMON—Confusion (mild); mental depression; unusual excitement (mild)

RARE—Bloody or black, tarry stools; bloody urine; pinpoint red spots on skin; swollen or painful glands; unusual bleeding or bruising; unusual tiredness or weakness (mild)

Side effects that usually do not require medical attention

These possible side effects may go away during treatment; however, if they continue or are bothersome, check with your doctor, nurse, or pharmacist.

MORE COMMON—Bloated or "gassy" feeling; dizziness or lightheadedness (mild); drowsiness (mild); nausea, vomiting, or stomach pain

Other side effects not listed above may also occur in some patients. If you notice any other effects, check with your doctor, nurse, or pharmacist.

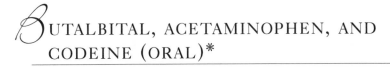BUTALBITAL, ACETAMINOPHEN, AND CODEINE (ORAL)*

ABOUT YOUR MEDICINE

Butalbital (byoo-TAL-bi-tal), **acetaminophen** (a-seat-a-MIN-oh-fen), and **codeine** (KOE-deen) combination is used to treat headaches. This medicine also contains caffeine (kaf-EEN).

If any of the information in this profile causes you special concern or if you want additional information about your medicine and its use, check with your doctor, nurse, or pharmacist. **Remember, keep this and all other medicines out of the reach of children and never share your medicines with others.**

BEFORE USING THIS MEDICINE

Tell your doctor, nurse, and pharmacist if you . . .
- are allergic to any medicine, either prescription or nonprescription (OTC);
- are pregnant or intend to become pregnant while using this medicine;
- are breast-feeding;
- are taking **any** other prescription or nonprescription (OTC) medicine;
- have **any** other medical problems.

PROPER USE OF THIS MEDICINE

Take this medicine only as directed by your doctor. Too much of this medicine may cause mental or physical dependence.

This medicine will relieve a headache best if you **take it as soon as the headache begins.** If you get warning signs of a migraine, take this medicine as soon as you are sure that the migraine is coming. **Lying down in a quiet, dark room for a while after taking the medicine also helps to relieve headaches.**

People who get a lot of headaches may need to take a different medicine to help prevent headaches. **It is important that you follow your doctor's directions about taking the other medicine, even if your headaches continue.**

PRECAUTIONS WHILE USING THIS MEDICINE

Check with your doctor if this medicine stops working as well as it did when you first started using it, or if your headaches are coming more often. Do not

*This profile has been developed by the USP based primarily on labeling provided by the manufacturer at the time of its approval. This information is intended for use as a temporary educational aid until the drug has been assessed by USP advisory panels. The information does not cover all possible uses, actions, precautions, side effects, or interactions of this medicine. It is not intended as medical advice for individual problems.

try to get better relief by increasing the amount of medicine you take. **Continuing to take this medicine will cause even more headaches later on.**

Check the labels of all prescription and nonprescription medicines you now take. If any contain a barbiturate, acetaminophen, or a narcotic, be especially careful, since taking them while taking this medicine may lead to overdose.

The butalbital and the codeine in this medicine will add to the effects of alcohol and other CNS depressants. Also, drinking large amounts of alcoholic beverages regularly may increase the chance of liver damage. **Check with your doctor before taking any such depressants while you are taking this medicine.**

This medicine may cause some people to become drowsy, dizzy, or lightheaded, or to feel a false sense of well-being. **Make sure you know how you react to this medicine before you drive, use machines, or do other jobs that require you to be alert and clearheaded.**

If you have been taking large amounts of this medicine, or if you have been taking it regularly for several weeks or more, **do not suddenly stop taking it without first checking with your doctor.**

If you think you or someone else in your home may have taken an overdose of this medicine, get emergency help at once. Taking an overdose of this medicine or taking alcohol or CNS depressants with this medicine may lead to unconsciousness or possibly death. Signs of overdose include severe drowsiness, confusion, or weakness; shortness of breath or unusually slow or troubled breathing; slurred speech; staggering; and unusually slow heartbeat.

POSSIBLE SIDE EFFECTS OF THIS MEDICINE

Side effects that should be reported to your doctor immediately
>MORE COMMON—Shortness of breath
>LESS COMMON—Fainting; seizures

Other side effects that should be reported to your doctor
>LESS COMMON—Earache; itching; fever; mental depression; ringing in ears; skin rash; stuffy nose; trouble in swallowing
>RARE—Black, tarry stools; blood in urine or stools; muscle cramps or pain; pinpoint red spots on skin; redness, tenderness, burning, or peeling of skin; sore throat; sores, ulcers, or white spots on lips or in mouth; unusual bleeding or bruising

Side effects that usually do not require medical attention
>These possible side effects may go away during treatment; however, if they continue or are bothersome, check with your doctor, nurse, or pharmacist.

>MORE COMMON—Dizziness; drowsiness; lightheadedness; nausea, vomiting, or stomach pain
>LESS COMMON—Confusion; constipation; excitement, nervousness, and restlessness; fast heartbeat; feeling numb; gas; heartburn; increased urination; shakiness; tingling

Other side effects not listed above may also occur in some patients. If you notice any other effects, check with your doctor, nurse, or pharmacist.

ℬUTALBITAL AND ASPIRIN (ORAL)

Including Butalbital and Aspirin; Butalbital, Aspirin, and Caffeine

ABOUT YOUR MEDICINE

Butalbital (byoo-TAL-bi-tal) and **aspirin** (AS-pir-in) is a combined pain reliever and relaxant. It is used to treat tension headaches. It may also be used for other conditions as determined by your doctor.

If any of the information in this profile causes you special concern or if you want additional information about your medicine and its use, check with your doctor, nurse, or pharmacist. **Remember, keep this and all other medicines out of the reach of children and never share your medicines with others.**

BEFORE USING THIS MEDICINE

Do not give a medicine containing aspirin to a child or a teenager with fever or other symptoms of a virus infection, especially flu or chickenpox, without first discussing its use with your child's doctor.

Tell your doctor, nurse, and pharmacist if you . . .
- are allergic to any medicine, either prescription or nonprescription (OTC);
- are pregnant or intend to become pregnant while using this medicine;
- are breast-feeding;
- are taking **any** other prescription or nonprescription (OTC) medicine;
- have **any** other medical problems.

PROPER USE OF THIS MEDICINE

Do not take this medicine if it has a strong vinegar-like odor.

Take this medicine only as directed. Too much of this medicine may cause mental or physical dependence. **This medicine may be taken with food or a full glass (8 ounces) of water** to lessen stomach irritation.

This medicine will relieve a headache best if you **take it as soon as the headache begins. Lying down in a quiet, dark room for a while after taking the medicine also helps to relieve headaches.**

People who get a lot of headaches may need to take a different medicine to help prevent headaches. **It is important that you follow your doctor's directions about taking the other medicine, even if your headaches continue.**

If you must take this medicine regularly and you miss a dose, take it as soon as possible. However, if it is almost time for your next dose, skip the missed dose and go back to your regular dosing schedule. Do not double doses.

PRECAUTIONS WHILE USING THIS MEDICINE

Check with your doctor if this medicine stops working as well as it did when you first started using it, or if your headaches are coming more often. Do not try to get better relief by increasing the amount of medicine you take. **Continuing to take this medicine will cause even more headaches later on.**

Check the labels of all prescription and nonprescription medicines you now take. If any contain a barbiturate, aspirin, or other salicylates, including diflunisal, be especially careful, since taking them while taking this medicine may lead to overdose.

This medicine will add to the effects of alcohol and other CNS depressants (medicines that slow down the nervous system). **Check with your doctor before taking any such depressants while you are using this medicine.**

This medicine may cause some people to become drowsy, dizzy, or lightheaded. **Make sure you know how you react to this medicine before you drive, use machines, or do other jobs that require you to be alert and clearheaded.**

If you have been taking this medicine regularly for several weeks, **do not suddenly stop taking it without checking with your doctor.**

If you think an overdose has been taken, get emergency help at once. Overdose or taking alcohol or CNS depressants with this medicine may lead to death. Signs include confusion; hearing loss; ringing in ears; severe nervousness, dizziness, drowsiness, or weakness; troubled breathing; or seizures.

POSSIBLE SIDE EFFECTS OF THIS MEDICINE

Side effects that should be reported to your doctor immediately
> LESS COMMON OR RARE—Bleeding or crusting sores on lips; bluish discoloration or flushing or redness of skin; chest pain; chills; coughing, shortness of breath, troubled breathing, tightness in chest, or wheezing; difficulty in swallowing; dizziness or feeling faint (severe); fever; hive-like swellings (large) on eyelids, face, lips, or tongue; red, thickened, or scaly skin; skin rash, itching, or hives; sores, ulcers, or white spots in mouth (painful); sore throat (unexplained); tenderness, burning, or peeling of skin

Other side effects that should be reported to your doctor
> LESS COMMON OR RARE—Bloody or black, tarry stools; bloody urine; confusion or mental depression; muscle pain; pinpoint red spots on skin; swollen or painful glands; unusual bleeding or bruising; unusual excitement (mild)

Side effects that usually do not require medical attention
> These possible side effects may go away during treatment; however, if they continue or are bothersome, check with your doctor, nurse, or pharmacist.

MORE COMMON—Bloated or "gassy" feeling; dizziness, drowsiness, or lightheadedness (mild); heartburn or indigestion; nausea, vomiting, or stomach pain

Other side effects not listed above may also occur in some patients. If you notice any other effects, check with your doctor, nurse, or pharmacist.

CALCITONIN (INJECTION)

ABOUT YOUR MEDICINE

Calcitonin (kal-si-TOE-nin) is used to treat Paget's disease of the bones. It also may be used to prevent continuing bone loss in women with postmenopausal osteoporosis and to treat hypercalcemia (too much calcium in the blood). This medicine may also be used for other conditions as determined by your doctor.

If any of the information in this profile causes you special concern or if you want additional information about your medicine and its use, check with your doctor, nurse, or pharmacist. **Remember, keep this and all other medicines out of the reach of children and never share your medicines with others.**

BEFORE USING THIS MEDICINE

Tell your doctor, nurse, and pharmacist if you . . .
- are allergic to any medicine, either prescription or nonprescription (OTC);
- are pregnant or intend to become pregnant while using this medicine;
- are breast-feeding;
- are taking any other prescription or nonprescription (OTC) medicine;
- have any other medical problems.

PROPER USE OF THIS MEDICINE

Some medicines given by injection may sometimes be given at home to patients who do not need to be in the hospital for the full time of treatment. If you are using this medicine at home, **make sure you clearly understand and carefully follow your doctor's instructions.**

Use the calcitonin only when the contents of the syringe are clear and colorless. Do not use the medicine if it looks grainy or discolored.

If you miss a dose of this medicine and your dosing schedule is:
- Two doses a day—If you remember within 2 hours of the missed dose, use it right away. Then go back to your regular dosing schedule. But if you do not remember the missed dose until later, skip it and go back to your regular dosing schedule. Do not double doses.

- One dose a day—Use the missed dose as soon as possible. Then go back to your regular dosing schedule. If you do not remember the missed dose until the next day, skip it and go back to your regular dosing schedule. Do not double doses.
- One dose every other day—Use the missed dose as soon as possible if you remember it on the day it should be used. Then go back to your regular dosing schedule. If you do not remember the missed dose until the next day, use it at that time. Then skip a day and start your dosing schedule again.
- One dose three times a week—Use the missed dose the next day. Then set each injection back a day for the rest of the week. Go back to your regular dosing schedule the following week. Do not double doses.

If you have any questions about this, check with your doctor.

PRECAUTIONS WHILE USING THIS MEDICINE

Your doctor should check your progress at regular visits to make sure that this medicine does not cause unwanted effects.

If you are using this medicine for hypercalcemia (too much calcium in the blood), your doctor may want you to follow a low-calcium diet. If you have any questions about this, check with your doctor.

POSSIBLE SIDE EFFECTS OF THIS MEDICINE

Side effects that should be reported to your doctor
RARE—Skin rash or hives

Side effects that usually do not require medical attention
These possible side effects may go away during treatment; however, if they continue or are bothersome, check with your doctor, nurse, or pharmacist.

MORE COMMON—Diarrhea; flushing or redness of face, ears, hands, or feet; loss of appetite; nausea or vomiting; pain, redness, soreness, or swelling at place of injection; stomach pain
LESS COMMON—Increased frequency of urination
RARE—Chills; dizziness; headache; pressure in chest; stuffy nose; tenderness or tingling of hands or feet; trouble in breathing; weakness

Other side effects not listed above may also occur in some patients. If you notice any other effects, check with your doctor, nurse, or pharmacist.

$\mathcal{C}$ALCIUM CHANNEL BLOCKERS (ORAL)

Including Amlodipine; Bepridil;
Diltiazem; Felodipine; Flunarizine; Isradipine;
Nicardipine; Nifedipine; Nimodipine; Verapamil

ABOUT YOUR MEDICINE

Calcium channel blockers are used to relieve and control angina (chest pain). Some are also used to treat high blood pressure (hypertension), prevent migraine headaches, or prevent and treat problems caused by a burst blood vessel in the head (also known as a ruptured aneurysm or subarachnoid hemorrhage). Channel blockers may also be used for other conditions as determined by your doctor.

If any of the information in this profile causes you special concern or if you want additional information about your medicine and its use, check with your doctor, nurse, or pharmacist. **Remember, keep this and all other medicines out of the reach of children and never share your medicines with others.**

BEFORE USING THIS MEDICINE

Tell your doctor, nurse, and pharmacist if you . . .
- are allergic to any medicine, either prescription or nonprescription (OTC);
- are pregnant or intend to become pregnant while using this medicine;
- are breast-feeding;
- are taking any other prescription or nonprescription (OTC) medicine, especially *any* other medicines for the heart, carbamazepine, corticosteroids, cyclosporine, or diuretics (water pills);
- have any other medical problems, especially other heart disease.

PROPER USE OF THIS MEDICINE

For patients taking bepridil:
- If bepridil causes upset stomach, it may be taken with meals or at bedtime.

For patients taking extended-release capsules or tablets or regular nifedipine:
- Swallow whole, without breaking, crushing, or chewing.

For patients taking diltiazem extended-release capsules:
- **Do not change to another brand without first checking with your doctor.**

For patients taking *Procardia XL*:
- You may notice what looks like a tablet in your stool. That is just the empty shell that is left after the medicine has been absorbed into your body.

For patients taking verapamil extended-release tablets:
- Your doctor may tell you to break the tablet in half. Do this only if you are instructed to do so. Also, take the tablets with food or milk.

Take exactly as directed even if you feel well. Do not take more of this medicine and do not take it more often than your doctor ordered. Do not miss any doses.

If you do miss a dose of this medicine, take it as soon as possible. However, if it is almost time for your next dose, skip the missed dose and go back to your regular dosing schedule. Do not double doses.

PRECAUTIONS WHILE USING THIS MEDICINE

If you have been using this medicine regularly for several weeks, do not suddenly stop using it. Stopping suddenly may bring on your previous problem. Check with your doctor for the best way to reduce gradually the amount you are taking before stopping completely.

Chest pain resulting from exercise or exertion is usually reduced or prevented by this medicine. This may tempt you to be overly active. **Make sure you discuss with your doctor a safe amount of exercise for your medical problem.**

In some patients, tenderness, swelling, or bleeding of the gums may occur. Brushing and flossing your teeth carefully and regularly and massaging your gums may help prevent this. **See your dentist regularly to have your teeth cleaned. Check with your physician or dentist if you notice any tenderness, swelling, or bleeding of your gums.**

For patients taking bepridil, diltiazem, or verapamil:
- **Ask your doctor or pharmacist how to count your pulse rate. Then, while you are taking this medicine, check your pulse regularly.** If it is much slower than your usual rate, or less than 50 beats per minute, check with your doctor.

For patients taking flunarizine:
- This medicine may cause some people to become drowsy or less alert than they are normally. **Make sure you know how you react before you drive, use machines, or do other jobs that require you to be alert.**

POSSIBLE SIDE EFFECTS OF THIS MEDICINE

Side effects that should be reported to your doctor

LESS COMMON—Breathing difficulty, coughing, or wheezing; dizziness; irregular or fast or slow heartbeat; skin rash; swelling of ankles, feet, or lower legs

RARE—Bleeding, tender, or swollen gums; chest pain; fainting; painful, swollen joints (nifedipine only); trouble in seeing (nifedipine only); unusual secretion of milk (flunarizine and verapamil only)

FOR FLUNARIZINE ONLY: LESS COMMON (IN ADDITION TO THE ABOVE)—Loss of balance control; mask-like face; mental depression; shuffling walk; stiff arms or legs; trembling of hands and fingers; trouble in speaking or swallowing

Side effects that usually do not require medical attention

These possible side effects may go away during treatment; however, if they continue or are bothersome, check with your doctor, nurse, or pharmacist.

FOR FLUNARIZINE: MORE COMMON—Drowsiness; increased appetite or weight
FOR AMLODIPINE, ISRADIPINE, AND NIFEDIPINE: MORE COMMON—Flushing
FOR AMLODIPINE, FELODIPINE, NICARDIPINE, NIFEDIPINE: MORE COMMON—
Headache

Other side effects not listed above may also occur in some patients. If you notice any other effects, check with your doctor, nurse, or pharmacist.

CALCIUM SUPPLEMENTS (ORAL)

Including Calcium Carbonate; Calcium Citrate; Calcium Glubionate; Calcium Gluceptate and Calcium Gluconate; Calcium Gluconate; Calcium Glycerophosphate and Calcium Lactate; Calcium Lactate; Calcium Lactate-Gluconate and Calcium Carbonate; Dibasic Calcium Phosphate; Tribasic Calcium Phosphate

ABOUT YOUR DIETARY SUPPLEMENT

Calcium supplements are taken by patients who are unable to get enough calcium in their regular diet or who have a need for more calcium. Pregnant women, nursing mothers, children, and adolescents may need more calcium than they normally get from eating calcium-rich foods. Adult women may take calcium supplements to help prevent a bone disease called osteoporosis.

Calcium supplements are also used to prevent or treat several conditions that may cause hypocalcemia (not enough calcium in the blood). These medicines may also be used for other conditions as determined by your doctor.

If any of the information in this profile causes you special concern or if you want additional information about your dietary supplement and its use, check with your doctor, nurse, or pharmacist. **Remember, keep this and all other medicines out of the reach of children and never share your medicines with others.**

BEFORE USING THIS DIETARY SUPPLEMENT

Follow carefully any diet program your doctor may recommend. For your specific vitamin and/or mineral needs, ask your doctor for a list of appropriate foods.

If you are taking this dietary supplement without a prescription, carefully read and follow any precautions on the label. You should be especially careful if you . . .

- are allergic to any medicine, either prescription or nonprescription (OTC);
- are pregnant, intend to become pregnant, or are breast-feeding;
- are taking any other prescription or nonprescription (OTC) medicine, especially cellulose sodium phosphate, digitalis glycosides (heart medicine), etidronate, gallium nitrate, magnesium sulfate (for injection), other calcium-containing medicines, phenytoin, or tetracyclines taken by mouth;
- have any other medical problems, especially heart disease, hypercalcemia, hypercalciuria, hyperparathyroidism, hypoparathyroidism, kidney disease or stones, or sarcoidosis.

If you have any questions, check with your doctor, nurse, or pharmacist.

PROPER USE OF THIS DIETARY SUPPLEMENT

Drink a full glass (8 ounces) of water or juice when taking a calcium supplement. However, if you are taking calcium carbonate as a phosphate binder in kidney dialysis, it is not necessary to drink a glass of water.

This medicine is best taken 1 to 1 and 1/2 hours after meals, unless otherwise directed by your doctor. However, patients with a condition known as achlorhydria may not absorb calcium supplements on an empty stomach and should take them with meals. If you are taking the syrup form of this dietary supplement, take it before meals. This will allow the dietary supplement to work faster. Mix the syrup in water or fruit juice for infants or children.

For patients taking the chewable tablet form of this dietary supplement:

- Chew the tablets completely before swallowing.

Take this dietary supplement only as directed. Do not take more of it and do not take it more often than recommended on the label.

If you are taking this dietary supplement on a regular schedule and you miss a dose, take it as soon as possible, then go back to your regular schedule.

PRECAUTIONS WHILE USING THIS DIETARY SUPPLEMENT

If this dietary supplement has been ordered for you by your doctor and you will be taking it in large doses or for a long time, your doctor should check your progress at regular visits. This is to make sure the dietary supplement is working properly and does not cause unwanted effects.

Do not take calcium supplements within 1 to 2 hours of taking other medicine by mouth. To do so may keep the other medicine from working properly.

When taking calcium, unless otherwise directed, it is best that you:

- **Do not take other medicines containing large amounts of calcium, phosphates, magnesium, or vitamin D.**
- **Do not take calcium supplements within 1 to 2 hours of eating large**

amounts of fiber-containing foods, such as bran and whole-grain cereals or breads, especially if you are being treated for hypocalcemia (not enough calcium in your blood).

- Do not drink large amounts of alcohol or caffeine-containing beverages, or use tobacco.

Recently, some calcium carbonate tablets have been shown to break up too slowly in the stomach to be properly absorbed into the body. If the calcium carbonate tablets you purchase are not specifically labeled as being "USP," check with your pharmacist. He or she may be able to help you determine which tablets are best.

POSSIBLE SIDE EFFECTS OF THIS DIETARY SUPPLEMENT

Side effects that should be reported to your doctor

RARE—Difficult or painful urination; drowsiness; nausea or vomiting (continuing); weakness

Other side effects not listed above may also occur in some patients. If you notice any other effects, check with your doctor, nurse, or pharmacist.

CAPSAICIN (TOPICAL)

ABOUT YOUR MEDICINE

Capsaicin (cap-SAY-sin) is used to help relieve a certain type of pain known as neuralgia (new-RAL-ja). Capsaicin is also used to temporarily help relieve the pain from osteoarthritis (OS-te-o-ar-THRI-tis) or rheumatoid arthritis (ROO-ma-toid ar-THRI-tis). This medicine will not cure any of these conditions. Capsaicin may also be used for neuralgias caused by other conditions as determined by your doctor.

If any of the information in this profile causes you special concern or if you want additional information about your medicine and its use, check with your doctor, nurse, or pharmacist. **Remember, keep this and all other medicines out of the reach of children and never share your medicines with others.**

BEFORE USING THIS MEDICINE

If you are taking this medicine without a prescription, carefully read and follow any precautions on the label. You should be especially careful if you . . .

- are allergic to any medicine, either prescription or nonprescription (OTC);
- are pregnant, intend to become pregnant, or are breast-feeding;
- are taking any other prescription or nonprescription (OTC) medicine;

- have any other medical problems, especially broken or irritated skin on area to be treated with capsaicin.

If you have any questions, check with your doctor, nurse, or pharmacist.

PROPER USE OF THIS MEDICINE

If you are using capsaicin for the treatment of neuralgia caused by herpes zoster, do not apply the medicine until the zoster sores have healed.

You do not need to wash the areas to be treated before you apply capsaicin, but doing so will not cause harm.

Apply a small amount of cream and use your fingers to rub it well into the affected area so that little or no cream is left on the surface of the skin afterwards.

Wash your hands with soap and water after applying capsaicin to avoid getting the medicine in your eyes or on other sensitive areas of the body. However, if you are using capsaicin for arthritis in your hands, do not wash your hands for at least 30 minutes after applying the cream.

If a bandage is being used on the treated area, it should not be applied tightly.

When you first begin to use capsaicin, a warm, stinging, or burning sensation (feeling) may occur. This is to be expected. Although this sensation usually disappears after the first several days of treatment, it may last 2 to 4 weeks or longer. Heat, humidity, clothing, bathing in warm water, or sweating may increase the sensation. However, the sensation usually occurs less often and is less severe the longer you use the medicine. Reducing the number of doses of capsaicin that you use each day will not lessen the sensation, and may lengthen the period of time that you get the sensation. Also, reducing the number of doses you use may reduce the amount of pain relief that you get.

Capsaicin must be used regularly every day as directed if it is to work properly. Even then, it may not relieve your pain right away. The length of time it takes to work depends on the type of pain you have. In persons with arthritis, pain relief usually begins within 1 to 2 weeks. In most persons with neuralgia, relief usually begins within 2 to 4 weeks, although with head and neck neuralgias, relief may take as long as 4 to 6 weeks.

Once capsaicin has begun to relieve pain, you must continue to use it regularly 3 or 4 times a day to keep the pain from returning. If you stop using capsaicin and your pain returns, you can begin using it again.

If you miss a dose of this medicine, use it as soon as possible. However, if it is almost time for your next dose, skip the missed dose and go back to your regular dosing schedule. Do not double doses.

PRECAUTIONS WHILE USING THIS MEDICINE

If capsaicin gets into your eyes or on other sensitive areas of the body, it will cause a burning sensation. If capsaicin gets into your eyes, flush your eyes with water. If capsaicin gets on other sensitive areas of your body, wash the areas with warm (not hot) soapy water.

If your condition gets worse, or does not improve after 1 month, stop using this medicine and check with your doctor.

POSSIBLE SIDE EFFECTS OF THIS MEDICINE

Side effects that usually do not require medical attention

> These possible side effects may go away during treatment; however, if they continue or are bothersome, check with your doctor, nurse, or pharmacist.

> MORE COMMON—Warm, stinging, or burning feeling at the place of treatment

> Other side effects not listed above may also occur in some patients. If you notice any other effects, check with your doctor, nurse, or pharmacist.

CARBAMAZEPINE (ORAL)

ABOUT YOUR MEDICINE

Carbamazepine (kar-ba-MAZ-e-peen) is used to control some types of seizures in the treatment of epilepsy. It is also used to relieve pain due to trigeminal neuralgia (tic douloureux). Carbamazepine may also be used for other conditions as determined by your doctor.

If any of the information in this profile causes you special concern or if you want additional information about your medicine and its use, check with your doctor, nurse, or pharmacist. **Remember, keep this and all other medicines out of the reach of children and never share your medicines with others.**

BEFORE USING THIS MEDICINE

Tell your doctor, nurse, and pharmacist if you . . .

- are allergic to any medicine, either prescription or nonprescription (OTC);
- are pregnant or intend to become pregnant while using this medicine;
- are breast-feeding;
- are taking **any** other prescription or nonprescription (OTC) medicine;
- have any other medical problems, especially anemia or other blood problems, or heart or blood vessel disease.

PROPER USE OF THIS MEDICINE

Take carbamazepine exactly as directed. It should be taken with meals to lessen the chance of stomach upset.

For patients taking this medicine for epilepsy: Do not suddenly stop taking it without first checking with your doctor.

If you miss a dose of this medicine, take it as soon as possible. However, if it is almost time for your next dose, skip the missed dose and go back to your regular dosing schedule. Do not double doses.

PRECAUTIONS WHILE USING THIS MEDICINE

It is very important that your doctor check your progress at regular visits.

This medicine will add to the effects of alcohol and other CNS depressants (medicines that may make you drowsy or less alert). **Check with your doctor before taking any such depressants while you are using this medicine.**

Oral contraceptives (birth control pills) containing estrogen may not work properly if you take them while you are taking carbamazepine. Unplanned pregnancies may occur. You should use a different or additional means of birth control while you are taking carbamazepine. If you have any questions about this, check with your doctor or pharmacist.

Some people who take carbamazepine may become more sensitive to sunlight than they are normally. **Avoid too much sun and do not use a sunlamp until you see how you react to the sun,** especially if you tend to burn easily. **If you have a severe reaction, check with your doctor.**

Before having any kind of surgery or dental or emergency treatment, tell the physician or dentist in charge that you are taking carbamazepine.

This medicine may cause some people to become drowsy, dizzy, lightheaded, or less alert than they are normally. It may also cause blurred or double vision, weakness, or loss of muscle control. **Make sure you know how you react before you drive or do jobs that require you to be alert and well-coordinated or able to see well.**

POSSIBLE SIDE EFFECTS OF THIS MEDICINE

Side effects that should be reported to your doctor immediately
>   **Check with your doctor immediately** if you notice black, tarry stools; blood in urine or stools; bone or joint pain; cough or hoarseness; darkening of urine; lower back or side pain; nosebleeds or other unusual bleeding or bruising; painful or difficult urination; pain, tenderness, swelling, or bluish color in leg or foot; pale stools; pinpoint red spots on skin; shortness of breath; sores, ulcers, or white spots on lips or in the mouth; sore throat, chills, and fever; swollen or painful glands; unusual tiredness or weakness; wheezing, tightness in chest, or troubled breathing; or yellow eyes or skin.

Other side effects that should be reported to your doctor
>   MORE COMMON—Blurred or double vision; continuous back-and-forth eye movements
>   LESS COMMON—Behavioral changes (especially in children); confusion, agitation, or hostility (especially in the elderly); diarrhea (severe); headache

(continuing); increase in seizures; nausea and vomiting (severe); skin rash, hives, or itching; unusual drowsiness

RARE—Buzzing or ringing in ears; chest pain; difficulty in speaking or slurred speech; fainting; frequent urination; irregular, pounding, or slow heartbeat; mental depression with restlessness; muscle or stomach cramps; numbness, tingling, pain, or weakness in hands and feet; rapid weight gain; rigidity; sudden decrease in amount of urine; swelling of face, hands, feet or lower legs; trembling; uncontrolled body movements; visual hallucinations

Side effects that usually do not require medical attention

These possible side effects may go away during treatment; however, if they continue or are bothersome, check with your doctor, nurse, or pharmacist.

MORE COMMON—Clumsiness or unsteadiness; dizziness or lightheadedness (mild); drowsiness (slight); nausea or vomiting (mild)

Other side effects not listed above may also occur in some patients. If you notice any other effects, check with your doctor, nurse, or pharmacist.

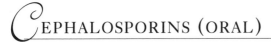

CEPHALOSPORINS (ORAL)

Including Cefaclor; Cefadroxil; Cefixime;
Cefpodoxime; Cefprozil; Cefuroxime; Cephalexin; Cephradine

ABOUT YOUR MEDICINE

Cephalosporins (sef-a-loe-SPOR-ins) are used to treat infections caused by bacteria. They will not work for colds, flu, or other virus infections.

If any of the information in this profile causes you special concern or if you want additional information about your medicine and its use, check with your doctor, nurse, or pharmacist. **Remember, keep this and all other medicines out of the reach of children and never share your medicines with others.**

BEFORE USING THIS MEDICINE

Tell your doctor, nurse, and pharmacist if you . . .

- are allergic to any medicine, either prescription or nonprescription (OTC);
- are pregnant or intend to become pregnant while using this medicine;
- are breast-feeding;
- are taking any other prescription or nonprescription (OTC) medicine, especially probenecid;
- have any other medical problems, especially history of stomach or intestinal disease, such as colitis, including colitis caused by antibiotics, or enteritis.

PROPER USE OF THIS MEDICINE

Cephalosporins may be taken on a full or empty stomach. If this medicine upsets your stomach, it may be taken with food. Cefuroxime axetil tablets and cefpodoxime should be taken with food to increase absorption of the medicine.

For patients taking the oral liquid form of this medicine:
- This medicine is to be taken by mouth even if it comes in a dropper bottle. If this medicine does not come in a dropper bottle, use a specially marked measuring spoon or other device to measure each dose accurately. The average household teaspoon may not hold the right amount of liquid.

For patients unable to swallow cefuroxime tablets whole:
- Cefuroxime tablets may be crushed and mixed with food (e.g., applesauce, ice cream) or drinks (apple, orange, or grape juice, or chocolate milk) to cover up the strong, lasting, bitter taste.

To help clear up your infection completely, **keep taking this medicine for the full time of treatment** even if you begin to feel better after a few days; **do not miss any doses.**

If you do miss a dose of this medicine, take it as soon as possible. This will help to keep a constant amount of medicine in the blood or urine. However, if it is almost time for your next dose, skip the missed dose and go back to your regular dosing schedule. Do not double doses.

PRECAUTIONS WHILE USING THIS MEDICINE

If your symptoms do not improve within a few days, or if they become worse, check with your doctor.

Diabetics—This medicine may cause false test results with some urine sugar tests. Check with your doctor before changing your diet or the dosage of your diabetes medicine.

For patients with phenylketonuria (PKU):
- Cefprozil oral suspension contains phenylalanine. Check with your doctor before taking this medicine.

If diarrhea occurs, do not take any diarrhea medicine without first checking with your doctor or pharmacist. Diarrhea medicines may make your diarrhea worse or make it last longer.

This medicine must not be given to other people or used for other infections unless you are otherwise directed by your doctor.

POSSIBLE SIDE EFFECTS OF THIS MEDICINE

Side effects that should be reported to your doctor immediately
>   LESS COMMON OR RARE—Abdominal or stomach cramps and pain (severe); diarrhea (watery and severe), which may also be bloody; fever

The above side effects may also occur up to several weeks after you stop taking this medicine.

> RARE—Convulsions (seizures); decrease in urine output; dizziness or lightheadedness; joint pain; loss of appetite; skin rash, itching, redness, or swelling; trouble in breathing

Side effects that usually do not require medical attention

> These possible side effects may go away during treatment; however, if they continue or are bothersome, check with your doctor, nurse, or pharmacist.

> MORE COMMON (LESS COMMON WITH SOME CEPHALOSPORINS)—Diarrhea (mild); nausea and vomiting; sore mouth or tongue; stomach cramps (mild)

> Other side effects not listed above may also occur in some patients. If you notice any other effects, check with your doctor, nurse, or pharmacist.

$\mathcal{C}$HOLESTEROL-LOWERING RESINS (ORAL)

Including Cholestyramine; Colestipol

ABOUT YOUR MEDICINE

Cholesterol-lowering resins are used to lower levels of cholesterol (a fat-like substance) in the blood. This may help prevent medical problems caused by cholesterol clogging the blood vessels. These medicines may also be used for other conditions as determined by your doctor.

If any of the information in this profile causes you special concern or if you want additional information about your medicine and its use, check with your doctor, nurse, or pharmacist. **Remember, keep this and all other medicines out of the reach of children and never share your medicines with others.**

BEFORE USING THIS MEDICINE

Importance of diet—Before prescribing medicine for your condition, your doctor will probably try to control your condition by prescribing a personal diet for you. Such a diet may be low in fats, sugars, and/or cholesterol. Many people are able to control their condition by carefully following their doctor's orders for proper diet and exercise. Medicine is prescribed only when additional help is needed and is effective only when a schedule of diet and exercise is properly followed.

Also, this medicine is less effective if you are greatly overweight. It may be very important for you to go on a reducing diet. However, check with your doctor before going on any diet.

Tell your doctor, nurse, and pharmacist if you . . .
- are allergic to any medicine, either prescription or nonprescription (OTC);
- are pregnant or intend to become pregnant while using this medicine;
- are breast-feeding;
- are taking any other prescription or nonprescription (OTC) medicine, especially anticoagulants (blood thinners), digitalis glycosides (heart medicine), diuretics (water pills), phenylbutazone, penicillins, propranolol, tetracyclines, thyroid hormones, or vancomycin;
- have any other medical problems, especially constipation or stomach problems;
- have phenylketonuria, since some brands of cholestyramine may contain aspartame.

PROPER USE OF THIS MEDICINE

This medicine should never be taken in its dry form, since it could cause you to choke. Instead, always mix as follows:
- For cholestyramine: Place the medicine in 2 ounces of any beverage and mix thoroughly. Then add an additional 2 to 4 ounces of beverage and again mix thoroughly (it will **not** dissolve) before drinking.
- For colestipol: Add this medicine to 3 ounces or more of water, milk, flavored drink, or your favorite juice or carbonated drink. If you use a carbonated drink, slowly mix in the powder in a large glass to prevent too much foaming.
- Stir until the medicine is completely mixed (it will **not** dissolve) before drinking. After drinking all the liquid, rinse the glass with a little more liquid and drink that also, to make sure you get the full dose.
- You may also mix this medicine with milk in hot or regular breakfast cereals, or in thin soups such as tomato or chicken noodle. Or you may add it to some pulpy fruits such as crushed pineapple, pears, peaches, or fruit cocktail.

Take this medicine exactly as directed by your doctor. Try not to miss any doses and do not take more medicine than your doctor ordered.

If you miss a dose of this medicine, take it as soon as possible. However, if it is almost time for your next dose, skip the missed dose and go back to your regular dosing schedule. Do not double doses.

PRECAUTIONS WHILE USING THIS MEDICINE

It is very important that your doctor check your progress at regular visits.

Do not take any other medicine unless prescribed by your doctor since cholesterol-lowering resins may change the effect of other medicines.

Do not stop taking this medicine without first checking with your doctor. When you stop taking this medicine, your blood cholesterol levels may increase again. Your doctor may want you to follow a special diet to help prevent this.

POSSIBLE SIDE EFFECTS OF THIS MEDICINE

Side effects that should be reported to your doctor immediately

RARE—Black, tarry stools; stomach pain (severe) with nausea and vomiting

Other side effects that should be reported to your doctor

MORE COMMON—Constipation

RARE—Loss of weight (sudden)

Side effects that usually do not require medical attention

These possible side effects may go away during treatment; however, if they continue or are bothersome, check with your doctor, nurse, or pharmacist.

MORE COMMON (LESS COMMON FOR COLESTIPOL)—Heartburn or indigestion; nausea or vomiting; stomach pain

Other side effects not listed above may also occur in some patients. If you notice any other effects, check with your doctor, nurse, or pharmacist.

CHORIONIC GONADOTROPIN (INJECTION)

ABOUT YOUR MEDICINE

Chorionic gonadotropin (kor-ee-ON-ik goe-NAD-oh-troe-pin) is a medicine whose actions are almost the same as those of luteinizing (loo-te-in-eye-ZING) hormone (LH), which is produced by the pituitary gland. Chorionic gonadotropin is a hormone also normally produced by the placenta in pregnancy. This medicine has different uses for females and males.

In females, chorionic gonadotropin is used to help conception occur. It is usually given in combination with other medicines such as menotropins and urofollitropin. Many women being treated with these medicines usually have already tried clomiphene alone and have not been able to conceive yet. Chorionic gonadotropin is also used in *in vitro* fertilization (IVF) programs.

In males, LH and chorionic gonadotropin stimulate the testes to produce male hormones such as testosterone. Testosterone causes the enlargement of the penis and testes and the growth of pubic and underarm hair. It also increases the production of sperm.

Although chorionic gonadotropin has been prescribed to help some patients lose weight, it should *never* be used this way. When used improperly, chorionic gonadotropin can cause serious problems.

If any of the information in this profile causes you special concern or if you want additional information about your medicine and its use, check with your doctor,

nurse, or pharmacist. **Remember, keep this and all other medicines out of the reach of children and never share your medicines with others.**

BEFORE USING THIS MEDICINE

Tell your doctor, nurse, and pharmacist if you . . .
- are allergic to any medicine, either prescription or nonprescription (OTC);
- are pregnant or intend to become pregnant while using this medicine;
- are breast-feeding;
- are taking any other prescription or nonprescription (OTC) medicine;
- have any other medical problems, especially cancer of the prostate, a cyst on an ovary, fibroid tumors of the uterus, pituitary gland enlargement or tumor, or unusual vaginal bleeding.

PRECAUTIONS WHILE USING THIS MEDICINE

It is very important that your doctor check your progress at regular visits to make sure that the medicine is working and to check for unwanted effects.

For women taking this medicine to become pregnant:
- Record your basal body temperature (BBT) every day if told to do so by your doctor, so that you will know if you have begun to ovulate. It is important that intercourse take place around the time of ovulation to give you the best chance of becoming pregnant. Your doctor will probably want to monitor the development of the ovarian follicle(s) by measuring the amount of estrogen in your bloodstream and by checking the size of the follicle(s) with ultrasound examinations.

POSSIBLE SIDE EFFECTS OF THIS MEDICINE

Side effects that should be reported to your doctor
  For females only—
  MORE COMMON—Bloating (mild); stomach or pelvic pain
  LESS COMMON OR RARE—Abdominal or stomach pain (severe); bloating (moderate to severe); decreased amount of urine; feeling of indigestion; nausea, vomiting, or diarrhea (continuing or severe); pelvic pain (severe); shortness of breath; swelling of feet or lower legs; weight gain (rapid)

  For boys only—
  LESS COMMON—Acne; enlargement of penis and testes; growth of pubic hair; increase in height (rapid)

Side effects that usually do not require medical attention
  These possible side effects may go away during treatment; however, if they continue or are bothersome, check with your doctor, nurse, or pharmacist.

  LESS COMMON—Enlargement of breasts; headache; irritability; mental depression; pain at place of injection; tiredness

After you stop using this medicine, it may continue to cause some side effects which require medical attention. During this time check with your doctor if you notice any of the following side effects:

For females only—

LESS COMMON OR RARE—Abdominal or stomach pain (severe); bloating (moderate to severe); decreased amount of urine; feeling of indigestion; nausea, vomiting, or diarrhea (continuing or severe); pelvic pain (severe); shortness of breath; weight gain (rapid)

Other side effects not listed above may also occur in some patients. If you notice any other effects, check with your doctor, nurse, or pharmacist.

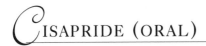

CISAPRIDE (ORAL)

ABOUT YOUR MEDICINE

Cisapride (SIS-a-pride) is used to treat symptoms such as heartburn caused by a backward flow of gastric acid into the esophagus. Cisapride may also be used for other conditions as determined by your doctor.

If any of the information in this profile causes you special concern or if you want additional information about your medicine and its use, check with your doctor, nurse, or pharmacist. **Remember, keep this and all other medicines out of the reach of children and never share your medicines with others.**

BEFORE USING THIS MEDICINE

Tell your doctor, nurse, and pharmacist if you . . .
- are allergic to any medicine, either prescription or nonprescription (OTC);
- are pregnant or intend to become pregnant while using this medicine;
- are breast-feeding;
- are taking any other prescription or nonprescription (OTC) medicine, especially anticholinergics (medicines for abdominal or stomach spasms or cramps), itraconazole, ketoconazole, miconazole, or troleandomycin;
- have any other medical problems, especially abdominal or stomach bleeding, or intestinal blockage.

PROPER USE OF THIS MEDICINE

Take this medicine 15 minutes before meals and at bedtime with a beverage, unless otherwise directed by your doctor.

If you miss a dose of this medicine, take it as soon as possible. However, if it is almost time for your next dose, skip the missed dose and go back to your regular dosing schedule. Do not double doses.

PRECAUTIONS WHILE USING THIS MEDICINE

This medicine may cause your body to absorb alcohol more quickly than you normally would. Therefore, you may notice the effects sooner. **Check with your doctor before drinking alcohol while you are using this medicine.**

This medicine may cause some people to become drowsy or less alert than they are normally. **Make sure you know how you react to this medicine before you drive, use machines, or do other jobs that require you to be alert.**

POSSIBLE SIDE EFFECTS OF THIS MEDICINE

Side effects that should be reported to your doctor immediately
     RARE—Convulsions (seizures)

Side effects that usually do not require medical attention
     These possible side effects may go away during treatment; however, if they continue or are bothersome, check with your doctor, nurse, or pharmacist.

     LESS COMMON—Abdominal cramping; constipation; diarrhea; drowsiness; headache; nausea; unusual tiredness or weakness

     Other side effects not listed above may also occur in some patients. If you notice any other effects, check with your doctor, nurse, or pharmacist.

CLARITHROMYCIN (ORAL)

ABOUT YOUR MEDICINE

Clarithromycin (kla-RITH-roe-mye-sin) is used to treat bacterial infections in many different parts of the body. It is also used to treat *Mycobacterium avium* complex (MAC) infection. However, this medicine will not work for colds, flu, or other virus infections. Clarithromycin may be used for other problems as determined by your doctor.

If any of the information in this profile causes you special concern or if you want additional information about your medicine and its use, check with your doctor, nurse, or pharmacist. **Remember, keep this and all other medicines out of the reach of children and never share your medicines with others.**

BEFORE USING THIS MEDICINE

Tell your doctor, nurse, and pharmacist if you . . .
- are allergic to any medicine, either prescription or nonprescription (OTC);
- are pregnant or intend to become pregnant while using this medicine;
- are breast-feeding;
- are taking any other prescription or nonprescription (OTC) medicine, especially carbamazepine, digoxin, rifabutin, rifampin, terfenadine, theophylline, warfarin, or zidovudine;
- have any other medical problems.

PROPER USE OF THIS MEDICINE

Clarithromycin may be taken with meals or milk or on an empty stomach.

To help clear up your infection completely, **keep taking clarithromycin for the full time of treatment,** even if you begin to feel better after a few days. If you stop taking this medicine too soon, your symptoms may return.

If you are using clarithromycin oral suspension, use a specially marked measuring spoon or other device to measure each dose accurately. The average household teaspoon may not hold the right amount of liquid.

If you miss a dose of this medicine, take it as soon as possible. However, if it is almost time for your next dose, skip the missed dose and go back to your regular dosing schedule. Do not double doses.

PRECAUTIONS WHILE USING THIS MEDICINE

If your symptoms do not improve within a few days, or if they become worse, check with your doctor.

POSSIBLE SIDE EFFECTS OF THIS MEDICINE

Side effects that should be reported to your doctor

RARE—Abdominal tenderness; fever; nausea and vomiting; severe abdominal or stomach cramps and pain; shortness of breath; skin rash and itching; unusual bleeding or bruising; watery and severe diarrhea, which may also be bloody; yellow eyes or skin

Side effects that usually do not require medical attention

These possible side effects may go away during treatment; however, if they continue or are bothersome, check with your doctor, nurse, or pharmacist.

LESS COMMON—Abnormal taste; diarrhea; headache

Other side effects not listed above may also occur in some patients. If you notice any other effects, check with your doctor, nurse, or pharmacist.

CLINDAMYCIN (VAGINAL)

ABOUT YOUR MEDICINE

Clindamycin (klin-da-MY-sin) is used to treat certain vaginal infections.

If any of the information in this profile causes you special concern or if you want additional information about your medicine and its use, check with your doctor, nurse, or pharmacist. **Remember, keep this and all other medicines out of the reach of children and never share your medicines with others.**

BEFORE USING THIS MEDICINE

Tell your doctor, nurse, and pharmacist if you . . .
- are allergic to any medicine, either prescription or nonprescription (OTC);
- are pregnant or intend to become pregnant while using this medicine;
- are breast-feeding;
- are taking any other prescription or nonprescription (OTC) medicine;
- have any other medical problems, especially history of stomach or intestinal disease (especially colitis, including colitis caused by antibiotics, or enteritis).

PROPER USE OF THIS MEDICINE

Vaginal clindamycin usually comes with patient directions. Read them carefully before using this medicine.

Wash your hands before and after using this medicine. Avoid getting this medicine in your eyes.

To help clear up your infection completely, **it is very important that you keep using this medicine for the full time of treatment,** even if your symptoms begin to clear up after a few days. If you stop using this medicine too soon, your symptoms may return. **Do not miss any doses. Also, continue using this medicine even if your menstrual period starts during treatment.**

If you do miss a dose of this medicine, use it as soon as possible. However, if it is almost time for your next dose, skip the missed dose and go back to your regular dosing schedule.

PRECAUTIONS WHILE USING THIS MEDICINE

If your symptoms do not improve within a few days, or if they become worse, check with your doctor.

This medicine may cause some people to become dizzy. **Make sure you know how to react to this medicine before you drive, use machines, or do anything else that could be dangerous if you are dizzy.**

Vaginal medicines usually leak out of the vagina during treatment. To keep the medicine from getting on your clothing, wear a minipad or sanitary napkin. Do not use tampons since they may soak up the medicine.

To help clear up your infection completely and to help make sure it does not return, good health habits are also required.

- Wear cotton panties (or panties or pantyhose with cotton crotches) instead of synthetic (for example, nylon or rayon) panties.
- Wear only freshly washed panties daily.

Do not have sexual intercourse while you are using this medicine. Having sexual intercourse may reduce the strength of the medicine. This may cause the medicine not to work as well.

Do not use latex (rubber) contraceptive products such as condoms, diaphragms, or cervical caps for 72 hours after stopping treatment with vaginal clindamycin cream. The cream contains oils that weaken or harm the latex products, causing them not to work properly to prevent pregnancy. If you have any questions about this, check with your doctor, nurse, or pharmacist.

POSSIBLE SIDE EFFECTS OF THIS MEDICINE

Side effects that should be reported to your doctor

MORE COMMON—Itching of the vagina or genital area; pain during sexual intercourse; thick, white vaginal discharge with no odor or with mild odor

LESS COMMON—Diarrhea; dizziness; headache; nausea or vomiting; stomach pain or cramps

RARE—Burning, itching, rash, redness, swelling or other signs of skin problems not present before use of this medicine

Other side effects not listed above may also occur in some patients. If you notice any other effects, check with your doctor, nurse, or pharmacist.

After you stop using this medicine, it may still cause side effects that need attention. During this time, check with your doctor if you notice itching of the vagina or genital area, pain during sexual intercourse, or thick, white vaginal discharge with or without odor.

C LOMIPHENE (ORAL)

ABOUT YOUR MEDICINE

Clomiphene (KLOE-mi-feen) is used as a fertility medicine in some women who are unable to become pregnant. It may also be used for other conditions in both females and males, as determined by your doctor. The following information applies only to female patients taking clomiphene. Check with your doctor if you are a male and have any questions about the use of clomiphene.

If any of the information in this profile causes you special concern or if you want additional information about your medicine and its use, check with your doctor, nurse, or pharmacist. **Remember, keep this and all other medicines out of the reach of children and never share your medicines with others.**

BEFORE USING THIS MEDICINE

If you become pregnant as a result of using this medicine, there is a chance of a multiple birth (for example, twins, triplets) occurring.

Tell your doctor, nurse, and pharmacist if you . . .
- are allergic to any medicine, either prescription or nonprescription (OTC);
- are taking any other prescription or nonprescription (OTC) medicine;
- have any other medical problems, especially cysts on the ovaries, endometriosis, fibroid tumors of the uterus, inflamed veins due to blood clots, liver disease (or history of), mental depression, or unusual vaginal bleeding.

PROPER USE OF THIS MEDICINE

Take this medicine only as directed by your doctor. If you are to begin on Day 5, count the first day of your menstrual period as Day 1. Beginning on Day 5, take the correct dose every day for as many days as your doctor ordered. To help you remember to take your dose of medicine, take it at the same time every day.

If you miss a dose of this medicine, take it as soon as possible. If you do not remember until it is time for the next dose, take both doses together. If you miss more than one dose, check with your doctor.

PRECAUTIONS WHILE USING THIS MEDICINE

It is very important that your doctor check your progress at regular visits to make sure this medicine is working and to check for unwanted effects.

If your doctor has asked you to record your temperature daily, make sure that you do this every day as soon as you awaken and before getting up. This will help you know if you have begun to ovulate. It is important that intercourse take place at the correct time to give you the best chance of becoming pregnant. **Follow your doctor's instructions carefully.**

There is a chance that clomiphene may cause birth defects if it is taken after you become pregnant. **Stop taking this medicine and tell your doctor immediately if you think you have become pregnant** while still taking clomiphene.

This medicine may cause blurred vision, difficulty in reading, or other changes in vision. It may also cause some people to become dizzy or lightheaded. **Make sure you know how you react to this medicine before you drive, use machines, or do other jobs that require you to see well or be clear-headed.**

POSSIBLE SIDE EFFECTS OF THIS MEDICINE

Side effects that should be reported to your doctor immediately
> MORE COMMON—Bloating; stomach or pelvic pain

Other side effects that should be reported to your doctor
> LESS COMMON OR RARE—Blurred vision; decreased or double vision or other vision problems; seeing flashes of light; sensitivity of eyes to light; yellow eyes or skin

Side effects that usually do not require medical attention
> These possible side effects may go away during treatment; however, if they continue or are bothersome, check with your doctor, nurse, or pharmacist.
>
> MORE COMMON—Hot flashes
>
> LESS COMMON OR RARE—Breast discomfort; dizziness or lightheadedness; headache, heavy menstrual periods or bleeding between periods; mental depression; nausea or vomiting; nervousness; restlessness; tiredness; trouble in sleeping
>
> Other side effects not listed above may also occur in some patients. If you notice any other effects, check with your doctor, nurse, or pharmacist.

CLONIDINE (ORAL)

ABOUT YOUR MEDICINE

Clonidine (KLOE-ni-deen) belongs to the general class of medicines called antihypertensives. It is used to treat high blood pressure (hypertension). Clonidine also may be prescribed for other conditions as determined by your doctor.

If any of the information in this profile causes you special concern or if you want additional information about your medicine and its use, check with your doctor, nurse, or pharmacist. **Remember, keep this and all other medicines out of the reach of children and never share your medicines with others.**

BEFORE USING THIS MEDICINE

Tell your doctor, nurse, and pharmacist if you . . .
- are allergic to any medicine, either prescription or nonprescription (OTC);
- are pregnant or intend to become pregnant while using this medicine;
- are breast-feeding;
- are taking any other prescription or nonprescription (OTC) medicine, especially beta-blockers or tricyclic antidepressants (medicine for depression);
- have any other medical problems.

PROPER USE OF THIS MEDICINE

For patients taking this medicine for high blood pressure:

- This medicine will not cure your high blood pressure but it does help control it. You must continue to take it—even if you feel well—if you expect to keep your blood pressure down. **You may have to take high blood pressure medicine for the rest of your life.**

If you miss a dose of this medicine, take it as soon as possible. Then go back to your regular dosing schedule. **If you miss 2 or more doses in a row, check with your doctor right away.** If your body goes without this medicine for too long, your blood pressure may go up to a dangerously high level and some unpleasant effects may occur.

PRECAUTIONS WHILE USING THIS MEDICINE

Check with your doctor before you stop taking this medicine. Your doctor may want you to reduce your dose gradually before stopping completely.

Make sure that you have enough medicine on hand to last through weekends, holidays, or vacations. You should not miss taking any doses. You may want to ask your doctor for another written prescription for clonidine to carry in your wallet or purse. You can then have it filled if you run out of medicine when you are away from home.

Clonidine will add to the depressant effects of alcohol and other CNS depressants (medicines that slow down the nervous system). **Check with your doctor before taking any such depressants while you are taking this medicine.**

Since clonidine may cause some people to become drowsy, **make sure you know how you react to it before you drive, use machines, or do other jobs that require you to be alert.**

Before having any kind of surgery or dental or emergency treatment, tell the physician or dentist in charge that you are using this medicine.

Dizziness, lightheadedness, or fainting may occur after you take this medicine, especially when you get up from a lying or sitting position. Getting up slowly may help. These effects are also more likely to occur if you drink alcohol, stand for long periods of time, exercise, or if the weather is hot.

POSSIBLE SIDE EFFECTS OF THIS MEDICINE

Side effects that should be reported to your doctor

LESS COMMON—Mental depression; swelling of feet and lower legs
RARE—Cold feeling or paleness in fingertips and toes; vivid dreams or
nightmares

Side effects that usually do not require medical attention

These possible side effects may go away during treatment; however, if they continue or are bothersome, check with your doctor, nurse, or pharmacist.

MORE COMMON—Constipation; dizziness; drowsiness; dryness of mouth; unusual tiredness or weakness

LESS COMMON—Decreased sexual ability; nausea or vomiting

Other side effects not listed above may also occur in some patients. If you notice any other effects, check with your doctor, nurse, or pharmacist.

After you stop taking clonidine, check with your doctor immediately if you notice anxiety or tenseness, chest pain, fast or pounding heartbeat, headache, increase in saliva, nausea or vomiting, nervousness, restlessness, shaking or trembling of hands and fingers, stomach cramps, sweating, or trouble in sleeping.

CLONIDINE (TRANSDERMAL)

ABOUT YOUR MEDICINE

Clonidine (KLOE-ni-deen) belongs to the general class of medicines called antihypertensives. It is used to treat high blood pressure (hypertension). Clonidine may also be used for other conditions as determined by your doctor.

If any of the information in this profile causes you special concern or if you want additional information about your medicine and its use, check with your doctor, nurse, or pharmacist. **Remember, keep this and all other medicines out of the reach of children and never share your medicines with others.**

BEFORE USING THIS MEDICINE

Tell your doctor, nurse, and pharmacist if you . . .
- are allergic to any medicine, either prescription or nonprescription (OTC);
- are pregnant or intend to become pregnant while using this medicine;
- are breast-feeding;
- are taking any other prescription or nonprescription (OTC) medicine, especially beta-blockers; tricyclic antidepressants (medicine for depression); or medicines for appetite control, asthma, colds, cough, hay fever, or sinus;
- have any other medical problems.

PROPER USE OF THIS MEDICINE

For patients using this medicine for high blood pressure:
- This medicine will not cure your high blood pressure but it does help control it. You must continue to use it as directed—even if you feel well—if you expect to lower your blood pressure and keep it down. **You may have to take high blood pressure medicine for the rest of your life.**

This medicine usually comes with patient instructions. Read them carefully before using this medicine.

Wash and dry your hands before and after handling the patch.

Do not trim or cut the patch to change the dose. Check with your doctor, instead.

Put the patch on a clean, dry area on your upper arm or chest that has little hair. Do not put it on scars, cuts, or irritation. Press the patch firmly in place. Put each patch on a different area of skin to prevent skin problems.

The patch will stay in place, even during showering, bathing, or swimming. If the patch becomes loose, cover it with the extra adhesive overlay provided. Apply a new patch if the first one becomes too loose or falls off.

After taking off a used patch, fold it in half with sticky sides together. Discard it carefully out of the reach of children.

If you forget to apply a new patch when you are supposed to, apply it as soon as possible. **If you miss changing the patch for three or more days, check with your doctor right away.**

PRECAUTIONS WHILE USING THIS MEDICINE

Check with your doctor before you stop using this medicine. Your doctor may want you to reduce your dose gradually before stopping completely.

Make sure you have enough clonidine on hand to last through weekends, holidays, or vacations. Ask your doctor for another prescription for clonidine that you can have filled if you run out of medicine when you are away from home.

Clonidine will add to the depressant effects of alcohol and other CNS depressants (medicines that slow down the nervous system). **Check with your doctor before taking any such depressants while you are using this medicine.**

Since clonidine may cause some people to become drowsy, **make sure you know how you react to it before you drive, use machines, or do other jobs that require you to be alert.**

Dizziness, lightheadedness, or fainting may occur, especially when you get up from a lying or sitting position. Getting up slowly may help. These effects are also more likely to occur if you drink alcohol, stand for long periods of time, exercise, or if the weather is hot.

POSSIBLE SIDE EFFECTS OF THIS MEDICINE

Side effects that should be reported to your doctor
>   MORE COMMON—Itching or redness of skin
>   LESS COMMON—Mental depression; swelling of feet and lower legs
>   RARE—Paleness or cold feeling in fingertips and toes; vivid dreams or
>   nightmares

Side effects that usually do not require medical attention

These possible side effects may go away during treatment; however, if they continue or are bothersome, check with your doctor, nurse, or pharmacist.

MORE COMMON—Constipation; dizziness; drowsiness; dry mouth; unusual tiredness or weakness

Other side effects not listed above may also occur in some patients. If you notice any other effects, check with your doctor, nurse, or pharmacist.

After you stop using clonidine, check with your doctor immediately if you notice anxiety or tenseness, chest pain, fast or irregular heartbeat, headache, increased salivation, nausea or vomiting, nervousness, restlessness, shaking or trembling of hands and fingers, stomach cramps, sweating, or trouble in sleeping.

CLOTRIMAZOLE (ORAL)

ABOUT YOUR MEDICINE

Clotrimazole (kloe-TRIM-a-zole) lozenges are dissolved slowly in the mouth to prevent and treat thrush. Thrush, also called candidiasis or white mouth, is a fungal infection of the mouth and throat. This medicine may also be used for other problems as determined by your doctor.

If any of the information in this profile causes you special concern or if you want additional information about your medicine and its use, check with your doctor, nurse, or pharmacist. **Remember, keep this and all other medicines out of the reach of children and never share your medicines with others.**

BEFORE USING THIS MEDICINE

Tell your doctor, nurse, and pharmacist if you . . .
- are allergic to any medicine, either prescription or nonprescription (OTC);
- are pregnant or intend to become pregnant while using this medicine;
- are breast-feeding;
- are taking any other prescription or nonprescription (OTC) medicine;
- have any other medical problems.

PROPER USE OF THIS MEDICINE

Clotrimazole lozenges should be held in the mouth and allowed to dissolve slowly and completely. This may take 15 to 30 minutes. **Do not chew or swallow the lozenges whole.**

Do not give clotrimazole lozenges to infants or children under 4 to 5 years of age. They may be too young to use the lozenges safely.

To help clear up your infection completely, **it is very important that you keep using clotrimazole for the full time of treatment** even if your symptoms begin to clear up after a few days. Since fungal infections may be very slow to clear up, you may have to continue using this medicine every day for 2 weeks or more. If you stop using this medicine too soon, your symptoms may return. **Do not miss any doses.**

If you do miss a dose of this medicine, take it as soon as possible. However, if it is almost time for your next dose, skip the missed dose and go back to your regular dosing schedule.

PRECAUTIONS WHILE USING THIS MEDICINE

If your symptoms do not improve within 1 week, or if they become worse, check with your doctor.

This medicine must not be given to other people or used for other infections unless you are otherwise directed by your doctor.

POSSIBLE SIDE EFFECTS OF THIS MEDICINE

Side effects that usually do not require medical attention
>   These possible side effects may go away during treatment; however, if they continue or are bothersome, check with your doctor, nurse, or pharmacist.

>   MORE COMMON (WHEN SWALLOWED)—Abdominal or stomach cramping or pain; diarrhea; nausea or vomiting

>   Other side effects not listed above may also occur in some patients. If you notice any other effects, check with your doctor, nurse, or pharmacist.

COPPER INTRAUTERINE DEVICES (IUDS)

Including Copper-T 200 IUD; Copper-T 200Ag IUD; Copper-T 380A IUD; Copper-T 380S IUD

ABOUT THIS PRODUCT

A **copper intrauterine** (IN-tra-YOU-ta-rin) **device** (also called an IUD) is inserted by a doctor or nurse into the uterus as a long-term contraceptive (birth control method).

Studies have shown that pregnancy can occur in 4 out of 100 women using copper IUDs during the first year of use. Talk with your doctor or nurse about the different kinds of birth control and the risks and benefits of each method.

IUDs do not protect a woman from sexually transmitted diseases (STDs), such as human immunodeficiency virus (HIV) or acquired immunodeficiency syndrome (AIDS). The use of latex (rubber) condoms or abstinence (no sex at all) is recommended for protection from these diseases.

Your lifestyle will determine how safe and reliable the copper IUD will be for you. Women who have a long-term relationship with only one sexual partner are much less likely to have problems while using an IUD. Also, it is important that your sexual partner not have any other sexual partners. If you or your partner has more than one sexual partner, it increases **your** chance of getting an infection in the vagina. If you have an infection in the vagina or uterus when the IUD is in place, it may make the infection worse. If your lifestyle changes while you are using a copper IUD or if you think you have been exposed to or have an STD, call your doctor or nurse.

Before Receiving

Tell your doctor or nurse if you . . .
- are allergic to copper;
- are pregnant or intend to become pregnant, or have recently had a baby;
- have **any** medical problems.

Proper Use

Copper IUDs come with patient information. Be sure you read and understand this information, especially about possible problems with the copper IUD. Keep this information for future use.

It is important that you check for the IUD threads after each menstrual period (or more often) to make sure that the copper IUD is still in place.

To check for the IUD threads:
- Wash your hands thoroughly.
- Squat and, using your middle finger, find the cervix high in the vagina.
- The IUD threads should hang down from the cervix. Do not pull on the threads.

Precautions

It is very important to keep all appointments with your doctor during the first year of IUD use. After that, your doctor will probably check that the device is still in place and working properly once a year.

Check with your doctor if you plan to have surgery of the uterus or fallopian tubes or have heat or radiation therapy, such as that used in sports medicine. Your doctor may take the IUD out before treatment.

Tell your doctor immediately if you think that the IUD has moved out of place. Do not try to put the IUD back into place or to remove it.

Also, check with your doctor and use another birth control method, such as condoms, if you think you are pregnant or if you miss a period; if you have unusual vaginal bleeding; if you are exposed to or get a sexually transmitted disease (STD); if you feel the tip of the IUD at the cervix or you or your partner feels pain during sexual intercourse; if you cannot find the threads from the IUD or think that the thread length is different; if you or your sexual partner's lifestyle changes and one or both of you have more than one sexual partner; if you have unusual lower abdominal pain or cramps, possibly with a fever; or if you have vaginal discharge or sores in the vaginal area.

You can use other products in the vagina, such as tampons or condoms, while you are using a copper IUD.

POSSIBLE SIDE EFFECTS

Get emergency help immediately if any of the following side effects occur:

RARE—Abdominal pain or cramps (severe); vaginal bleeding (unexpected and heavy)

Other side effects that should be reported to your doctor immediately

MORE COMMON—Faintness, dizziness, or sharp pain at time of IUD insertion; increased amount of menstrual bleeding at regular monthly periods; normal menstrual bleeding occurring earlier or lasting longer than expected

LESS COMMON—Abnormal vaginal bleeding (mild to moderate) not associated with a menstrual period; abdominal pain (dull or aching), odorous vaginal discharge, pain on urination with increased urge to urinate, and unusual vaginal bleeding

RARE—Abdominal pain or cramps, fever, nausea, and vomiting; painful intercourse; unusual tiredness or weakness

Side effects that usually do not require medical attention

These possible side effects may go away as your body adjusts to the device; however, if they continue or are bothersome, check with your doctor or nurse.

MORE COMMON—Increased abdominal pain and cramping at menstrual periods

Other side effects not listed above may also occur in some patients. If you notice any other effects, check with your doctor or nurse.

After you stop using this device, you may become pregnant. If you stop using an IUD and still do not want to become pregnant, you should begin using another contraceptive method immediately to prevent pregnancy.

Corticosteroids (inhalation)

Including Beclomethasone;
Dexamethasone; Flunisolide; Triamcinolone

About Your Medicine

Inhalation corticosteroids (kor-ti-koe-STER-oids) are used every day to decrease the number and severity of asthma attacks. They will not relieve an attack that has already started.

This medicine may be used with other asthma medicines.

If any of the information in this profile causes you special concern or if you want additional information about your medicine and its use, check with your doctor, nurse, or pharmacist. **Remember, keep this and all other medicines out of the reach of children and never share your medicines with others.**

Before Using This Medicine

Tell your doctor, nurse, and pharmacist if you . . .
- are allergic to any medicine, either prescription or nonprescription (OTC);
- are pregnant or intend to become pregnant while using this medicine;
- are breast-feeding;
- are taking any other prescription or nonprescription (OTC) medicine;
- have any other medical problems.

Proper Use of This Medicine

Inhaled corticosteroids will not relieve an asthma attack that has already started. However, your doctor may want you to continue taking this medicine at the usual time, even if you use another medicine to relieve the asthma attack.

Use this medicine only as directed. Do not use more of it and do not use it more often than your doctor ordered. To do so may increase the chance of side effects.

In order for this medicine to help you, it must be used every day in regularly spaced doses as ordered by your doctor. Up to four weeks may pass before you begin to notice improvement in your condition. It may take several months before you feel the full effects of this medicine.

Gargling and rinsing your mouth with water after each dose may help prevent hoarseness, throat irritation, and infection. However, do not swallow the water after rinsing. Your doctor may also want you to use a spacer device to lessen these problems.

This medicine usually comes with patient directions. **Read the directions carefully before using.** If you do not understand the directions or you are not sure how to use the inhaler, ask your doctor, nurse, or pharmacist to show you what to do. Also, **ask** your doctor, nurse, or pharmacist, to check regularly how you use the inhaler to make sure you are using it properly.

If you miss a dose of this medicine, use it as soon as possible. Then use any remaining doses for that day at regularly spaced times.

PRECAUTIONS WHILE USING THIS MEDICINE

Check with your doctor if:
- You go through a period of unusual stress to your body, such as surgery, injury, or infection.
- You have an asthma attack that does not improve after you take a bronchodilator medicine.
- Signs of mouth, throat, or lung infection occur.
- Your symptoms do not improve or if your condition gets worse.

Before you have any kind of surgery (including dental surgery) or emergency treatment, tell the medical doctor or dentist in charge that you are using this medicine.

If you are also regularly taking a corticosteroids by mouth in tablet or liquid form:
- **Do not stop taking the corticosteroid taken by mouth without your doctor's advice, even if your asthma seems better.** Your doctor may want you to reduce gradually the amount you are taking before stopping completely.
- When your doctor tells you to reduce the dose, or to stop taking the corticosteroid taken by mouth, follow the directions carefully. **It is especially important that your doctor check your progress at regular visits during this time.** Ask your doctor if there are special directions you should follow if you have a severe asthma attack, if you need any other medical or surgical treatment, or if certain side effects occur. Be certain that you understand these directions, and follow them carefully.

POSSIBLE SIDE EFFECTS OF THIS MEDICINE

Side effects that should be reported to your doctor immediately
> RARE—Troubled breathing, tightness in chest, or wheezing

Other side effects that should be reported to your doctor
> LESS COMMON—Creamy white, curd-like patches in mouth or throat and/or pain when eating or swallowing
> RARE—Behavior changes; mental depression; nervousness; restlessness; pain or burning in the chest

Side effects that usually do not require medical attention
> These possible side effects may go away during treatment; however, if they continue or are bothersome, check with your doctor, nurse, or pharmacist.

> MORE COMMON—Cough; dry mouth; hoarseness or voice changes; sore throat

Other side effects not listed above may also occur in some patients. If you notice any other effects, check with your doctor, nurse, or pharmacist.

CORTICOSTEROIDS (NASAL)

Including Beclomethasone; Budesonide; Dexamethasone; Flunisolide; Triamcinolone

ABOUT YOUR MEDICINE

Nasal corticosteroids (kor-ti-koh-STER-oids) are cortisone-like medicines. They belong to the family of medicines called steroids. These medicines are sprayed or inhaled into the nose to help relieve the stuffy nose, irritation, and discomfort of hay fever, other allergies, and other nasal problems. These medicines are also used to prevent nasal polyps from growing back after they have been removed by surgery.

If any of the information in this profile causes you special concern or if you want additional information about your medicine and its use, check with your doctor, nurse, or pharmacist. **Remember, keep this and all other medicines out of the reach of children and never share your medicines with others.**

BEFORE USING THIS MEDICINE

Children using this medicine should have their progress checked by their doctor at regular visits. Also, if used in high doses or too often, this medicine may get into the bloodstream through the lining of the nose and may affect growth. It is important to follow your doctor's directions carefully.

Tell your doctor, nurse, and pharmacist if you . . .
- are allergic to any medicine, either prescription or nonprescription (OTC);
- are pregnant or intend to become pregnant while using this medicine;
- are breast-feeding;
- have **any** other medical problems.

PROPER USE OF THIS MEDICINE

This medicine usually comes with patient directions. **Read them carefully before using the medicine.** Beclomethasone, budesonide, dexamethasone and triamcinolone are used with a special inhaler. If you do not understand the directions, or if you are not sure how to use the inhaler, check with your doctor, nurse, or pharmacist.

Before using this medicine, clear the nasal passages by blowing your nose. Then, with the nosepiece inserted into the nostril, aim the spray towards the inner corner of the eye.

In order for this medicine to help you, it must be used regularly as ordered by your doctor. This medicine usually begins to work in about 1 week, but up to 3 weeks may pass before you feel its full effects.

Use this medicine only as directed. Do not use more of it and do not use it more often than your doctor ordered. To do so may increase the chance of unwanted effects.

Check with your doctor before using this medicine for nasal problems other than the one for which it was prescribed, since it should not be used on many types of nasal infections.

Save the inhaler that comes with beclomethasone or dexamethasone, since refill units may be available at lower cost.

If you miss a dose of this medicine and remember within an hour or so, use it right away. However, if you do not remember until later, skip the missed dose and go back to your regular dosing schedule. Do not double doses.

PRECAUTIONS WHILE USING THIS MEDICINE

If you will be using this medicine for more than a few weeks, your doctor should check your progress at regular visits.

Check with your doctor:
—if signs of a nose, sinus, or throat infection occur.
—if your symptoms do not improve within 7 days (for dexamethasone) or within 3 weeks (for beclomethasone, budesonide, flunisolide, or triamcinolone).
—if your condition gets worse.

POSSIBLE SIDE EFFECTS OF THIS MEDICINE

Side effects that should be reported to your doctor
> LESS COMMON OR RARE—Bad smell; bloody mucus or unexplained nosebleeds; burning or stinging after use of spray or irritation inside nose (continuing); crusting, white patches, or sores inside nose; eye pain; gradual loss of vision; headache; hives; lightheadedness or dizziness; loss of sense of taste or smell; nausea or vomiting; shortness of breath, troubled breathing, tightness in chest, or wheezing; skin rash; sore throat, cough, or hoarseness; stomach pains; stuffy, dry, or runny nose or watery eyes (continuing); swelling of eyelids, face, or lips; unusual tiredness or weakness; white patches in throat

Side effects that usually do not require medical attention
> These possible side effects may go away during treatment; however, if they continue or are bothersome, check with your doctor, nurse, or pharmacist.

MORE COMMON—Burning, dryness, or other irritation inside the nose (mild, lasting only a short time); increase in sneezing; irritation of throat

Other side effects not listed above may also occur in some patients. If you notice any other effects, check with your doctor, nurse, or pharmacist.

CORTICOSTEROIDS (ORAL)

Including Betamethasone;
Cortisone Dexamethasone; Hydrocortisone;
Methylprednisolone; Prednisolone; Prednisone; Triamcinolone

ABOUT YOUR MEDICINE

Corticosteroids (kor-ti-koh-STER-oids) are produced naturally by the body and are necessary for good health. If your body does not make enough, your doctor may prescribe this medicine to help make up the difference. These medicines are used also to relieve inflamed areas of the body or for severe allergies or skin problems, asthma, or arthritis. Corticosteroids may also be used for other conditions as determined by your doctor.

If any of the information in this profile causes you special concern or if you want additional information about your medicine and its use, check with your doctor, nurse, or pharmacist. **Remember, keep this and all other medicines out of the reach of children and never share your medicines with others.**

BEFORE USING THIS MEDICINE

Tell your doctor, nurse, and pharmacist if you . . .
- are allergic to any medicine, either prescription or nonprescription (OTC);
- are pregnant or intend to become pregnant while using this medicine;
- are breast-feeding;
- are taking **any** other prescription or nonprescription (OTC) medicine;
- have **any** other medical problems.

PROPER USE OF THIS MEDICINE

Take this medicine with food to help prevent upset stomach.

Use this medicine only as directed.

If you miss a dose of this medicine, and your dosing schedule is:
- One dose every other day—Take the missed dose as soon as possible if you remember it the same morning, then go back to your regular schedule. If

you do not remember until later, wait and take it the following morning. Then skip a day and start your regular dosing schedule again.

- One dose a day—Take the missed dose as soon as possible, then go back to your regular dosing schedule. If you do not remember until the next day, skip the missed dose and do not double the next one.
- Several doses a day—Take the missed dose as soon as possible, then go back to your regular dosing schedule. If you do not remember until your next dose is due, double the next dose.

PRECAUTIONS WHILE USING THIS MEDICINE

Do not stop using this medicine without first checking with your doctor.

Your doctor may want you to follow a low-salt or potassium-rich diet.

Tell the doctor in charge that you are using this medicine before having skin tests, before having any kind of surgery (including dental surgery) or emergency treatment, or if you get a serious infection or injury.

While you are being treated with this medicine, and after you stop taking it, **do not have any immunizations without your doctor's approval.**

Diabetic patients: Check with your doctor if you notice a change in your blood sugar levels.

Avoid close contact with anyone who has chickenpox or measles. This is especially important for children. **Tell the doctor right away if you think you have been exposed to chickenpox or measles.**

POSSIBLE SIDE EFFECTS OF THIS MEDICINE

Side effects that should be reported to your doctor

LESS COMMON—Decreased or blurred vision; frequent urination; increased thirst

RARE—Confusion; excitement; false sense of well-being; hallucinations; mental depression; mistaken feelings of self-importance or being mistreated; mood swings; restlessness

WITH LONG-TERM USE—Abdominal or stomach pain or burning (continuing); acne or other skin problems; bloody or black, tarry stools; filling or rounding out of face; irregular heartbeat; menstrual problems; muscle cramps, pain, or weakness; nausea; pain in back, hips, ribs, arms, shoulders, or legs; reddish purple lines on skin; swelling of feet or lower legs; thin, shiny skin; unusual bruising; unusual tiredness or weakness; vomiting; weight gain (rapid); wounds that will not heal

Side effects that usually do not require medical attention

These possible side effects may go away during treatment; however, if they continue or are bothersome, check with your doctor, nurse, or pharmacist.

MORE COMMON—Increased appetite; indigestion; loss of appetite (triamcinolone only); nervousness or restlessness; trouble in sleeping

After you stop using this medicine, your body may need time to adjust. During this time, **check with your doctor immediately if any of the following side effects occur:** Abdominal, stomach, or back pain; dizziness; fainting; fever; loss of appetite (continuing); muscle or joint pain; nausea; reappearance of disease symptoms; shortness of breath; unexplained headaches (frequent or continuing); unusual tiredness or weakness; vomiting; weight loss (rapid).

Other side effects not listed above may also occur in some patients. If you notice any other effects, check with your doctor, nurse, or pharmacist.

CORTICOSTEROIDS (TOPICAL—LOW POTENCY)

Including Alclometasone; Clocortolone; Desonide; Dexamethasone; Flumethasone; Flurandrenolide (0.125%); Hydrocortisone; Hydrocortisone Acetate; Methylprednisolone

ABOUT YOUR MEDICINE

Corticosteroids (kor-ti-koh-STER-oids) are used to help relieve redness, swelling, itching, and discomfort of many skin problems. These medicines are like cortisone. They belong to the general family of medicines called steroids.

If any of the information in this profile causes you special concern or if you want additional information about your medicine and its use, check with your doctor, nurse, or pharmacist. **Remember, keep this and all other medicines out of the reach of children and never share your medicines with others.**

BEFORE USING THIS MEDICINE

If you are using the 1/2% or 1% hydrocortisone product without a prescription, carefully read and follow any precautions on the label.

Tell your doctor, nurse, and pharmacist if you . . .
- are allergic to any medicine, either prescription or nonprescription (OTC);
- are pregnant, intend to become pregnant, or are breast-feeding;
- are taking any other prescription or nonprescription (OTC) medicine;
- have any other medical problems.

PROPER USE OF THIS MEDICINE

Do not use more often or for a longer time than ordered. To do so may increase absorption through the skin and the chance of side effects. In addition, too much use, especially on areas with thinner skin (for example, face, armpits, groin), may result in thinning of the skin and stretch marks.

Do not bandage or otherwise wrap the area of the skin being treated unless directed to do so by your doctor.

If this medicine has been prescribed for you, it is meant to treat a specific skin problem. **Do not use it for other skin problems without first checking with your doctor.** Topical—Low Potency corticosteroids should not be used on many kinds of bacterial, virus, or fungus skin infections.

If you miss a dose of this medicine, apply it as soon as possible. Then go back to your regular dosing schedule. However, if it is almost time for your next dose, do not apply the missed dose at all. Instead, go back to your regular dosing schedule.

PRECAUTIONS WHILE USING THIS MEDICINE

Children and teenagers who must use this medicine should be followed closely by their doctor since this medicine may be absorbed through the skin and rarely can slow growth.

If this medicine is to be used on the diaper area of a child, avoid using tight-fitting diapers or plastic pants. Wearing these may increase the chance of absorption of the medicine through the skin and the chance of side effects.

POSSIBLE SIDE EFFECTS OF THIS MEDICINE

Side effects that should be reported to your doctor

LESS COMMON OR RARE—Lack of healing of skin condition; skin pain, redness, itching, or pus-containing blisters; severe burning and continued itching of skin

When the gel, solution, lotion, or aerosol form of this medicine is applied, a mild, temporary stinging may be expected.

Other side effects not listed above may also occur in some patients. If you notice any other effects, check with your doctor, nurse, or pharmacist.

Corticosteroids (topical—medium to very high potency)

Including Amcinonide; Beclomethasone;
Betamethasone; Clobetasol; Clobetasone; Desoximetasone;
Diflorasone; Diflucortolone; Fluocinolone; Fluocinonide;
Flurandrenolide (0.25% or 0.5%); Halcinonide; Hydrocortisone
Butyrate; Hydrocortisone Valerate; Mometasone; Triamcinolone

About Your Medicine

Corticosteroids (kor-ti-koh-STER-oids) are used to help relieve redness, swelling, itching, and discomfort of many skin problems. These medicines are like cortisone. They belong to the general family of medicines called steroids.

If any of the information in this profile causes you special concern or if you want additional information about your medicine and its use, check with your doctor, nurse, or pharmacist. **Remember, keep this and all other medicines out of the reach of children and never share your medicines with others.**

Before Using This Medicine

Tell your doctor, nurse, and pharmacist if you . . .
  • are allergic to any medicine, either prescription or nonprescription (OTC);
  • are pregnant or intend to become pregnant while using this medicine;
  • are breast-feeding;
  • are taking any other prescription or nonprescription (OTC) medicine;
  • have any other medical problems.

Proper Use of This Medicine

Do not use more often or for a longer time than ordered. To do so may increase absorption through the skin and the chance of side effects. In addition, too much use, especially on areas with thinner skin (for example, face, armpits, groin), may result in thinning of the skin and stretch marks.

Do not bandage or otherwise wrap the area of the skin being treated unless directed to do so by your doctor.

This medicine was prescribed for a specific skin problem. **Do not use any leftover medicine on other skin problems without first checking with your doctor** since the medicine should not be used on many kinds of bacterial, virus, or fungus skin infections.

If you miss a dose of this medicine, apply it as soon as possible. Then go back to your regular dosing schedule. However, if it is almost time for your next dose, do not apply the missed dose at all. Instead, go back to your regular dosing schedule.

PRECAUTIONS WHILE USING THIS MEDICINE

Children and teenagers who must use this medicine should be followed closely by their doctor since this medicine may be absorbed through the skin and rarely can slow growth.

If this medicine is to be used on the diaper area of a child, avoid using tight-fitting diapers or plastic pants. Wearing these may increase the chance of absorption of the medicine through the skin and the chance of side effects.

POSSIBLE SIDE EFFECTS OF THIS MEDICINE

Side effects that should be reported to your doctor

LESS COMMON OR RARE—Blood-containing blisters on skin; increased skin sensitivity (for some brands of betamethasone lotion); lack of healing of skin condition; loss of top skin layer (for tape dosage forms); numbness in fingers; raised, dark red, wart-like spots on skin; skin pain, redness, itching, or pus-containing blisters; thinning of skin with easy bruising

WITH LONG-TERM OR IMPROPER USE—Acne or oily skin; backache; burning or itching of skin with pinhead-sized red blisters; changes in vision or eye pain (occurs gradually if certain products have been used near the eye); filling out of face; increased blood pressure; irregular heartbeat; irregular menstrual periods; irritability; irritation of skin around the mouth; loss of appetite (continuing); mental depression; muscle cramps, pain, or weakness; nausea; rapid weight gain or loss; reddish purple lines (stretch marks) on arms, legs, trunk, or groin; skin color changes; softening of skin; stomach bloating, pain, cramping, or burning; swelling of feet or lower legs; tearing of the skin; unusual decrease in sexual desire or ability (in men); unusual increase in hair growth; unusual loss of hair; unusual tiredness or weakness; vomiting; weakness of the arms, legs, or trunk (severe); worsening of infections

When the gel, solution, lotion, or aerosol form of this medicine is applied, a mild, temporary stinging may be expected.

Other side effects not listed above may also occur in some patients. If you notice any other effects, check with your doctor, nurse, or pharmacist.

Cough/cold combinations (oral)

About Your Medicine

Cough/cold combinations are used mainly to relieve the cough due to colds, influenza, or hay fever.

Cough/cold combination products contain more than one ingredient. For example, some products may contain an antihistamine, a decongestant, and an analgesic, in addition to a medicine for coughing. If you are treating yourself, it is important to choose a product that is best for your symptoms. Also, in general, it is best to buy a product that includes only those medicines you really need. If you have questions about which product to buy, check with your pharmacist.

If any of the information in this profile causes you special concern or if you want additional information about your medicine and its use, check with your doctor, nurse, or pharmacist. **Remember, keep this and all other medicines out of the reach of children and never share your medicines with others.**

Before Using This Medicine

Do not give medicine containing aspirin or other salicylates to a child or a teenager with a fever or other symptoms of a virus infection, especially flu or chickenpox, without first discussing its use with your child's doctor.

If you are taking this medicine without a prescription, carefully read and follow any precautions on the label. You should be especially careful if you . . .

- are allergic to any medicine, either prescription or nonprescription (OTC);
- are pregnant, intend to become pregnant, or are breast-feeding;
- are taking **any** other prescription or nonprescription (OTC) medicine;
- have **any** other medical problems.

If you have any questions, check with your doctor, nurse, or pharmacist.

Proper Use of This Medicine

To help loosen mucus or phlegm in the lungs, **drink a glass of water after each dose of this medicine**, unless otherwise directed by your doctor.

Take this medicine only as directed. Do not take more of it and do not take it more often than recommended on the label, unless otherwise directed by your doctor. To do so may increase the chance of side effects. Also, if you are taking an extended-release form of this medicine, swallow the capsule or tablet whole without breaking it or chewing it.

If you must take this medicine regularly and you miss a dose, take it as soon as possible. However, if it is almost time for your next dose, skip the missed dose and go back to your regular dosing schedule. Do not double doses.

PRECAUTIONS WHILE USING THIS MEDICINE

For patients taking an antihistamine- or narcotic-containing combination:

- This medicine will add to the effects of alcohol and other CNS depressants. **Check with your doctor before taking any other CNS depressants while you are taking this medicine.**
- This medicine may cause some people to become drowsy, dizzy, or less alert than they are normally. **Make sure you know how you react to this medicine before you drive, use machines, or do other jobs that require you to be alert and clearheaded.**

For patients taking an analgesic-containing combination:

- **Check the labels of all over-the-counter (OTC) and prescription medicines you now take.** Avoid any that contain acetaminophen or aspirin or other salicylates, since taking them while taking a cough/cold combination medicine that already contains them may lead to overdose.

For patients taking a decongestant-containing combination:

- This medicine may add to the central nervous system (CNS) stimulant and other effects of phenylpropanolamine (PPA)-containing diet aids. **Do not use medicines for diet or appetite control while taking this medicine unless you have checked with your doctor.**
- **This medicine may cause some people to be nervous or restless or to have trouble in sleeping. If you have trouble in sleeping, take the last dose of this medicine for each day a few hours before bedtime.**

POSSIBLE SIDE EFFECTS OF THIS MEDICINE

Side effects that should be reported to your doctor

The side effects that may occur with cough/cold combinations will differ, depending on the ingredients. **Ask your doctor, nurse, or pharmacist if there are any serious side effects that may occur with the medicine you are taking.**

CROMOLYN (INHALATION)

ABOUT YOUR MEDICINE

Cromolyn (KROE-moe-lin) is taken by oral inhalation to prevent the symptoms of asthma. It is also used to prevent bronchospasm (wheezing or difficulty in breathing) caused by things such as allergens, chemicals, cold air, or air pollution. In addition, cromolyn is used to prevent bronchospasm following exercise. This medicine will not help an asthma or bronchospasm attack that has already started.

Cromolyn may be used alone or with other asthma medicines, such as bronchodilators (medicines that open up narrowed breathing passages) or corticosteroids (cortisone-like medicines).

If any of the information in this profile causes you special concern or if you want additional information about your medicine and its use, check with your doctor, nurse, or pharmacist. **Remember, keep this and all other medicines out of the reach of children and never share your medicines with others.**

BEFORE USING THIS MEDICINE

Tell your doctor, nurse, and pharmacist if you . . .
- are allergic to any medicine, either prescription or nonprescription (OTC);
- are pregnant or intend to become pregnant while using this medicine;
- are breast-feeding;
- are taking any other prescription or nonprescription (OTC) medicine;
- have any other medical problems.

PROPER USE OF THIS MEDICINE

Cromolyn oral inhalation is used to help prevent symptoms of asthma or bronchospasm. It will not relieve an attack that has already started.

Use cromolyn oral inhalation only as directed. Do not use more of it and do not use it more often than your doctor ordered. To do so may increase the chance of side effects.

Cromolyn inhalation usually comes with patient directions. Read them carefully before using this medicine. If you do not understand the directions or if you are not sure how to use the inhaler, ask your doctor, nurse, or pharmacist to show you how to use it. Also, ask your doctor, nurse, or pharmacist to check regularly how you use the inhaler to make sure you are using it properly.

For patients using cromolyn capsules for inhalation:
- **Do not swallow the capsules. The medicine will not work this way.**
- This medicine is used with a special inhaler, either the *Spinhaler* or the *Halermatic*. Follow directions for use.

For patients using cromolyn inhalation solution:
- Use this medicine only in a power-operated nebulizer that has an adequate flow rate and is equipped with a face mask or mouthpiece. Make sure you understand exactly how to use it. Hand-squeezed bulb nebulizers cannot be used with this medicine.

In order for cromolyn to work properly, it must be inhaled every day in regularly spaced doses as ordered by your doctor. Up to 4 weeks may pass before you feel the full effects of the medicine.

If you are using cromolyn regularly and you miss a dose, use it as soon as possible. Then use any remaining doses for that day at regularly spaced times.

PRECAUTIONS WHILE USING THIS MEDICINE

If your symptoms do not improve within 4 weeks, check with your doctor. Also check with your doctor if your condition becomes worse.

You may also be taking a corticosteroid or a bronchodilator for asthma along with this medicine. **Do not stop taking the corticosteroid or bronchodilator even if your asthma seems better, unless you are told to do so by your doctor.**

Dryness of the mouth or throat, throat irritation, and hoarseness may occur after you use this medicine. Gargling and rinsing your mouth or taking a drink of water after each dose may help prevent these effects.

POSSIBLE SIDE EFFECTS OF THIS MEDICINE

Side effects that should be reported to your doctor
> LESS COMMON—Increased wheezing, tightness in chest, or difficulty in breathing
> RARE—Chest pain; chills; difficult or painful urination; difficulty in swallowing; dizziness; frequent urge to urinate; headache (severe or continuing); joint pain or swelling; muscle pain or weakness; skin rash, hives, or itching; sweating; swelling of the face, lips, eyelids, hands, feet, or inside of mouth

Side effects that usually do not require medical attention
> These possible side effects may go away during treatment; however, if they continue or are bothersome, check with your doctor, nurse, or pharmacist.
>
> MORE COMMON—Cough; dryness of the mouth or throat; nausea; stuffy nose; throat irritation
>
> Other side effects not listed above may also occur in some patients. If you notice any other effects, check with your doctor, nurse, or pharmacist.

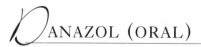

DANAZOL (ORAL)

ABOUT YOUR MEDICINE

Danazol (DA-na-zole) may be used for a number of different medical problems. These include treatment of:
- pain and/or infertility due to endometriosis;
- a tendency for females to develop cysts in the breasts (fibrocystic breast disease);
- hereditary angioedema, which causes swelling of the face, arms, legs, throat, windpipe, bowels, or sexual organs.

Danazol may also be used for other conditions as determined by your doctor.

If any of the information in this profile causes you special concern or if you want additional information about your medicine and its use, check with your doctor, nurse, or pharmacist. **Remember, keep this and all other medicines out of the reach of children and never share your medicines with others.**

BEFORE USING THIS MEDICINE

Tell your doctor, nurse, and pharmacist if you . . .
- are allergic to any medicine, either prescription or nonprescription (OTC);
- are pregnant or intend to become pregnant while using this medicine;
- are breast-feeding;
- are taking any other prescription or nonprescription (OTC) medicine, especially anticoagulants (blood thinners);
- have any other medical problems, especially diabetes mellitus (sugar diabetes); epilepsy; heart, kidney, or liver disease; or migraine headaches.

PROPER USE OF THIS MEDICINE

In order for danazol to help you, **it must be taken regularly for the full time of treatment** as ordered by your doctor.

If you miss a dose of this medicine, take it as soon as possible. Then go back to your regular dosing schedule. However, if it is almost time for your next dose, skip the missed dose and go back to your regular dosing schedule. Do not double doses.

PRECAUTIONS WHILE USING THIS MEDICINE

For patients taking danazol for endometriosis or fibrocystic breast disease:
- During the time you are taking danazol, you should use birth control methods that do not contain hormones. **If you suspect that you may have become pregnant, stop taking this medicine and check with your doctor.** Continued use may cause male-like changes in female babies.

Some people who take danazol may become more sensitive to sunlight than they are normally. **When you first begin taking this medicine, avoid too much sun and do not use a sunlamp until you see how you react to the sun. If you have a severe reaction, check with your doctor.**

POSSIBLE SIDE EFFECTS OF THIS MEDICINE

Side effects that should be reported to your doctor
  For both males and females
    LESS COMMON—Acne or increased oiliness of skin or hair; muscle cramps or spasms; rapid weight gain; swelling of feet or lower legs; unusual tiredness or weakness
    RARE—Bleeding gums; bloating, pain, or tenderness of abdomen or stomach; blood in urine; changes in vision; chest pain; chills; cough; dark-colored

urine; diarrhea; discharge from nipple; eye pain; fast heartbeat; fever; headache; hives or other skin rashes; joint pain; light-colored stools; loss of appetite (continuing); more frequent nosebleeds; muscle aches; nausea; pain, numbness, tingling, or burning in all fingers except the smallest finger; purple- or red-colored, or other spots on body or inside the mouth or nose; sore throat; tingling, numbness, or weakness in legs, which may move upward to arms, trunk or face; unusual bruising or bleeding; unusual tiredness, weakness, or general feeling of illness; vomiting; yellow eyes or skin

For females only
MORE COMMON—Decrease in breast size; irregular menstrual periods; weight gain
RARE—Enlarged clitoris; hoarseness or deepening of voice; unnatural hair growth

For males only
RARE—Decrease in size of testicles

Side effects that usually do not require medical attention
These possible side effects may go away during treatment; however, if they continue or are bothersome, check with your doctor, nurse, or pharmacist.

For both males and females
LESS COMMON—Flushing or redness of skin; mood or mental changes; nervousness; sweating
RARE—Increased sensitivity of skin to sunlight

For females only
LESS COMMON—Burning, dryness, or itching of vagina or vaginal bleeding

Other side effects not listed above may also occur in some patients. If you notice any other effects, check with your doctor, nurse, or pharmacist.

DECONGESTANTS AND ANALGESICS (ORAL)

Including Phenylephrine and Acetaminophen; Phenylpropanolamine and Acetaminophen; Phenylpropanolamine, Acetaminophen, and Aspirin; Phenylpropanolamine, Acetaminophen, Aspirin, and Caffeine; Phenylpropanolamine, Acetaminophen, and Caffeine; Phenylpropanolamine, Acetaminophen, Salicylamide, and Caffeine; Phenylpropanolamine and Aspirin; Pseudoephedrine and Acetaminophen; Pseudoephedrine, Acetaminophen, a

Caffeine; Pseudoephedrine and Aspirin; Pseudoephedrine,
Aspirin, and Caffeine; Pseudoephedrine and Ibuprofen

About Your Medicine

Decongestant and **analgesic** combinations are taken by mouth to relieve sinus and nasal congestion (stuffy nose) and headache of colds, allergy, and hay fever.

If any of the information in this profile causes you special concern or if you want additional information about your medicine and its use, check with your doctor, nurse, or pharmacist. **Remember, keep this and all other medicines out of the reach of children and never share your medicines with others.**

Before Using This Medicine

If you are taking this medicine without a prescription, carefully read and follow any precautions on the label. You should be especially careful if you . . .

- are allergic to any medicine, either prescription or nonprescription (OTC);
- are pregnant, intend to become pregnant, or are breast-feeding;
- are taking **any** other prescription or nonprescription (OTC) medicine;
- have **any** other medical problems.

If you have any questions, check with your doctor, nurse, or pharmacist.

Proper Use of This Medicine

For aspirin or salicylate-containing products:

- Use of aspirin in children or teenagers with fever due to a virus infection (especially flu or chickenpox) has been associated with a serious illness called Reye's syndrome. **Do not give medicines containing aspirin or other salicylates to a child or a teenager with symptoms of flu or chickenpox** unless you have first discussed this with your child's doctor.

Take this medicine only as directed. Do not take more of it or take it more often than recommended on the label, unless otherwise directed by your doctor.

If this medicine irritates your stomach, you may take it with food or a glass of water or milk to lessen the irritation.

If you must take this medicine regularly and you miss a dose, take it as soon as possible. However, if it is almost time for your next dose, skip the missed dose and go back to your regular dosing schedule. Do not double doses.

Precautions While Using This Medicine

Check with your doctor if your symptoms do not improve or become worse, or if you have a high fever.

This medicine may cause some people to become nervous or restless or to have trouble in sleeping. If you have trouble in sleeping, **take the last dose of this medicine for each day a few hours before bedtime.**

Do not drink alcoholic beverages while taking this medicine.

If you think that you or anyone else may have taken an overdose of this medicine, get emergency help at once.

For patients taking **ibuprofen-containing medicine:**

- This medicine may cause some people to become confused, drowsy, dizzy, lightheaded, or less alert than they are normally. It may also cause blurred vision or other vision problems in some people. **Make sure you know how you react to this medicine before you drive, use machines, or do other jobs that require you to be alert and clearheaded.**

POSSIBLE SIDE EFFECTS OF THIS MEDICINE

Side effects that should be reported to your doctor

MORE COMMON—Nausea, vomiting, or stomach pain (mild—for combinations containing aspirin or ibuprofen)

LESS COMMON OR RARE—Bloody, or black, tarry stools; bloody or cloudy urine; blurred vision or any changes in vision or eyes; changes in facial skin color; changes in hearing; difficult or painful urination; fever; headache (severe), with fever and stiff neck; increased blood pressure; muscle cramps or pain; skin rash, hives, or itching; sores, ulcers, or white spots on lips or in mouth; swelling of face, fingers, feet, or lower legs; swollen or painful glands; unexplained sore throat and fever; unusual bleeding or bruising; unusual tiredness or weakness; vomiting of blood or material that looks like coffee grounds; weight gain (unusual); yellow eyes or skin

Side effects that usually do not require medical attention

These possible side effects may go away during treatment; however, if they continue or are bothersome, check with your doctor, nurse, or pharmacist.

MORE COMMON—Heartburn or indigestion (for medicines containing salicylates or ibuprofen); nervousness or restlessness

Other side effects not listed above may also occur in some patients. If you notice any other effects, check with your doctor, nurse, or pharmacist.

DECONGESTANTS/EXPECTORANTS (ORAL)

ABOUT YOUR MEDICINE

Decongestant/expectorant combinations are used mainly to relieve the cough and nasal congestion due to colds, influenza, or hay fever. They are not to be used for the chronic cough that occurs with smoking, asthma, or emphysema or when there is an unusually large amount of mucus or phlegm (pronounced flem) with the cough.

If any of the information in this profile causes you special concern or if you want additional information about your medicine and its use, check with your doctor, nurse, or pharmacist. **Remember, keep this and all other medicines out of the reach of children and never share your medicines with others.**

BEFORE USING THIS MEDICINE

If you are taking this medicine without a prescription, carefully read and follow any precautions on the label. You should be especially careful if you . . .
- are allergic to any medicine, either prescription or nonprescription (OTC);
- are pregnant, intend to become pregnant, or are breast-feeding;
- are taking any other prescription or nonprescription (OTC) medicine, especially antihypertensives, beta-blockers, CNS stimulants, MAO inhibitors, rauwolfia alkaloids, or tricyclic antidepressants;
- have any other medical problems, especially heart or blood vessel disease, diabetes, hypertension, or thyroid disease.

If you have any questions, check with your doctor, nurse, or pharmacist.

PROPER USE OF THIS MEDICINE

To help loosen mucus or phlegm in the lungs, **drink a glass of water after each dose of this medicine**, unless otherwise directed by your doctor.

Take this medicine only as directed. Do not take more of it and do not take it more often than recommended on the label, unless otherwise directed by your doctor. To do so may increase the chance of side effects.

For patients **taking extended-release capsules or tablets:**
- Swallow the capsule or tablet whole.
- Do not crush, break, or chew before swallowing.
- If the capsule is too large to swallow, you may mix the contents with applesauce, jelly, honey, or syrup and swallow without chewing.

If you must take this medicine regularly and you miss a dose, take it as soon as possible. However, if it is almost time for your next dose, skip the missed dose and go back to your regular dosing schedule. Do not double doses.

PRECAUTIONS WHILE USING THIS MEDICINE

This medicine may add to the CNS stimulant and other effects of phenylpropanolamine (PPA)-containing diet aids. **Do not use medicines for diet or appetite control while taking this medicine unless you have checked with your doctor.**

This medicine may cause some people to be nervous or restless or to have trouble in sleeping. If you have trouble in sleeping, take the last dose of this medicine for each day a few hours before bedtime.

POSSIBLE SIDE EFFECTS OF THIS MEDICINE

Side effects that should be reported to your doctor

The side effects that may occur with decongestant/expectorant combinations will differ, depending on the ingredients. **Ask your doctor, nurse, or pharmacist if there are any serious side effects that may occur with the medicine you are taking.**

Side effects that usually do not require medical attention

These possible side effects may go away during treatment; however, if they continue or are bothersome, check with your doctor, nurse, or pharmacist.

Headache; nausea or vomiting; trouble in sleeping; unusual excitement, nervousness, restlessness, or irritability

Other side effects not listed above may also occur in some patients. If you notice any other effects, check with your doctor, nurse, or pharmacist.

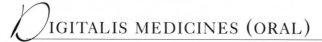

$\mathcal{D}$IGITALIS MEDICINES (ORAL)

Including Digitoxin; Digoxin

ABOUT YOUR MEDICINE

Digitalis (di-ji-TAL-iss) **medicines** are used to improve the strength and efficiency of the heart or to control the rate and rhythm of the heartbeat. This leads to better blood circulation and reduced swelling of hands and ankles in patients with heart problems.

If any of the information in this profile causes you special concern or if you want additional information about your medicine and its use, check with your doctor, nurse, or pharmacist. **Remember, keep this and all other medicines out of the reach of children and never share your medicines with others.**

BEFORE USING THIS MEDICINE

Tell your doctor, nurse, and pharmacist if you . . .
- are allergic to any medicine, either prescription or nonprescription (OTC);
- are pregnant or intend to become pregnant while using this medicine;
- are breast-feeding;
- are taking any other prescription or nonprescription (OTC) medicine, especially any other heart medicines, calcium channel blockers, cholestyramine, colestipol, cortisone-like medicines, diarrhea medicine, diuretics (water pills), ephedrine, epinephrine, medicine for colds or sinus,

potassium-containing medicines or supplements, propafenone, quinidine, reducing or diet medicine, or sucralfate;

- have any other medical problems, especially heart disease, heart rhythm problems, severe lung disease, or if you have had a recent heart attack.

PROPER USE OF THIS MEDICINE

To keep your heart working properly, **take this medicine exactly as directed even though you may feel well.** Do not miss taking any of the doses and do not take more medicine than ordered.

Ask your doctor about checking your pulse rate. Then, while you are taking this medicine, check your pulse regularly. If it is much slower, or faster, than usual (or less than 60 beats per minute), or if it changes in rhythm or force, check with your doctor. Such changes may mean that side effects are developing.

After you begin taking digitalis medicine, your doctor may sometimes check your blood level of digitalis medicine to find out if your dose needs to be changed. **Do not change your dose** unless your doctor tells you to do so.

If you miss a dose of this medicine, and you remember it within 12 hours, take it as soon as you remember. However, if you do not remember until later, do not take the missed dose at all and do not double the next one. Instead, go back to your regular dosing schedule. If you have any questions about this or if you miss doses for 2 or more days in a row, check with your doctor.

PRECAUTIONS WHILE USING THIS MEDICINE

Do not suddenly stop taking this medicine without first checking with your doctor.

Watch for signs of overdose (too much medicine) while you are taking digitalis medicine. The amount of medicine needed to help most people is very close to the amount that could cause serious problems from overdose. Follow directions carefully and watch for the early warning signs of overdose.

Before having any kind of surgery or dental or emergency treatment, tell the physician or dentist in charge that you are using this medicine.

Do not take any other medicine unless ordered by your doctor. Many nonprescription medicines contain ingredients which may interfere with digitalis medicines or which may make your condition worse. They include antacids; asthma remedies; cold, cough, or sinus preparations; laxatives; medicine for diarrhea; and reducing or diet medicines.

POSSIBLE SIDE EFFECTS OF THIS MEDICINE

Side effects that should be reported to your doctor
RARE—Skin rash or hives
POSSIBLE SIGNS OF OVERDOSE (IN THE ORDER IN WHICH THEY MAY OCCUR)—
Loss of appetite; nausea or vomiting; lower stomach pain; diarrhea; unusual

tiredness or weakness (extreme); slow or uneven heartbeat (may be fast in children); blurred vision or "yellow, green, or white vision" (a yellow, green, or white halo seen around objects); drowsiness; confusion or mental depression; headache; fainting

Other side effects not listed above may also occur in some patients. If you notice any other effects, check with your doctor, nurse, or pharmacist.

ERGOLOID MESYLATES (ORAL)

ABOUT YOUR MEDICINE

Ergoloid mesylates (ER-goe-loid MESS-i-lates) belongs to the group of medicines known as ergot alkaloids. It is used to treat some mood, behavior, or other problems that may be due to changes in the brain from Alzheimer's disease or several small strokes. This medicine is different from other ergot alkaloids such as ergotamine and methysergide. It is not useful for treating migraine headache.

If any of the information in this profile causes you special concern or if you want additional information about your medicine and its use, check with your doctor, nurse, or pharmacist. **Remember, keep this and all other medicines out of the reach of children and never share your medicines with others.**

BEFORE USING THIS MEDICINE

Tell your doctor, nurse, and pharmacist if you . . .
- are allergic to any medicine, either prescription or nonprescription (OTC);
- are pregnant or intend to become pregnant while using this medicine;
- are breast-feeding;
- are taking any other prescription or nonprescription (OTC) medicine;
- have any other medical problems, especially low blood pressure, other mental problems, or slow heartbeat.

PROPER USE OF THIS MEDICINE

Take this medicine only as directed by your doctor. Do not take more or less of it, and do not take it more often or for a longer period of time than your doctor ordered. To do so may increase the chance of unwanted effects.

For patients taking the sublingual (under-the-tongue) tablets:
- Dissolve the tablet under your tongue. The sublingual tablet should not be chewed or swallowed since it works much faster when absorbed through the lining of the mouth. Do not eat, drink, or smoke while a tablet is dissolving.

If you miss a dose of this medicine, skip the missed dose and go back to your regular dosing schedule. Do not double doses. If you have any questions about this, or if you miss two or more doses in a row, check with your doctor.

Precautions While Using This Medicine

It is important that your doctor check your progress at regular visits to make sure this medicine is working and to check for unwanted effects.

It may take several weeks for this medicine to work. **However, do not stop taking this medicine without first checking with your doctor.**

Possible Side Effects of This Medicine

Side effects that should be reported to your doctor

LESS COMMON OR RARE—Dizziness or lightheadedness when getting up from a lying or sitting position; drowsiness; skin rash; slow pulse

Side effects that usually do not require medical attention

These possible side effects may go away during treatment; however, if they continue or are bothersome, check with your doctor, nurse, or pharmacist.

LESS COMMON OR RARE—Soreness under tongue (with sublingual use)

Other side effects not listed above may also occur in some patients. If you notice any other effects, check with your doctor, nurse, or pharmacist.

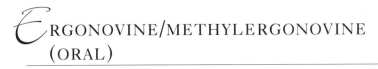

Ergonovine/Methylergonovine (Oral)

Including Ergonovine; Methylergonovine

About Your Medicine

Ergonovine (er-goe-NOE-veen) and **methylergonovine** (meth-ill-er-goe-NOE-veen) belong to the group of medicines known as ergot alkaloids. These medicines are usually given to stop heavy bleeding that sometimes occurs after the birth of a baby. Ergonovine and methylergonovine may also be used for other conditions as determined by your doctor.

If any of the information in this profile causes you special concern or if you want additional information about your medicine and its use, check with your doctor, nurse, or pharmacist. **Remember, keep this and all other medicines out of the reach of children and never share your medicines with others.**

BEFORE USING THIS MEDICINE

Tell your doctor, nurse, and pharmacist if you . . .
- are allergic to any medicine, either prescription or nonprescription (OTC);
- are pregnant or intend to become pregnant while using this medicine;
- are breast-feeding;
- are taking any other prescription or nonprescription (OTC) medicine, especially bromocriptine, nitrates or other medicines for angina, or other ergot alkaloids;
- have any other medical problems, especially angina (chest pain), blood vessel disease, high blood pressure, infection, kidney disease, liver disease, Raynaud's phenomenon, or stroke (history of).

PROPER USE OF THIS MEDICINE

Take this medicine only as directed by your doctor. Do not take more of it, do not take it more often, and do not take it for a longer time than your doctor ordered. If too much is taken or if it is taken for a longer time than your doctor ordered, it may cause serious effects.

If you miss a dose of this medicine, do not take the missed dose at all and do not double the next one. Instead, go back to your regular dosing schedule.

PRECAUTIONS WHILE USING THIS MEDICINE

If you have an infection or illness of any kind, check with your doctor before taking this medicine, since you may be more sensitive to the effects of it.

POSSIBLE SIDE EFFECTS OF THIS MEDICINE

Side effects that should be reported to your doctor immediately
LESS COMMON—Chest pain
RARE—Blurred vision; convulsions (seizures); crushing chest pain; headache (sudden and severe); irregular heartbeat; unexplained shortness of breath

Other side effects that should be reported to your doctor
LESS COMMON—Slow heartbeat
RARE—Itching of skin; pain in arms, legs, or lower back; pale or cold hands or feet; weakness in legs
WITH LONG-TERM USE—Dry, shriveled-looking skin on hands, lower legs, or feet; false feeling of insects crawling on the skin; pain and redness in an arm or leg; paralysis of one side of the body

Side effects that usually do not require medical attention
These possible side effects may go away during treatment; however, if they continue or are bothersome, check with your doctor, nurse, or pharmacist.

MORE COMMON—Cramping of the uterus; nausea; vomiting

Other side effects not listed above may also occur in some patients. If you notice any other effects, check with your doctor, nurse, or pharmacist.

ERGOT MEDICINES (ORAL)

Including Ergotamine; Ergotamine, Belladonna Alkaloids, and Phenobarbital; Ergotamine and Caffeine; Ergotamine, Caffeine, Belladonna Alkaloids, and Pentobarbital

ABOUT YOUR MEDICINE

Ergot medicines are used to treat migraine headaches and some kinds of throbbing headaches. They are not used to prevent headaches but are used to relieve a headache once it has started. Some of these medicines may also be used for other conditions as determined by your doctor.

If any of the information in this profile causes you special concern or if you want additional information about your medicine and its use, check with your doctor, nurse, or pharmacist. **Remember, keep this and all other medicines out of the reach of children and never share your medicines with others.**

BEFORE USING THIS MEDICINE

Tell your doctor, nurse, and pharmacist if you . . .
- are allergic to any medicine, either prescription or nonprescription (OTC);
- are pregnant or intend to become pregnant while using this medicine;
- are breast-feeding;
- are taking **any** other prescription or nonprescription (OTC) medicine;
- have **any** other medical problems;
- use cocaine;
- regularly drink large amounts of caffeine-containing beverages such as coffee, tea, soft drinks, or cocoa.

PROPER USE OF THIS MEDICINE

Take this medicine only as directed by your doctor. If the amount you are to take does not relieve your headache, do not take more than your doctor ordered. Instead, check with your doctor. Taking too much of this medicine or taking it too often may cause serious effects such as nausea and vomiting; cold, painful hands or feet; or even gangrene, especially in elderly patients.

This medicine works best if you:
- **Take it at the first sign of headache or migraine attack.**
- **Lie down in a quiet, dark room for at least 2 hours after taking it.**

PRECAUTIONS WHILE USING THIS MEDICINE

Since drinking alcoholic beverages may make headaches worse, it is best to avoid use of alcohol while you are suffering from them.

Since smoking may increase some of the harmful effects of this medicine, it is best to avoid smoking while you are using it.

If you have a serious infection or illness of any kind, check with your doctor before taking this medicine, since you may be more sensitive to its effects.

This medicine may make you more sensitive to cold temperatures, especially if you have blood circulation problems. Dress warmly during cold weather and be careful during prolonged exposure to cold, such as in winter sports. This is especially important for elderly people.

Belladonna alkaloids (may be contained in this medicine) also may cause your eyes to become more sensitive to light than they are normally. Wearing sunglasses may help lessen the discomfort from bright light.

The caffeine in this combination medicine may interfere with the results of a test that uses dipyridamole (e.g., Persantine) to help find out how well your blood is flowing through certain blood vessels. You should not have any caffeine for at least 4 hours before the test.

POSSIBLE SIDE EFFECTS OF THIS MEDICINE

Side effects that should be reported to your doctor immediately
> Changes in vision; confusion; convulsions (seizures); fever; mental depression; muscle twitching; numbness and tingling of fingers, toes, or face; red or violet blisters on skin of hands or feet; ringing or other sounds in ears; seeing flashes of "zig-zag" lights; shortness of breath; stomach pain or bloating; tiredness or weakness; slurred speech; unusually fast, irregular, or slow heartbeat

Other side effects that should be reported to your doctor
> MORE COMMON—Headaches, more often and/or more severe than before; swelling of feet and lower legs
> LESS COMMON OR RARE—Anxiety; chest pain; eye pain; hives or itching of skin; pain in arms, legs, or lower back; pale or cold hands or feet; sore throat and fever; unusual bleeding or bruising; yellow eyes or skin

Side effects that usually do not require medical attention
> These possible side effects may go away during treatment; however, if they continue or are bothersome, check with your doctor, nurse, or pharmacist.
> MORE COMMON—Decreased sweating; diarrhea; dizziness; dryness of mouth, nose, throat, or skin; nausea or vomiting

Other side effects not listed above may also occur in some patients. If you notice any other effects, check with your doctor, nurse, or pharmacist.

After you stop using this medicine, your body may need time to adjust. The length of time this takes depends on the amount of medicine you were using and how long you used it. During this time check with your doctor if your headaches begin again or worsen.

$\mathcal{E}$RYTHROMYCINS (ORAL)

Including Erythromycin; Erythromycin Estolate;
Erythromycin Ethylsuccinate; Erythromycin Stearate

ABOUT YOUR MEDICINE

Erythromycins (eh-rith-roe-MYE-sins) are used to treat infections caused by bacteria. They will not work for colds, flu, or other virus infections. Erythromycins are also used to prevent "strep" infections in patients with a history of rheumatic heart disease who may be allergic to penicillin. These medicines may also be used in Legionnaires' disease and for other problems as determined by your doctor.

If any of the information in this profile causes you special concern or if you want additional information about your medicine and its use, check with your doctor, nurse, or pharmacist. **Remember, keep this and all other medicines out of the reach of children and never share your medicines with others.**

BEFORE USING THIS MEDICINE

Tell your doctor, nurse, and pharmacist if you . . .
- are allergic to any medicine, either prescription or nonprescription (OTC);
- are pregnant or intend to become pregnant while using this medicine;
- are breast-feeding;
- are taking **any** other prescription or nonprescription (OTC) medicine;
- are taking astemizole, terfenadine, or terfenadine-containing medicines;
- have any other medical problems, especially liver disease.

PROPER USE OF THIS MEDICINE

Generally, erythromycins are best taken with a full glass (8 ounces) of water on an empty stomach (at least 1 hour before or 2 hours after meals). If stomach upset occurs, erythromycins may be taken with food. If you have any questions about this, check with your doctor or pharmacist.

To help clear up your infection completely, **keep taking this medicine for the full time of treatment** even if you begin to feel better after a few days; **do not miss any doses. This is especially important if you have a "strep" infection since serious heart problems could develop later** if your infection is not cleared up completely.

If you do miss a dose of this medicine, take it as soon as possible. This will help to keep a constant amount of medicine in the blood. However, if it is almost time for your next dose, skip the missed dose and go back to your regular dosing schedule. Do not double doses.

PRECAUTIONS WHILE USING THIS MEDICINE

If your symptoms do not improve within a few days, or if they become worse, check with your doctor.

This medicine must not be given to other people or used for other infections unless you are otherwise directed by your doctor.

POSSIBLE SIDE EFFECTS OF THIS MEDICINE

Side effects that should be reported to your doctor immediately
> LESS COMMON—Fever; nausea; skin rash, redness, or itching; stomach pain (severe); unusual tiredness or weakness; vomiting; yellow eyes or skin— with erythromycin estolate (rare with other erythromycins)

Side effects that usually do not require medical attention
> These possible side effects may go away during treatment; however, if they continue or are bothersome, check with your doctor, nurse, or pharmacist.

> MORE COMMON—Diarrhea; nausea or vomiting; stomach cramping and discomfort
> LESS COMMON—Sore mouth or tongue; vaginal itching or discharge

> Other side effects not listed above may also occur in some patients. If you notice any other effects, check with your doctor, nurse, or pharmacist.

ESTRADIOL (TRANSDERMAL)

ABOUT YOUR MEDICINE

Estradiol (es-tra-DYE-ol) is an estrogen (a type of female hormone). It is necessary for sexual development of the female and regulation of the menstrual cycle during childbearing years.

Transdermal estradiol is used as a skin patch and is prescribed to provide additional hormone when the body does not produce enough of its own, as after menopause or certain kinds of surgery in females. Estradiol may also be used for other conditions as determined by your doctor.

If any of the information in this profile causes you special concern or if you want additional information about your medicine and its use, check with your doctor, nurse, or pharmacist. **Remember, keep this and all other medicines out of the reach of children and never share your medicines with others.**

BEFORE USING THIS MEDICINE

Tell your doctor, nurse, and pharmacist if you . . .
- are allergic to any medicine, either prescription or nonprescription (OTC);
- are pregnant or intend to become pregnant while using this medicine;
- are breast-feeding;
- are taking **any** other prescription or nonprescription (OTC) medicine;
- have any other medical problems, especially blood clots (or history of), breast cancer (active or suspected), or changes in vaginal bleeding;
- are a smoker.

PROPER USE OF THIS MEDICINE

This medicine usually comes with patient instructions. Read them carefully before using this medicine.

Wash and dry your hands thoroughly before and after handling the patch.

Do not trim or cut the patch to change the dose.

Put the patch on a clean, dry area of your abdomen (stomach) or buttocks that has little hair. Do not put it on scars, cuts, or irritations. **Do not apply the patch to the breasts** or to areas where clothes may rub it loose. Press the patch firmly in place to make sure it sticks. Put each patch on a different area of skin to prevent skin problems. Wait at least 1 week before you use the same area again.

With normal activity, the patch will stay in place, even during swimming, showering, or bathing. If a patch becomes loose or falls off, reapply it or discard it and apply a new one.

After taking off a used patch, fold it in half with sticky sides together. Discard carefully out of the reach of children.

If you forget to apply a new patch when you are supposed to, apply it as soon as possible. However, if it is almost time for the next patch, skip the missed one and go back to your regular schedule. Do not apply more than one patch at a time.

PRECAUTIONS WHILE USING THIS MEDICINE

It is very important that your doctor check your progress at regular visits to make sure this medicine does not cause unwanted effects.

It is not yet known whether the use of estrogens increases the risk of breast cancer in women. Check your breasts regularly for any unusual lumps or discharge and have a mammogram done if your doctor recommends it.

If you think that you may be pregnant, stop using the medicine immediately and check with your doctor. Continued use of some estrogens during pregnancy may cause birth defects in the child.

POSSIBLE SIDE EFFECTS OF THIS MEDICINE

Side effects that should be reported to your doctor

> MORE COMMON—Breast pain; increased breast size; swelling of feet and lower legs; weight gain (rapid)
>
> LESS COMMON OR RARE—Changes in vaginal bleeding; lumps in, or discharge from, breast; pains in stomach, side, or abdomen; uncontrolled jerky muscle movements; yellow eyes or skin

Side effects that usually do not require medical attention

> These possible side effects may go away during treatment; however, if they continue or are bothersome, check with your doctor, nurse, or pharmacist.
>
> MORE COMMON—Bloating of stomach; cramps of lower stomach; loss of appetite; nausea; skin irritation or redness where skin patch was worn
>
> LESS COMMON—Diarrhea (mild); dizziness (mild); headaches (mild); migraine headaches; problems in wearing contact lenses; unusual increase in sexual desire; vomiting (usually with high doses)

Many women who take estrogens with a progestin (another female hormone) start having monthly vaginal bleeding, similar to menstrual periods again. This effect continues for as long as the medicine is taken. However, monthly bleeding will not occur if the uterus has been removed by surgery (total hysterectomy).

Other side effects not listed above may also occur in some patients. If you notice any other effects, check with your doctor, nurse, or pharmacist.

ESTROGENS (INJECTION)

Including Diethylstilbestrol;
Estradiol; Estrogens, Conjugated; Estrone

ABOUT YOUR MEDICINE

Estrogens (ESS-troe-jenz) are produced by the body and are necessary for the normal sexual development of the female and for the regulation of the menstrual cycle. They are prescribed for several reasons:

- to provide additional hormone when the body does not produce enough of its own, as during the menopause or following certain kinds of surgery.

- in the treatment of selected cases of breast cancer in men and women.
- in the treatment of men with certain kinds of cancer of the prostate.
- to help prevent osteoporosis in women past menopause.

Estrogens may also be used for other conditions as determined by your doctor.

If any of the information in this profile causes you special concern or if you want additional information about your medicine and its use, check with your doctor, nurse, or pharmacist. **Remember, keep this and all other medicines out of the reach of children and never share your medicines with others.**

BEFORE USING THIS MEDICINE

Tell your doctor, nurse, and pharmacist if you . . .
- are allergic to any medicine, either prescription or nonprescription (OTC);
- are pregnant or intend to become pregnant while using this medicine;
- are breast-feeding;
- are taking **any** other prescription or nonprescription (OTC) medicine;
- have any other medical problems, especially blood clots (or history of during estrogen therapy), breast cancer (active or suspected), changes in vaginal bleeding, heart or circulation disease, or stroke (for men); or if you smoke.

PROPER USE OF THIS MEDICINE

Most patients will receive an information sheet regarding the benefits and risks of this medicine. **Be sure you have read and understand that information.** This profile is not intended to replace that information sheet.

PRECAUTIONS WHILE USING THIS MEDICINE

It is very important that your doctor check your progress at regular visits. These visits will usually be every year.

It is not yet known whether the use of estrogens increases the risk of breast cancer in women. Breast cancer has occurred rarely in men using estrogens.

Cigarette smoking when using birth control pills containing estrogen has been found to increase the risk of serious side effects affecting the heart or circulation. **To reduce the risk, do not smoke cigarettes while using estrogens.**

If you think that you may be pregnant, stop using the medicine immediately and check with your doctor. Continued use of some estrogens during pregnancy may cause birth defects in the child. Diethylstilbestrol may also increase the risk of vaginal cancer developing in daughters when they reach childbearing age.

POSSIBLE SIDE EFFECTS OF THIS MEDICINE

Along with their wanted effects, **estrogens sometimes cause some serious unwanted effects.** Rarely, they have caused blood clots, stroke, and heart attack in men being treated with high doses for cancer. The prolonged use of estrogens has been reported to increase the risk of endometrial cancer (cancer of the lining of the uterus) in women after menopause. When estrogens are used in low doses for less than 1 year, there is less risk. The risk is also reduced if a progestin (another female hormone) is added to, or replaces part of, the estrogen dose. If the uterus has been removed, there is no risk of endometrial cancer.

Side effects that should be reported to your doctor immediately

Stop using this medicine and get emergency help immediately if any of the following side effects occur:

RARE (FOR MALES BEING TREATED FOR BREAST OR PROSTATE CANCER ONLY)— Change in vision (sudden); headache (sudden or severe); loss of coordination; pains in chest, groin, or leg, especially in calf of leg; shortness of breath; slurring of speech; weakness or numbness in arm or leg

Other side effects that should be reported to your doctor

MORE COMMON—Breast pain (in females and males); increased breast size (in females and males); swelling of feet and lower legs; weight gain (rapid)

LESS COMMON OR RARE—Changes in vaginal bleeding; lumps in, or discharge from, breast (in females and males); pains in stomach, side, or abdomen; uncontrolled, jerky muscle movements; yellow eyes or skin

Also, many women who are using estrogens with a progestin (another female hormone) and have not had their uterus removed will start having monthly vaginal bleeding, similar to menstrual periods, again.

Other side effects not listed above may also occur in some patients. If you notice any other effects, check with your doctor, nurse, or pharmacist.

$\mathcal{E}$STROGENS (ORAL)

Including Chlorotrianisene; Diethylstilbestrol;
Estradiol; Estrogens, Conjugated; Estrogens,
Esterified; Estropipate; Ethinyl Estradiol; Quinestrol

ABOUT YOUR MEDICINE

Estrogens (ESS-troe-jenz) are produced by the body and are necessary for the normal sexual development of the female and for the regulation of the menstrual cycle. They are prescribed for several reasons:

- to provide additional hormone when the body does not produce enough of its own, as during the menopause or following certain kinds of surgery.
- in the treatment of selected cases of breast cancer in men and women.
- in the treatment of men with certain kinds of cancer of the prostate.
- to help prevent osteoporosis in women past menopause.

Estrogens may also be used for other conditions as determined by your doctor.

If any of the information in this profile causes you special concern or if you want additional information about your medicine and its use, check with your doctor, nurse, or pharmacist. **Remember, keep this and all other medicines out of the reach of children and never share your medicines with others.**

BEFORE USING THIS MEDICINE

Tell your doctor, nurse, and pharmacist if you . . .
- are allergic to any medicine, either prescription or nonprescription (OTC);
- are pregnant or intend to become pregnant while using this medicine;
- are breast-feeding;
- are taking **any** other prescription or nonprescription (OTC) medicine;
- have any other medical problems, especially blood clots (or history of during estrogen therapy); breast cancer (active or suspected); changes in vaginal bleeding; heart or circulation disease or stroke (for men); or if you smoke.

PROPER USE OF THIS MEDICINE

Most patients will receive an information sheet regarding the benefits and risks of this medicine. **Be sure you have read and understand that information.** This profile is not intended to replace that information sheet.

Take this medicine only as directed. Do not take more of it and do not take it for a longer time than your doctor ordered. Try to take the medicine at the same time each day to reduce the possibility of side effects.

If you miss a dose of this medicine, take it as soon as possible. However, if it is almost time for your next dose, skip the missed dose. Do not double doses.

PRECAUTIONS WHILE USING THIS MEDICINE

It is very important that your doctor check your progress at regular visits. These visits will usually be every year.

It is not yet known whether the use of estrogens increases the risk of breast cancer in women. Breast cancer has occurred rarely in men taking estrogens.

Cigarette smoking when using birth control pills containing estrogen has been found to increase the risk of serious side effects affecting the heart or circulation. **To reduce the risk, do not smoke cigarettes while using estrogens.**

If you think that you may be pregnant, stop using the medicine immediately and check with your doctor. Continued use of some estrogens during pregnancy may cause birth defects in the child. Diethylstilbestrol may also increase the risk of vaginal cancer developing in daughters when they reach childbearing age.

POSSIBLE SIDE EFFECTS OF THIS MEDICINE

Along with their wanted effects, **estrogens sometimes cause some serious unwanted effects.** Rarely, they have caused blood clots, stroke, and heart attack in men being treated with high doses for cancer. The prolonged use of estrogens has been reported to increase the risk of endometrial cancer (cancer of the lining of the uterus) in women after menopause. When estrogens are used in low doses for less than 1 year, there is less risk. The risk is also reduced if a progestin (another female hormone) is added to, or replaces part of, the estrogen dose. If the uterus has been removed, there is no risk of endometrial cancer.

Side effects that should be reported to your doctor immediately

Stop taking this medicine and get emergency help immediately if any of the following side effects occur:

RARE (FOR MALES BEING TREATED FOR BREAST OR PROSTATE CANCER ONLY)—
Headache (sudden or severe); loss of coordination; change in vision (sudden); pains in chest, groin, or leg, especially in calf of leg; shortness of breath; slurring of speech; weakness or numbness in arm or leg

Other side effects that should be reported to your doctor

MORE COMMON—Breast pain (in females and males); increased breast size (in females and males); swelling of feet and lower legs; weight gain (rapid)

LESS COMMON OR RARE—Changes in vaginal bleeding; lumps in, or discharge from, breast (in females and males); pains in stomach, side, or abdomen; uncontrolled, jerky muscle movements; yellow eyes or skin

Also, many women who are taking estrogens with a progestin (another female hormone) and have not had their uterus removed will start having monthly vaginal bleeding, similar to menstrual periods, again.

Other side effects not listed above may also occur in some patients. If you notice any other effects, check with your doctor, nurse, or pharmacist.

ESTROGENS (VAGINAL)

Including Dienestrol; Estradiol;
Estrogens, Conjugated; Estrone; Estropipate

ABOUT YOUR MEDICINE

Estrogens (ESS-troe-jenz) are female hormones. They are produced by the body and are necessary for the normal sexual development of the female and for the regulation of the menstrual cycle during the childbearing years.

Uncomfortable changes may occur in vaginal tissues when the body does not produce enough estrogens, as during the menopause. In order to relieve such uncomfortable conditions, estrogens are prescribed for vaginal use.

If any of the information in this profile causes you special concern or if you want additional information about your medicine and its use, check with your doctor, nurse, or pharmacist. **Remember, keep this and all other medicines out of the reach of children and never share your medicines with others.**

BEFORE USING THIS MEDICINE

Since vaginal estrogens may be absorbed into the body, the following should be kept in mind:

- Most patients will receive an information sheet regarding the benefits and risks of this medicine. **Be sure you have read and understand that information.** This profile is not intended to replace that information sheet.
- The prolonged use of estrogens has been reported to increase the risk of endometrial cancer (cancer of the lining of the uterus) in women after the menopause. When estrogens are used in low doses for less than 1 year, there is less risk. The risk is also reduced if a progestin (another female hormone) is added to, or replaces part of, the estrogen dose. If the uterus has been removed by surgery (hysterectomy), there is no risk of endometrial cancer.
- Cigarette smoking when using birth control pills containing estrogen has been found to increase the risk of serious side effects affecting the heart or circulation. **To reduce the risk, do not smoke cigarettes while using estrogens.**

Tell your doctor, nurse, and pharmacist if you . . .

- are allergic to any medicine, either prescription or nonprescription (OTC);
- are pregnant or intend to become pregnant while using this medicine;
- are breast-feeding;
- are taking **any** other prescription or nonprescription (OTC) medicine;
- have any other medical problems, especially blood clots (or history of during estrogen therapy), breast cancer (active or suspected), or changes in vaginal bleeding.

PROPER USE OF THIS MEDICINE

Use this medicine only as directed. Do not use more of it and do not use it for a longer time than your doctor ordered.

If you miss a dose of this medicine and do not remember it until the next day, do not use the missed dose at all. Instead, go back to your regular schedule.

PRECAUTIONS WHILE USING THIS MEDICINE

It is very important that your doctor check your progress at regular visits. These visits will usually be every year.

Certain brands of vaginal estrogens contain oils that can weaken latex (rubber) condoms, diaphragms, or cervical caps. This increases the chance of a condom breaking during sexual intercourse. The rubber in cervical caps or diaphragms may break down faster and wear out sooner. Check with your doctor, nurse, or pharmacist to make sure the vaginal estrogen product you are using can be used with latex (rubber) birth control devices.

It is not yet known whether the use of estrogens increases the risk of breast cancer in women.

If you think that you may be pregnant, stop using the medicine immediately and check with your doctor. Continued use of some estrogens during pregnancy may cause birth defects in the child.

POSSIBLE SIDE EFFECTS OF THIS MEDICINE

Side effects that should be reported to your doctor

MORE COMMON—Pain, tenderness, or enlargement of breasts; swelling of feet and lower legs; weight gain (rapid)

LESS COMMON OR RARE—Changes in vaginal bleeding; lumps in, or discharge from, breast; pains in stomach, side, or abdomen; swelling, redness, or itching around vaginal area; uncontrolled, jerky muscle movements; yellow eyes or skin

Side effects that usually do not require medical attention

These possible side effects may go away during treatment; however, if they continue or are bothersome, check with your doctor, nurse, or pharmacist.

MORE COMMON—Bloating of stomach; cramps of lower stomach; loss of appetite

Also, many women who are using estrogens with a progestin (another female hormone) and have not had their uterus removed will start having monthly vaginal bleeding, similar to menstrual periods, again.

Other side effects not listed above may also occur in some patients. If you notice any other effects, check with your doctor, nurse, or pharmacist.

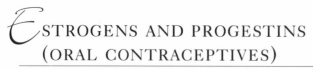

ℰSTROGENS AND PROGESTINS (ORAL CONTRACEPTIVES)

ABOUT YOUR MEDICINE

Most **oral contraceptives** (birth control pills) contain two types of female hormones, **estrogens** (ESS-troe-jenz) and **progestins** (proe-JESS-tins). They are taken by mouth on a regular schedule to prevent pregnancy. Some brands may also be used for other conditions as determined by your doctor. Oral contraceptives do not prevent venereal or sexually transmitted diseases (VD or STDs).

If any of the information in this profile causes you special concern or if you want additional information about your medicine and its use, check with your doctor, nurse, or pharmacist. **Remember, keep this and all other medicines out of the reach of children and never share your medicines with others.**

BEFORE USING THIS MEDICINE

Tell your doctor, nurse, and pharmacist if you . . .
- are allergic to any medicine, either prescription or nonprescription (OTC);
- suspect that you are pregnant;
- are breast-feeding;
- are taking **any** other prescription or nonprescription (OTC) medicine;
- smoke cigarettes;
- have **any** other medical problems.

PROPER USE OF THIS MEDICINE

You should get a paper (package insert) about the use of this medicine as well as risks of using it. **Be sure you have read and understand that information.** This profile does not replace that information.

Oral contraceptives must be taken exactly on schedule to prevent pregnancy. Take them at the same time each day, not more than 24 hours apart.

If you miss a dose of this medicine:
- **For one day**—Take the missed tablet as soon as you remember. If it is not remembered until the next day, take the missed tablet plus the tablet that is regularly scheduled for that day. With some products, you will need to use a second method of birth control to make sure that you are protected for the rest of the cycle (pill packet). The package insert you got with your prescription should tell you if you need to take this extra precaution. If you have any questions about this, check with your doctor, nurse, or pharmacist.
- **For more than one day—Check with your doctor or the package insert for your product.** With certain brands, your doctor may need to tell you how to get back on a regular dosing schedule and how to avoid pregnancy.

PRECAUTIONS WHILE USING THIS MEDICINE

It is very important that your doctor check your progress at regular visits to make sure this medicine does not cause unwanted effects.

Tell the physician or dentist in charge that you are taking this medicine before having any kind of surgery or dental or emergency treatment.

Certain medicines may reduce the effectiveness of oral contraceptives. **Use a second method of birth control during each cycle (pill packet) in which any of the following medicines are used:** ampicillin, bacampicillin, barbiturates, carbamazepine, chloramphenicol, corticosteroids (cortisone-like medicine), dihydroergotamine, griseofulvin, mineral oil, neomycin (oral), penicillin V, phenylbutazone, phenytoin, primidone, rifampin, sulfonamides (sulfa medicine), tetracyclines, tranquilizers, valproic acid.

When you begin to use oral contraceptives, your body needs at least 7 days to adjust before pregnancy will be prevented. **Use a second method of birth control for the first cycle (pill packet) to be sure you are protected.**

Cigarette smoking when using oral contraceptives has been found to increase the risk of serious side effects affecting the heart and circulation. **To reduce the risk, do not smoke cigarettes while using oral contraceptives.**

If you think that you are pregnant, stop taking this medicine immediately and check with your doctor.

POSSIBLE SIDE EFFECTS OF THIS MEDICINE

Rarely, birth control pills cause serious effects such as benign (not cancerous) liver tumors, liver cancer, blood clots, heart attack and stroke, and problems of the gallbladder, liver, and uterus. These effects can be very serious and may cause death. **Carefully read the package insert you received with this medicine and discuss these effects with your doctor.**

Side effects that should be reported to your doctor immediately

The following side effects may be caused by blood clots but rarely occur. However, **if they do occur, they require immediate medical attention. Get emergency help immediately if you have** abdominal or stomach pain (sudden, severe, or continuing); coughing up blood; headache (severe); loss of coordination; loss of or change in vision (sudden); shortness of breath (sudden or unexplained); slurring of speech; pains in chest, groin, or leg (especially in calf); unexplained weakness, numbness, or pain in arm or leg.

Other side effects that should be reported to your doctor

LESS COMMON OR RARE—Bulging eyes; changes in vaginal bleeding; double vision; fainting; frequent urge to urinate or painful urination; increased blood pressure; loss of vision; lumps in, or discharge from, breast; mental depression; skin rash, redness, or other skin irritation; swelling, pain, or tenderness in stomach, side, or abdomen; unusual or dark-colored mole; vaginal discharge (thick, white, or curd-like); vaginal itching or irritation; yellow eyes or skin

Side effects that usually do not require medical attention

These possible side effects may go away during treatment; however, if they continue or are bothersome, check with your doctor, nurse, or pharmacist.

MORE COMMON—Acne; bloating of stomach; changes in appetite; cramps of lower stomach; nausea; swelling of ankles and feet; swelling and increased tenderness of breasts; unusual tiredness or weakness; unusual weight gain

Other side effects not listed above may also occur in some patients. If you notice any other effects, check with your doctor, nurse, or pharmacist.

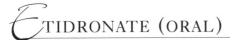TIDRONATE (ORAL)

ABOUT YOUR MEDICINE

Etidronate (e-TID-roh-nate) is used to treat Paget's disease of bone. It may also be used to treat or prevent a certain type of bone problem that may occur after hip replacement surgery or spinal injury.

Etidronate is also used to treat hypercalcemia (too much calcium in the blood) that may occur with some types of cancer.

If any of the information in this profile causes you special concern or if you want additional information about your medicine and its use, check with your doctor, nurse, or pharmacist. **Remember, keep this and all other medicines out of the reach of children and never share your medicines with others.**

BEFORE USING THIS MEDICINE

Tell your doctor, nurse, and pharmacist if you . . .
- are allergic to any medicine, either prescription or nonprescription (OTC);
- are pregnant or intend to become pregnant while using this medicine;
- are breast-feeding;
- are taking any other prescription or nonprescription (OTC) medicine, especially antacids containing calcium, magnesium, or aluminum; or mineral supplements or other medicines containing calcium, iron, magnesium, or aluminum;
- have any other medical problems, especially bone fracture, intestinal or bowel disease, or kidney disease.

PROPER USE OF THIS MEDICINE

Take etidronate with water on an empty stomach at least 2 hours before or after food (midmorning is best) or at bedtime. Food may decrease the amount of etidronate absorbed by your body.

Take etidronate only as directed. Do not take more of it, do not take it more often, and do not take it for a longer time than your doctor ordered. To do so may increase the chance of side effects.

In some patients, etidronate takes up to 3 months to work. If you feel that the medicine is not working, do not stop taking it on your own. Instead, check with your doctor.

It is important that you eat a well-balanced diet with an adequate amount of calcium and vitamin D (found in milk or other dairy products). Too much or too little of either may increase the chance of side effects while you are taking etidronate. Your doctor can help you choose the meal plan that is best for you. **However, do not take any food, especially milk, milk formulas, or other dairy products, or antacids, mineral supplements, or other medicines that are high in calcium or iron (high amounts of these minerals may also be in some vitamin preparations), magnesium, or aluminum** within 2 hours of taking etidronate. To do so may keep this medicine from working properly.

If you miss a dose of this medicine, take it as soon as possible. However, if it is almost time for your next dose, skip the missed dose and go back to your regular dosing schedule. Do not double doses.

PRECAUTIONS WHILE USING THIS MEDICINE

It is important that your doctor check your progress at regular visits even if you are between treatments and are not taking this medicine. If your condition has improved and your doctor has told you to stop taking etidronate, your progress must still be checked. The results of laboratory tests or the occurrence of certain symptoms will tell your doctor if more medicine must be taken. Your doctor may want you to begin another course of treatment after you have been off the medicine for at least 3 months.

If this medicine causes you to have nausea or diarrhea and it continues, check with your doctor. The dose may need to be changed.

If bone pain occurs or worsens during treatment, check with your doctor.

POSSIBLE SIDE EFFECTS OF THIS MEDICINE

Side effects that should be reported to your doctor

> MORE COMMON—Bone pain or tenderness (increased, continuing, or returning—in patients with Paget's disease)
> LESS COMMON—Bone fractures, especially of the thigh bone
> RARE—Hives; skin rash or itching; swelling of the arms, legs, face, lips, tongue, or throat

Side effects that usually do not require medical attention

> These possible side effects may go away during treatment; however, if they continue or are bothersome, check with your doctor, nurse, or pharmacist.
>
> MORE COMMON—AT HIGHER DOSES—Diarrhea; nausea

> Other side effects not listed above may also occur in some patients. If you notice any other effects, check with your doctor, nurse, or pharmacist.

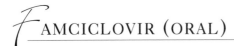AMCICLOVIR (ORAL)

ABOUT YOUR MEDICINE

Famciclovir (fam-SYE-kloe-veer) is used to treat the symptoms of herpes zoster (also known as shingles), a herpes virus infection of the skin. Although famciclovir will not cure herpes zoster, it does help relieve the pain and discomfort and helps the sores heal faster.

If any of the information in this profile causes you special concern or if you want additional information about your medicine and its use, check with your doctor, nurse, or pharmacist. **Remember, keep this and all other medicines out of the reach of children and never share your medicines with others.**

BEFORE USING THIS MEDICINE

Tell your doctor, nurse, and pharmacist if you . . .
- are allergic to any medicine, either prescription or nonprescription (OTC);
- are pregnant or intend to become pregnant while using this medicine;
- are breast-feeding;
- are taking any other prescription or nonprescription (OTC) medicine;
- have any other medical problems, especially kidney disease.

PROPER USE OF THIS MEDICINE

Famciclovir is best used within 48 hours after the symptoms of herpes infection (for example, pain, burning, blisters) begin to appear.

Famciclovir may be taken with meals.

To help clear up your herpes infection, **keep taking famciclovir for the full time of treatment,** even if your symptoms begin to clear up after a few days. **Do not miss any doses.** However, **do not use this medicine more often or for a longer time than your doctor ordered.**

If you do miss a dose of this medicine, take it as soon as possible. However, if it is almost time for your next dose, skip the missed dose and go back to your regular dosing schedule. Do not double doses.

PRECAUTIONS WHILE USING THIS MEDICINE

If your symptoms do not improve within a few days, or if they become worse, check with your doctor.

The areas affected by herpes should be kept as clean and dry as possible. Also, wear loose-fitting clothing to avoid irritating the sores (blisters).

POSSIBLE SIDE EFFECTS OF THIS MEDICINE

Side effects that usually do not require medical attention

These possible side effects may go away during treatment; however, if they continue or are bothersome, check with your doctor, nurse, or pharmacist.

MORE COMMON—Headache

LESS COMMON—Diarrhea; dizziness; nausea; unusual tiredness or weakness; vomiting

Other side effects not listed above may also occur in some patients. If you notice any other effects, check with your doctor, nurse, or pharmacist.

FENTANYL (TRANSDERMAL)*

ABOUT YOUR MEDICINE

Fentanyl (FEN-ta-nil) transdermal system (stick-on patch) belongs to the group of medicines known as narcotic analgesics (nar-KOT-ik an-al-JEE-zicks). This medicine is used to relieve severe, chronic (long-lasting) pain.

If any of the information in this profile causes you special concern or if you want additional information about your medicine and its use, check with your doctor, nurse, or pharmacist. **Remember, keep this and all other medicines out of the reach of children and never share your medicines with others.**

BEFORE USING THIS MEDICINE

Tell your doctor, nurse, and pharmacist if you . . .
- are allergic to any medicine, either prescription or nonprescription (OTC);
- are pregnant or intend to become pregnant while using this medicine;
- are breast-feeding;
- are taking any other prescription or nonprescription (OTC) medicine, especially CNS depressants;
- have any other medical problems.

*This profile has been developed by the USP based primarily on labeling provided by the manufacturer at the time of its approval. This information is intended for use as a temporary educational aid until the drug has been assessed by USP advisory panels. The information does not cover all possible uses, actions, precautions, side effects, or interactions of this medicine. It is not intended as medical advice for individual problems.

PROPER USE OF THIS MEDICINE

Use this medicine only as directed by your medical doctor. Do not use more of it and do not use it more often than directed. Using too much of this medicine may lead to medical problems because of an overdose.

This medicine comes with directions on how to apply and remove the skin patch. Check with your pharmacist if you have not received these directions, or if you have any questions about how this medicine is to be used.

If you miss a dose of this medicine, use it as soon as you remember.

PRECAUTIONS WHILE USING THIS MEDICINE

Fentanyl will add to the effects of alcohol and other CNS depressants (medicines that slow down the nervous system). Check with your doctor before taking any such depressants while you are using this medicine.

This medicine may cause some people to become drowsy, dizzy, or lightheaded, or to feel a false sense of well-being. Make sure you know how you react to this medicine before you drive, use machines, or do other jobs that require you to be alert and clearheaded.

If you have been using this medicine regularly for several weeks or more, do not suddenly stop using it without first checking with your doctor. Your doctor may want you to reduce your dose gradually.

Check with your doctor if you get a fever while you are using this medicine. A fever may cause fentanyl to be absorbed through the skin faster. This increases the chance of side effects.

If you think an overdose has been taken, get emergency help at once. Taking an overdose or taking alcohol or CNS depressants with this medicine may lead to unconsciousness or death. Signs of overdose include confusion; seizures; severe nervousness or restlessness, dizziness, drowsiness, or weakness; and unusually slow or troubled breathing.

POSSIBLE SIDE EFFECTS OF THIS MEDICINE

Side effects that should be reported to your doctor

> MORE COMMON—Decreased urination; difficulty in breathing; hallucinations; itching of skin; mental depression
> LESS COMMON—Chest pain; fainting; irregular heartbeat; mood changes; problems with coordination, speech, or walking; skin rash or redness at place of application
> RARE—Double vision; frequent urge to urinate; pain in bladder; red, thickened, scaly, or peeling skin; slow heartbeat; wheezing

Side effects that usually do not require medical attention

> These possible side effects may go away during treatment; however, if they continue or are bothersome, check with your doctor, nurse, or pharmacist.

MORE COMMON—Confusion; constipation; diarrhea; headache; indigestion; loss of appetite; nausea or vomiting; sleepiness; stomach pain; weakness

LESS COMMON OR RARE—Dizziness or lightheadedness; feeling of burning, crawling, tingling, or prickling in the skin; memory loss; unusual dreams; unusual nervousness or restlessness

Other side effects not listed above may also occur in some patients. If you notice any other effects, check with your doctor, nurse, or pharmacist.

FLUOROQUINOLONES (ORAL)

Including Ciprofloxacin; Enoxacin;
Lomefloxacin; Norfloxacin; Ofloxacin

ABOUT YOUR MEDICINE

Fluoroquinolones (flu-roe-KWIN-a-lones) are used to treat bacterial infections in many different parts of the body. These medicines will not work for colds, flu, or other virus infections. Fluoroquinolones may also be used for other problems as determined by your doctor.

If any of the information in this profile causes you special concern or if you want additional information about your medicine and its use, check with your doctor, nurse, or pharmacist. **Remember, keep this and all other medicines out of the reach of children and never share your medicines with others.**

BEFORE USING THIS MEDICINE

Tell your doctor, nurse, and pharmacist if you . . .
- are allergic to any medicine, either prescription or nonprescription (OTC);
- are pregnant or intend to become pregnant while using this medicine;
- are breast-feeding;
- are taking any other prescription or nonprescription (OTC) medicine, especially aminophylline, antacids, anticoagulants (blood thinners), oxtriphylline, sucralfate, or theophylline;
- have any other medical problems, especially brain or spinal cord damage, history of convulsive disorders (seizures, epilepsy), or kidney disease.

PROPER USE OF THIS MEDICINE

This medicine should not be used in infants, children, adolescents, or pregnant or breast-feeding women unless otherwise directed by your doctor.

This medicine is best taken with a full glass (8 ounces) of water on an empty stomach (either 1 hour before or 2 hours after meals). However, if this medicine upsets your stomach, your doctor may want you to take it with food; **but do not take milk or other dairy products within 1 or 2 hours of the time you take this medicine. Several additional glasses of water should be taken every day,** unless otherwise directed.

To help clear up your infection completely, **keep taking this medicine for the full time of treatment,** even if you begin to feel better after a few days.

This medicine works best when there is a constant amount in the blood or urine. **To help keep the amount constant, do not miss any doses. Also, it is best to take the doses at evenly spaced times, day and night.**

If you do miss a dose of this medicine, take it as soon as possible. However, if it is almost time for your next dose, skip the missed dose and go back to your regular dosing schedule. Do not double doses.

PRECAUTIONS WHILE USING THIS MEDICINE

If your symptoms do not improve within a few days, check with your doctor.

If you are taking antacids or sucralfate, do not take them at the same time that you take this medicine. It is best to take antacids or sucralfate 2 to 3 hours before or after taking this medicine.

Some people who take fluoroquinolones may become more sensitive to sunlight than they are normally. When you first begin taking this medicine, avoid too much sun and do not use a sunlamp until you see how you react to the sun, especially if you tend to burn easily. **If you have a severe reaction, check with your doctor.**

This medicine may cause vision problems. It may also cause some people to become dizzy, lightheaded, drowsy, or less alert than they are normally. **Make sure you know how you react before you drive, use machines, or do other jobs that could be dangerous if you are not alert or able to see well.**

This medicine must not be given to other people or used for other infections unless you are otherwise directed by your doctor.

POSSIBLE SIDE EFFECTS OF THIS MEDICINE

Side effects that should be reported to your doctor immediately
> RARE—Agitation; confusion; fever; hallucinations; peeling of the skin; shakiness or tremors; shortness of breath; skin rash, itching, or redness; swelling of face or neck

Side effects that usually do not require medical attention
> These possible side effects may go away during treatment; however, if they continue or are bothersome, check with your doctor, nurse, or pharmacist.

MORE COMMON—Abdominal or stomach pain or discomfort; diarrhea; dizziness; drowsiness; headache; lightheadedness; nausea or vomiting; nervousness; trouble in sleeping

LESS COMMON OR RARE—Increased sensitivity of skin to sunlight

Other side effects not listed above may also occur in some patients. If you notice any other effects, check with your doctor, nurse, or pharmacist.

$\mathcal{F}$LUOXETINE (ORAL)

ABOUT YOUR MEDICINE

Fluoxetine (floo-OX-uh-teen) is used to treat mental depression. It is also used to treat obsessive-compulsive disorder.

If any of the information in this profile causes you special concern or if you want additional information about your medicine and its use, check with your doctor, nurse, or pharmacist. **Remember, keep this and all other medicines out of the reach of children and never share your medicines with others.**

BEFORE USING THIS MEDICINE

Tell your doctor, nurse, and pharmacist if you . . .
- are allergic to any medicine, either prescription or nonprescription (OTC);
- are pregnant or intend to become pregnant while using this medicine;
- are breast-feeding;
- are taking any other prescription or nonprescription (OTC) medicine, especially anticoagulants (blood thinners), CNS depressants, digitalis glycosides (heart medicine), MAO inhibitors, phenytoin, or tryptophan;
- have any other medical problems, especially kidney disease or liver disease, or a history of seizure disorders.

PROPER USE OF THIS MEDICINE

Take this medicine only as directed by your doctor, to benefit your condition as much as possible. Do not take more of it, do not take it more often, and do not take it for a longer time than your doctor ordered.

If this medicine upsets your stomach, it may be taken with food.

Sometimes fluoxetine must be taken for up to 4 weeks or longer before you begin to feel better. Your doctor should check your progress at regular visits during this time.

If you miss a dose of this medicine, it is not necessary to make up the missed dose. Skip the missed dose and continue with your next scheduled dose. Do not double doses.

PRECAUTIONS WHILE USING THIS MEDICINE

It is important that your doctor check your progress at regular visits, to allow dosage adjustments and help reduce any side effects.

This medicine will add to the effects of alcohol and other CNS depressants (medicines that slow down the nervous system). **Check with your doctor before taking any such depressants while you are using this medicine.**

If you develop a skin rash or hives, stop taking fluoxetine and check with your doctor as soon as possible.

This medicine may cause some people to become drowsy. **Make sure you know how you react to fluoxetine before you drive, use machines, or do other jobs that could be dangerous if you are not alert.**

Dizziness, lightheadedness, or fainting may occur, especially when you get up from a lying or sitting position. Getting up slowly may help. If this problem continues or gets worse, check with your doctor.

This medicine may cause dryness of the mouth. For temporary relief, use sugarless gum or candy, melt bits of ice in your mouth, or use a saliva substitute. However, if your mouth continues to feel dry for more than 2 weeks, check with your physician or dentist. Continuing dryness of the mouth may increase the chance of dental disease, including tooth decay, gum disease, and fungus infections.

POSSIBLE SIDE EFFECTS OF THIS MEDICINE

Side effects that should be reported to your doctor
>   LESS COMMON—Chills or fever; joint or muscle pain; skin rash, hives, or itching; trouble in breathing
>   RARE—Anxiety or nervousness; burning or tingling in fingers, hands, or arms; cold sweats; confusion; convulsions (seizures); cool, pale skin; difficulty in concentration; drowsiness; excessive hunger; fast heartbeat; headache; shakiness or unsteady walk; swelling of feet or lower legs; swollen glands; unusual tiredness or weakness

Side effects that usually do not require medical attention
>   These possible side effects may go away during treatment; however, if they continue or are bothersome, check with your doctor, nurse, or pharmacist.

>   MORE COMMON—Anxiety and nervousness; diarrhea; drowsiness; headache; increased sweating; nausea; trouble in sleeping
>   LESS COMMON—Abnormal dreams; change in taste; changes in vision; chest pain; constipation; cough; decreased appetite or weight loss; decreased sexual drive or ability; decrease in concentration; dizziness or

lightheadedness; dryness of mouth; fast or irregular heartbeat; feeling of warmth or heat; flushing or redness of skin, especially on face and neck; frequent urination; increased appetite; menstrual pain; stomach cramps, gas, or pain; stuffy nose; tiredness or weakness; tremor; vomiting

Other side effects not listed above may also occur in some patients. If you notice any other effects, check with your doctor, nurse, or pharmacist.

Fluvastatin (Oral)

About Your Medicine

Fluvastatin (FLOO-va-stat-in) is used to lower levels of cholesterol and other fats in the blood. This may help prevent medical problems caused by cholesterol clogging the blood vessels.

Fluvastatin belongs to the group of medicines called HMG-CoA reductase inhibitors.

If any of the information in this profile causes you special concern or if you want additional information about your medicine and its use, check with your doctor, nurse, or pharmacist. **Remember, keep this and all other medicines out of the reach of children and never share your medicines with others.**

Before Using This Medicine

Importance of diet—Before prescribing medicine to lower your cholesterol, your doctor will probably try to control your condition by prescribing a personal diet for you. Such a diet may be low in fats, sugars, and/or cholesterol. Many people are able to control their condition by carefully following their doctor's orders for proper diet and exercise. **Medicine is prescribed only when additional help is needed** and is effective only when a schedule of diet and exercise is properly followed.

Also, this medicine is less effective if you are greatly overweight. It may be very important for you to go on a reducing diet. However, check with your doctor before going on any diet.

Tell your doctor, nurse, and pharmacist if you . . .
- are allergic to any medicine, either prescription or nonprescription (OTC);
- **are pregnant or intend to become pregnant while using this medicine;**
- are breast-feeding;
- are taking any other prescription or nonprescription (OTC) medicine, especially cyclosporine, gemfibrozil, or niacin;

- have had major surgery, especially a heart transplant;
- have any other medical problems, especially convulsions (seizures) or liver disease.

PROPER USE OF THIS MEDICINE

Use this medicine only as directed by your doctor. Do not use more or less of it, and do not use it more often or for a longer time than ordered.

Remember that this medicine will not cure your condition but it does help control it. Therefore, you must continue to take it as directed if you expect to keep your cholesterol levels down.

If you miss a dose of this medicine, take it as soon as possible. However, if it is almost time for your next dose, skip the missed dose and go back to your regular dosing schedule. Do not double doses.

PRECAUTIONS WHILE USING THIS MEDICINE

It is very important that your doctor check your progress at regular visits. This will allow your doctor to see if the medicine is working properly to lower your cholesterol levels and that it does not cause unwanted effects.

Check with your doctor immediately if you think that you may be pregnant. This medicine may cause birth defects or other problems in the baby if taken during pregnancy.

Do not stop taking this medicine without first checking with your doctor. When you stop taking this medicine, your blood cholesterol levels may increase again. Your doctor may want you to follow a special diet to help prevent this from happening.

Before having any kind of surgery or dental or emergency treatment, tell the physician or dentist in charge that you are taking this medicine.

POSSIBLE SIDE EFFECTS OF THIS MEDICINE

Side effects that should be reported to your doctor immediately
> LESS COMMON OR RARE—Fever; muscle aches or cramps; stomach pain (severe); unusual tiredness or weakness

Other side effects that should be reported to your doctor
> MORE COMMON—Constipation; diarrhea; dizziness; gas; headache; heartburn; nausea; skin rash; stomach pain
> RARE—Decreased sexual ability; trouble in sleeping

> Other side effects not listed above may also occur in some patients. If you notice any other effects, check with your doctor, nurse, or pharmacist.

FOLIC ACID (VITAMIN B9) (ORAL)

ABOUT YOUR DIETARY SUPPLEMENT

Vitamins (VYE-ta-mins) are compounds that you *must* have for growth and health. They are needed in small amounts only and are usually available in the foods that you eat. **Folic acid** (FOE-lik) (**vitamin B9**) is necessary for strong blood.

Lack of folic acid may lead to anemia (weak blood). Your doctor may treat this by prescribing folic acid for you.

Patients with the following conditions may be more likely to have a deficiency of folic acid: alcoholism; continuing diarrhea or stress; hemodialysis; hemolytic anemia; intestine disease; liver disease; prolonged fever or illness; or surgical removal of the stomach. In addition, infants smaller than normal, breast-fed infants, or those receiving unfortified formulas (such as evaporated milk or goat's milk) may need additional folic acid. If any of the above apply to you, you should take folic acid supplements only on the advice of your doctor after need has been established.

Some studies have found that folic acid taken by women before they become pregnant and during early pregnancy may reduce the chances of certain birth defects (neural tube defects).

If any of the information in this profile causes you special concern or if you want additional information about your dietary supplement and its use, check with your doctor, nurse, or pharmacist. **Remember, keep this and all other medicines out of the reach of children and never share your medicines with others.**

BEFORE USING THIS DIETARY SUPPLEMENT

Importance of diet—Vitamin supplements should be taken only if you cannot get enough vitamins in your diet; however, some diets may not contain all the vitamins you need. A balanced diet should provide all the vitamins you normally need. Folic acid is found in various foods, including vegetables, fruits, potatoes, cereal and cereal products, and organ meats (for example, liver or kidney).

In some cases, it may not be possible for you to get enough food to supply you with the proper vitamins. In other cases, the amount of vitamins you need may be increased above normal. Therefore, a vitamin supplement may be needed.

If you are taking this dietary supplement without a prescription, carefully read and follow any precautions on the label. However, it may be a good idea to check with your doctor before taking folic acid on your own. You should be especially careful if you . . .

- are allergic to any medicine, either prescription or nonprescription (OTC);
- are pregnant, intend to become pregnant, or are breast-feeding;
- are taking any other prescription or nonprescription (OTC) medicine;
- have any other medical problems, especially pernicious anemia (a special blood problem).

If you have any questions, check with your doctor, nurse, or pharmacist.

Proper Use of This Dietary Supplement

Some people believe that taking very large doses of vitamins (called megadoses or megavitamin therapy) is useful for treating certain medical problems. Studies have not proven this. Large doses should be taken only under the direction of your doctor after need has been identified.

If you miss taking a vitamin for one or more days there is no cause for concern, since it takes some time for your body to become seriously low in vitamins. However, if your doctor has recommended that you take this vitamin, try to remember to take it as directed every day.

Possible Side Effects of This Dietary Supplement

Side effects that should be reported to your doctor

RARE—Fever; reddened skin; shortness of breath; skin rash; tightness in chest; troubled breathing; wheezing

Other side effects not listed above may also occur in some patients. If you notice any other effects, check with your doctor, nurse, or pharmacist.

Gemfibrozil (Oral)

About Your Medicine

Gemfibrozil (gem-FI-broe-zil) is used to lower levels of cholesterol and triglyceride (fat-like substances) in the blood. This may help prevent medical problems caused by such substances clogging the blood vessels.

If any of the information in this profile causes you special concern or if you want additional information about your medicine and its use, check with your doctor, nurse, or pharmacist. **Remember, keep this and all other medicines out of the reach of children and never share your medicines with others.**

Before Using This Medicine

In addition to its helpful effects in treating your medical problem, this type of medicine may have some harmful effects.

Results of a large study using gemfibrozil seem to show that it may cause a higher rate of some cancers in humans. In addition, the action of gemfibrozil is similar to that of another medicine called clofibrate. Studies with clofibrate have suggested that it may increase the patient's risk of cancer, liver disease, and pancreatitis (inflammation of the pancreas), gallstones, and problems from gallbladder surgery.

However, it may also decrease the risk of heart attacks. Other studies have not found all of these effects. Be sure you have discussed this with your doctor before taking this medicine.

Importance of diet—Your doctor will probably try to control your condition by prescribing a personal diet for you. Such a diet may be low in fats, sugars, and/or cholesterol. Also, it may be very important for you to go on a reducing diet. **Medicine is prescribed only when additional help is needed** and is effective only when a schedule of diet and exercise is properly followed. However, check with your doctor before going on any diet.

Tell your doctor, nurse, and pharmacist if you . . .
- are allergic to any medicine, either prescription or nonprescription (OTC);
- are pregnant or intend to become pregnant while using this medicine;
- are breast-feeding;
- are taking any other prescription or nonprescription (OTC) medicine, especially anticoagulants (blood thinners) or lovastatin;
- have any other medical problems, especially kidney disease or liver disease.

PROPER USE OF THIS MEDICINE

Use this medicine only as directed by your doctor. Do not use more or less of it, and do not use it more often or for a longer time than your doctor ordered.

This medicine is usually taken twice a day. If you are taking 2 doses a day, it is best to take the medicine 30 minutes before your breakfast and evening meals.

If you miss a dose of this medicine, take it as soon as possible. However, if it is almost time for your next dose, skip the missed dose and go back to your regular dosing schedule. Do not double doses.

PRECAUTIONS WHILE USING THIS MEDICINE

It is very important that your doctor check your progress at regular visits. This will allow your doctor to see if the medicine is working properly to lower your cholesterol and triglyceride levels and if you should continue to take it.

Do not stop taking this medication without first checking with your doctor. When you stop taking this medicine, your blood cholesterol levels may increase again. Your doctor may want you to follow a special diet to help prevent this from happening.

POSSIBLE SIDE EFFECTS OF THIS MEDICINE

Side effects that should be reported to your doctor immediately
RARE—Cough or hoarseness; fever or chills; lower back or side pain; painful or difficult urination; stomach pain (severe) with nausea and vomiting

Other side effects that should be reported to your doctor
RARE—Muscle pain; unusual tiredness or weakness

Side effects that usually do not require medical attention

These possible side effects may go away during treatment; however, if they continue or are bothersome, check with your doctor, nurse, or pharmacist.

MORE COMMON—Stomach pain, gas, or heartburn
LESS COMMON—Diarrhea; nausea or vomiting; skin rash

Other side effects not listed above may also occur in some patients. If you notice any other effects, check with your doctor, nurse, or pharmacist.

H_2-BLOCKERS (ORAL)
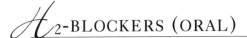

Including Cimetidine; Famotidine; Nizatidine; Ranitidine

ABOUT YOUR MEDICINE

H_2-blockers are used in the treatment and prevention of duodenal ulcers. Some of the H_2-blockers are used also to treat gastric ulcers. In addition, H_2-blockers are used in some conditions in which the stomach produces too much acid. These medicines may also be used for other conditions as determined by your doctor.

If any of the information in this profile causes you special concern or if you want additional information about your medicine and its use, check with your doctor, nurse, or pharmacist. **Remember, keep this and all other medicines out of the reach of children and never share your medicines with others.**

BEFORE USING THIS MEDICINE

Tell your doctor, nurse, and pharmacist if you . . .
- are allergic to any medicine, either prescription or nonprescription (OTC);
- are pregnant or intend to become pregnant while using this medicine;
- are breast-feeding;
- are taking any other prescription or nonprescription (OTC) medicine, especially ketoconazole;
- are taking cimetidine and are also taking aminophylline, amitriptyline, amoxapine, anticoagulants (blood thinners), caffeine, clomipramine, desipramine, doxepin, imipramine, metoprolol, nortriptyline, oxtriphylline, phenytoin, propranolol, protriptyline, theophylline, or trimipramine;
- are taking ranitidine and are also taking anticoagulants (blood thinners), caffeine, metoprolol, phenytoin, or theophylline;
- have any other medical problems, especially severe kidney disease.

PROPER USE OF THIS MEDICINE

It may take several days for this medicine to begin to relieve stomach pain. To help relieve pain, antacids may be taken with this medicine, unless your doctor has told you not to use them. However, you should wait one-half to one hour between taking the antacid and this medicine.

Take this medicine for the full time of treatment, even if you begin to feel better. Also, it is important that you keep your doctor's appointments for checkups so that your doctor will be better able to tell you when to stop taking this medicine.

For patients taking:
- One dose a day—Take it at bedtime, unless otherwise directed.
- Two doses a day—Take one in the morning and one at bedtime.
- Several doses a day—Take them with meals and at bedtime for best results.

If you miss a dose of this medicine, take it as soon as possible. However, if it is almost time for your next dose, skip the missed dose and go back to your regular dosing schedule. Do not double doses.

PRECAUTIONS WHILE USING THIS MEDICINE

Some tests may be affected by this medicine. Tell the doctor in charge that you are taking this medicine before:
- You have any skin tests for allergies.
- You have any tests to determine how much acid your stomach produces.

Remember that certain medicines, such as aspirin, as well as certain foods and drinks (e.g., citrus products, carbonated drinks, etc.) irritate the stomach and may make your problem worse.

Cigarette smoking tends to decrease the effect of H_2-blockers by increasing the amount of acid produced by the stomach. This is more likely to affect the stomach's nighttime production of acid. While taking this medicine, stop smoking completely, or at least do not smoke after the last dose of the day.

Be careful of the amount of alcohol you drink while taking this medicine. H_2-blockers have been shown to increase alcohol levels in the blood. You should consult your doctor, nurse, or pharmacist for guidance.

Check with your doctor if your ulcer pain continues or gets worse.

POSSIBLE SIDE EFFECTS OF THIS MEDICINE

Side effects that should be reported to your doctor

RARE—Burning, itching, redness, skin rash; confusion; fast, pounding, or irregular heartbeat; fever; slow heartbeat; sore throat and fever; swelling; tightness in chest; unusual bleeding or bruising; unusual tiredness or weakness

Other side effects not listed above may also occur in some patients. If you notice any other effects, check with your doctor, nurse, or pharmacist.

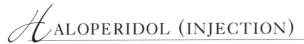ALOPERIDOL (INJECTION)

ABOUT YOUR MEDICINE

Haloperidol (ha-loe-PER-i-dole) is used to treat nervous, mental, and emotional conditions. It may also be used for other conditions as determined by your doctor.

If any of the information in this profile causes you special concern or if you want additional information about your medicine and its use, check with your doctor, nurse, or pharmacist. **Remember, keep this and all other medicines out of the reach of children and never share your medicines with others.**

BEFORE USING THIS MEDICINE

Discuss with your doctor possible side effects of this medicine. Some may be serious and/or permanent. For example, tardive dyskinesia (a movement disorder) may occur and may not go away after you stop using the medicine.

Tell your doctor, nurse, and pharmacist if you . . .

- are allergic to any medicine, either prescription or nonprescription (OTC);
- are pregnant or intend to become pregnant while using this medicine;
- are breast-feeding;
- are taking **any** other prescription or nonprescription (OTC) medicine;
- have any other medical problems, especially difficult urination, epilepsy, heart or blood vessel disease, or Parkinson's disease.

PROPER USE OF THIS MEDICINE

Do not use more of this medicine and do not use it more often than ordered.

Sometimes haloperidol must be used for several days to several weeks before its full effect is reached.

If you miss a dose of this medicine, use it as soon as possible. Then use any remaining doses for that day at regularly spaced intervals. Do not double doses.

PRECAUTIONS WHILE USING THIS MEDICINE

Your doctor should check your progress at regular visits, especially during the first few months of treatment with this medicine.

Do not stop using this medicine without first checking with your doctor.

This medicine will add to the effects of alcohol and other CNS depressants (medicines that may make you drowsy or less alert). **Check with your doctor before taking any such depressants while you are taking this medicine.**

Haloperidol may cause some people to become drowsy or less alert than they are normally. Even if you use this medicine at bedtime, you may feel drowsy or less alert on arising. **Make sure you know how you react before you drive or do jobs that require you to be alert.**

Some people who use haloperidol may become more sensitive to sunlight than they are normally. **When you first begin using this medicine, avoid too much sun** and do not use a sunlamp until you see how you react to the sun. If you have a severe reaction, check with your doctor.

Use extra care not to become overheated during exercise or hot weather. Also, hot baths or saunas may make you feel dizzy or faint while you are using this medicine.

Before having any kind of surgery or dental or emergency treatment, tell the physician or dentist in charge that you are using this medicine.

The effect of the long-acting injection form of this medicine may last for up to 6 weeks. The precaution and side effects information for this medicine applies during this time.

POSSIBLE SIDE EFFECTS OF THIS MEDICINE

Side effects that should be reported to your doctor immediately

Stop taking this medicine and get emergency help immediately if any of the following side effects occur:

RARE—Convulsions; fast or irregular heartbeat; fever (high); high or low blood pressure; increased sweating; loss of bladder control; muscle stiffness (severe); tiredness or weakness; troubled breathing; unusually pale skin

Other side effects that should be reported to your doctor

MORE COMMON—Difficulty speaking or swallowing; inability to move eyes; loss of balance control; muscle spasms of neck and back; restlessness; shuffling walk; stiff or weak arms and legs; trembling hands

LESS COMMON—Difficult urination; dizziness, lightheadedness, or fainting; hallucinations; skin rash; uncontrolled movements of mouth, tongue, and jaw

RARE—Hot, dry skin, or lack of sweating; increased blinking or spasms of eyelids; muscle weakness; sore throat and fever; uncontrolled twisting movements of neck, trunk, arms, or legs; unusual bleeding or bruising; unusual facial expressions or body positions; yellow eyes or skin

Side effects that usually do not require medical attention

These possible side effects may go away during treatment; however, if they continue or are bothersome, check with your doctor, nurse, or pharmacist.

MORE COMMON—Blurred vision; changes in menstrual period; constipation; dryness of mouth; swelling or pain in breasts in females; unusual secretion of milk; weight gain

Other side effects not listed above may also occur in some patients. If you notice any other effects, check with your doctor, nurse, or pharmacist.

After you stop using this medicine, your body may need time to adjust. Check with your doctor if you experience trembling of fingers and hands, or uncontrolled movements of mouth, tongue, and jaw.

$\mathscr{H}$ALOPERIDOL (ORAL)

ABOUT YOUR MEDICINE

Haloperidol (ha-loe-PER-i-dole) is used to treat nervous, mental, and emotional conditions. It is used also to control the effects of Tourette's disorder. Haloperidol may also be used for other conditions as determined by your doctor.

If any of the information in this profile causes you special concern or if you want additional information about your medicine and its use, check with your doctor, nurse, or pharmacist. **Remember, keep this and all other medicines out of the reach of children and never share your medicines with others.**

BEFORE USING THIS MEDICINE

Discuss with your doctor possible side effects of this medicine. Some may be serious and/or permanent. For example, tardive dyskinesia (a movement disorder) may occur and may not go away after you stop using the medicine.

Tell your doctor, nurse, and pharmacist if you . . .
- are allergic to any medicine, either prescription or nonprescription (OTC);
- are pregnant or intend to become pregnant while using this medicine;
- are breast-feeding;
- are taking any other prescription or nonprescription (OTC) medicine, especially CNS depressants; epinephrine; levodopa; lithium; other medicines for nervous, mental, and emotional conditions; metoclopramide; metyrosine; promethazine; rauwolfia alkaloids; or trimeprazine;
- have any other medical problems, especially difficult urination, epilepsy, heart or blood vessel disease, or Parkinson's disease.

PROPER USE OF THIS MEDICINE

Do not take more of this medicine and do not take it more often than ordered. To lessen stomach upset, it may be taken with food or milk.

Sometimes haloperidol must be taken for several days to several weeks before its full effect is reached.

If you miss a dose of this medicine, take it as soon as possible. Then take any remaining doses for that day at regularly spaced intervals. Do not double doses.

PRECAUTIONS WHILE USING THIS MEDICINE

Your doctor should check your progress at regular visits, especially during the first few months of treatment with this medicine.

Do not stop taking this medicine without first checking with your doctor.

This medicine will add to the effects of alcohol and other CNS depressants (medicines that slow down the nervous system). **Check with your doctor before taking any such depressants while you are taking this medicine.**

Haloperidol may cause some people to become drowsy or less alert than they are normally. Even if you take this medicine at bedtime, you may feel drowsy or less alert on arising. **Make sure you know how you react before you drive or do jobs that require you to be alert.**

Some people who take haloperidol may become more sensitive to sunlight than they are normally. **When you first begin taking this medicine, avoid too much sun and do not use a sunlamp until you see how you react to the sun. If you have a severe reaction, check with your doctor.**

Use extra care not to become overheated during exercise or hot weather since overheating may result in heat stroke. Also, hot baths or saunas may make you feel dizzy or faint while you are taking this medicine.

If you are taking the liquid form of this medicine, avoid getting it on your skin because it may cause a skin rash or other irritation.

Before having any kind of surgery or dental or emergency treatment, tell the physician or dentist in charge that you are using this medicine.

POSSIBLE SIDE EFFECTS OF THIS MEDICINE

Side effects that should be reported to your doctor immediately
  Stop taking this medicine and get emergency help immediately if any of the following side effects occur:

  RARE—Convulsions; fast or irregular heartbeat; fever (high); high or low blood pressure; increased sweating; loss of bladder control; muscle stiffness (severe); tiredness or weakness; troubled breathing; unusually pale skin

Other side effects that should be reported to your doctor
  MORE COMMON—Difficulty speaking or swallowing; inability to move eyes; loss of balance control; mask-like face; muscle spasms of neck and back; restlessness; shuffling walk; stiff or weak arms and legs; trembling hands
  LESS COMMON—Difficult urination; dizziness, lightheadedness, or fainting; hallucinations; skin rash; uncontrolled movements of mouth, tongue, and jaw
  RARE—Hot, dry skin, or lack of sweating; increased blinking or spasms of eyelids; muscle weakness; sore throat and fever; uncontrolled twisting movements of neck, trunk, arms, or legs; unusual bleeding or bruising; unusual facial expressions or body positions; yellow eyes or skin

Side effects that usually do not require medical attention
  These possible side effects may go away during treatment; however, if they continue or are bothersome, check with your doctor, nurse, or pharmacist.

  MORE COMMON—Blurred vision; changes in menstrual period; constipation; dryness of mouth; swelling or pain in breasts in females; unusual secretion of milk; weight gain

Other side effects not listed above may also occur in some patients. If you notice any other effects, check with your doctor, nurse, or pharmacist.

After you stop taking this medicine, your body may need time to adjust. Check with your doctor if you experience trembling of fingers and hands, or uncontrolled movements of mouth, tongue, and jaw.

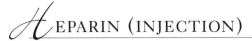EPARIN (INJECTION)

ABOUT YOUR MEDICINE

Heparin (HEP-a-rin) is an anticoagulant. It is used to decrease the clotting ability of the blood and therefore help prevent harmful clots from forming in the blood vessels.

If any of the information in this profile causes you special concern or if you want additional information about your medicine and its use, check with your doctor, nurse, or pharmacist. **Remember, keep this and all other medicines out of the reach of children and never share your medicines with others.**

BEFORE USING THIS MEDICINE

Tell your doctor, nurse, and pharmacist if you . . .
- are allergic to any medicine, either prescription or nonprescription (OTC);
- are pregnant or intend to become pregnant while using this medicine;
- are breast-feeding;
- have received heparin before and had a reaction to it called thrombocytopenia, or if new blood clots formed while you were receiving this medicine;
- are taking **any** other prescription or nonprescription (OTC) medicine;
- have **any** other medical problems.

PROPER USE OF THIS MEDICINE

If you are using these injections at home, make sure your doctor has explained exactly how this medicine is to be given.
In order to obtain the best results without causing serious bleeding, **use this medicine exactly as directed by your doctor. Be certain that you are using the right amount of heparin, and that you use it according to schedule.**

Your doctor should check your progress at regular visits. A blood test must be taken regularly to see how fast your blood is clotting.

If you miss a dose of this medicine, use it as soon as possible. However, if it is almost time for your next dose, do not use the missed dose at all and do not double the next one. **Doubling the dose may cause bleeding.** Instead, go back to your regular dosing schedule. It is best to keep a record of each injection. Be sure to give your doctor a record of any doses you miss.

PRECAUTIONS WHILE USING THIS MEDICINE

Do not take aspirin or ibuprofen while using this medicine. Many over-the-counter (OTC) or nonprescription medicines and some prescription medicines contain aspirin or ibuprofen.

Tell all physicians and dentists you visit that you are using this medicine.

While you are using this medicine, it is very important that you report to your doctor any falls, blows to the body or head, or other injuries.

Take special care in brushing your teeth and in shaving. Use a soft toothbrush and floss gently. Also, it is best to use an electric shaver rather than a blade.

POSSIBLE SIDE EFFECTS OF THIS MEDICINE

Side effects that should be reported to your doctor immediately

SIGNS OF BLEEDING INSIDE THE BODY—Abdominal or stomach pain or swelling; back pain or backaches; blood in urine; bloody or black tarry stools; constipation; coughing up blood; dizziness; headache (severe or continuing); joint pain, stiffness, or swelling; vomiting blood or material that looks like coffee grounds

SIGNS OF A SERIOUS ALLERGIC REACTION—Changes in the skin color of the face; fast or irregular breathing; puffiness or swelling of the eyelids or around the eyes; shortness of breath, troubled breathing, tightness in chest, and/or wheezing; skin rash, hives, and/or itching

Other side effects that should be reported to your doctor

LESS COMMON OR RARE—Back or rib pain (with long-term use); change in skin color, especially near the place of injection or in the fingers, toes, arms, or legs; chest pain; chills and/or fever; collection of blood under skin (blood blister) at place of injection; decrease in height (with long-term use); frequent or persistent erection; irritation, pain, redness, or ulcers at place of injection; itching and burning feeling, especially at the bottom of the feet; nausea and/or vomiting; numbness or tingling in hands or feet; pain, coldness, or blue color of skin of arms or legs; peeling of skin; tearing of eyes; unusual hair loss (with long-term use); unusual runny nose

POSSIBLE SIGNS OF OVERDOSE—Bleeding from gums when brushing teeth; unexplained bruising or purplish areas on skin; unexplained nosebleeds; unusually heavy bleeding or oozing from cuts or wounds; unusually heavy or unexpected menstrual bleeding

Other side effects not listed above may also occur in some patients. If you notice any other effects, check with your doctor, nurse, or pharmacist.

$\mathscr{H}$YDANTOIN ANTICONVULSANTS (ORAL)

Including Ethotoin; Mephenytoin; Phenytoin

ABOUT YOUR MEDICINE

Hydantoin anticonvulsants (hye-DAN-toyn an-tye-kon-VUL-sants) are used to control certain types of seizures in the treatment of epilepsy. Phenytoin may also be used for other conditions as determined by your doctor.

If any of the information in this profile causes you special concern or if you want additional information about your medicine and its use, check with your doctor, nurse, or pharmacist. **Remember, keep this and all other medicines out of the reach of children and never share your medicines with others.**

BEFORE USING THIS MEDICINE

Tell your doctor, nurse, and pharmacist if you . . .
- are allergic to any medicine, either prescription or nonprescription (OTC);
- are pregnant or intend to become pregnant while using this medicine;
- are breast-feeding;
- are taking **any** other prescription or nonprescription (OTC) medicine;
- have any other medical problems, especially blood, heart, kidney, or liver disease; or porphyria.

PROPER USE OF THIS MEDICINE

Take this medicine every day exactly as ordered by your doctor in order to control your medical problem. If it upsets your stomach, take it with food.

If you miss a dose of this medicine and your schedule is:
- One dose a day—Take it as soon as possible. However, if you do not remember until the next day, skip the missed dose. Do not double doses.
- More than one dose a day—Take it as soon as possible unless your next scheduled dose is within 4 hours. Do not double doses.

If you miss doses for 2 or more days in a row, check with your doctor.

PRECAUTIONS WHILE USING THIS MEDICINE

Your doctor should check your progress at regular visits, especially during the first few months of treatment with this medicine since your dose may have to be adjusted. Also, do not change brands or dosage forms of phenytoin without first checking with your doctor. Different products may not work the same way.

If you have been taking this medicine for several weeks or more, do not suddenly stop taking it. Your doctor may want you to reduce your dose gradually.

Before having any kind of surgery or dental or emergency treatment, tell the physician or dentist in charge that you are taking this medicine.

Taking other medicines or drinking alcohol may change the way this medicine works. Check with your doctor before you stop or start taking other medicines or before drinking alcoholic beverages while you are taking this medicine.

Oral contraceptives containing estrogen may not work as well if you take them while taking this medicine. Unplanned pregnancies may occur. Use different or additional birth control while taking this medicine.

Do not take this medicine within 2 to 3 hours of taking antacids or medicine for diarrhea. Taking them too close together may make this medicine less effective.

This medicine may cause some people to become dizzy, drowsy, lightheaded, or less alert than they are normally. **Make sure you know how you react before you drive or do jobs that require you to be alert.**

In some patients (usually younger ones), tenderness, swelling, or bleeding of the gums (gingival hyperplasia) may appear soon after taking phenytoin. Brushing and flossing your teeth carefully and regularly and massaging your gums may help prevent this. **If you have questions about how to take care of your teeth and gums or if you notice problems,** check with your physician or dentist.

POSSIBLE SIDE EFFECTS OF THIS MEDICINE

Side effects that should be reported to your doctor

MORE COMMON—Bleeding, tender, or enlarged gums; clumsiness or unsteadiness; confusion; enlarged glands in neck or underarms; fever; increase in seizures; mood or mental changes; muscle weakness; skin rash or itching; slurred speech; stuttering; trembling of hands; unusual excitement, nervousness, or irritability

RARE—Bone malformations; chest discomfort; dark urine; frequent breaking of bones; headache; joint pain; learning difficulties (in children taking high doses for a long time); light-colored stools; loss of appetite; pain of penis on erection; restlessness or agitation; slowed growth; soreness of muscles; sore throat, chills, and fever; stomach pain (severe); troubled or quick, shallow breathing; uncontrolled jerking or twisting movements of hands, arms, or legs; uncontrolled movements of lips, tongue, or cheeks; unusual bleeding (such as nosebleeds) or bruising; unusual weight loss; unusual tiredness or weakness; yellow eyes or skin

SIGNS OF OVERDOSE—Blurred or double vision; continuous, uncontrolled back and forth and/or rolling eye movements; dizziness or drowsiness (severe); staggering walk; trembling

Side effects that usually do not require medical attention

These possible side effects may go away during treatment; however, if they continue or are bothersome, check with your doctor, nurse, or pharmacist.

MORE COMMON—Constipation; dizziness or drowsiness; nausea and vomiting

Other side effects not listed above may also occur in some patients. If you notice any other effects, check with your doctor, nurse, or pharmacist.

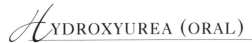YDROXYUREA (ORAL)

ABOUT YOUR MEDICINE

Hydroxyurea (hye-DROX-ee-yoo-REE-ah) belongs to the group of medicines called antimetabolites. It is used to treat some kinds of cancer.

If any of the information in this profile causes you special concern or if you want additional information about your medicine and its use, check with your doctor, nurse, or pharmacist. **Remember, keep this and all other medicines out of the reach of children and never share your medicines with others.**

BEFORE USING THIS MEDICINE

Discuss with your doctor the possible side effects that may be caused by this medicine. Some of them may be serious and/or long-term.

Tell your doctor, nurse, and pharmacist if you . . .
- are allergic to any medicine, either prescription or nonprescription (OTC);
- are pregnant or intend to have children;
- are breast-feeding;
- are taking **any** other prescription or nonprescription (OTC) medicine;
- have any other medical problems, especially anemia, chicken pox (including recent exposure), herpes zoster (shingles), infection, or kidney disease;
- have ever been treated with radiation or cancer medicines.

PROPER USE OF THIS MEDICINE

Take hydroxyurea only as directed by your doctor. Do not use more or less of it, and do not use it more often than your doctor ordered.

For patients who cannot swallow the capsules:
- The contents of the capsule may be emptied into a glass of water and then taken immediately. Some powder may float on the surface of the water, but that is just filler from the capsule.

While you are using this medicine, your doctor may want you to drink extra fluids so that you will pass more urine. This will help prevent kidney problems and keep your kidneys working well.

This medicine commonly causes nausea, vomiting, and diarrhea. However, it is very important that you continue to use the medicine, even if you begin to feel ill. Ask your doctor, nurse, or pharmacist for ways to lessen these effects.

If you vomit shortly after taking a dose of hydroxyurea, check with your doctor.

If you miss a dose of this medicine, do not take the missed dose at all and do not double the next one. Instead, go back to your regular dosing schedule and check with your doctor.

Precautions While Using This Medicine

It is very important that your doctor check your progress at regular visits to make sure this medicine is working properly and to check for unwanted effects.

While you are being treated with hydroxyurea, and after you stop treatment, **do not have any immunizations (vaccinations) without your doctor's approval.**

Hydroxyurea can lower the number of white blood cells in your blood, increasing the chance of getting an infection. It can also lower the number of platelets, which are necessary for proper blood clotting. If this occurs:

- Avoid people with infections.
- Be careful when using a regular toothbrush, dental floss, or toothpick.
- Do not touch your eyes or the inside of your nose unless you have just washed your hands and have not touched anything else in the meantime.
- Be careful not to cut, bruise, or injure yourself.

Possible Side Effects of This Medicine

Side effects that should be reported to your doctor immediately

LESS COMMON—Cough or hoarseness; fever or chills; lower back or side pain; painful or difficult urination

RARE—Black, tarry stools; blood in urine or stools; pinpoint red spots on skin; unusual bleeding or bruising

Other side effects that should be reported to your doctor

LESS COMMON—Sores in mouth and on lips

RARE—Confusion; convulsions (seizures); dizziness; hallucinations; headache; joint pain; swelling of feet or lower legs

Side effects that usually do not require medical attention

These possible side effects may go away during treatment; however, if they continue or are bothersome, check with your doctor, nurse, or pharmacist.

MORE COMMON—Diarrhea; drowsiness; loss of appetite; nausea or vomiting

LESS COMMON—Constipation; redness of skin; skin rash and itching

Other side effects not listed above may also occur in some patients. If you notice any other effects, check with your doctor, nurse, or pharmacist.

After you stop taking hydroxyurea, it may still produce some side effects that need attention. During this time, check with your doctor as soon as possible if you notice black, tarry stools; blood in urine or stools; cough or hoarseness; fever or chills; lower back or side pain; painful or difficult urination; pinpoint red spots on skin; or unusual bleeding or bruising.

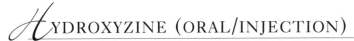Hydroxyzine (oral/injection)

About Your Medicine

Hydroxyzine (hye-DROX-i-zeen) is used in the treatment of nervous and emotional conditions to help control anxiety. It can also be used to help control anxiety and induce sleep before surgery.

Because hydroxyzine has antihistamine action, it is used to relieve the itching caused by allergic conditions.

If any of the information in this profile causes you special concern or if you want additional information about your medicine and its use, check with your doctor, nurse, or pharmacist. **Remember, keep this and all other medicines out of the reach of children and never share your medicines with others.**

Before Using This Medicine

Tell your doctor, nurse, and pharmacist if you . . .
- are allergic to any medicine, either prescription or nonprescription (OTC);
- are pregnant or intend to become pregnant while using this medicine;
- are breast-feeding;
- are taking any other prescription or nonprescription (OTC) medicine, especially CNS depressants, MAO inhibitors, or anticholinergics (medicine for abdominal or stomach spasms or cramps);
- have any other medical problems, especially difficult urination, enlarged prostate, glaucoma, or urinary tract blockage.

Proper Use of This Medicine

Use hydroxyzine only as directed. Do not use more of it and do not use it more often than your doctor ordered. To do so may increase the chance of side effects.

For patients using the injection form of this medicine:
- If you will be giving yourself the injections, make sure you understand exactly how to give them. If you have any questions about this, check with your doctor, nurse, or pharmacist.

If you miss a dose of this medicine, use it as soon as possible. However, if it is almost time for your next dose, skip the missed dose and go back to your regular dosing schedule. Do not double doses.

Precautions While Using This Medicine

Hydroxyzine will add to the effects of alcohol and other CNS depressants (medicines that may make you drowsy or less alert). **Check with your doctor before taking any such depressants while you are using this medicine.**

This medicine may cause some people to become drowsy or less alert than they are normally. Even if used at bedtime, it may cause some people to feel drowsy or less alert on arising. **Make sure you know how you react to this medicine before you drive, use machines, or do other jobs that require you to be alert.**

POSSIBLE SIDE EFFECTS OF THIS MEDICINE

Side effects that should be reported to your doctor

> LESS COMMON OR RARE—Sore throat and fever; unusual bleeding or bruising; unusual tiredness or weakness

Side effects that usually do not require medical attention

> These possible side effects may go away during treatment; however, if they continue or are bothersome, check with your doctor, nurse, or pharmacist.

> MORE COMMON—Drowsiness; thickening of mucus

> Other side effects not listed above may also occur in some patients. If you notice any other effects, check with your doctor, nurse, or pharmacist.

INSULIN (INJECTION)

ABOUT YOUR MEDICINE

Insulin (IN-su-lin) helps the body turn food into energy. This occurs whether we make our own insulin in the pancreas gland or take it by injection. Diabetes mellitus (sugar diabetes) is a condition in which the body does not make enough insulin or does not properly use the insulin it makes. Your doctor will discuss the number of injections you will need, the kind of insulin to use, the correct dose, and the right time to take it.

If any of the information in this profile causes you special concern or if you want additional information about your medicine and its use, check with your doctor, nurse, or pharmacist. **Remember, keep this and all other medicines out of the reach of children and never share your medicines with others.**

BEFORE USING THIS MEDICINE

Tell your doctor, nurse, and pharmacist if you . . .
- are allergic to insulins made from beef or pork;
- are pregnant or intend to become pregnant while using this medicine;
- are taking **any** other prescription or nonprescription (OTC) medicine;
- have **any** other medical problems.

Proper Use of This Medicine

Do not change the strength, brand, or type of insulin you are using unless told to do so by your doctor.

Each package of insulin contains a patient information sheet. Read this sheet carefully.

Follow carefully the special meal plan your doctor gave you. This is the most important part of controlling your condition. Also, **test for sugar in your blood or urine as directed and follow directions for exercise and care of your feet.**

An unopened bottle of insulin should be refrigerated without freezing until needed. However, insulin you are now using regularly may be kept at room temperature if it will be used up within a month. Insulin that has been kept at room temperature for longer than a month should be thrown away. Do not expose insulin to very hot temperatures or sunlight.

Precautions While Using This Medicine

Drinking alcohol while you are using insulin may cause you to have dangerously low blood sugar. **Avoid alcoholic beverages until you have discussed this with your doctor.**

Eat or drink something containing sugar and check with your doctor right away if mild symptoms of low blood sugar (hypoglycemia) appear. Good sources of sugar are glucose tablets or gel, fruit juice, corn syrup, honey, regular (non-diet) soft drinks, or sugar dissolved in water.

If severe symptoms such as convulsions (seizures) or unconsciousness occur, diabetics should not eat or drink anything. There is a chance that they could choke from not swallowing correctly. Emergency medical help should be obtained immediately. Glucagon is also used in emergency situations such as unconsciousness. Have a glucagon kit available, along with a syringe and needle. Make sure you and people in your household know how and when to prepare and use it.

Low blood sugar may occur if you use too much insulin, skip or delay meals, exercise more than usual, have any sickness, especially with vomiting or diarrhea, take certain medicines, or drink a significant amount of alcohol.

Symptoms of low blood sugar can include anxious feeling; behavior change similar to being drunk; blurred vision; cold sweats; confusion; cool pale skin; difficulty in concentrating; drowsiness; excessive hunger; headache; nausea; nervousness; rapid heartbeat; shakiness; unusual tiredness or weakness;.

High blood sugar symptoms may occur if you do not take enough insulin; if you skip a dose of insulin; if you overeat or do not follow your meal plan; if you have a fever or infection; or do not exercise as much as usual.

Symptoms of high blood sugar appear more slowly than those for low blood sugar, and can include blurred vision; drowsiness; dry mouth; flushed, dry skin;

fruit-like breath odor; increased urination; loss of appetite; nausea or vomiting; stomachache; tiredness; troubled breathing (rapid and deep); or unusual thirst.

Symptoms of both low blood sugar and high blood sugar must be corrected before they progress to a more serious condition. In either situation, you should check with your doctor immediately. Also, **if you become sick,** especially with nausea, vomiting, or fever, call your doctor for instructions.

POSSIBLE SIDE EFFECTS OF THIS MEDICINE

Side effects that should be reported to your doctor

> RARE—Depressed skin at the place of injection; swelling of face, fingers, feet, or ankles; thickening of the skin layers at the place of injection

> Side effects not listed above may also occur in some patients. If you notice any other effects, check with your doctor, nurse, or pharmacist.

$\mathcal{I}$PRATROPIUM (INHALATION)

ABOUT YOUR MEDICINE

Ipratropium (i-pra-TROE-pee-um) is a bronchodilator (medicine that opens up narrowed breathing passages). It is taken by inhalation to help control the symptoms of lung diseases, such as bronchial asthma, chronic bronchitis, and emphysema. When ipratropium is used every day, it may be used alone or with other brochodilators to help decrease coughing, wheezing, shortness of breath, and troubled breathing.

When ipratropium inhalation is used to treat acute attacks of asthma, it is used only in a nebulizer and must be used together with other bronchodilators.

If any of the information in this profile causes you special concern or if you want additional information about your medicine and its use, check with your doctor, nurse, or pharmacist. **Remember, keep this and all other medicines out of the reach of children and never share your medicines with others.**

BEFORE USING THIS MEDICINE

Tell your doctor, nurse, and pharmacist if you . . .

- are allergic to any medicine, either prescription or nonprescription (OTC);
- are pregnant or intend to become pregnant while using this medicine;
- are breast-feeding;
- are taking any other prescription or nonprescription (OTC) medicine;
- have any other medical problems.

PROPER USE OF THIS MEDICINE

Ipratropium is used to help control the symptoms of lung diseases, such as chronic bronchitis, emphysema, and asthma. However, for treatment of bronchospasm or asthma attacks that have already started, ipratropium inhalation solution is used only in a nebulizer and in combination with other bronchodilators.

It is very important that you use ipratropium only as directed. Do not use more of it and do not use it more often than your doctor ordered. To do so may increase the chance of serious side effects.

Keep the spray or solution away from the eyes because this medicine may cause irritation or blurred vision. Closing your eyes while you are inhaling ipratropium may help keep the medicine out of your eyes. Rinsing your eyes with cool water may help if any medicine does get in your eyes.

Ipratropium usually comes with patient directions. Read them carefully before using this medicine.

For patients using ipratropium inhalation aerosol:
- If you do not understand the directions or you are not sure how to use the inhaler, ask your doctor, nurse, or pharmacist to show you how to use it. Also, ask your doctor, nurse, or pharmacist to check regularly how you use the inhaler to make sure you are using it properly.

For patients using ipratropium inhalation solution:
- Use this medicine only in a power-operated nebulizer with an adequate flow rate and equipped with a face mask or mouthpiece. Your doctor will tell you which nebulizer to use. Make sure you understand exactly how to use it. If you have any questions about this, check with your doctor.

For patients using ipratropium regularly (for example, every day):
- **In order for ipratropium to work properly, it must be inhaled every day in regularly spaced doses as directed by your doctor.**

If you use ipratropium inhalation regularly and you miss a dose, use it as soon as possible. Then use any remaining doses for that day at regularly spaced times.

PRECAUTIONS WHILE USING THIS MEDICINE

Check with your doctor at once if your symptoms do not improve within 30 minutes after using a dose of this medicine or if your condition gets worse.

For patients using ipratropium inhalation solution:
- **If you are also using cromolyn inhalation solution, do not mix that solution with the ipratropium inhalation solution from the 20-mL multiple-dose vial for use in a nebulizer.** To do so will cause the solution to become cloudy and prevent the cromolyn from working as well as it should. However, if your doctor has told you to use cromolyn inhalation solution with ipratropium inhalation solution, it may be mixed with ipratropium inhalation solution from the 2-mL single-dose vial.

POSSIBLE SIDE EFFECTS OF THIS MEDICINE

Side effects that should be reported to your doctor

> LESS COMMON—Increased wheezing, tighness in chest, or difficulty breathing
>
> RARE—Difficulty in swallowing, eye pain (severe); skin rash or hives; swelling of tongue or lips; ulcers or sores in mouth and on lips

Side effects that usually do not require medical attention

> These possible side effects may go away during treatment; however, if they continue or are bothersome, check with your doctor, nurse, or pharmacist.
>
> MORE COMMON—Cough or dryness of mouth or throat; headache or dizziness; nervousness; stomach upset or nausea
>
> LESS COMMON OR RARE—Blurred vision or other changes in vision; constipation (continuing); difficult urination; metallic or unpleasant taste; pounding heartbeat; stuffy nose; trembling; trouble in sleeping; unusual tiredness or weakness
>
> Other side effects not listed above may also occur in some patients. If you notice any other effects, check with your doctor, nurse, or pharmacist.

IRON SUPPLEMENTS (ORAL)

Including Ferrous Fumarate; Ferrous Gluconate; Ferrous Sulfate; Iron-Polysaccharide

ABOUT YOUR DIETARY SUPPLEMENT

Iron is a mineral that the body needs to produce red blood cells. When the body does not get enough iron, it cannot produce the number of normal red blood cells needed to keep you in good health. This condition is called iron-deficiency (iron shortage) or iron-deficiency anemia.

Although many people in the U.S. get enough iron from their diet, some must take additional amounts to meet their needs. Only your doctor can determine if you have an iron deficiency, and if an iron supplement is necessary.

Lack of iron may lead to unusual tiredness, shortness of breath, a decrease in physical performance, learning problems in children, and may increase your chance of getting an infection. The best sources of absorbable iron are lean red meat, chicken, turkey, and fish.

If any of the information in this profile causes you special concern or if you want additional information about your dietary supplement and its use, check with your doctor, nurse, dietitian, or pharmacist. **Remember, keep this and all other** medicines out of the reach of children and never share your medicines with others.

BEFORE USING THIS DIETARY SUPPLEMENT

Tell your doctor, nurse, and pharmacist if you . . .
- are allergic to any medicine, either prescription or nonprescription (OTC);
- are pregnant or intend to become pregnant while using this medicine;
- are breast-feeding;
- are taking any other prescription or nonprescription (OTC) medicine, especially acetohydroxamic acid, dimercaprol, etidronate, or tetracyclines;
- have any other medical problems, especially blood disease.

PROPER USE OF THIS DIETARY SUPPLEMENT

After you start using this dietary supplement, continue to visit your doctor to see if you are benefitting from the iron. Some blood tests may be necessary.

Iron is best taken on an empty stomach, with water or fruit juice, about 1 hour before or 2 hours after meals. However, to lessen the possibility of stomach upset, iron may be taken with food or immediately after meals. If this is done, certain foods should not be taken at the same time as iron. These include cheese, eggs, milk, tea, coffee, spinach, whole-grain breads and cereals, bran, and yogurt.

If you miss a dose of this medicine, skip the missed dose and go back to your regular dosing schedule. Do not double doses.

PRECAUTIONS WHILE USING THIS DIETARY SUPPLEMENT

Do not take iron supplements and antacids or calcium supplements at the same time. It is best to space doses of these two products 1 to 2 hours apart.

Keep iron supplements out of the reach of children since overdose is very dangerous in children and may cause death. As few as 3 adult iron tablets can cause serious poisoning in small children. **If you think an overdose has been taken:**
- **Immediate medical attention is very important. Call your doctor, a poison control center, or the nearest hospital emergency room at once.**
- **Follow any instructions given to you.** If ipecac syrup has been ordered and given, do not delay going to the emergency room while waiting for the ipecac to empty the stomach. It may require 20 to 30 minutes to show results.
- **Go to the emergency room without delay, taking the container of iron medicine with you.** Early signs of iron overdose may not occur for up to 60 minutes or more after the overdose was taken. By this time emergency treatment should be obtained.

POSSIBLE SIDE EFFECTS OF THIS DIETARY SUPPLEMENT

Side effects that should be reported to your doctor

MORE COMMON—Abdominal or stomach pain or cramping

LESS COMMON OR RARE—Chest or throat pain, especially when swallowing; stools with signs of blood

Early signs of iron poisoning include diarrhea (may contain blood), nausea, stomach pain (sharp), and severe vomiting (may contain blood).

Late signs of iron poisoning include bluish-colored lips, fingernails, and palms; convulsions (seizures); drowsiness; pale, clammy skin; unusual weakness; and weak and fast heartbeat.

Side effects that usually do not require medical attention

These possible side effects may go away during treatment; however, if they continue or are bothersome, check with your doctor, nurse, or pharmacist.

MORE COMMON—Constipation; diarrhea; nausea; vomiting

LESS COMMON—Dark urine; heartburn; staining of teeth (liquid dosage forms)

Stools commonly become dark green or black when iron preparations are taken by mouth. However, in rare cases, black stools of a sticky consistency may occur along with other symptoms such as red streaks in the stool, cramping, soreness, or sharp pains in the stomach or abdominal area. **Check with your doctor immediately** if these signs appear.

Other side effects not listed above may also occur in some patients. If you notice any other effects, check with your doctor, nurse, or pharmacist.

$\mathcal{I}$SONIAZID (ORAL)

ABOUT YOUR MEDICINE

Isoniazid (eye-soe-NYE-a-zid) is used to prevent or treat tuberculosis (TB). It may be given alone to prevent, or, in combination with other medicines, to treat TB. This medicine may also be used for other problems as determined by your doctor.

If you are being treated for active tuberculosis (TB): To help clear up your TB completely, you must keep taking this medicine for the full time of treatment, even if you begin to feel better. This is very important. It is also important that you do not miss any doses.

If any of the information in this profile causes you special concern or if you want additional information about your medicine and its use, check with your doctor,

nurse, or pharmacist. **Remember, keep this and all other medicines out of the reach of children and never share your medicines with others.**

BEFORE USING THIS MEDICINE

This medicine may cause some serious side effects, including damage to the liver. Liver damage is more likely to occur in patients over 50 years of age. **You and your doctor should talk about the good this medicine will do, as well as the risks of taking it.**

Tell your doctor, nurse, and pharmacist if you . . .
- are allergic to any medicine, either prescription or nonprescription (OTC);
- are pregnant or intend to become pregnant while using this medicine;
- are breast-feeding;
- are taking **any** other prescription or nonprescription (OTC) medicine;
- have any other medical problems, especially alcohol abuse (or history of) or liver disease.

PROPER USE OF THIS MEDICINE

If isoniazid upsets your stomach, take it with food. Antacids may also help. However, do not take aluminum-containing antacids within 1 hour of taking isoniazid. They may keep this medicine from working properly.

To help clear up your tuberculosis (TB) completely, **it is very important that you keep taking this medicine for the full time of treatment** even if you begin to feel better after a few weeks. You may have to take it every day for as long as 6 months to 2 years. **It is important that you do not miss any doses.**

Your doctor may also want you to take pyridoxine (e.g., Hexa-Betalin, vitamin B$_6$) every day to help prevent or lessen some of the side effects of isoniazid. If it is needed, **it is very important to take pyridoxine every day along with this medicine. Do not miss any doses.**

If you do miss a dose of this medicine, take it as soon as possible. However, if it is almost time for your next dose, skip the missed dose and go back to your regular dosing schedule. Do not double doses.

PRECAUTIONS WHILE USING THIS MEDICINE

It is very important that your doctor check your progress at regular visits. Also, **check with your doctor immediately if blurred vision or loss of vision, with or without eye pain, occurs during treatment.** Your doctor may want you to have your eyes checked by an ophthalmologist (eye doctor).

If your symptoms do not improve within 2 to 3 weeks, or if they become worse, check with your doctor.

Liver problems may be more likely to occur if you drink alcoholic beverages regularly while you are taking isoniazid. Also, the regular use of alcohol may keep this medicine from working properly. **Therefore, you should strictly** limit the amount of alcoholic beverages you drink while you are taking isoniazid.

If isoniazid causes you to feel very tired or very weak, or causes clumsiness; unsteadiness; loss of appetite; nausea; numbness, tingling, burning, or pain in the hands and feet; or vomiting, check with your doctor immediately. These may be early warning signs of more serious liver or nerve problems that could develop later.

Diabetics—This medicine may cause false test results with some urine sugar tests. Check with your doctor before changing your diet or the dosage of your diabetes medicine.

POSSIBLE SIDE EFFECTS OF THIS MEDICINE

Side effects that should be reported to your doctor immediately

MORE COMMON—Clumsiness or unsteadiness; dark urine; loss of appetite; nausea or vomiting; numbness, tingling, burning, or pain in hands and feet; unusual tiredness or weakness; yellow eyes or skin

RARE—Blurred vision or loss of vision, with or without eye pain; convulsions (seizures); fever and sore throat; joint pain; mood or other mental changes; skin rash; unusual bleeding or bruising

Side effects that usually do not require medical attention

These possible side effects may go away during treatment; however, if they continue or are bothersome, check with your doctor, nurse, or pharmacist.

MORE COMMON—Diarrhea; stomach pain

Other side effects not listed above may also occur in some patients. If you notice any other effects, check with your doctor, nurse, or pharmacist.

*I*SOTRETINOIN (ORAL)

ABOUT YOUR MEDICINE

Isotretinoin (eye-soe-TRET-i-noyn) is taken by mouth to treat severe, disfiguring nodular acne. It should be used only after other acne medicines have been tried and have failed to help the acne. Isotretinoin also may be used to treat other skin diseases as determined by your doctor.

Isotretinoin must not be used in women who are able to bear children unless other forms of treatment have been tried first and have failed. Isotretinoin must not be taken during pregnancy, because it causes birth defects in humans. If you are able to bear children, it is very important that you read, understand, and follow the pregnancy warnings for isotretinoin.

If any of the information in this profile causes you special concern or if you want additional information about your medicine and its use, check with your doctor, nurse, or pharmacist. **Remember, keep this and all other medicines out of the reach of children and never share your medicines with others.**

BEFORE USING THIS MEDICINE

Isotretinoin comes with patient information. It is very important that you read and understand this information. Be sure to ask your doctor about anything you do not understand.

Isotretinoin causes birth defects in humans. It must not be taken during pregnancy or if there is a chance that you may become pregnant during treatment or within one month following treatment. Isotretinoin must not be taken unless an effective form of contraception (birth control) is used for at least 1 month before the beginning of treatment. Contraception must be continued during the period of treatment, which is up to 20 weeks, and for 1 month after isotretinoin is stopped. Be sure you have discussed this information with your doctor. In addition, you will be asked to sign an informed consent form stating that you understand the above information.

Tell your doctor, nurse, and pharmacist if you . . .
- are allergic to any medicine, either prescription or nonprescription (OTC);
- **are pregnant or may become pregnant while using this medicine;**
- are breast-feeding;
- are taking any other prescription or nonprescription (OTC) medicine, especially etretinate, tetracyclines, tretinoin, or vitamin A;
- have any other medical problems.

PROPER USE OF THIS MEDICINE

It is very important that you take isotretinoin only as directed. Do not take more of it, do not take it more often, and do not take it for a longer time than your doctor ordered. To do so may increase the chance of side effects.

If you miss a dose of this medicine, take it as soon as possible. However, if it is almost time for your next dose, skip the missed dose and go back to your regular dosing schedule. Do not double doses.

PRECAUTIONS WHILE USING THIS MEDICINE

Isotretinoin causes birth defects in humans if taken during pregnancy. Therefore, if you suspect that you may have become pregnant, stop taking this medicine immediately and check with your doctor.

Do not donate blood to a blood bank while you are taking isotretinoin or for 30 days after you stop taking it. This is to prevent the possibility of a pregnant patient receiving the blood.

Do not take vitamin A or any vitamin supplement containing vitamin A while taking this medicine, unless otherwise directed by your doctor.

Drinking too much alcohol while taking isotretinoin may increase the chance of unwanted effects on the heart and blood vessels. **It is best that you do not drink alcoholic beverages or that you at least reduce the amount you usually drink.**

In some patients, isotretinoin may cause a decrease in night vision. This decrease may occur suddenly. If it does occur, **do not drive, use machines, or do other jobs that require you to see well.** Also, check with your doctor.

POSSIBLE SIDE EFFECTS OF THIS MEDICINE

Side effects that should be reported to your doctor

MORE COMMON—Burning, redness, itching, or other sign of eye inflammation; nosebleeds; scaling, redness, burning, pain, or other sign of inflammation of lips

LESS COMMON—Mental depression; skin infection or rash

RARE—Abdominal or stomach pain (severe); bleeding or inflammation of gums; blurred vision or other changes in vision; diarrhea (severe); headache (severe or continuing); mood changes; nausea and vomiting; pain or tenderness of eyes; rectal bleeding; yellow eyes or skin

Side effects that usually do not require medical attention

These possible side effects may go away during treatment; however, if they continue or are bothersome, check with your doctor, nurse, or pharmacist.

MORE COMMON—Dryness of mouth or nose; dryness or itching of skin

Other side effects not listed above may also occur in some patients. If you notice any other effects, check with your doctor, nurse, or pharmacist.

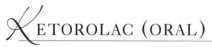

KETOROLAC (ORAL)

ABOUT YOUR MEDICINE

Ketorolac (kee-TOE-role-ak) is used to relieve pain. It belongs to the group of medicines called anti-inflammatory analgesics. Ketorolac is not a narcotic and is not habit-forming. It will not cause physical or mental dependence, as narcotics can. However, ketorolac is sometimes used together with a narcotic to provide better pain relief than either medicine used alone.

If any of the information in this profile causes you special concern or if you want additional information about your medicine and its use, check with your doctor, nurse, or pharmacist. **Remember, keep this and all other medicines out of the reach of children and never share your medicines with others.**

Before Using This Medicine

Tell your doctor, nurse, and pharmacist if you . . .
- are allergic to any medicine, either prescription or nonprescription (OTC);
- are pregnant or intend to become pregnant while using this medicine;
- are breast-feeding;
- are taking any other prescription or nonprescription (OTC) medicine, especially anticoagulants; aspirin or other salicylates or other medicines for pain or inflammation, except narcotics; cefamandole; cefoperazone; cefotetan; heparin; lithium; methotrexate; moxalactam; plicamycin; probenecid; or valproic acid;
- have any other medical problems, especially colitis, stomach ulcer, or other stomach problems; hemophilia or other bleeding problems; or kidney disease;
- smoke tobacco.

Proper Use of This Medicine

To lessen stomach upset, ketoralac tablets should be taken with food (a meal or a snack) or with an antacid. However, your doctor may want you to take the first few doses 30 minutes before meals or 2 hours after meals. This helps the medicine work a little faster when you first begin to take it.

Take this medicine with a full glass of water. Also, do not lie down for about 15 to 30 minutes after taking it. This helps to prevent irritation that may lead to trouble in swallowing.

For safe and effective use of this medicine, do not take more of it, do not take it more often, and do not take it for a longer time than ordered by your doctor. Taking too much of this medicine increases the chance of unwanted effects, especially in elderly patients.

If you have been directed to take this medicine according to a regular schedule, and you miss a dose, take it as soon as possible. However, if it is almost time for your next dose, skip the missed dose and go back to your regular dosing schedule. Do not double doses.

Precautions While Using This Medicine

Ketorolac may cause some people to become dizzy or drowsy. If either of these side effects occurs, **do not drive, use machines, or do other jobs that require you to be alert.**

Possible Side Effects of This Medicine

Side effects that should be reported to your doctor immediately
> RARE—Bleeding or crusting sores on lips; blue lips and fingernails; chest pain; convulsions; fainting; shortness of breath, fast, irregular, noisy, or troubled breathing, tightness in chest, or wheezing; vomiting of blood or material that looks like coffee grounds

Other side effects that should be reported to your doctor

LESS COMMON—Swelling of face, fingers, lower legs, ankles, and/or feet; weight gain (unusual)

RARE—Abdominal or stomach pain, cramping, or burning (severe); bleeding from rectum or bloody or black, tarry stools; bloody or cloudy urine; bruising or small red spots on skin; burning, red, tender, thick, scaly, or peeling skin; decrease in amount of urine (sudden); fever with or without chills or sore throat; hallucinations; hives or itching of skin; increased blood pressure; muscle cramps or pain; nausea, heartburn, or indigestion (severe and continuing); nosebleeds; pain in lower back or side; puffiness or swelling of the eyelids or around eyes; skin rash; sores, ulcers, or white spots on lips or in mouth; swollen or painful glands; swollen tongue; thirst (continuing); unusual tiredness or weakness

Side effects that usually do not require medical attention

These possible side effects may go away during treatment; however, if they continue or are bothersome, check with your doctor, nurse, or pharmacist.

MORE COMMON—Abdominal or stomach pain (mild or moderate); drowsiness; indigestion; nausea

LESS COMMON—Bloating or gas; constipation; diarrhea; dizziness; feeling of fullness in abdominal or stomach area; headache; increased sweating; vomiting

Other side effects not listed above may also occur in some patients. If you notice any other effects, check with your doctor, nurse, or pharmacist.

ℒAXATIVES, BULK-FORMING (ORAL)

Including Malt Soup Extract; Malt
Soup Extract and Psyllium; Methylcellulose;
Polycarbophil; Psyllium; Psyllium Hydrophilic Mucilloid;
Psyllium Hydrophilic Mucilloid and Carboxymethylcellulose

ABOUT YOUR MEDICINE

Oral **bulk-forming laxatives** are medicines taken by mouth to encourage bowel movements and relieve constipation.

Bulk-forming laxatives may be used to provide relief:

- during pregnancy.
- for a few days after giving birth.
- for constipation of bedfast patients.

- for constipation caused by other medicines.
- following surgery when straining should be avoided.
- for some medical conditions that may be made worse by straining, for example, heart disease, hemorrhoids, hernia (rupture), high blood pressure, or history of stroke.

Laxative products are overused by many people. Such a practice (the "laxative habit") often leads to dependence on the laxative action to produce a bowel movement. In severe cases, overuse of some laxatives has caused damage to the nerves, muscles, and tissues of the intestines and bowel. If you have any questions about the use of laxatives, check with your doctor or pharmacist.

If any of the information in this profile causes you special concern or if you want additional information about your medicine and its use, check with your doctor, nurse, or pharmacist. **Remember, keep this and all other medicines out of the reach of children and never share your medicines with others.**

BEFORE USING THIS MEDICINE

Laxatives should not be given to young children (up to 6 years of age) unless prescribed by their doctor. The child may have a condition that needs other treatment. If so, laxatives will not help, and may even cause unwanted effects or make the condition worse.

If you are taking this medicine without a prescription, carefully read and follow any precautions on the label. You should be especially careful if you . . .
- are allergic to any medicine, either prescription or nonprescription (OTC);
- are pregnant, intend to become pregnant, or are breast-feeding;
- are taking any other prescription or nonprescription (OTC) medicine, especially tetracyclines (for polycarbophil);
- have any other medical problems, especially appendicitis (or signs of), diabetes mellitus (sugar diabetes), heart disease, high blood pressure, intestinal blockage, rectal bleeding of unknown cause, or swallowing difficulty.

If you have any questions, check with your doctor, nurse, or pharmacist.

PROPER USE OF THIS MEDICINE

In order for this medicine to work properly it should be taken with a full glass (8 ounces) of water. You should drink at least 6 to 8 full glasses of water every day while you are using this medicine.

Do not try to swallow this medicine in the dry form. Mix with liquid.

Results usually occur within 12 hours, but may not occur for some individuals until after 2 or 3 days.

PRECAUTIONS WHILE USING THIS MEDICINE

Do not take a laxative:
- if you have signs of appendicitis or inflamed bowel.
- for more than 1 week.
- within 2 hours of taking other medicine.
- if you do not need it.
- if you miss a bowel movement for a day or two.
- if you develop a skin rash.

If you notice a sudden change in bowel habits or function that lasts longer than 2 weeks, or that keeps returning off and on, check with your doctor before using a laxative. This will allow the cause of your problem to be determined before it may become more serious.

Many laxatives contain large amounts of sugars, carbohydrates, and sodium. If you are on a low-sugar, low-calorie, or low-sodium diet, check with your doctor or pharmacist before using a laxative.

POSSIBLE SIDE EFFECTS OF THIS MEDICINE

Side effects that should be reported to your doctor

Difficulty in breathing; intestinal blockage; skin rash or itching; swallowing difficulty (feeling of lump in throat)

Other side effects not listed above may also occur in some patients. If you notice any other effects, check with your doctor, nurse, or pharmacist.

LAXATIVES, BULK-FORMING AND STIMULANT COMBINATION (ORAL)

Including Psyllium and Senna; Psyllium Hydrophilic Mucilloid and Senna; Psyllium Hydrophilic Mucilloid and Sennosides

ABOUT YOUR MEDICINE

Oral **bulk-forming** and **stimulant combination laxatives** are taken by mouth to encourage bowel movements and relieve constipation.

Laxative products are overused by many people. Such a practice often leads to dependence on the laxative action to produce a bowel movement. In severe cases, overuse of some laxatives has caused damage to the nerves, muscles, and tissues of the intestines and bowel.

If any of the information in this profile causes you special concern or if you want additional information about your medicine and its use, check with your doctor, nurse, or pharmacist. **Remember, keep this and all other medicines out of the reach of children and never share your medicines with others.**

BEFORE USING THIS MEDICINE

Laxatives should not be given to young children (up to 6 years of age) unless prescribed by their doctor. The child may have a condition that needs other treatment. If so, laxatives will not help, and may even cause unwanted effects or make the condition worse.

If you are taking this medicine without a prescription, carefully read and follow any precautions on the label. You should be especially careful if you . . .
- are allergic to any medicine, either prescription or nonprescription (OTC);
- are pregnant, intend to become pregnant, or are breast-feeding;
- are taking any other prescription or nonprescription (OTC) medicine;
- have any other medical problems, especially appendicitis (or signs of), diabetes mellitus (sugar diabetes), heart disease, high blood pressure, intestinal blockage, rectal bleeding of unknown cause, or swallowing difficulty.

PROPER USE OF THIS MEDICINE

Do not try to swallow this medicine in the dry form. Take with liquid.

To allow this laxative to work properly and to prevent intestinal blockage, it is necessary to drink plenty of fluids during its use. Each dose should be taken in or with a full glass (8 ounces) or more of cold water or fruit juice. This will provide enough liquid for the laxative to work properly. A second glass of water or juice by itself is often recommended with each dose. In addition, at least 6 to 8 full glasses of liquids should be taken each day.

Stimulant-containing laxatives are often taken at bedtime to produce results the next morning.

PRECAUTIONS WHILE USING THIS MEDICINE

Do not take a laxative:
- **if you have signs of appendicitis or inflamed bowel.**
- **for more than 1 week.**
- **within 2 hours of taking other medicine.**
- **if you do not need it.**
- **if you miss a bowel movement for a day or two.**
- **if you develop a skin rash.**

If you notice a sudden change in bowel habits or function that lasts longer than 2 weeks, or that keeps returning off and on, check with your doctor before using a laxative. This will allow the cause of your problem to be determined before it may become more serious.

Many laxatives contain large amounts of sugars, carbohydrates, and sodium. If you are on a low-sugar, low-calorie, or low-sodium diet, check with your doctor or pharmacist before using a laxative.

POSSIBLE SIDE EFFECTS OF THIS MEDICINE

Side effects that should be reported to your doctor

Confusion; difficulty in breathing; intestinal blockage; irregular heartbeat; muscle cramps; pink to red, red to violet, or red to brown coloration of alkaline urine (for senna only); skin rash or itching; swallowing difficulty (feeling of lump in throat); unusual tiredness or weakness; yellow to brown coloration of acid urine (for senna only)

Side effects that usually do not require medical attention

These possible side effects may go away during treatment; however, if they continue or are bothersome, check with your doctor, nurse, or pharmacist.

Belching; cramping; diarrhea; nausea

Other side effects not listed above may also occur in some patients. If you notice any other effects, check with your doctor, nurse, or pharmacist.

LAXATIVES, STIMULANT (ORAL)

Including Bisacodyl; Casanthranol; Cascara Sagrada; Cascara Sagrada and Aloe; Cascara Sagrada and Phenolphthalein; Castor Oil; Dehydrocholic Acid; Phenolphthalein; Phenolphthalein and Senna; Senna; Sennosides

ABOUT YOUR MEDICINE

Oral **stimulant laxatives** are taken by mouth to encourage bowel movements and relieve constipation. Stimulant laxatives are a popular type of laxative for self-treatment. However, they also are more likely to cause side effects. One of the stimulant laxatives, dehydrocholic acid, may also be used for treating certain conditions of the biliary tract.

Stimulant laxatives may cause unwanted effects in the expectant mother if improperly used. Castor oil in particular should not be used as it may cause contractions of the womb.

Laxative products are overused by many people. Such a practice often leads to dependence on the laxative action to produce a bowel movement. In severe cases, overuse of some laxatives has caused damage to the nerves, muscles, and tissues of the intestines and bowel.

If any of the information in this profile causes you special concern or if you want additional information about your medicine and its use, check with your doctor, nurse, or pharmacist. **Remember, keep this and all other medicines out of the reach of children and never share your medicines with others.**

BEFORE USING THIS MEDICINE

Laxatives should not be given to young children (up to 6 years of age) unless prescribed by their doctor. The child may have a condition that needs other treatment. If so, laxatives will not help and may even cause unwanted effects or make the condition worse.

If you are taking this medicine without a prescription, carefully read and follow any precautions on the label. You should be especially careful if you . . .

- are allergic to any medicine, either prescription or nonprescription (OTC);
- are pregnant, intend to become pregnant, or are breast-feeding;
- are taking any other prescription or nonprescription (OTC) medicine;
- have any other medical problems, especially appendicitis (or signs of), diabetes mellitus (sugar diabetes), heart disease, high blood pressure, intestinal blockage, or rectal bleeding of unknown cause.

PROPER USE OF THIS MEDICINE

Stimulant laxatives are usually taken on an empty stomach for rapid effect. Results are slowed if taken with food. Also, at least 6 to 8 glasses (8 ounces each) of liquids should be taken each day. This will help make the stool softer.

Many stimulant laxatives (but not castor oil) are taken at bedtime to produce results the next morning (some may require 24 hours or more). **Castor oil** is not usually taken late in the day because its results occur within 2 to 6 hours.

The unpleasant taste of **castor oil** may be improved by chilling in the refrigerator for at least an hour and then stirring the dose into a full glass of cold orange juice just before it is taken. Also, flavored preparations of castor oil are available.

Bisacodyl tablets are specially coated to prevent irritation. Do not chew or crush the tablets or take them within an hour of milk or antacids.

Because of the way **phenolphthalein** works in the body, a single dose may cause a laxative effect in some people for up to 3 days.

PRECAUTIONS WHILE USING THIS MEDICINE

Do not take a laxative:
- **if you have signs of appendicitis or inflamed bowel.**
- **for more than 1 week.**
- **within 2 hours of taking other medicine.**
- **if you do not need it.**

- if you miss a bowel movement for a day or two.
- if you develop a skin rash.

If you notice a sudden change in bowel habits or function that lasts longer than 2 weeks, or that keeps returning off and on, check with your doctor before using a laxative. This will allow the cause of your problem to be determined before it may become more serious.

Many laxatives contain large amounts of sugars, carbohydrates, and sodium. If you are on a low-sugar, low-calorie, or low-sodium diet, check with your doctor or pharmacist before using a laxative.

POSSIBLE SIDE EFFECTS OF THIS MEDICINE

Side effects that should be reported to your doctor

Confusion; irregular heartbeat; muscle cramps; pink to red coloration of alkaline urine and stools (for phenolphthalein only); pink to red, red to violet, or red to brown coloration of alkaline urine (for cascara or senna only); skin rash; unusual tiredness or weakness; yellow to brown coloration of acid urine (for cascara, phenolphthalein, or senna only)

Side effects that usually do not require medical attention

These possible side effects may go away during treatment; however, if they continue or are bothersome, check with your doctor, nurse, or pharmacist.

Belching; cramping; diarrhea; nausea

Other side effects not listed above may also occur in some patients. If you notice any other effects, check with your doctor, nurse, or pharmacist.

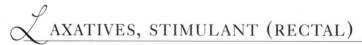

LAXATIVES, STIMULANT (RECTAL)

Including Bisacodyl; Senna

ABOUT YOUR MEDICINE

Rectal **stimulant laxatives** are used as enemas or suppositories to produce bowel movements in a short time.

Rectal laxatives may provide relief in a number of situations such as:
- before giving birth.
- for a few days after giving birth.
- preparation for examination or surgery.
- following surgery when straining should be avoided.
- constipation caused by other medicines.

Laxative products are overused by many people. Such a practice often leads to dependence on the laxative action to produce a bowel movement. In severe cases, overuse of some laxatives has caused damage to the nerves, muscles, and tissues of the intestines and bowel.

If any of the information in this profile causes you special concern or if you want additional information about your medicine and its use, check with your doctor, nurse, or pharmacist. **Remember, keep this and all other medicines out of the reach of children and never share your medicines with others.**

BEFORE USING THIS MEDICINE

Laxatives should not be given to young children (up to 6 years of age) unless prescribed by their doctor. The child may have a condition that needs other treatment. If so, laxatives will not help and may even cause unwanted effects or make the condition worse.

If you are using this medicine without a prescription, carefully read and follow any precautions on the label. You should be especially careful if you . . .
- are allergic to any medicine, either prescription or nonprescription (OTC);
- are pregnant, intend to become pregnant, or are breast-feeding;
- are taking any other prescription or nonprescription (OTC) medicine;
- have any other medical problems, especially appendicitis (or signs of), intestinal blockage, or rectal bleeding of unknown causes.

If you have any questions, check with your doctor, nurse, or pharmacist.

PROPER USE OF THIS MEDICINE

For patients using the enema or rectal solution form of this medicine:
- This medicine usually comes with patient directions. Read them carefully before using this medicine.
- Lubricate the anus with petroleum jelly before inserting the applicator.
- Gently insert the rectal tip of the enema applicator to prevent damage to the rectal wall.

For patients using the suppository form of this medicine:
- If the suppository is too soft to insert, chill the suppository in the refrigerator for 30 minutes or run cold water over it, before removing the foil wrapper.
- To insert suppository: First remove the foil wrapper and moisten the suppository with cold water. Lie down on your side and use your finger to push the suppository well up into the rectum.

Results often may be obtained with bisacodyl enemas or suppositories in 15 minutes to 1 hour, or with senna enemas or suppositories in 30 minutes, but results may not occur in some individuals for up to 2 hours.

PRECAUTIONS WHILE USING THIS MEDICINE

Do not use a laxative:
- if you have signs of appendicitis or inflamed bowel.
- more often than your doctor prescribed. This is true even when you have had no results from the laxative.
- if you do not need it.
- if you miss a bowel movement for a day or two.

If you notice a sudden change in bowel habits or function that lasts longer than 2 weeks, or keeps returning off and on, check with your doctor before using a laxative. This will allow the cause of your problem to be determined before it becomes more serious.

For patients using the enema or rectal solution form of this medicine:
- Check with your doctor if you notice rectal bleeding, blistering, pain, burning, itching, or other sign of irritation not present before you started using this medicine.

POSSIBLE SIDE EFFECTS OF THIS MEDICINE

Side effects that should be reported to your doctor

LESS COMMON—Rectal bleeding, blistering, burning, itching, or pain (with enemas only)

Side effects that usually do not require medical attention

These possible side effects may go away during treatment; however, if they continue or are bothersome, check with your doctor, nurse, or pharmacist.

LESS COMMON—Skin irritation surrounding rectal area

Other side effects not listed above may also occur in some patients. If you notice any other effects, check with your doctor, nurse, or pharmacist.

LAXATIVES, STIMULANT AND STOOL SOFTENER COMBINATION (ORAL)

Including Bisacodyl and Docusate; Casanthranol and Docusate; Danthron and Docusate; Dehydrocholic Acid and Docusate; Dehydrocholic Acid, Docusate, and Phenolphthalein; Docusate and Phenolphthalein; Senna and Docusate

ABOUT YOUR MEDICINE

Oral **stimulant and stool softener combination laxatives** are taken by mouth to encourage bowel movements and relieve constipation.

Laxative products are overused by many people. Such a practice often leads to dependence on the laxative action to produce a bowel movement. In severe cases, overuse of some laxatives has caused damage to the nerves, muscles, and tissues of the intestines and bowel.

If any of the information in this profile causes you special concern or if you want additional information about your medicine and its use, check with your doctor, nurse, or pharmacist. **Remember, keep this and all other medicines out of the reach of children and never share your medicines with others.**

BEFORE USING THIS MEDICINE

Laxatives should not be given to young children (up to 6 years of age) unless prescribed by their doctor. The child may have a condition that needs other treatment. If so, laxatives will not help, and may even cause unwanted effects or make the condition worse.

If you are taking this medicine without a prescription, carefully read and follow any precautions on the label. You should be especially careful if you . . .
- are allergic to any medicine, either prescription or nonprescription (OTC);
- are pregnant, intend to become pregnant, or are breast-feeding;
- are taking any other prescription or nonprescription (OTC) medicine;
- have any other medical problems, especially appendicitis (or signs of), diabetes mellitus (sugar diabetes), heart disease, high blood pressure, intestinal blockage, or rectal bleeding of unknown cause.

PROPER USE OF THIS MEDICINE

At least 6 to 8 glasses (8 ounces each) of liquids should be taken each day. This will help make the stool softer.

Stimulant-containing laxatives are often taken at bedtime to produce results the next morning.

Liquid forms of stool softener–containing laxatives may be taken in milk or fruit juice to improve flavor.

Bisacodyl-containing tablets are specially coated to prevent irritation. Do not chew, crush, or take the tablets within an hour of milk or antacids.

PRECAUTIONS WHILE USING THIS MEDICINE

Do not take a laxative:
- **if you have signs of appendicitis or inflamed bowel.**
- **for more than 1 week.**
- **within 2 hours of taking other medicine.**
- **if you do not need it.**
- **if you miss a bowel movement for a day or two.**
- **if you develop a skin rash.**

Many laxatives contain large amounts of sugars, carbohydrates, and sodium. If you are on a low-sugar, low-calorie, or low-sodium diet, check with your doctor or pharmacist before using a laxative.

If you notice a sudden change in bowel habits or function that lasts longer than 2 weeks, or that keeps returning off and on, check with your doctor before using a laxative. This will allow the cause of your problem to be determined before it may become more serious.

POSSIBLE SIDE EFFECTS OF THIS MEDICINE

Side effects that should be reported to your doctor

Confusion; irregular heartbeat; muscle cramps; pink to red coloration of alkaline urine and stools (for phenolphthalein only); pink to red, red to violet, or red to brown coloration of alkaline urine (for danthron and/or senna only); skin rash; unusual tiredness or weakness; yellow to brown coloration of acid urine (for phenolphthalein or senna only)

Side effects that usually do not require medical attention

These possible side effects may go away during treatment; however, if they continue or are bothersome, check with your doctor, nurse, or pharmacist.

Belching; diarrhea; nausea; stomach or intestinal cramping; throat irritation (liquid forms only)

Other side effects not listed above may also occur in some patients. If you notice any other effects, check with your doctor, nurse, or pharmacist.

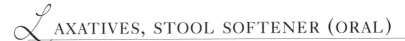 AXATIVES, STOOL SOFTENER (ORAL)

Including Docusate; Poloxamer 188

About Your Medicine

Oral **stool softeners** are medicines taken by mouth to *allow* the patient to have a bowel movement without straining. They do not *cause* a bowel movement.

Stool softeners may be used to provide relief:
- during pregnancy.
- for a few days after giving birth.
- for constipation of bedfast patients.
- for constipation caused by other medicines.
- following surgery when straining should be avoided.
- for some medical conditions that may be made worse by straining, for example, heart disease, hemorrhoids, hernia (rupture), high blood pressure, or history of stroke.

If any of the information in this profile causes you special concern or if you want additional information about your medicine and its use, check with your doctor, nurse, or pharmacist. **Remember, keep this and all other medicines out of the reach of children and never share your medicines with others.**

Before Using This Medicine

Laxatives should not be given to young children (up to 6 years of age) unless prescribed by their doctor. The child may have a condition that needs other treatment. If so, laxatives will not help and may even cause unwanted effects or make the condition worse.

If you are taking this medicine without a prescription, carefully read and follow any precautions on the label. You should be especially careful if you . . .
- are allergic to any medicine, either prescription or nonprescription (OTC);
- are pregnant, intend to become pregnant, or are breast-feeding;
- are taking any other prescription or nonprescription (OTC) medicine;
- have any other medical problems, especially appendicitis (or signs of), diabetes mellitus (sugar diabetes), heart disease, high blood pressure, intestinal blockage, or rectal bleeding of unknown cause.

If you have any questions, check with your doctor, nurse, or pharmacist.

Broper Use of This Medicine

At least 6 to 8 glasses (8 ounces each) of liquids should be taken each day. This will help make the stool softer.

Liquid forms may be taken in milk or fruit juice to improve flavor.

Results usually occur 1 to 2 days after the first dose. However, this may not occur for some individuals until after 3 to 5 days.

PRECAUTIONS WHILE USING THIS MEDICINE

Do not take a laxative:
- if you have signs of appendicitis or inflamed bowel.
- for more than 1 week.
- within 2 hours of taking other medicine.
- if you do not need it.
- if you miss a bowel movement for a day or two.
- if you develop a skin rash.

If you notice a sudden change in bowel habits or function that lasts longer than 2 weeks, or that keeps returning off and on, check with your doctor before using a laxative. This will allow the cause of your problem to be determined before it may become more serious.

Laxative products are overused by many people. Such a practice (the "laxative habit") often leads to dependence on the laxative action to produce a bowel movement. In severe cases, overuse of some laxatives has caused damage to the nerves, muscles, and tissues of the intestines and bowel. If you have any questions about the use of laxatives, check with your doctor or pharmacist.

Many laxatives contain large amounts of sugars, carbohydrates, and sodium. If you are on a low-sugar, low-calorie, or low-sodium diet, check with your doctor or pharmacist before using a laxative.

POSSIBLE SIDE EFFECTS OF THIS MEDICINE

Side effects that should be reported to your doctor
Skin rash

Side effects that usually do not require medical attention
These possible side effects may go away during treatment; however, if they continue or are bothersome, check with your doctor, nurse, or pharmacist.

Stomach and/or intestinal cramping; throat irritation (liquid forms only)

Other side effects not listed above may also occur in some patients. If you notice any other effects, check with your doctor, nurse, or pharmacist.

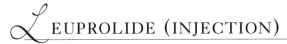EUPROLIDE (INJECTION)

ABOUT YOUR MEDICINE

Leuprolide (loo-PROE-lide) may be used for treatment of cancer of the prostate gland in men, and pain and/or infertility caused by endometriosis in women. It may also be used for other conditions as determined by your doctor.

If any of the information in this profile causes you special concern or if you want additional information about your medicine and its use, check with your doctor, nurse, or pharmacist. **Remember, keep this and all other medicines out of the reach of children and never share your medicines with others.**

BEFORE USING THIS MEDICINE

Discuss with your doctor the possible side effects that may be caused by this medicine. Some of them may be serious and/or long-term.

Tell your doctor, nurse, and pharmacist if you . . .
- are allergic to any medicine, either prescription or nonprescription (OTC);
- are pregnant or intend to become pregnant while using this medicine or if you intend to have children (for men and women);
- are breast-feeding;
- are taking any other prescription or nonprescription (OTC) medicine;
- have any other medical problems, especially bleeding from the vagina with unknown cause (in females) or problems in passing urine (in males).

PROPER USE OF THIS MEDICINE

Leuprolide comes with patient directions. Read these instructions carefully.

Use the syringes provided in the kit. Other syringes may not provide the correct dose. These disposable syringes and needles are already sterilized and designed to be used one time only and then discarded. If you have any questions about the use of disposable syringes, check with your doctor, nurse, or pharmacist.

Use this medicine only as directed by your doctor. Do not use more or less of it, and do not use it more often than your doctor ordered.

For patients using leuprolide for endometriosis:
- Leuprolide sometimes causes unwanted effects such as hot flashes or decreased interest in sex. It may also cause a temporary increase in pain when you first begin to use it. However, it is very important that you continue to use the medicine, even after you begin to feel better. **Do not stop using this medicine without first checking with your doctor.**

For patients using leuprolide for cancer of the prostate:
- Leuprolide sometimes causes unwanted effects such as hot flashes or decreased sexual ability. It may also cause a temporary increase in pain or difficulty in urinating, as well as temporary numbness or tingling of hands or feet, or weakness when you first begin to use it. However, it is very

important that you continue to use the medicine, even after you begin to feel better. **Do not stop using this medicine without first checking with your doctor.**

If you are using this medicine every day and miss a dose, use it as soon as possible. However, if you do not remember until the next day, skip the missed dose and go back to your regular dosing schedule. Do not double doses.

PRECAUTIONS WHILE USING THIS MEDICINE

For patients using leuprolide for endometriosis:
- While you are using leuprolide, your menstrual period may not be regular or you may not have a period at all. This is to be expected when being treated with this medicine. If regular menstruation does not begin 90 days after you stop receiving this medicine, check with your doctor.
- During the time you are using leuprolide, you should use birth control methods that do not contain hormones. If you have any questions about this, check with your doctor, nurse, or pharmacist.
- **If you think you may have become pregnant, stop using this medicine and check with your doctor.** There is a chance that continued use of leuprolide during pregnancy could cause birth defects or a miscarriage.

POSSIBLE SIDE EFFECTS OF THIS MEDICINE

Side effects that should be reported to your doctor immediately
Get emergency help immediately if any of the following side effects occur:

FOR MALES ONLY—RARE—Pains in groin or legs (especially in calves of legs); shortness of breath (sudden)

Other side effects that should be reported to your doctor
FOR BOTH FEMALES AND MALES—LESS COMMON—Fast or irregular heartbeat
FOR FEMALES ONLY—LESS COMMON—Deepening of voice; increased hair growth
FOR MALES ONLY—LESS COMMON—Chest pain

Side effects that usually do not require medical attention
These possible side effects may go away during treatment; however, if they continue or are bothersome, check with your doctor, nurse, or pharmacist.

FOR BOTH FEMALES AND MALES—MORE COMMON—Sudden sweating and feelings of warmth ("hot flashes")
FOR FEMALES ONLY—MORE COMMON—Light, irregular vaginal bleeding; stopping of menstrual periods

Other side effects not listed above may also occur in some patients. If you notice any other effects, check with your doctor, nurse, or pharmacist.

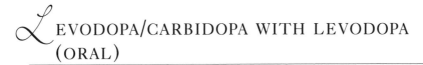EVODOPA/CARBIDOPA WITH LEVODOPA (ORAL)

Including Carbidopa with Levodopa; Levodopa

ABOUT YOUR MEDICINE

Levodopa (LEE-voe-doe-pa) is a medicine used alone or in combination with **carbidopa** (KAR-bi-doe-pa) to treat Parkinson's disease, sometimes referred to as shaking palsy or paralysis agitans.

If any of the information in this profile causes you special concern or if you want additional information about your medicine and its use, check with your doctor, nurse, or pharmacist. **Remember, keep this and all other medicines out of the reach of children and never share your medicines with others.**

BEFORE USING THIS MEDICINE

Tell your doctor, nurse, and pharmacist if you . . .
- are allergic to any medicine, either prescription or nonprescription (OTC);
- are pregnant or intend to become pregnant while using this medicine;
- are breast-feeding;
- are taking any other prescription or nonprescription (OTC) medicine, especially anticonvulsants, haloperidol, MAO inhibitors, phenothiazines, pyridoxine (vitamin B$_6$), or selegiline;
- have any other medical problems, especially asthma, bronchitis, emphysema, or other chronic lung disease; glaucoma; heart or blood vessel disease; kidney disease or difficult urination; mental illness; skin cancer; or stomach ulcer;
- use cocaine.

PROPER USE OF THIS MEDICINE

Take this medicine only as directed. Do not take more or less of it, do not take it more often, and do not stop taking it unless ordered by your doctor. Some people must take this medicine for several weeks before full benefit is received.

Your doctor may want you to take food shortly after taking this medicine (about 15 minutes after) to lessen possible stomach upset. If stomach upset is severe or continues, check with your doctor.

For patients taking carbidopa and levodopa extended-release tablets:
- Swallow the tablet whole without crushing or chewing, unless your doctor tells you not to. If your doctor tells you to, you may break the tablet in half.

If you miss a dose of this medicine, take it as soon as possible. However, if your next scheduled dose is within 2 hours, skip the missed dose and go back to your regular dosing schedule. Do not double doses.

PRECAUTIONS WHILE USING THIS MEDICINE

This medicine may cause some people to become drowsy or less alert than they are normally. **Make sure you know how you react to this medicine before you drive, use machines, or do other jobs that require you to be alert.**

Dizziness, lightheadedness, or fainting may occur, especially when you get up from a lying or sitting position. Getting up slowly may help.

Pyridoxine (vitamin B_6) has been found to reduce the effects of levodopa when taken alone (not in combination with carbidopa). If you are taking levodopa, do not take vitamin products containing vitamin B_6 unless prescribed. Also remember that certain foods contain large amounts of vitamin B_6.

As your condition improves and your body movements become easier, **be careful not to overdo physical activities. Injuries resulting from falls may occur.**

POSSIBLE SIDE EFFECTS OF THIS MEDICINE

Side effects that should be reported to your doctor

MORE COMMON—Mental depression; mood changes; unusual and uncontrolled movements of the upper body (such as the tongue, arms, head)

LESS COMMON (MORE COMMON WHEN LEVODOPA IS USED ALONE)—Difficult urination; dizziness or lightheadedness when getting up from a lying or sitting position; irregular heartbeat; nausea and vomiting (severe or continuing); spasm or closing of eyelids

RARE—High blood pressure; stomach pain; unusual tiredness or weakness

After taking this medicine for long periods of time, such as one to several years, some patients suddenly lose the ability to move. This may last from a few minutes to hours. The patient is then able to move as before until the condition unexpectedly occurs again. If you should have this problem, check with your doctor.

Side effects that usually do not require medical attention

These possible side effects may go away during treatment; however, if they continue or are bothersome, check with your doctor, nurse, or pharmacist.

MORE COMMON—Anxiety

LESS COMMON—Constipation or diarrhea; dryness of mouth

This medicine sometimes causes the urine and sweat to be darker than usual. The urine may at first be reddish, then turn to nearly black after being exposed to air. This effect is not important and is to be expected.

Other side effects not listed above may also occur in some patients. If you notice any other effects, check with your doctor, nurse, or pharmacist.

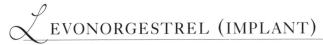EVONORGESTREL (IMPLANT)

About Your Medicine

Levonorgestrel (LEE-voe-nor-jes-trel) implant is used to prevent pregnancy. Levonorgestrel belongs to the general group of medicines called progestins.

If any of the information in this profile causes you special concern of if you want additional information about your medicine and its use, check with your doctor, nurse, or pharmacist.

Before Receiving This Medicine

Tell your doctor, nurse, and pharmacist if you . . .
- are allergic to any medicine, either prescription or nonprescription (OTC);
- are taking **any** other prescription or nonprescription (OTC) medicine;
- have any other medical problems, especially breast disease, such as breast lumps or cysts (history of); heart or circulation problems, or liver disease.

Proper Use of This Medicine

Levonorgestrel implant usually comes with patient directions. Read them carefully before receiving the implant.

Levonorgestrel implant will not protect a woman from sexually transmitted diseases (STDs), including human immunodeficiency virus (HIV), or acquired immunodeficiency syndrome (AIDS). The use of latex (rubber) condoms or abstinence is recommended for protection from these diseases.

For insertion of levonorgestrel implants:
- Six implants are inserted under the skin of your upper arm by a doctor or nurse. This usually takes about 15 minutes. You will be given an injection to prevent pain during the insertion of the implant.

For care of insertion site:
- Keep the gauze wrap on for 24 hours after the insertion. Then, you should remove it. The sterile strips of tape should be left over the area for 3 days.
- Be careful not to bump the site or get that area wet for at least 3 days after the insertion. Do not do any heavy lifting for 24 hours. Swelling and bruising are common for a few days.

For contraceptive protection:
- Full protection from pregnancy begins within 24 hours, if the insertion is done within 7 days of the beginning of your menstrual period. Otherwise, use another birth control method for the rest of your first cycle. Protection using this method lasts for 5 years or until removal, whichever comes first.

For removal:
- Implants need to be removed after 5 years. However, you may have them removed by a doctor or nurse at any time before that.
- Keep the gauze wrap on for 24 hours after the removal. The sterile strips of

tape underneath the gauze wrap should be left over the area for 3 days. Be careful not to bump the site or get that area wet until the area is healed.

- If you want to continue using this form of birth control, your doctor or nurse may insert new implants in the same area as the old ones were or into the other arm.
- If the inserts are hard to remove, your doctor or nurse may want you to return another day before the removal process is completed.

PRECAUTIONS WHILE USING THIS MEDICINE

It is very important that your doctor check your progress at regular visits. Your doctor will want to check the area where your implants were placed within 30 days after they are put in or removed from your arm. After that, a visit every 12 months is usually all that is needed.

Vaginal bleeding (called spotting when bleeding is slight and breakthrough bleeding when it is heavier) may occur between your regular periods during the first 3 months of use. Having vaginal bleeding or a delayed or missed period can be normal. **Check with your doctor** if bleeding continues for an unusually long time or if your period has not started within 45 days of your last period. **If you think you may be pregnant, call your doctor immediately.**

If you are scheduled for any laboratory tests, tell your doctor or nurse that you are using levonorgestrel implants. Levonorgestrel can change certain test results.

Use a second method of birth control during and for 4 weeks (a full cycle) after stopping medicines that reduce the contraceptive effects of progestins. These medicines include aminoglutethimide, carbamazepine, phenobarbital, phenytoin, rifabutin, and rifampin. Your doctor may ask that you use one or more of these medicines with levonorgestrel but will give you special directions to make sure your progestin works properly.

POSSIBLE SIDE EFFECTS OF THIS MEDICINE

Side effects that should be reported to your doctor
MORE COMMON—Changes in uterine bleeding (increased amounts of menstrual bleeding at regular monthly periods; lighter or heavier bleeding between periods; stopping of menstrual periods)
LESS COMMON OR RARE—Mental depression; skin rash; unexpected or increased flow of breast milk

Side effects that usually do not require medical attention
These possible side effects may go away during treatment; however, if they continue or are bothersome, check with your doctor, nurse, or pharmacist.

MORE COMMON—Abdominal pain or cramping; headache (mild); swelling of face, ankles, or feet; mood changes; nervousness; pain or irritation at place of implantation; unusual tiredness or weakness; weight gain
LESS COMMON—Acne; breast pain or tenderness; brown spots on exposed skin,

possibly long-lasting; hot flashes; loss or gain of body, face, or scalp hair; loss of sexual desire; nausea; trouble in sleeping

Other side effects not listed above may also occur in some patients. If you notice any other effects, check with your doctor, nurse, or pharmacist.

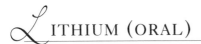ITHIUM (ORAL)

ABOUT YOUR MEDICINE

Lithium (LITH-ee-um) is used to treat the manic stage of bipolar disorder (manic-depressive illness). It may also help reduce the frequency and severity of depression in bipolar disorder. Lithium may also be used for other conditions as determined by your doctor.

It is important that you and your family understand the effects of lithium. These depend on your individual condition and response and the amount of lithium you use. You also must know when to contact your doctor if there are problems.

If any of the information in this profile causes you special concern or if you want additional information about your medicine and its use, check with your doctor, nurse, or pharmacist. **Remember, keep this and all other medicines out of the reach of children and never share your medicines with others.**

BEFORE USING THIS MEDICINE

Tell your doctor, nurse, and pharmacist if you . . .
- are allergic to any medicine, either prescription or nonprescription (OTC);
- are pregnant or intend to become pregnant while using this medicine;
- are breast-feeding;
- are taking **any** other prescription or nonprescription (OTC) medicine;
- have any other medical problems, especially epilepsy, heart disease, kidney disease, leukemia (history of), Parkinson's disease, problems with urination, severe infections, or severe water loss.

PROPER USE OF THIS MEDICINE

During treatment with lithium, drink 2 or 3 quarts of water or other fluids each day, and use a normal amount of salt, unless otherwise directed.

Take this medicine exactly as directed. Do not take more or less of it, do not take it more or less often, and do not take it for a longer time than your doctor ordered. To do so may increase the chance of unwanted effects. **Sometimes lithium must be taken for 1 to several weeks before you begin to feel better.**

In order for lithium to work properly, it must be taken every day in regularly spaced doses as ordered by your doctor. This is necessary to keep a constant amount of lithium in your blood. Do not miss any doses and do not stop taking the medicine even if you feel better.

If you do miss a dose, take it as soon as possible. However, if it is within 2 hours (6 hours for the long-acting tablets or capsules) of your next dose, skip the missed dose and go back to your regular schedule. Do not double doses.

PRECAUTIONS WHILE USING THIS MEDICINE

Your doctor should check your progress at regular visits to make sure that the medicine is working properly and that possible side effects are avoided. Laboratory tests may be necessary.

Lithium may not work properly if you drink large amounts of caffeine-containing coffee, tea, or colas.

Lithium may cause some people to become dizzy, drowsy, or less alert than they are normally. **Make sure you know how you react to this medicine before you drive, use machines, or do other jobs that require you to be alert.**

The loss of too much water and salt from your body may lead to serious side effects from lithium. **Use extra care in hot weather and during activities that cause you to sweat heavily, such as hot baths, saunas, or exercising. Also, check with your doctor before going on a diet to lose weight, or if you have an illness that causes sweating, vomiting, or diarrhea.**

POSSIBLE SIDE EFFECTS OF THIS MEDICINE

Side effects that should be reported to your doctor immediately
> EARLY SIGNS OF OVERDOSE OR TOXICITY—Diarrhea; drowsiness; loss of appetite; muscle weakness; nausea or vomiting; slurred speech; trembling
> LATE SIGNS OF OVERDOSE OR TOXICITY—Blurred vision; clumsiness or unsteadiness; confusion; convulsions (seizures); dizziness; trembling (severe); unusual increase in amount of urine

Other side effects that should be reported to your doctor
> LESS COMMON—Fainting; fast, slow, or irregular heartbeat; troubled breathing (especially during hard work or exercise); unusual tiredness or weakness; weight gain
> RARE—Blue color and pain in fingers and toes; cold arms and legs; dizziness; eye pain; headache; unusual noises in the ears; vision problems
> SIGNS OF LOW THYROID FUNCTION—Dry, rough skin; hair loss; hoarseness; mental depression; sensitivity to cold; swelling of feet or lower legs; swelling of neck; unusual excitement

Side effects that usually do not require medical attention
> These possible side effects may go away during treatment; however, if they continue or are bothersome, check with your doctor, nurse, or pharmacist.

MORE COMMON—Increased frequency of urination or loss of bladder control—more common in women, usually beginning 2 to 7 years after start of treatment; increased thirst; nausea (mild); trembling of hands (slight)

Other side effects not listed above may also occur in some patients. If you notice any other effects, check with your doctor, nurse, or pharmacist.

$\mathcal{L}$OOP DIURETICS (ORAL)

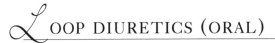

Including Bumetanide; Ethacrynic Acid; Furosemide

ABOUT YOUR MEDICINE

Loop diuretics help reduce the amount of water in the body by increasing the flow of urine. Furosemide is also used to treat high blood pressure (hypertension) in certain patients. These medicines may also be used for other conditions as determined by your doctor.

If any of the information in this profile causes you special concern or if you want additional information about your medicine and its use, check with your doctor, nurse, or pharmacist. **Remember, keep this and all other medicines out of the reach of children and never share your medicines with others.**

BEFORE USING THIS MEDICINE

Tell your doctor, nurse, and pharmacist if you . . .
- are allergic to any medicine, either prescription or nonprescription (OTC);
- are pregnant or intend to become pregnant while using this medicine;
- are breast-feeding;
- are taking **any** other prescription or nonprescription (OTC) medicine;
- have any other medical problems, especially inflammation of the pancreas or severe kidney disease.

PROPER USE OF THIS MEDICINE

This medicine may cause an unusual feeling of tiredness when you begin to take it. You may also notice an increase in urine or in your frequency of urination. To keep this from affecting sleep:
- if you are to take a single dose a day, take it in the morning after breakfast.
- if you are to take more than one dose, take the last one no later than 6 p.m.

For patients taking this medicine for high blood pressure:
- This medicine will not cure your high blood pressure but it does help control it. You must continue to take it—even if you feel well—if you

expect to keep your blood pressure down. **You may have to take high blood pressure medicine for the rest of your life.**

If you miss a dose of this medicine, take it as soon as possible. However, if it is almost time for your next dose, skip the missed dose and go back to your regular dosing schedule. Do not double doses.

PRECAUTIONS WHILE USING THIS MEDICINE

This medicine may cause a loss of potassium from your body. To help prevent this, your doctor **may** want you to eat or drink foods that have a high potassium content, take a potassium supplement, or take another medicine to help prevent loss of potassium in the first place. It is very important to follow these directions. Also, it is important not to change your diet on your own and to check with your doctor if you become sick and have severe or continuing vomiting or diarrhea.

Dizziness, lightheadedness, or fainting may occur, especially when you get up from a lying or sitting position. Getting up slowly may help. **Also, drinking alcohol may make these effects worse and may cause a serious drop in blood pressure.** Check with your doctor before drinking alcohol.

POSSIBLE SIDE EFFECTS OF THIS MEDICINE

Side effects that should be reported to your doctor

RARE—Black, tarry stools; blood in urine or stools; cough or hoarseness; fever or chills; joint pain; lower back or side pain; painful or difficult urination; pinpoint red spots on skin; ringing or buzzing in ears or any loss of hearing; skin rash or hives; stomach pain (severe) with nausea and vomiting; unusual bleeding or bruising; yellow eyes or skin; yellow vision (furosemide only)

SIGNS OF TOO MUCH POTASSIUM LOSS—Dryness of mouth; increased thirst; irregular heartbeat; mood or mental changes; muscle cramps or pain; nausea or vomiting; unusual tiredness or weakness; weak pulse

Side effects that usually do not require medical attention

These possible side effects may go away during treatment; however, if they continue or are bothersome, check with your doctor, nurse, or pharmacist.

MORE COMMON—Dizziness or lightheadedness when getting up from a lying or sitting position

Other side effects not listed above may also occur in some patients. If you notice any other effects, check with your doctor, nurse, or pharmacist.

$\mathscr{M}$AO INHIBITOR ANTIDEPRESSANTS (ORAL)

Including Isocarboxazid; Phenelzine; Tranylcypromine

ABOUT YOUR MEDICINE

Monoamine oxidase (MAO) inhibitors are used to relieve certain types of mental depression. These medicines may also be used for other conditions as determined by your doctor.

If any of the information in this profile causes you special concern or if you want additional information about your medicine and its use, check with your doctor, nurse, or pharmacist. **Remember, keep this and all other medicines out of the reach of children and never share your medicines with others.**

BEFORE USING THIS MEDICINE

Tell your doctor, nurse, and pharmacist if you . . .
- are allergic to any medicine, either prescription or nonprescription (OTC);
- are pregnant or intend to become pregnant while using this medicine;
- are breast-feeding;
- are taking **any** other prescription or nonprescription (OTC) medicine;
- have **any** other medical problems.

PROPER USE OF THIS MEDICINE

MAO inhibitors may be taken with or without food. Take them as directed. **Sometimes this medicine must be taken for several weeks before you begin to feel better. Your doctor should check your progress at regular visits to make sure that this medicine is working properly.**

Take this medicine only as directed. Do not take more of it, do not take it more often, and do not take it for a longer time than ordered.

If you miss a dose of this medicine, take it as soon as possible. However, if it is within 2 hours of your next dose, skip the missed dose and go back to your regular dosing schedule. Do not double doses.

PRECAUTIONS WHILE USING THIS MEDICINE

Do not stop taking this medicine without checking with your doctor. You may have to reduce gradually the amount you are using before stopping completely.

This medicine may cause blurred vision or make some people drowsy or less alert than they are normally. **Make sure you know how you react before you drive, use machines, or do other jobs that require you to be alert.**

Before having any kind of surgery or dental or emergency treatment, tell the physician or dentist in charge that you are using this medicine or have used it within the past 2 weeks.

When taken with certain foods, drinks, or other medicines, **MAO inhibitors can cause very dangerous reactions such as sudden high blood pressure** (also called hypertensive crisis). **To help avoid such reactions:**
- Do not eat foods that are aged or fermented to increase their flavor, such as cheeses; fava or broad bean pods; yeast or meat extracts; smoked or pickled meat, poultry, or fish; fermented sausage (bologna, pepperoni, salami, and summer sausage) or other fermented meat; sauerkraut; or any overripe fruit. Ask your doctor, nurse, or pharmacist for a list of these foods and beverages.
- Do not drink alcoholic beverages or alcohol-free or reduced-alcohol beer and wine or eat or drink large amounts of caffeine-containing food or beverages such as coffee, tea, cola, or chocolate.
- Do not take any other medicine unless prescribed by your doctor.

After you stop using this medicine, you must continue to obey the rules of caution concerning food, drink, and other medicine for at least 2 weeks since those substances may continue to react with MAO inhibitors.

POSSIBLE SIDE EFFECTS OF THIS MEDICINE

Side effects that should be reported to your doctor immediately
Stop taking this medicine and get emergency help immediately if any of the following signs of unusually high blood pressure (hypertensive crisis) occur:

Chest pain (severe); enlarged pupils; fast or slow heartbeat; headache (severe); increased sensitivity of eyes to light; increased sweating (possibly with fever or cold, clammy skin); nausea and vomiting; stiff or sore neck

Other side effects that should be reported to your doctor
MORE COMMON—Dizziness or lightheadedness (severe)
LESS COMMON—Diarrhea; fast or pounding heartbeat; swelling of feet or lower legs; unusual excitement or nervousness
RARE—Dark urine; fever; skin rash; slurred speech; sore throat; staggering walk; yellow eyes or skin

Side effects that usually do not require medical attention
These possible side effects may go away during treatment; however, if they continue or are bothersome, check with your doctor, nurse, or pharmacist.

MORE COMMON—Blurred vision; decreased amount of urine; decreased sexual ability; dizziness or lightheadedness (mild); drowsiness; headache (mild); increased appetite (especially for sweets) or weight gain; increased sweating; muscle twitching during sleep; restlessness; shakiness or trembling; tiredness and weakness; trouble in sleeping

Other side effects not listed above may also occur in some patients. If you notice any other effects, check with your doctor, nurse, or pharmacist.

$\mathcal{M}$ECLIZINE/BUCLIZINE/ CYCLIZINE (ORAL)

Including Meclizine; Buclizine; Cyclizine

ABOUT YOUR MEDICINE

Meclizine (MEK-li-zeen), **buclizine** (BYOO-kli-zeen), and **cyclizine** (SYE-kli-zeen) are used to prevent and treat nausea, vomiting, and dizziness associated with motion sickness, and vertigo (dizziness caused by other medical problems).

If any of the information in this profile causes you special concern or if you want additional information about your medicine and its use, check with your doctor, nurse, or pharmacist. **Remember, keep this and all other medicines out of the reach of children and never share your medicines with others.**

BEFORE USING THIS MEDICINE

If you are taking this medicine without a prescription, carefully read and follow any precautions on the label. You should be especially careful if you . . .
- are allergic to any medicine, either prescription or nonprescription (OTC);
- are pregnant, intend to become pregnant, or are breast-feeding;
- are taking any other prescription or nonprescription (OTC) medicine, especially other CNS depressants;
- have any other medical problems.

If you have any questions, check with your doctor, nurse, or pharmacist.

PROPER USE OF THIS MEDICINE

This medicine is used to relieve or prevent the symptoms of motion sickness or vertigo (dizziness caused by other medical problems). Take it only as directed. Do not take more of it or take it more often than stated on the label or ordered by your doctor. To do so may increase the chance of side effects.

For patients taking this medicine for motion sickness:
—take buclizine or cyclizine at least 30 minutes before you begin to travel.
—take meclizine at least 1 hour before you begin to travel.

If you must take this medicine regularly and you miss a dose, take the missed dose as soon as possible. However, if it is almost time for your next dose, skip the missed dose and go back to your regular dosing schedule. Do not double doses.

PRECAUTIONS WHILE USING THIS MEDICINE

This medicine will add to the effects of alcohol and other CNS depressants (medicines that may make you drowsy or less alert). **Check with your doctor before taking any such depressants while you are taking this medicine.**

This medicine may cause some people to become drowsy or less alert than they are normally. **Make sure you know how you react to this medicine before you drive, use machines, or do other jobs that require you to be alert.**

Buclizine, cyclizine, and meclizine may cause dryness of the mouth. For temporary relief use sugarless candy or gum, dissolve bits of ice in your mouth, or use a saliva substitute. However, if your mouth continues to feel dry for more than 2 weeks, check with your physician or dentist. Continuing dryness of the mouth may increase the chance of dental disease, including tooth decay, gum disease, and fungus infections.

POSSIBLE SIDE EFFECTS OF THIS MEDICINE

Side effects that usually do not require medical attention
These possible side effects may go away during treatment; however, if they continue or are bothersome, check with your doctor, nurse, or pharmacist.

MORE COMMON—Drowsiness
LESS COMMON OR RARE—Blurred or double vision; constipation; diarrhea; difficult or painful urination; dizziness; dryness of mouth, nose, and throat; fast heartbeat; headache; loss of appetite; nervousness, restlessness, or trouble in sleeping; skin rash; upset stomach

Other side effects not listed above may also occur in some patients. If you notice any other effects, check with your doctor, nurse, or pharmacist.

MEDROXYPROGESTERONE (FOR CONTRACEPTIVE USE—INJECTION)

ABOUT YOUR MEDICINE

Medroxyprogesterone (me-droks-ee-proh-JES-te-rone) is used to prevent pregnancy. Medroxyprogesterone belongs to the general group of medicines called progestins.

If any of the information in this profile causes you special concern of if you want additional information about your medicine and its use, check with your doctor, nurse, or pharmacist.

BEFORE RECEIVING THIS MEDICINE

Tell your doctor, nurse, and pharmacist if you . . .
- are allergic to any medicine, either prescription or nonprescription (OTC);
- are pregnant or intend to become pregnant while using this medicine;
- are breast-feeding;
- are taking **any** other prescription or nonprescription (OTC) medicine;
- have any other medical problems, especially breast disease, such as breast lumps or cysts (history of), heart or circulation problems, or liver disease.

PROPER USE OF THIS MEDICINE

Medroxyprogesterone usually comes with patient directions. Read them carefully before receiving this medicine.

Medroxyprogesterone will not protect a woman from sexually transmitted diseases (STDs), including human immunodeficiency virus (HIV), or acquired immunodeficiency syndrome (AIDS). The use of latex (rubber) condoms or abstinence is recommended for protection from these diseases.

Your injection is given by a doctor or nurse **every** 3 months (13 weeks).

To stop using medroxyprogesterone injection for contraception, simply do not have another injection.

Full protection from pregnancy begins immediately if you receive the first injection within the first 5 days of your menstrual period, or within 5 days after delivering a baby if you are not going to breast-feed. If you are breast-feeding, your doctor may ask you to wait before having your first injection. If you follow this schedule, you do not need to use another method of birth control. Protection from that one injection ends after 3 months (13 weeks). You will need another injection every 3 months (13 weeks) to have full protection from becoming pregnant. However, if another schedule for giving the injection is followed, you will need to use another method of birth control as directed by your doctor.

If you miss having your next injection and it has been longer than 13 weeks since your last injection, your doctor may want you to stop receiving the medicine. Use another method of birth control until your period begins or until your doctor determines that you are not pregnant.

PRECAUTIONS WHILE USING THIS MEDICINE

It is very important that your doctor check your progress at regular visits. A physical exam is only needed every 12 months, but you need an injection every 3 months (13 weeks).

Vaginal bleeding (called spotting when bleeding is slight and breakthrough bleeding when it is heavier) may occur between your regular periods during the first 3 months of use. Having vaginal bleeding or a delayed or missed period can be normal. **Check with your doctor** if bleeding continues for an unusually long time or if your period has not started within 45 days of your last period. **If you think you may be pregnant, call your doctor immediately.**

If you are scheduled for any laboratory tests, tell your doctor or nurse that you are using this medicine. Medroxyprogesterone can change certain test results.

Use a second method of birth control while taking medicines that reduce the contraceptive effects of progestins. These medicines include aminoglutethimide, carbamazepine, phenobarbital, phenytoin, rifabutin, and rifampin. Continue to use another method of birth control until you have your next injection. Your doctor may ask that you use one or more of these medicines with medroxyprogesterone but will give you special directions to make sure your birth control works properly.

POSSIBLE SIDE EFFECTS OF THIS MEDICINE

Side effects that should be reported to your doctor
MORE COMMON—Changes in uterine bleeding (increased amounts of menstrual bleeding at regular monthly periods; lighter or heavier bleeding between periods; stopping of menstrual periods)

LESS COMMON OR RARE—Mental depression; skin rash; unexpected or increased flow of breast milk

Side effects that usually do not require medical attention
These possible side effects may go away during treatment; however, if they continue or are bothersome, check with your doctor, nurse, or pharmacist.

MORE COMMON—Abdominal pain or cramping; headache (mild); swelling of face, ankles, or feet; mood changes; nervousness; pain at place of injection; unusual tiredness or weakness; weight gain

LESS COMMON—Acne; breast pain or tenderness; brown spots on exposed skin, possibly long-lasting; hot flashes; loss or gain of body, face, or scalp hair; loss of sexual desire; nausea; trouble in sleeping

Other side effects not listed above may also occur in some patients. If you notice any other effects, check with your doctor, nurse, or pharmacist.

$\mathcal{M}$ENOTROPINS (INJECTION)

ABOUT YOUR MEDICINE

Menotropins (men-oh-TROE-pins) are used in combination with another medicine to treat infertility. They are used in some women who are unable to become pregnant. Menotropins are also used to stimulate the production of sperm in some forms of male infertility.

If any of the information in this profile causes you special concern or if you want additional information about your medicine and its use, check with your doctor, nurse, or pharmacist. **Remember, keep this and all other medicines out of the reach of children and never share your medicines with others.**

BEFORE USING THIS MEDICINE

Tell your doctor, nurse, and pharmacist if you . . .
- are allergic to any medicine, either prescription or nonprescription (OTC);
- are pregnant or intend to become pregnant while using this medicine;
- are breast-feeding;
- are taking any other prescription or nonprescription (OTC) medicine;
- have any other medical problems, especially a cyst on an ovary or unusual vaginal bleeding.

PRECAUTIONS WHILE USING THIS MEDICINE

It is very important that your doctor check your progress at regular visits to make sure that the medicine is working properly and to check for unwanted effects. Your doctor will probably want to follow the development of the ovarian follicle(s) by measuring the amount of estrogen in your bloodstream and by checking the size of the follicle(s) with ultrasound examination.

For females only:
- If your doctor has asked you to record your basal body temperatures (BBTs) daily, make sure that you do this every day. It is important that intercourse take place around the time of ovulation to give you the best chance of becoming pregnant. **Follow your doctor's instructions carefully.**

POSSIBLE SIDE EFFECTS OF THIS MEDICINE

Side effects that should be reported to your doctor
   For females only
   MORE COMMON—Bloating (mild); pain, swelling, or irritation at place of
      injection; rash at place of injection or on body; stomach or pelvic pain
   LESS COMMON OR RARE—Abdominal or stomach pain (severe); bloating
      (moderate to severe); decreased amount of urine; feeling of indigestion;
      nausea, vomiting, or diarrhea (continuing or severe); pelvic pain (severe);
      shortness of breath; swelling of lower legs; weight gain (rapid)

For males only

MORE COMMON—Dizziness; fainting; headache; irregular heartbeat; loss of appetite; more frequent nosebleeds; shortness of breath

Side effects that usually do not require medical attention

These possible side effects may go away during treatment; however, if they continue or are bothersome, check with your doctor, nurse, or pharmacist.

For males only

LESS COMMON—Enlargement of breasts

For females only: After you stop using this medicine, your body may need time to adjust. The length of time this takes depends on the amount of medicine you were using and how long you used it. During this time check with your doctor if you notice abdominal or stomach pain (severe); bloating (moderate to severe); decreased amount of urine; feeling of indigestion; nausea, vomiting, or diarrhea (continuing or severe); pelvic pain (severe); shortness of breath or weight gain (rapid).

Other side effects not listed above may also occur in some patients. If you notice any other effects, check with your doctor, nurse, or pharmacist.

$\mathcal{M}$ESALAMINE (ORAL)

ABOUT YOUR MEDICINE

Mesalamine (me-SAL-a-meen) is used to treat inflammatory bowel disease, such as ulcerative colitis.

If any of the information in this profile causes you special concern or if you want additional information about your medicine and its use, check with your doctor, nurse, or pharmacist. **Remember, keep this and all other medicines out of the reach of children and never share your medicines with others.**

BEFORE USING THIS MEDICINE

Tell your doctor, nurse, and pharmacist if you . . .
- are allergic to any medicine, either prescription or nonprescription (OTC);
- are pregnant or intend to become pregnant while using this medicine;
- are breast-feeding;
- are taking any other prescription or nonprescription (OTC) medicine;
- have any other medical problems, especially kidney disease.

PROPER USE OF THIS MEDICINE

Swallow the capsule or tablet whole. Do not break, crush, or chew it before swallowing.

Take this medicine before meals and at bedtime with a full glass (8 ounces) of water, unless otherwise directed by your doctor.

Keep taking this medicine for the full time of treatment, even if you begin to feel better after a few days. **Do not miss any doses.**

Do not change to another brand without checking with your doctor. The doses are different for different brands. If you refill your medicine and it looks different, check with your pharmacist.

For patients taking the capsule form of this medicine:
- You may sometimes notice what looks like small beads in your stools. These are just the empty shells that are left after the medicine has been absorbed into your body.

For patients taking the tablet form of this medicine:
- You may sometimes notice what looks like a tablet in your stool. This is just the empty shell that is left after the medicine has been absorbed into your body.

If you do miss a dose of this medicine, take it as soon as possible. However, if it is almost time for your next dose, skip the missed dose and go back to your regular dosing schedule. Do not double doses.

PRECAUTIONS WHILE USING THIS MEDICINE

It is important that your doctor check your progress at regular visits.

POSSIBLE SIDE EFFECTS OF THIS MEDICINE

Side effects that should be reported to your doctor immediately
Stop using this medicine and check with your doctor immediately if any of the following side effects occur:

LESS COMMON—Abdominal or stomach cramps or pain (severe); bloody diarrhea; fever; headache (severe); skin rash and itching

RARE—Anxiety; back pain (severe); blue or pale skin; chest pain, possibly moving to the left arm, neck, or shoulder; chills; fast heartbeat; nausea or vomiting; shortness of breath; swelling of the stomach; unusual tiredness or weakness; yellow eyes or skin

Side effects that usually do not require medical attention
These possible side effects may go away during treatment; however, if they continue or are bothersome, check with your doctor, nurse, or pharmacist.

MORE COMMON—Abdominal or stomach cramps or pain (mild); diarrhea (mild); dizziness; headache (mild); runny or stuffy nose or sneezing

LESS COMMON—Acne; back or joint pain; gas or flatulence; indigestion; loss of appetite; loss of hair

Other side effects not listed above may also occur in some patients. If you notice any other effects, check with your doctor, nurse, or pharmacist.

$\mathcal{M}$ESALAMINE (RECTAL)

ABOUT YOUR MEDICINE

Mesalamine (me-SAL-a-meen) is used to treat inflammatory bowel disease, such as ulcerative colitis.

If any of the information in this profile causes you special concern or if you want additional information about your medicine and its use, check with your doctor, nurse, or pharmacist. **Remember, keep this and all other medicines out of the reach of children and never share your medicines with others.**

BEFORE USING THIS MEDICINE

Tell your doctor, nurse, and pharmacist if you . . .
- are allergic to any medicine, either prescription or nonprescription (OTC);
- are pregnant or intend to become pregnant while using this medicine;
- are breast-feeding;
- are taking any other prescription or nonprescription (OTC) medicine;
- have any other medical problems.

PROPER USE OF THIS MEDICINE

For best results, empty your bowel just before using this medicine.

Mesalamine usually comes with patient directions. Read them carefully before using this medicine.

For patients using **the enema form** of this medicine:
- Remove the bottles from the protective foil pouch, being careful not to squeeze or puncture them. The enema is an off-white to tan color. Slight darkening will not affect the strength of the enema. However, enemas that appear dark brown should be discarded.
- Shake the bottle well. Remove the protective cover from the applicator tip. Hold bottle at the neck so that no medicine spills out.
- Lie on your left side with your left leg straight and your right knee bent in front of you for balance.
- Gently insert the tip of the enema pointed slightly toward your naval to

prevent damage to the rectal wall. Tilt the nozzle slightly toward the back. Slowly squeeze the medicine into your rectum. Withdraw the bottle and discard.

- Stay on your left side for at least 30 minutes. If you can, keep the medicine inside the rectum all night.

For patients using **the suppository form** of this medicine:

- Avoid excessive handling of the suppository, which is designed to melt at body temperature.
- Remove the foil wrapper. Use your finger to push the suppository (pointed end first) well up into the rectum. If you can, keep the suppository inside the rectum for 3 hours or longer.

Keep using this medicine for the full time of treatment even if you begin to feel better after a few days. **Do not miss any doses.**

If you miss a dose of mesalamine enema, use it as soon as possible if you remember it that same night. However, if you do not remember it until the next morning, skip the missed dose and go back to your regular dosing schedule. If you miss a dose of mesalamine suppository, use it as soon as possible unless it is almost time for your next dose. Do not double doses.

Precautions While Using This Medicine

It is important that your doctor check your progress at regular visits.

Check with your doctor if you notice rectal bleeding, blistering, pain, burning, itching, or other irritation not present before you started using this medicine.

Mesalamine rectal enema may stain clothing, fabrics, painted surfaces, marble, granite, vinyl, or other surfaces it touches.

Possible Side Effects of This Medicine

Side effects that should be reported to your doctor immediately
Stop using this medicine and check with your doctor immediately if any of the following side effects occur:

Rare—Abdominal or stomach cramps or pain (severe); anxiety; back pain (severe); bloody diarrhea; blue or pale skin; chest pain, possibly moving to the left arm, neck, or shoulder; chills; fast heartbeat; fever; headache (severe); nausea or vomiting; shortness of breath; skin rash; swelling of the stomach; unusual tiredness or weakness; yellow eyes or skin

Other side effects that should be reported to your doctor
Rare—Rectal irritation

Side effects that usually do not require medical attention
These possible side effects may go away during treatment; however, if they continue or are bothersome, check with your doctor, nurse, or pharmacist.

MORE COMMON—Abdominal or stomach cramps or pain (mild); gas or flatulence; headache (mild); nausea (mild)

Other side effects not listed above may also occur in some patients. If you notice any other effects, check with your doctor, nurse, or pharmacist.

$\mathscr{M}$ETHOTREXATE (FOR CANCER— ORAL/INJECTION)

ABOUT YOUR MEDICINE

Methotrexate (meth-o-TREX-ate) is used to treat some kinds of cancer.

If any of the information in this profile causes you special concern or if you want additional information about your medicine and its use, check with your doctor, nurse, or pharmacist. **Remember, keep this and all other medicines out of the reach of children and never share your medicines with others.**

BEFORE USING THIS MEDICINE

Discuss with your doctor the possible side effects that may be caused by this medicine. Some of them may be serious and/or long-term.

Tell your doctor, nurse, and pharmacist if you . . .
- are allergic to any medicine, either prescription or nonprescription (OTC);
- are pregnant or intend to have children;
- are breast-feeding an infant;
- are taking **any** other prescription or nonprescription (OTC) medicine;
- have any other medical problems, especially chickenpox (including recent exposure), alcoholism, colitis, disease of the immune system, herpes zoster (shingles), infection, kidney disease, mouth sores or inflammation, or stomach ulcer;
- have ever been treated with radiation or cancer medicines.

PROPER USE OF THIS MEDICINE

Take this medicine only as directed by your doctor. Do not take more or less, and do not take it more often than ordered.

While you are using methotrexate, your doctor may want you to drink extra fluids so that you will pass more urine.

Methotrexate commonly causes nausea and vomiting. Ask your doctor, nurse, or pharmacist for ways to lessen these effects. If you vomit shortly after taking a dose, check with your doctor.

If you miss a dose of this medicine, do not take the missed dose at all and do not double the next one. Instead, go back to your regular dosing schedule and check with your doctor.

PRECAUTIONS WHILE USING THIS MEDICINE

It is very important that your doctor check your progress at regular visits.

Do not drink alcohol while using this medicine.

When you begin using methotrexate, avoid too much sun and do not use a sunlamp since you may become more sensitive than usual.

Do not take aspirin or other medicine for inflammation or pain without first checking with your doctor.

While you are taking methotrexate, and after you stop treatment, **do not have any immunizations (vaccinations) without your doctor's approval.**

Methotrexate can temporarily lower the number of white blood cells in your blood, increasing the chance of getting an infection. It can also lower the number of platelets, which are necessary for proper blood clotting. If this occurs:
- Avoid people with infections.
- Be careful when using a regular toothbrush, dental floss, or toothpick.
- Do not touch your eyes or the inside of your nose unless you have just washed your hands and have not touched anything else in the meantime.
- Be careful not to cut, bruise, or injure yourself.

POSSIBLE SIDE EFFECTS OF THIS MEDICINE

Side effects that should be reported to your doctor immediately

MORE COMMON—Black, tarry stools; bloody vomit; diarrhea; reddening of skin; sores in mouth and on lips; stomach pain

LESS COMMON—Blood in urine or stools; blurred vision; confusion; convulsions (seizures); cough or hoarseness; fever or chills; lower back or side pain; painful or difficult urination; pinpoint red spots on skin; shortness of breath; swelling of feet or lower legs; unusual bleeding or bruising

Other side effects that should be reported to your doctor

LESS COMMON—Back pain; dark urine; dizziness; drowsiness; headache; joint pain; unusual tiredness or weakness; yellow eyes or skin

Side effects that usually do not require medical attention

These possible side effects may go away during treatment; however, if they continue or are bothersome, check with your doctor, nurse, or pharmacist.

MORE COMMON—Loss of appetite; nausea or vomiting

This medicine may cause a temporary loss of hair in some people. After treatment with methotrexate has ended, normal hair growth should return.

Other side effects not listed above may also occur in some patients. If you notice any other effects, check with your doctor, nurse, or pharmacist.

After you stop methotrexate, check with your doctor as soon as possible if you notice back pain, blurred vision, confusion, convulsions, dizziness, drowsiness, fever, headache, or unusual tiredness or weakness.

METHOTREXATE (FOR NONCANCEROUS CONDITIONS—ORAL/INJECTION)

ABOUT YOUR MEDICINE

Methotrexate (meth-o-TREX-ate) is used to treat psoriasis and rheumatoid arthritis. It may also be used for other conditions as determined by your doctor.

If any of the information in this profile causes you special concern or if you want additional information about your medicine and its use, check with your doctor, nurse, or pharmacist. **Remember, keep this and all other medicines out of the reach of children and never share your medicines with others.**

BEFORE USING THIS MEDICINE

Discuss with your doctor the possible side effects that may be caused by this medicine. Some of them may be serious and/or long-term.

Tell your doctor, nurse, and pharmacist if you . . .
- are allergic to any medicine, either prescription or nonprescription (OTC);
- are pregnant or intend to have children;
- are breast-feeding;
- are taking **any** other prescription or nonprescription (OTC) medicine;
- have any other medical problems, especially chickenpox (including recent exposure), alcohol abuse (or history of), colitis, disease of the immune system, herpes zoster (shingles), infection, kidney disease, liver disease, mouth sores or inflammation, or stomach ulcer;
- have ever been treated with radiation or cancer medicines.

PROPER USE OF THIS MEDICINE

Use this medicine only as directed by your doctor. Do not use more or less, and do not use it more often than ordered.

Methotrexate may cause nausea. Even if you begin to feel ill, **do not stop using this medicine without first checking with your doctor.** Ask your doctor, nurse, or pharmacist for ways to lessen this effect.

If you vomit shortly after using a dose, check with your doctor.

If you miss a dose of this medicine, do not use the missed dose at all and do not double the next one. Instead, go back to your regular dosing schedule and check with your doctor.

PRECAUTIONS WHILE USING THIS MEDICINE

It is very important that your doctor check your progress at regular visits.

Do not drink alcohol while using this medicine.

When you first begin using methotrexate, avoid too much sun and do not use a sunlamp since you may become more sensitive than usual. In case of a severe burn, check with your doctor. This is especially important if you are using this medicine for psoriasis because sunlight can make the psoriasis worse.

Do not take aspirin or other medicine for inflammation or pain without first checking with your doctor.

While you are using methotrexate, and for several weeks after you stop treatment, **do not have any immunizations (vaccinations) without your doctor's approval.**

POSSIBLE SIDE EFFECTS OF THIS MEDICINE

Side effects that should be reported to your doctor immediately
> LESS COMMON—Diarrhea; reddening of skin; sores in mouth and on lips; stomach pain
> RARE—Black, tarry stools; blood in urine or stools; blurred vision; convulsions (seizures); cough or hoarseness; fever or chills; lower back or side pain; painful or difficult urination; pinpoint red spots on skin; shortness of breath; unusual bleeding or bruising

Other side effects that should be reported to your doctor
> RARE—Back pain; dark urine; dizziness; drowsiness; headache; unusual tiredness or weakness; yellow eyes or skin

Side effects that usually do not require medical attention
> These possible side effects may go away during treatment; however, if they continue or are bothersome, check with your doctor, nurse, or pharmacist.

> LESS COMMON OR RARE—Acne; boils; loss of appetite; nausea or vomiting; pale skin; skin rash or itching

> This medicine may cause a temporary loss of hair in some people. After treatment with methotrexate has ended, normal hair growth should return.

> Other side effects not listed above may also occur in some patients. If you notice any other effects, check with your doctor, nurse, or pharmacist.

METHYLDOPA (ORAL)

ABOUT YOUR MEDICINE

Methyldopa (meth-ill-DOE-pa) belongs to the general class of medicines called antihypertensives. It is used to treat high blood pressure (hypertension).

If any of the information in this profile causes you special concern or if you want additional information about your medicine and its use, check with your doctor, nurse, or pharmacist. **Remember, keep this and all other medicines out of the reach of children and never share your medicines with others.**

BEFORE USING THIS MEDICINE

Tell your doctor, nurse, and pharmacist if you . . .
- are allergic to any medicine, either prescription or nonprescription (OTC);
- are pregnant or intend to become pregnant while using this medicine;
- are breast-feeding;
- are taking any other prescription or nonprescription (OTC) medicine, especially MAO inhibitors or medicines for appetite control, asthma, colds, cough, hay fever, or sinus;
- have any other medical problems, especially liver disease or pheochromocytoma (PCC).

PROPER USE OF THIS MEDICINE

This medicine will not cure your high blood pressure but it does help control it. You must continue to take it—even if you feel well—if you expect to keep your blood pressure down. **You may have to take high blood pressure medicine for the rest of your life.**

If you miss a dose of this medicine, take it as soon as possible. However, if it is almost time for your next dose, skip the missed dose and go back to your regular dosing schedule. Do not double doses.

PRECAUTIONS WHILE USING THIS MEDICINE

It is important that your doctor check your progress at regular visits while you are taking this medicine.

If you have a fever and there seems to be no reason for it, check with your doctor immediately. This is especially important the first few weeks you take methyldopa.

Methyldopa may cause some people to become drowsy or less alert than they are normally. **Make sure you know how you react to this medicine before you drive, use machines, or do other jobs that require you to be alert.**

Tell the doctor in charge that you are taking this medicine before you have any medical tests. The results of some tests may be affected by this medicine.

POSSIBLE SIDE EFFECTS OF THIS MEDICINE

Side effects that should be reported to your doctor immediately

LESS COMMON—Fever shortly after starting to take this medicine

Other side effects that should be reported to your doctor

MORE COMMON—Swelling of feet or lower legs

LESS COMMON—Mental depression or anxiety; nightmares or unusually vivid dreams

RARE—Continuing tiredness or weakness after having taken this medicine for several weeks; dark or amber urine; fever, chills, troubled breathing, and fast heartbeat; general feeling of discomfort, illness, or weakness; joint pain; pale stools; severe or continuing diarrhea or stomach cramps; severe stomach pain with nausea and vomiting; skin rash or itching; yellow eyes or skin

Side effects that usually do not require medical attention

These possible side effects may go away during treatment; however, if they continue or are bothersome, check with your doctor, nurse, or pharmacist.

MORE COMMON—Drowsiness; dryness of mouth; headache

LESS COMMON—Decreased sexual ability or interest in sex; dizziness or lightheadedness when getting up from a lying or sitting position; nausea or vomiting; numbness, tingling, pain or weakness in hands or feet; slow heartbeat; stuffy nose; swelling of breasts or unusual milk production

Other side effects not listed above may also occur in some patients. If you notice any other effects, check with your doctor, nurse, or pharmacist.

METOCLOPRAMIDE (ORAL)

ABOUT YOUR MEDICINE

Metoclopramide (met-oh-KLOE-pra-mide) is a medicine that increases the movements or contractions of the stomach and intestines. When taken by mouth, metoclopramide is used to treat the symptoms of a certain type of stomach problem called diabetic gastroparesis. It relieves symptoms such as nausea, vomiting, continued feeling of fullness after meals, and loss of appetite. Metoclopramide is also used to treat symptoms such as heartburn caused by a backward flow of gastric acid into the esophagus. Metoclopramide may also be used for other conditions as determined by your doctor.

If any of the information in this profile causes you special concern or if you want additional information about your medicine and its use, check with your doctor,

nurse, or pharmacist. **Remember, keep this and all other medicines out of the reach of children and never share your medicines with others.**

BEFORE USING THIS MEDICINE

Tell your doctor, nurse, and pharmacist if you . . .
- are allergic to any medicine, either prescription or nonprescription (OTC);
- are pregnant or intend to become pregnant while using this medicine;
- are breast-feeding;
- are taking any other prescription or nonprescription (OTC) medicine, especially CNS depressants;
- have any other medical problems, especially abdominal or stomach bleeding, epilepsy, intestinal blockage, pheochromocytoma (PCC), or severe kidney disease.

PROPER USE OF THIS MEDICINE

Take this medicine 30 minutes before meals and at bedtime, unless otherwise directed by your doctor.

Take metoclopramide only as directed. Do not take more of it, do not take it more often, and do not take it for a longer period of time than your doctor ordered. To do so may increase the chance of side effects.

If you miss a dose of this medicine, take it as soon as possible. However, if it is almost time for your next dose, skip the missed dose and go back to your regular dosing schedule. Do not double doses.

PRECAUTIONS WHILE USING THIS MEDICINE

This medicine will add to the effects of alcohol and other CNS depressants (medicines that make you drowsy or less alert). **Check with your doctor before taking any such depressants while you are using this medicine.**

This medicine may cause some people to become dizzy, lightheaded, drowsy, or less alert than they are normally. **Make sure you know how you react to this medicine before you drive, use machines, or do other jobs that require you to be alert.**

POSSIBLE SIDE EFFECTS OF THIS MEDICINE

Side effects that should be reported to your doctor
> RARE—Chills; difficulty in speaking or swallowing; dizziness or fainting; fast or irregular heartbeat; fever; general feeling of tiredness or weakness; headache (severe or continuing); increase in blood pressure; lip smacking or puckering; loss of balance control; mask-like face; rapid or worm-like movements of tongue; shuffling walk; sore throat; stiffness of arms or legs; trembling and shaking of hands and fingers; uncontrolled chewing movements; uncontrolled movements of arms and legs

WITH HIGH DOSES (MAY OCCUR WITHIN MINUTES OF RECEIVING A DOSE OF
METOCLOPRAMIDE AND LAST FOR 2 TO 24 HOURS)—Aching or discomfort in
lower legs; panic-like sensation; sensation of crawling in legs; unusual
nervousness, restlessness, or irritability

Side effects that usually do not require medical attention

These possible side effects may go away during treatment; however, if they
continue or are bothersome, check with your doctor, nurse, or pharmacist.

MORE COMMON—Diarrhea (with high doses); drowsiness; restlessness

Other side effects not listed above may also occur in some patients. If you
notice any other effects, check with your doctor, nurse, or pharmacist.

METRONIDAZOLE (ORAL)

ABOUT YOUR MEDICINE

Metronidazole (me-troe-NI-da-zole) is used to treat infections. It may also be used
for other problems as determined by your doctor. It will not work for colds, flu, or
other virus infections.

If any of the information in this profile causes you special concern or if you want
additional information about your medicine and its use, check with your doctor,
nurse, or pharmacist. **Remember, keep this and all other medicines out of the
reach of children and never share your medicines with others.**

BEFORE USING THIS MEDICINE

Tell your doctor, nurse, and pharmacist if you . . .

- are allergic to any medicine, either prescription or nonprescription (OTC);
- are pregnant or intend to become pregnant while using this medicine;
- are breast-feeding;
- are taking any other prescription or nonprescription (OTC) medicine,
  especially anticoagulants (blood thinners) or disulfiram;
- have any other medical problems, especially blood disease or a history of
  blood disease; central nervous system (CNS) disease, including epilepsy; or
  severe liver disease.

PROPER USE OF THIS MEDICINE

If this medicine upsets your stomach, it may be taken with meals or a snack. If
stomach upset continues, check with your doctor.

To help clear up your infection completely, **keep taking this medicine for the full time of treatment** even if you begin to feel better after a few days; **do not miss any doses.**

If you do miss a dose of this medicine, take it as soon as possible. This will help to keep a constant amount of medicine in the blood. However, if it is almost time for your next dose, skip the missed dose and go back to your regular dosing schedule. Do not double doses.

PRECAUTIONS WHILE USING THIS MEDICINE

If your symptoms do not improve within a few days, or if they become worse, check with your doctor.

Drinking alcoholic beverages while taking this medicine may cause stomach pain, nausea, vomiting, headache, or flushing or redness of the face. Other alcohol-containing preparations (for example, elixirs, cough syrups, tonics) may also cause problems. Therefore, **you should not drink alcoholic beverages or use other alcohol-containing preparations while taking this medicine and for at least one day after stopping it.**

This medicine may cause some people to become dizzy or lightheaded. **Make sure you know how you react to this medicine before you drive, use machines, or do other jobs that require you to be alert.** If these reactions are especially bothersome, check with your doctor.

This medicine must not be given to other people or used for other infections unless you are otherwise directed by your doctor.

POSSIBLE SIDE EFFECTS OF THIS MEDICINE

Side effects that should be reported to your doctor immediately
    LESS COMMON—Numbness, tingling, pain, or weakness in hands or feet
    RARE—Convulsions (seizures)

Other side effects that should be reported to your doctor
    LESS COMMON—Any vaginal irritation, discharge, or dryness not present before
        use of this medicine; clumsiness or unsteadiness; mood or other mental
        changes; skin rash, hives, redness, or itching; sore throat and fever; stomach
        and back pain (severe)

Side effects that usually do not require medical attention
    These possible side effects may go away during treatment; however, if they
    continue or are bothersome, check with your doctor, nurse, or pharmacist.

    MORE COMMON—Diarrhea; dizziness or lightheadedness; headache; loss of
        appetite; nausea; stomach pain or cramps; vomiting

    In some patients metronidazole may cause dark urine. This is only temporary
    and will go away when you stop taking this medicine.

Other side effects not listed above may also occur in some patients. If you notice any other effects, check with your doctor, nurse, or pharmacist.

METRONIDAZOLE (TOPICAL)

ABOUT YOUR MEDICINE

Topical **metronidazole** (me-troe-NI-da-zole) is applied to the skin in adults to help control rosacea (roe-ZAY-she-ah), also known as acne rosacea and "adult acne." This medicine helps to reduce the redness of the skin and the number of pimples, usually found on the face, in patients with rosacea.

If any of the information in this profile causes you special concern or if you want additional information about your medicine and its use, check with your doctor, nurse, or pharmacist. **Remember, keep this and all other medicines out of the reach of children and never share your medicines with others.**

BEFORE USING THIS MEDICINE

Tell your doctor, nurse, and pharmacist if you . . .
- are allergic to any medicine, either prescription or nonprescription (OTC);
- are pregnant or intend to become pregnant while using this medicine;
- are breast-feeding;
- are taking any other prescription or nonprescription (OTC) medicine;
- have any other medical problems.

PROPER USE OF THIS MEDICINE

Do not use this medicine in or near the eyes. Watering of the eyes may occur when the medicine is used too close to the eyes.

If this medicine does get into your eyes, wash them out immediately, but carefully, with large amounts of cool tap water. If your eyes still burn or are painful, check with your doctor.

Before applying this medicine, thoroughly wash the affected area(s) with a mild, nonirritating cleanser, rinse well, and gently pat dry.

To use:
- After washing the affected area(s), apply this medicine with your fingertips.
- Apply and rub in a thin film of medicine, using enough to cover the affected area(s) lightly. **You should apply the medicine to the whole area usually affected by rosacea, not just to the pimples themselves.**
- Wash the medicine off your hands.

To help keep your rosacea under control, **keep using this medicine for the full time of treatment.** You may have to continue using this medicine every day for 9 weeks or longer. **Do not miss any doses.**

If you do miss a dose of this medicine, apply it as soon as possible. However, if it is almost time for your next dose, skip the missed dose and go back to your regular dosing schedule.

PRECAUTIONS WHILE USING THIS MEDICINE

If your rosacea does not improve within 3 weeks, or if it becomes worse, check with your doctor. However, treatment of rosacea may take up to 9 weeks or longer before you see full improvement.

Stinging or burning of the skin may be expected after this medicine is applied. These effects may last up to a few minutes or more. If irritation continues, check with your doctor. You may have to use the medicine less often or stop using it altogether. Follow your doctor's directions.

You may continue to use cosmetics (make-up) while you are using this medicine for rosacea. However, it is best to use only "oil-free" cosmetics. Also, it is best not to use cosmetics too heavily or too often. They may make your rosacea worse. If you have any questions about this, check with your doctor.

POSSIBLE SIDE EFFECTS OF THIS MEDICINE

Side effects that usually do not require medical attention
> These possible side effects may go away during treatment; however, if they continue or are bothersome, check with your doctor, nurse, or pharmacist.

> LESS COMMON—Dry skin; redness or other sign of skin irritation not present before use of this medicine; stinging or burning of the skin; watering of eyes

> Other side effects not listed above may also occur in some patients. If you notice any other effects, check with your doctor, nurse, or pharmacist.

METRONIDAZOLE (VAGINAL)

ABOUT YOUR MEDICINE

Metronidazole (me-troe-NI-da-zole) is used to treat certain vaginal infections. This medicine will not work for vaginal fungus or yeast infections.

If any of the information in this profile causes you special concern or if you want additional information about your medicine and its use, check with your doctor,

nurse, or pharmacist. **Remember, keep this and all other medicines out of the reach of children and never share your medicines with others.**

BEFORE USING THIS MEDICINE

Tell your doctor, nurse, and pharmacist if you . . .
- are allergic to any medicine, either prescription or nonprescription (OTC);
- are pregnant or intend to become pregnant while using this medicine;
- are breast-feeding;
- are taking any other prescription or nonprescription (OTC) medicine, especially alcohol or alcohol-containing medicines, anticoagulants (blood thinners), or disulfiram;
- have any other medical problems, especially central nervous system (CNS) disease, including epilepsy; liver disease (severe); or low white blood cell count (or history of).

PROPER USE OF THIS MEDICINE

Wash your hands before and after using the medicine.

Vaginal metronidazole products usually comes with patient directions. Read them carefully before using this medicine.

To help you clear up your infection completely, **it is very important that you keep using this medicine for the full time of treatment,** even if your symptoms begin to clear up after a few days. If you stop using this medicine too soon, your symptoms may return. **Do not miss any doses. Also, continue using this medicine even if your menstrual period starts during treatment.**

If you do miss a dose of this medicine, use it as soon as possible. However, if it is almost time for your next dose, skip the missed dose and go back to your regular dosing schedule.

PRECAUTIONS WHILE USING THIS MEDICINE

If your symptoms do not improve within a few days, or if they become worse, check with your doctor.

Do not drink alcoholic beverages or use other alcohol-containing preparations while using this medicine and for at least one day after stopping it.

This medicine may cause some people to become dizzy or lightheaded. **Make sure you know how you react to this medicine before you drive, use machines, or do anything else that requires you to be alert or clearheaded.** If these reactions are especially bothersome, check with your doctor.

Vaginal medicines usually leak out of the vagina during treatment. To keep the medicine from getting on your clothing, wear a minipad or sanitary napkin. **Do not use tampons** since they may soak up the medicine.

To help clear up your infection completely and to help make sure it does not return, good health habits are also required.
- Wear cotton panties (or panties or pantyhose with cotton crotches) instead of synthetic (for example, nylon or rayon) panties.
- Wear only freshly washed panties daily.

Do not have sexual intercourse while you are using this medicine. Having sexual intercourse may reduce the strength of the medicine.

Many vaginal infections (for example, trichomoniasis) are spread by having sexual intercourse. You can give the infection to your sexual partner, and he can give the infection back to you later. Your partner may also need to be treated for some infections. **Until you are sure that the infection is completely cleared up after your treatment with this medicine, your partner should wear a condom during sexual intercourse.** If you have any questions about this, check with your doctor, nurse, or pharmacist.

POSSIBLE SIDE EFFECTS OF THIS MEDICINE

Side effects that should be reported to your doctor

MORE COMMON—Itching in the vagina; pain during sexual intercourse; thick, white vaginal discharge with or without odor

LESS COMMON—Abdominal or stomach cramping or pain; burning or irritation of penis of sexual partner; burning on urination or need to urinate more often; itching, stinging or redness of the genital area

Metronidazole may cause your urine to become dark. This is harmless and will go away when you stop using this medicine.

Other side effects not listed above may also occur in some patients. If you notice any other effects, check with your doctor, nurse, or pharmacist.

After you stop using this medicine, your body may need time to adjust. The length of time this takes depends on the amount of medicine you were using and how long you used it. During this time check with your doctor if you notice any vaginal or genital irritation or itching; pain during intercourse; or thick, white discharge not present before treatment, with or without odor.

MIDAZOLAM (INJECTION)

ABOUT YOUR MEDICINE

Midazolam (mid-AY-zoe-lam) is used to produce sleepiness or drowsiness and to relieve anxiety before surgery or certain procedures. It is also used to produce loss of consciousness before and during surgery.

If any of the information in this profile causes you special concern or if you want additional information about your medicine and its use, check with your doctor, nurse, or pharmacist.

BEFORE USING THIS MEDICINE

Tell your doctor, nurse, and pharmacist if you . . .
- are allergic to any medicine, either prescription or nonprescription (OTC);
- are pregnant;
- are breast-feeding;
- are taking any other prescription or nonprescription (OTC) medicine, especially CNS depressants;
- have any other medical problems, especially lung disease, or myasthenia gravis or other muscle and nerve disease.

PRECAUTIONS AFTER RECEIVING THIS MEDICINE

For patients going home within 24 hours after receiving midazolam:
- Midazolam may cause some people to feel drowsy, tired, or weak for one or two days after it has been given. It may also cause problems with coordination and one's ability to think. Therefore, **do not drive, use machines, or do other jobs that require you to be alert,** until the effects of the medicine have disappeared or until the day after you receive midazolam, whichever period of time is longer.
- **Do not drink alcoholic beverages or take other CNS depressants (medicines that slow down the nervous system) for about 24 hours after you have received midazolam, unless otherwise directed by your doctor.** To do so may add to the effects of the medicine.

POSSIBLE SIDE EFFECTS OF THIS MEDICINE

Side effects that usually do not require medical attention
These possible side effects may go away; however, if they continue or are bothersome, check with your doctor, nurse, or pharmacist.

LESS COMMON OR RARE—Blurred vision or other changes in vision; dizziness, lightheadedness, or feeling faint; drowsiness (prolonged); headache; nausea or vomiting; numbness, tingling, pain, or weakness in hands or feet; redness, pain, lump or hardness, or muscle stiffness at place of injection

Other side effects not listed above may also occur in some patients. If you notice any other effects, check with your doctor, nurse, or pharmacist.

$\mathcal{M}$ISOPROSTOL (ORAL)

ABOUT YOUR MEDICINE

Misoprostol (mye-soe-PROST-ole) is taken to prevent stomach ulcers in patients taking anti-inflammatory drugs, including aspirin. Misoprostol may also be used for other conditions as determined by your doctor.

If any of the information in this profile causes you special concern or if you want additional information about your medicine and its use, check with your doctor, nurse, or pharmacist. **Remember, keep this and all other medicines out of the reach of children and never share your medicines with others.**

BEFORE USING THIS MEDICINE

Tell your doctor, nurse, and pharmacist if you . . .
- are allergic to any medicine, either prescription or nonprescription (OTC);
- are pregnant or intend to become pregnant while using this medicine;
- are breast-feeding;
- are taking any other prescription or nonprescription (OTC) medicine;
- have any other medical problems.

PROPER USE OF THIS MEDICINE

Misoprostol is best taken with or after meals and at bedtime, unless otherwise directed by your doctor.

Antacids may be taken with misoprostol, if needed, to help relieve stomach pain, unless you are otherwise directed by your doctor. However, do not take magnesium-containing antacids, since they may worsen the diarrhea that is sometimes caused by misoprostol.

Take this medicine for the full time of treatment, even if you begin to feel better. Also, it is important that you keep your appointments with your doctor so that he or she will be better able to tell you when to stop taking this medicine.

If you miss a dose of this medicine, take it as soon as possible. However, if it is almost time for your next dose, skip the missed dose and go back to your regular dosing schedule. Do not double doses.

PRECAUTIONS WHILE USING THIS MEDICINE

Misoprostol may cause miscarriage if taken during pregnancy. Therefore, if you suspect that you may have become pregnant, stop taking this medicine immediately and check with your doctor.

This medicine may cause diarrhea in some people. The diarrhea will usually disappear within a few days as your body adjusts to the medicine. However, check with your doctor if the diarrhea is severe and/or does not stop after a week. Your doctor may need to lower the dose of misoprostol you are taking.

POSSIBLE SIDE EFFECTS OF THIS MEDICINE

Side effects that usually do not require medical attention

These possible side effects may go away during treatment; however, if they continue or are bothersome, check with your doctor, nurse, or pharmacist.

MORE COMMON—Abdominal or stomach pain (mild); diarrhea

LESS COMMON OR RARE—Bleeding from vagina; constipation; cramps in lower abdomen or stomach area; gas; headache; nausea and/or vomiting

Other side effects not listed above may also occur in some patients. If you notice any other effects, check with your doctor, nurse, or pharmacist.

MULTIVITAMINS (ORAL)

Vitamins (VYE-ta-mins) are compounds that you *must* have for growth and health. They are needed in small amounts only and are usually available in the foods that you eat. Vitamins are sometimes taken as a dietary supplement to prevent a vitamin deficiency (lack of a certain vitamin).

Most vitamin supplements are available without a prescription. However, it may be a good idea to check with your doctor before taking vitamins on your own. Taking too much of some vitamins (especially vitamins A and D) over a period of time may cause unwanted effects.

If any of the information in this profile causes you special concern or if you want additional information about your dietary supplement and its uses, check with your doctor, nurse, dietitian, or pharmacist. **Remember, keep this and all medicines out of the reach of children and never share your medicines with others.**

BEFORE USING THIS DIETARY SUPPLEMENT

Importance of diet—Vitamin supplements should be taken only if you cannot get enough vitamins in your diet; however, some diets may not contain all of the vitamins you need. Follow carefully any diet program your doctor recommends. For your specific vitamin and/or mineral needs, ask your doctor for a list of appropriate foods. A balanced diet should provide all the vitamins you normally need.

In some cases, it may not be possible for you to get enough food to supply you with the proper vitamins. In other cases, the amount of vitamins you need may be increased above normal. Therefore, a vitamin supplement may be needed. People who may need a vitamin supplement include those who:

- are pregnant, intend to become pregnant, or are breast-feeding;
- are not able to get a diet that contains all of the vitamins needed (e.g., with

rapid weight loss, unusual diets, prolonged intravenous feeding, or malnutrition);
- do heavy manual labor, have been under a lot of stress for a long time, or have had a long illness, a serious injury, or surgery.

If you have any questions, check with your doctor, nurse, or pharmacist.

PROPER USE OF THIS DIETARY SUPPLEMENT

Do not take more than the recommended daily amount. Most vitamins are water soluble. Water soluble vitamins are not stored in the body; if you take more than you need, the extra will pass into your urine. However, some vitamins are fat soluble (e.g., vitamins A, D, and E). Fat soluble vitamins are stored in the body. **Taking too much of a fat soluble vitamin over a period of time can cause very serious side effects.**

Some people believe that taking very large doses of vitamins (called megadoses or megavitamin therapy) is useful for treating certain medical problems. Studies have not proven this. Large doses should be taken only under the direction of your doctor after need has been identified.

If you miss taking a multivitamin for one or more days, there is no cause for concern, since it takes some time for your body to become seriously low in vitamins. However, if your doctor has recommended that you take a multivitamin, try to remember to take it as directed every day.

POSSIBLE SIDE EFFECTS OF THIS MEDICINE

When multivitamins are used at recommended doses, side effects usually are rare. However, if you notice any effects, check with your doctor, nurse, or pharmacist.

NAFARELIN (NASAL)

ABOUT YOUR MEDICINE

Nafarelin (NAF-a-re-lin) is used to treat endometriosis.

Nafarelin is usually only used in those women who cannot or do not want to take danazol, oral contraceptives (birth control pills), or progestin, or choose not to have surgery. Treatment with nafarelin is usually only for a few months and is generally not repeated.

If any of the information in this profile causes you special concern or if you want additional information about your medicine and its use, check with your doctor, nurse, or pharmacist. **Remember, keep this and all other medicines out of the reach of children and never share your medicines with others.**

BEFORE USING THIS MEDICINE

Discuss with your doctor the possible side effects that may be caused by this medicine. Some of them may be serious and/or long-term.

Tell your doctor, nurse, and pharmacist if you . . .
- are allergic to any medicine, either prescription or nonprescription (OTC);
- are pregnant or intend to become pregnant while using this medicine;
- are breast-feeding;
- are taking any other prescription or nonprescription (OTC) medicine;
- have any other medical problems.

PROPER USE OF THIS MEDICINE

You will be given a fact sheet with your prescription for nafarelin that explains how to use the pump spray bottle. If you have any questions about using the pump spray, ask your doctor, nurse, or pharmacist.

To use nafarelin spray:
- Before you use each new bottle of nafarelin, the spray pump needs to be started. Point the bottle away from you and pump it firmly about 7 times. A spray should come out by the seventh pump. **This only needs to be done once for each new bottle of nafarelin.** Do not breathe in this spray, because you could inhale extra medicine.
- Before you use nafarelin, blow your nose gently. Hold your head forward a little. Put the spray tip into one nostril. Aim the tip toward the back and outside of your nostril. Do not put the tip too far into your nose.
- Close your other nostril off by pressing on the outside of your nose with a finger. Then, sniff in the spray as you pump the bottle once.
- Take the spray bottle out of your nose. Tilt your head back for a few seconds, to let the spray get onto the back of your nose.
- Repeat these steps for each dose of medicine.
- Each time you use the spray bottle, wipe off the tip with a clean tissue or cloth. Keep the blue safety clip and plastic cap on the bottle when you are not using it.
- Every 3 or 4 days you should clean the tip of the spray bottle. To do this, hold the bottle sideways. Rinse the tip with warm water, while wiping the tip with your finger or soft cloth for about 15 seconds. Dry the tip with a soft cloth or tissue. Replace the cap right after use. Be careful not to get water into the bottle, since this could dilute the medicine.

If you miss a dose of this medicine, use it as soon as possible. However, if it is almost time for your next dose, skip the missed dose and go back to your regular dosing schedule. Do not double doses.

PRECAUTIONS WHILE USING THIS MEDICINE

Your doctor should check your progress at regular visits to make sure that this medicine is working properly and to check for unwanted effects.

Using nafarelin can cause dryness of the vagina. If this is uncomfortable, especially during sex, there are several water-based vaginal lubricant products that you can use. Using a lubricant may also help to prevent soreness or damage to the vagina from sex. If you decide to use a lubricant during sex and you are using condoms, a cervical cap, or a diaphragm, make sure the lubricant you choose will not damage the birth control device. Some lubricants contain oils, which can break down latex rubber and cause any of these types of birth control devices to rip or tear.

POSSIBLE SIDE EFFECTS OF THIS MEDICINE

Side effects that should be reported to your doctor
> MORE COMMON—Longer or heavier menstrual periods; vaginal bleeding between regular menstrual periods
> RARE—Chest pain; hives; joint pain; lower abdomen bloating or tenderness (mild); shortness of breath; unexpected or excess flow of milk

Side effects that usually do not require medical attention
> These possible side effects may go away during treatment; however, if they continue or are bothersome, check with your doctor, nurse, or pharmacist.

> MORE COMMON—Acne; decreased breast size; decreased sex drive; dryness of the vagina; hot flashes; oily skin; pain during sex; pounding heartbeat; stopping of menstrual periods

> Other side effects not listed above may also occur in some patients. If you notice any other effects, check with your doctor, nurse, or pharmacist.

NARCOTIC ANALGESICS (INJECTION)

Including Buprenorphine; Butorphanonl; Codeine; Dezocine; Hydromorphone; Levorphanol; Meperidine; Methadone; Morphine; Nalbuphine; Opium; Oxymorphone; Pentazocine

ABOUT YOUR MEDICINE

Narcotic analgesics (nar-KOT-ik an-al-JEE-zicks) are medicines used to relieve pain. Narcotic analgesics may also be used for other purposes as determined by your doctor.

If any of the information in this profile causes you special concern or if you want additional information about your medicine and its use, check with your doctor, nurse, or pharmacist. **Remember, keep this and all other medicines out of the reach of children and never share your medicines with others.**

Before Using This Medicine

Tell your doctor, nurse, and pharmacist if you . . .

- are allergic to any medicine, either prescription or nonprescription (OTC);
- are pregnant or intend to become pregnant while using this medicine;
- are breast-feeding;
- are taking any other prescription or nonprescription (OTC) medicine, especially CNS depressants, MAO inhibitors, naltrexone, rifampin, tricyclic antidepressants, or zidovudine;
- have any other medical problems, especially asthma, chronic lung disease, colitis, or drug dependence (or history of).

Proper Use of This Medicine

Some narcotic analgesics given by injection may be given at home to patients who do not need to be in the hospital. If you are using this medicine at home, **make sure you clearly understand and carefully follow your doctor's instructions.**

Use this medicine only as directed by your doctor. Do not use more of it and do not use it more often or for a longer time than directed. If too much is used, the medicine may become habit-forming or lead to medical problems because of an overdose.

If you must use this medicine regularly and you miss a dose, use it as soon as you remember. However, if it is almost time for your next dose, skip the missed dose and go back to your regular schedule. **Do not double doses.**

Precautions While Using This Medicine

Narcotic analgesics will add to the effects of alcohol and other CNS depressants (medicines that slow down the nervous system). **Check with your doctor before taking any such depressants while you are using this medicine.**

This medicine may cause some people to become drowsy, dizzy, or lightheaded, or to feel a false sense of well-being. **Make sure you know how you react to this medicine before you drive, use machines, or do other jobs that require you to be alert and clearheaded.**

If you have been using this medicine regularly for several weeks or more, **do not suddenly stop using it without first checking with your doctor.** Your doctor may want you to reduce your dose gradually.

If you think an overdose has been used, get emergency help at once. Using an overdose or taking alcohol or CNS depressants with this medicine may lead to unconsciousness or death. Signs of overdose include confusion; seizures; severe nervousness or restlessness, dizziness, drowsiness, or weakness; and unusually slow or troubled breathing.

POSSIBLE SIDE EFFECTS OF THIS MEDICINE

Side effects that should be reported to your doctor

LESS COMMON OR RARE—Chest pain; coughing occurring together with breathing problems; difficult, decreased, or frequent urination; difficult, slow, or shallow breathing; feelings of unreality; hallucinations; hives, itching, or skin rash; increase or decrease in blood pressure; increased sweating; irregular heartbeat; mental depression or other mood changes; redness or flushing of face; ringing or buzzing in ears; shortness of breath or wheezing; swelling of face, fingers, lower legs, or feet; trembling or uncontrolled muscle movements; unusual excitement or restlessness, especially in children; unusually fast or pounding heartbeat; weight gain

Side effects that usually do not require medical attention

These possible side effects may go away during treatment; however, if they continue or are bothersome, check with your doctor, nurse, or pharmacist.

MORE COMMON—Dizziness; drowsiness; feeling faint; lightheadedness; nausea or vomiting

Other side effects not listed above may also occur in some patients. If you notice any other effects, check with your doctor, nurse, or pharmacist.

After you stop using this medicine, your body may need time to adjust. **Check with your doctor if you notice any unusual effects,** especially body aches; diarrhea; fast heartbeat; fever; gooseflesh; large pupils of eyes; loss of appetite; nausea or vomiting; nervousness or restlessness; runny nose; sneezing; shivering or trembling; stomach cramps; trouble in sleeping; unusual sweating, yawning, or irritability; unusually fast heartbeat; or weakness.

$\mathcal{N}$ARCOTIC ANALGESICS (ORAL)

*Including Codeine; Hydrocodone; Hydromorphone;
Levorphanol; Meperidine; Methadone; Morphine;
Oxycodone; Pentazocine; Pentazocine and Naloxone; Propoxyphene*

ABOUT YOUR MEDICINE

Narcotic analgesics (nar-KOT-ik an-al-JEE-zicks) are medicines used to relieve pain. Codeine and hydrocodone are also used to relieve coughing. Methadone is also used to help some people control their dependence on heroin or other narcotics.

Narcotic analgesics may also be used for other purposes as determined by your doctor.

If any of the information in this profile causes you special concern or if you want additional information about your medicine and its use, check with your doctor, nurse, or pharmacist. **Remember, keep this and all other medicines out of the reach of children and never share your medicines with others.**

BEFORE USING THIS MEDICINE

Tell your doctor, nurse, and pharmacist if you . . .
- are allergic to any medicine, either prescription or nonprescription (OTC);
- are pregnant or intend to become pregnant while using this medicine;
- are breast-feeding;
- are taking any other prescription or nonprescription (OTC) medicine, especially carbamazepine, CNS depressants, MAO inhibitors, rifampin, or zidovudine;
- have any other medical problems, especially asthma, chronic lung disease, or colitis.

PROPER USE OF THIS MEDICINE

Take this medicine only as directed by your medical doctor or dentist. Do not take more of it and do not take it more often or for a longer period of time than directed. If too much is taken, the medicine may become habit-forming or lead to medical problems because of an overdose.

If you must take this medicine regularly and you miss a dose, take it as soon as you remember. However, if it is almost time for your next dose, skip the missed dose and go back to your regular schedule. **Do not double doses.**

PRECAUTIONS WHILE USING THIS MEDICINE

Narcotic analgesics will add to the effects of alcohol and other CNS depressants (medicines that slow down the nervous system). **Check with your doctor before taking any such depressants while you are using this medicine.**

This medicine may cause some people to become drowsy, dizzy, or lightheaded, or to feel a false sense of well-being. **Make sure you know how you react to this medicine before you drive, use machines, or do other jobs that require you to be alert and clearheaded.**

If you have been taking this medicine regularly for several weeks or more, **do not suddenly stop taking it without first checking with your doctor.** Your doctor may want you to reduce your dose gradually.

If you think an overdose has been taken, get emergency help at once. Taking an overdose or taking alcohol or CNS depressants with this medicine may lead to unconsciousness or death. Signs of overdose include confusion; seizures; severe nervousness or restlessness, dizziness, drowsiness, or weakness; and unusually slow or troubled breathing.

POSSIBLE SIDE EFFECTS OF THIS MEDICINE

Side effects that should be reported to your doctor

LESS COMMON OR RARE—Feelings of unreality; hallucinations; hives, itching, or skin rash; increased sweating; mental depression or other mood changes; redness or flushing of face; ringing or buzzing in ears; shortness of breath or wheezing; swelling of face; trembling or uncontrolled muscle movements; unusual excitement or restlessness, especially in children; unusually fast or pounding heartbeat

If you are taking propoxyphene, you should also tell your doctor if you notice darkening of your urine, pale stools, or yellow eyes or skin.

Side effects that usually do not require medical attention

These possible side effects may go away during treatment; however, if they continue or are bothersome, check with your doctor, nurse, or pharmacist.

MORE COMMON—Dizziness; drowsiness; feeling faint; lightheadedness; nausea or vomiting

Other side effects not listed above may also occur in some patients. If you notice any other effects, check with your doctor, nurse, or pharmacist.

After you stop using this medicine, your body may need time to adjust. **Check with your doctor if you notice any unusual effects,** especially body aches; diarrhea; fever; gooseflesh; large pupils of eyes; loss of appetite; nausea or vomiting; nervousness or restlessness; runny nose; sneezing; shivering or trembling; stomach cramps; trouble in sleeping; unusual sweating, yawning, or irritability; unusually fast heartbeat; or weakness.

NARCOTIC ANALGESICS AND ACETAMINOPHEN (ORAL)

Including Acetaminophen and Codeine;
Acetaminophen, Codeine, and Caffeine; Dihydrocodeine,
Acetaminophen, and Caffeine; Hydrocodone and Acetaminophen;
Meperidine and Acetaminophen; Oxycodone and Acetaminophen;
Pentazocine and Acetaminophen; Propoxyphene and Acetaminophen

ABOUT YOUR MEDICINE

Combination medicines containing **narcotic analgesics** (nar-KOT-ik an-al-JEE-zicks) and **acetaminophen** (a-seat-a-MIN-oh-fen) are used to relieve pain.

If any of the information in this profile causes you special concern or if you want additional information about your medicine and its use, check with your doctor, nurse, or pharmacist. **Remember, keep this and all other medicines out of the reach of children and never share your medicines with others.**

BEFORE USING THIS MEDICINE

Tell your doctor, nurse, and pharmacist if you . . .
- are allergic to any medicine, either prescription or nonprescription (OTC);
- are pregnant or intend to become pregnant while using this medicine;
- are breast-feeding;
- are taking any other prescription or nonprescription (OTC) medicine, especially carbamazepine, CNS depressants, MAO inhibitors, or naltrexone;
- have any other medical problems, especially colitis; emphysema, asthma, or chronic lung disease; heart disease; or hepatitis or other liver disease.

PROPER USE OF THIS MEDICINE

Take this medicine only as directed by your medical doctor or dentist. Do not take more of it and do not take it more often or for a longer period of time than ordered. If too much of a narcotic analgesic is taken, it may become habit-forming or lead to medical problems because of an overdose.

If you must take this medicine regularly and you miss a dose, take it as soon as possible. However, if it is almost time for your next dose, skip the missed dose and go back to your regular dosing schedule. **Do not double doses.**

PRECAUTIONS WHILE USING THIS MEDICINE

Check the labels of all nonprescription (OTC) and prescription medicines you now take. If any contain acetaminophen or a narcotic, be especially careful, since taking them while taking this medicine may lead to overdose.

This medicine will add to the effects of alcohol and other CNS depressants (medicines that slow down the nervous system). **Check with your doctor before taking any such depressants while you are using this medicine.**

This medicine may cause some people to become drowsy, dizzy, or lightheaded, or to feel a false sense of well-being. **Make sure you know how you react to this medicine before you drive, use machines, or do other jobs that require you to be alert and clearheaded.**

If you have been taking this medicine regularly for several weeks, **do not suddenly stop using it without checking with your doctor.** Your doctor may want you to reduce gradually the amount you are taking before stopping completely.

If you think you or someone else may have taken an overdose, get emergency help at once. Taking an overdose or taking alcohol or CNS depressants with this medicine may lead to unconsciousness or death. Signs of overdose include confusion; convulsions (seizures); severe nervousness or restlessness, dizziness, drowsiness, or weakness; or unusually slow or troubled breathing.

POSSIBLE SIDE EFFECTS OF THIS MEDICINE

Side effects that should be reported to your doctor

LESS COMMON OR RARE—Black, tarry stools; bloody or cloudy urine; confusion; difficult or painful urination; fast, slow, or pounding heartbeat; frequent urge to urinate; hallucinations; irregular breathing; mental depression; pale stools; pinpoint red spots on skin; ringing or buzzing in ears; shortness of breath or troubled breathing; skin rash, hives, or itching; sore throat and fever; sudden decrease in amount of urine; swelling of face; trembling or uncontrolled muscle movements; unusual bleeding or bruising; unusual excitement, especially in children; yellow eyes or skin

Side effects that usually do not require medical attention

These possible side effects may go away during treatment; however, if they continue or are bothersome, check with your doctor, nurse, or pharmacist.

MORE COMMON—Dizziness or lightheadedness; drowsiness; feeling faint; nausea or vomiting; unusual tiredness or weakness

Other side effects not listed above may also occur in some patients. If you notice any other effects, check with your doctor, nurse, or pharmacist.

After you stop using this medicine, your body may need time to adjust. This may take several days or more. **Check with your doctor if you notice any unusual effects,** especially body aches; diarrhea; gooseflesh; nausea or vomiting; shivering or trembling; stomach cramps; fever, runny nose, or sneezing; unusual sweating, nervousness, restlessness or irritability; unusually fast heartbeat; or weakness.

NARCOTIC ANALGESICS AND ASPIRIN (ORAL)

Including Aspirin and Codeine; Aspirin, Codeine, and Caffeine; Aspirin, Caffeine, and Dihydrocodeine; Buffered Aspirin, Codeine, and Caffeine; Hydrocodone and Aspirin; Oxycodone and Aspirin; Pentazocine and Aspirin; Propoxyphene and Aspirin; Propoxyphene, Aspirin, and Caffeine

ABOUT YOUR MEDICINE

Combination medicines containing **narcotic analgesics** (nar-KOT-ik an-al-JEE-zicks) and **aspirin** (AS-pir-in) are used to relieve pain.

If any of the information in this profile causes you special concern or if you want additional information about your medicine and its use, check with your doctor,

nurse, or pharmacist. **Remember, keep this and all other medicines out of the reach of children and never share your medicines with others.**

Before Using This Medicine

Do not give a medicine containing aspirin to a child or teenager with flu or chickenpox without first discussing its use with your child's doctor.
Tell your doctor, nurse, and pharmacist if you . . .

- are allergic to any medicine, either prescription or nonprescription (OTC);
- are pregnant or intend to become pregnant while using this medicine;
- are breast-feeding;
- are taking any other prescription or nonprescription (OTC) medicine;
- have any other medical problems, especially asthma, allergies, and nasal polyps (history of); chronic lung disease; colitis; hemophilia or other bleeding problems; kidney disease; or stomach ulcer or other stomach problems.

Proper Use of This Medicine

Take this medicine with food and a full glass (8 ounces) of water as directed. Do not take more or for a longer time than ordered.

Do not take this medicine if it has a strong vinegar-like odor. This odor means the aspirin in it is breaking down.

If you must take this medicine regularly and you miss a dose, take it as soon as possible. However, if it is almost time for your next dose, skip the missed dose and go back to your regular dosing schedule. **Do not double doses.**

Precautions While Using This Medicine

Check the labels of all over-the-counter (OTC) and prescription medicines you now take. If any contain a narcotic or a salicylate, be especially careful, since taking them while taking this medicine may lead to overdose.

This medicine will add to the effects of alcohol and other CNS depressants. **Check with your physician or dentist before taking any such depressants while you are using this medicine.**

This medicine may cause some people to become drowsy, dizzy, or lightheaded, or to feel a false sense of well-being. **Make sure you know how you react before you drive, use machines, or do jobs that require you to be alert.**

If you have been taking this medicine regularly for several weeks, do not suddenly stop using it without checking with your doctor. Your doctor may want you to reduce gradually the amount you are taking before stopping completely.

If you think an overdose has been taken, get emergency help at once. Taking an overdose or taking alcohol or CNS depressants with this medicine may lead to unconsciousness or death. Signs of overdose include hearing loss; ringing in the ear; hallucinations; severe confusion, excitement, nervousness, restlessness, dizziness, drowsiness, or weakness; shortness of breath or troubled breathing; or convulsions (seizures).

POSSIBLE SIDE EFFECTS OF THIS MEDICINE

Side effects that should be reported to your doctor

LESS COMMON OR RARE—Bloody or black tarry stools; dark or bloody urine; fast, slow, or pounding heartbeat; increased sweating (more common with hydrocodone); mental depression; pale stools; redness or flushing of face (more common with hydrocodone); skin rash, hives, or itching; swelling of face; tightness in chest or wheezing; trembling or uncontrolled muscle movements; unusual excitement; unusual tiredness or weakness; vomiting of blood or material that looks like coffee grounds; yellow eyes or skin

Side effects that usually do not require medical attention

These effects may go away during treatment or if you lie down; however, if they continue or are bothersome, check with your doctor, nurse, or pharmacist.

MORE COMMON—Dizziness or lightheadedness; drowsiness; feeling faint; heartburn or indigestion; nausea or vomiting; stomach pain (mild)

Other side effects not listed above may also occur in some patients. If you notice any other effects, check with your doctor, nurse, or pharmacist.

After you stop using this medicine, your body may need time to adjust. **Check with your doctor if you notice any unusual effects,** especially body aches; diarrhea; gooseflesh; nausea or vomiting; shivering or trembling; stomach cramps; fever, runny nose, or sneezing; increased sweating; nervousness, restlessness, irritability, or weakness.

NIACIN (FOR HIGH CHOLESTEROL—ORAL)

ABOUT YOUR MEDICINE

Niacin (NYE-a-sin) is used to help lower high cholesterol and fat levels in the blood. This may help prevent medical problems caused by cholesterol and fat clogging the blood vessels.

Some strengths of niacin are available only with your doctor's prescription. Others are available without a prescription, since niacin is also a vitamin. However, it is best to take it only under your doctor's direction so that you can be sure you are taking the correct dose.

If any of the information in this profile causes you special concern or if you want additional information about your medicine and its use, check with your doctor,

nurse, or pharmacist. **Remember, keep this and all other medicines out of the reach of children and never share your medicines with others.**

BEFORE USING THIS MEDICINE

Importance of diet—Before prescribing medicine for your condition, your doctor will probably try to control it by prescribing a personal diet for you. Such a diet may be low in fats, sugars, and/or cholesterol. Many people are able to control their condition by carefully following their doctor's orders for proper diet and exercise. Medicine is prescribed only when additional help is needed and is effective only when a schedule of diet and exercise is properly followed.

Also, this medicine is less effective if you are greatly overweight. It may be very important for you to go on a reducing diet. However, check with your doctor before going on any diet.

If you are taking this medicine without a prescription, carefully read and follow any precautions on the label. You should be especially careful if you . . .
- are allergic to any medicine, either prescription or nonprescription (OTC);
- are pregnant, intend to become pregnant, or are breast-feeding;
- are taking any other prescription or nonprescription (OTC) medicine;
- have any other medical problems, especially bleeding problems, diabetes mellitus (sugar diabetes), liver disease, low blood pressure, or stomach ulcer.

PROPER USE OF THIS MEDICINE

Use this medicine only as directed by your doctor. Do not use more or less of it, do not use it more often, and do not use it for a longer time than your doctor ordered. To do so may increase the chance of unwanted effects.

If this medicine upsets your stomach, it may be taken with meals or milk. If stomach upset (nausea or diarrhea) continues, check with your doctor.

For patients taking the extended-release capsule form of this medicine:
- Swallow the capsule whole. Do not crush, break, or chew before swallowing. However, if the capsule is too large to swallow, you may mix the contents of the capsule with jam or jelly and swallow without chewing.

For patients taking the extended-release tablet form of this medicine:
- Swallow the tablet whole. If the tablet is scored, it may be broken, but not crushed or chewed, before being swallowed.

If you miss a dose of this medicine, take it as soon as possible. However, if it is almost time for your next dose, skip the missed dose and go back to your regular dosing schedule. Do not double doses.

PRECAUTIONS WHILE USING THIS MEDICINE

It is very important that your doctor check your progress at regular visits. This will allow your doctor to see if the medicine is working properly to lower your cholesterol and triglyceride (fat) levels and if you should continue to take it.

Do not stop taking niacin without first checking with your doctor. When you stop taking this medicine, your blood cholesterol levels may increase again. Your doctor may want you to follow a special diet to help prevent this from happening.

This medicine may cause you to feel dizzy or faint, especially when you get up from a lying or sitting position. Getting up slowly may help. This effect should lessen after a week or two as your body gets used to the medicine. However, if the problem continues or gets worse, check with your doctor.

POSSIBLE SIDE EFFECTS OF THIS MEDICINE

Side effects that should be reported to your doctor immediately
> LESS COMMON (WITH PROLONGED USE OF EXTENDED-RELEASE NIACIN)—
> Darkening of urine; light gray-colored stools; loss of appetite; stomach pain (severe); yellow eyes or skin

Side effects that usually do not require medical attention
> These possible side effects may go away during treatment; however, if they continue or are bothersome, check with your doctor, nurse, or pharmacist.
>
> LESS COMMON—Feeling of warmth; flushing or redness of skin, especially on face and neck; headache
> WITH HIGH DOSES—Diarrhea; dizziness or faintness; dryness of skin; fever; frequent urination; itching of skin; joint pain; muscle aching or cramping; nausea or vomiting; side, lower back, or stomach pain; swelling of feet or lower legs; unusual thirst; unusual tiredness or weakness; unusually fast, slow, or irregular heartbeat

> Other side effects not listed above may also occur in some patients. If you notice any other effects, check with your doctor, nurse, or pharmacist.

$\mathcal{N}$ICOTINE (TRANSDERMAL)

ABOUT YOUR MEDICINE

Nicotine (NIK-o-teen) in a skin patch is used to help you stop smoking. It is used for up to 12 to 20 weeks as part of a supervised stop-smoking program. These programs may include education, counseling, and psychological support. It is best to use nicotine patches while taking part in such a program.

If any of the information in this profile causes you special concern or if you want additional information about your medicine and its use, check with your doctor, nurse, or pharmacist. **Remember, keep this and all other medicines out of the reach of children and never share your medicines with others.**

BEFORE USING THIS MEDICINE

Tell your doctor, nurse, and pharmacist if you . . .

- are allergic to any medicine, either prescription or nonprescription (OTC);
- are pregnant or intend to become pregnant while using this medicine;
- are breast-feeding;
- are taking any other prescription or nonprescription (OTC) medicine, especially asthma medicines (such as aminophylline, oxtriphylline, and theophylline), insulin, propoxyphene, or propranolol;
- have any other medical problems, especially heart or blood vessel disease.

PROPER USE OF THIS MEDICINE

Use this medicine exactly as directed by your doctor. It will work only if applied correctly. **This medicine usually comes with patient instructions. Read them carefully before using this product.**

Do not remove the patch from its pouch until you are ready to put it on.

Apply the patch to a clean, dry area of skin on your upper arm, chest, or back. Choose an area that is not very oily, has little or no hair, and is free of scars, cuts, burns, or any other skin irritations.

Press the patch firmly in place with the palm of your hand for about 10 seconds. Make sure there is good contact with your skin, especially around the edges of the patch.

The patch should stay in place even when you are showering, bathing, or swimming. Apply a new patch if one falls off.

Rinse your hands with plain water without soap after you have finished applying the patch to your skin. Nicotine on your hands could get into your eyes and nose and cause stinging, redness, or more serious problems.

After 16 or 24 hours, depending on which product you are using, remove the patch. Choose a different place on your skin to apply the next patch. Do not put a new patch in the same place for at least one week. Do not leave the patch on for more than 24 hours.

After removing a used patch, fold the patch in half with the sticky sides together. Place the folded, used patch in its protective pouch or in aluminum foil. Be sure to dispose of it out of the reach of children and pets.

PRECAUTIONS WHILE USING THIS MEDICINE

Your doctor should check your progress at regular visits to make sure nicotine patches are working properly and that possible side effects are avoided.

Do not smoke during treatment with nicotine patches because of the risk of nicotine overdose.

Nicotine patches must be kept out of the reach of children and pets. Even used nicotine patches contain enough nicotine to cause problems in children. If a child handles a patch that is out of the sealed pouch, take it away from the child and contact your doctor or poison control center at once.

Nicotine should not be used during pregnancy. If there is a possibility you might become pregnant, you may want to use some type of birth control. If you think you may have become pregnant, stop using this medicine immediately and check with your doctor.

Mild itching, burning, or tingling may occur when the patch is first applied, and should go away within an hour. After a patch is removed, the skin underneath it may be somewhat red. It should not remain red for more than a day. **If you get a skin rash from the patch, or if the skin becomes swollen or very red, call your doctor.** Do not put on a new patch. If you become allergic to the nicotine in the patch, you could get sick from using cigarettes.

Do not use nicotine patches for longer than 12 to 20 weeks (depending on the product) if you have stopped smoking.

POSSIBLE SIDE EFFECTS OF THIS MEDICINE

Side effects that should be reported to your doctor
RARE—Hives, itching, rash, redness, or swelling; irregular heartbeat

Side effects that usually do not require medical attention
These possible side effects may go away during treatment; however, if they continue or are bothersome, check with your doctor, nurse, or pharmacist.

MORE COMMON—Fast heartbeat; headache (mild); increased appetite; redness, itching, or burning at site of application—usually stops within an hour

Other side effects not listed above may also occur in some patients. If you notice any other effects, check with your doctor, nurse, or pharmacist.

NITRATES (ORAL)

Including Erythrityl Tetranitrate; Isosorbide Dinitrate; Isosorbide Mononitrate; Nitroglycerin; Pentaerythritol Tetranitrate

ABOUT YOUR MEDICINE

Nitrates improve the supply of blood and oxygen to the heart. When taken by mouth and swallowed, these medicines are used to reduce the number of angina (chest pain) attacks. Nitrates may also be used for other conditions as determined by your doctor.

If any of the information in this profile causes you special concern or if you want additional information about your medicine and its use, check with your doctor, nurse, or pharmacist. **Remember, keep this and all other medicines out of the reach of children and never share your medicines with others.**

BEFORE USING THIS MEDICINE

Tell your doctor, nurse, and pharmacist if you . . .
- are allergic to any medicine, either prescription or nonprescription (OTC);
- are pregnant or intend to become pregnant while using this medicine;
- are breast-feeding;
- are taking any other prescription or nonprescription (OTC) medicine, especially high blood pressure medicine or other heart medicine;
- have any other medical problems, especially severe anemia; glaucoma; overactive thyroid; or a recent heart attack, stroke, or head injury.

PROPER USE OF THIS MEDICINE

Take this medicine exactly as directed by your doctor. It will work only if taken correctly.

This form of nitrate is used to reduce the number of angina attacks. In most cases, it will not relieve an attack that has already started, because it works too slowly. Check with your doctor if you need a fast-acting medicine to relieve the pain of an angina attack.

Take this medicine with a full glass (8 ounces) of water on an empty stomach. If taken either 1 hour before or 2 hours after meals, it will start working sooner.

Extended-release capsules and tablets are not to be broken, crushed, or chewed before they are swallowed. If broken up, they will not release the medicine properly.

If you are taking this medicine regularly and you miss a dose, take it as soon as possible. However, if your next scheduled dose is within 2 hours (or within 6 hours for extended-release capsules or tablets), skip the missed dose and go back to your regular dosing schedule. Do not double doses.

PRECAUTIONS WHILE USING THIS MEDICINE

If you have been using this medicine regularly for several weeks or more, do not suddenly stop using it. Stopping suddenly may bring on attacks of angina. Check with your doctor for the best way to reduce gradually the amount you are taking before stopping completely.

Dizziness, lightheadedness, or faintness may occur, especially when you get up quickly from a lying or sitting position. Getting up slowly may help. **Be careful to limit the amount of alcohol you drink and during exercise, hot weather, or if standing for a long time.**

After taking a dose of this medicine you may get a headache that lasts for a short time. This is a common side effect, which should become less noticeable after you have taken the medicine for a while. If this effect continues or if the headaches are severe, check with your doctor.

POSSIBLE SIDE EFFECTS OF THIS MEDICINE

Side effects that should be reported to your doctor

RARE—Blurred vision; dryness of mouth; headache (severe or prolonged); skin rash

Side effects that usually do not require medical attention

These possible side effects may go away during treatment; however, if they continue or are bothersome, check with your doctor, nurse, or pharmacist.

MORE COMMON—Dizziness, lightheadedness, or fainting when standing up; fast pulse; flushing of face and neck; headache; nausea or vomiting; restlessness

Other side effects not listed above may also occur in some patients. If you notice any other effects, check with your doctor, nurse, or pharmacist.

NITRATES (SUBLINGUAL)

Including Erythrityl Tetranitrate;
Isosorbide Dinitrate; Nitroglycerin

ABOUT YOUR MEDICINE

Nitrates improve the supply of blood and oxygen to the heart. Sublingual nitroglycerin and isosorbide dinitrate are used either to relieve the pain of angina (chest pain) attacks or to reduce the number of such attacks. Sublingual erythrityl tetranitrate is used only to reduce the number of angina attacks.

If any of the information in this profile causes you special concern or if you want additional information about your medicine and its use, check with your doctor, nurse, or pharmacist. **Remember, keep this and all other medicines out of the reach of children and never share your medicines with others.**

Before Using This Medicine

Tell your doctor, nurse, and pharmacist if you . . .
- are allergic to any medicine, either prescription or nonprescription (OTC);
- are pregnant or intend to become pregnant while using this medicine;
- are breast-feeding;
- are taking any other prescription or nonprescription (OTC) medicine, especially high blood pressure medicine or other heart medicine;
- have any other medical problems, especially severe anemia; glaucoma; overactive thyroid; or a recent heart attack, stroke, or head injury.

Proper Use of This Medicine

Make sure you understand the proper way to use this medicine. Follow your doctor's instructions. **Sublingual tablets should not be chewed, crushed, or swallowed.** Do not eat, drink, smoke, or use chewing tobacco while a tablet is dissolving.

For patients using nitroglycerin or isosorbide dinitrate to relieve the pain of an angina attack:
- When you begin to feel an attack of angina starting (chest pains or a tightness or squeezing in the chest), sit down. Then place a tablet under your tongue and let it dissolve. Do not chew or swallow the tablet. If you become dizzy or feel faint while sitting, take several deep breaths and bend forward with your head between your knees.
- This medicine usually gives relief in 1 to 5 minutes. However, if the pain is not relieved, dissolve a second tablet under the tongue. If the pain continues for another 5 minutes, a third tablet may be used. **If you still have chest pains after a total of 3 tablets in a 15-minute period, contact your doctor or go to a hospital emergency room without delay.**

For patients using erythrityl tetranitrate or isosorbide dinitrate regularly to prevent angina attacks: If you miss a dose of this medicine, use it as soon as possible. However, if the next scheduled dose is within 2 hours, skip the missed dose and go back to your regular dosing schedule. Do not double doses.

For patients using nitroglycerin tablets: It is important to store nitroglycerin properly in order for it to keep its strength. Carefully follow any directions for storage that are on the bottle.

Precautions While Using This Medicine

If you have been using this medicine regularly for several weeks, do not suddenly stop using it. Stopping suddenly may bring on attacks of angina. Check with your doctor for the best way to reduce gradually the amount you are taking before stopping completely.

Dizziness, lightheadedness, or faintness may occur, especially when you get up quickly from a lying or sitting position. Getting up slowly may help. **Be careful to**

limit the amount of alcohol you drink and during exercise, hot weather, or if standing for a long time.

After using a dose of this medicine you may get a headache that lasts for a short time. This is a common side effect, which should become less noticeable after you have used the medicine for a while. If this effect continues, or if the headaches are severe, check with your doctor.

POSSIBLE SIDE EFFECTS OF THIS MEDICINE

Side effects that should be reported to your doctor

> RARE—Blurred vision; dryness of mouth; headache (severe or prolonged); skin rash

Side effects that usually do not require medical attention

> These possible side effects may go away during treatment; however, if they continue or are bothersome, check with your doctor, nurse, or pharmacist.

> MORE COMMON—Dizziness or lightheadedness when standing up; fast pulse; flushing of face and neck; headache; nausea or vomiting; restlessness

> Other side effects not listed above may also occur in some patients. If you notice any other effects, check with your doctor, nurse, or pharmacist.

$\mathcal{N}$YSTATIN (VAGINAL)

ABOUT YOUR MEDICINE

Nystatin (nye-STAT-in) belongs to the group of medicines called antifungals. Vaginal nystatin is used to treat fungus infections of the vagina. Nystatin may also be used for other problems as determined by your doctor.

If any of the information in this profile causes you special concern or if you want additional information about your medicine and its use, check with your doctor, nurse, or pharmacist. **Remember, keep this and all other medicines out of the reach of children and never share your medicines with others.**

BEFORE USING THIS MEDICINE

Tell your doctor, nurse, and pharmacist if you . . .
- are allergic to any medicine, either prescription or nonprescription (OTC);
- are pregnant or intend to become pregnant while using this medicine;
- are breast-feeding;

- are taking any other prescription or nonprescription (OTC) medicine;
- have any other medical problems.

PROPER USE OF THIS MEDICINE

Nystatin usually comes with patient directions. Read them carefully before using this medicine.

This medicine is usually inserted into the vagina with an applicator. However, if you are pregnant, check with your doctor before using the applicator to insert the vaginal tablet.

To help clear up your infection completely, **keep using this medicine for the full time of treatment** even if your condition has improved. Also, keep using this medicine even if you begin to menstruate during the time of treatment. **Do not miss any doses.**

If you do miss a dose of this medicine, insert it as soon as possible. But if it is almost time for your next dose, skip the missed dose and go back to your regular dosing schedule.

PRECAUTIONS WHILE USING THIS MEDICINE

To help cure the infection and to help prevent reinfection, good health habits are required:
- Wear cotton panties (or panties or pantyhose with cotton crotches) instead of synthetic (for example, nylon, rayon) underclothes.
- Wear freshly laundered underclothes.

If you have any questions about this, check with your doctor, nurse, or pharmacist.

If you have any questions about douching or intercourse during the time of treatment with nystatin, check with your doctor.

Since there may be some vaginal drainage while you are using this medicine, a sanitary napkin may be worn to protect your clothing.

This medicine must not be given to other people or used for other infections unless you are otherwise directed by your doctor.

POSSIBLE SIDE EFFECTS OF THIS MEDICINE

Side effects that should be reported to your doctor
RARE—Vaginal irritation not present before use of this medicine

Other side effects not listed above may also occur in some patients. If you notice any other effects, check with your doctor, nurse, or pharmacist.

OLSALAZINE (ORAL)

ABOUT YOUR MEDICINE

Olsalazine (ole-SAL-a-zeen) is used in patients who have had ulcerative colitis to prevent the condition from occurring again.

If any of the information in this profile causes you special concern or if you want additional information about your medicine and its use, check with your doctor, nurse, or pharmacist. **Remember, keep this and all other medicines out of the reach of children and never share your medicines with others.**

BEFORE USING THIS MEDICINE

Tell your doctor, nurse, and pharmacist if you . . .
- are allergic to any medicine, either prescription or nonprescription (OTC);
- are pregnant or intend to become pregnant while using this medicine;
- are breast-feeding;
- are taking any other prescription or nonprescription (OTC) medicine;
- have any other medical problems.

PROPER USE OF THIS MEDICINE

Olsalazine is best taken with food, to lessen stomach upset. If stomach or intestinal problems continue or are bothersome, check with your doctor.

Keep taking this medicine for the full time of treatment, even if you begin to feel better after a few days. **Do not miss any doses.**

If you do miss a dose of this medicine, take it as soon as possible. However, if it is almost time for your next dose, skip the missed dose and go back to your regular dosing schedule. Do not double doses.

PRECAUTIONS WHILE USING THIS MEDICINE

It is very important that your doctor check your progress at regular visits, especially if you will be taking this medicine for a long time.

POSSIBLE SIDE EFFECTS OF THIS MEDICINE

Side effects that should be reported to your doctor
> RARE—Back or stomach pain (severe); bloody diarrhea; fast heartbeat; fever; nausea or vomiting; skin rash; swelling of the stomach; yellow eyes or skin

Side effects that usually do not require medical attention
> These possible side effects may go away during treatment; however, if they continue or are bothersome, check with your doctor, nurse, or pharmacist.

> MORE COMMON—Abdominal or stomach pain or upset; diarrhea; loss of appetite

LESS COMMON—Aching joints and muscles; acne; anxiety or depression; drowsiness or dizziness; headache; trouble in sleeping

Other side effects not listed above may also occur in some patients. If you notice any other effects, check with your doctor, nurse, or pharmacist.

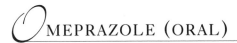MEPRAZOLE (ORAL)

ABOUT YOUR MEDICINE

Omeprazole (o-MEP-ra-zole) is used to treat certain conditions in which there is too much acid in the stomach. It is used to treat duodenal ulcers and gastroesophageal reflux disease, a condition in which the acid in the stomach washes back up into the esophagus. Omeprazole is also used to treat Zollinger-Ellison disease, a condition in which the stomach produces too much acid. It may also be used for other conditions as determined by your doctor.

If any of the information in this profile causes you special concern or if you want additional information about your medicine and its use, check with your doctor, nurse, or pharmacist. **Remember, keep this and all other medicines out of the reach of children and never share your medicines with others.**

BEFORE USING THIS MEDICINE

Tell your doctor, nurse, and pharmacist if you . . .
- are allergic to any medicine, either prescription or nonprescription (OTC);
- are pregnant or intend to become pregnant while using this medicine;
- are breast-feeding;
- are taking any other prescription or nonprescription (OTC) medicine, especially anticoagulants, diazepam, or phenytoin;
- have any other medical problems, especially liver disease.

PROPER USE OF THIS MEDICINE

Take omeprazole immediately before a meal, preferably in the morning.

It may take several days before this medicine begins to relieve stomach pain. To help relieve this pain, antacids may be taken with omeprazole, unless your doctor has told you not to use them.

Swallow the capsule whole. Do not crush, break, chew, or open the capsule.

Take this medicine for the full time of treatment, even if you begin to feel better. Also, keep your appointments with your doctor for check-ups so that your doctor will be better able to tell you when to stop taking this medicine.

If you miss a dose of this medicine, take it as soon as possible. However, if it is almost time for your next dose, skip the missed dose and go back to your regular dosing schedule. Do not double doses.

PRECAUTIONS WHILE USING THIS MEDICINE

If your condition does not improve, or if it becomes worse, check with your doctor.

POSSIBLE SIDE EFFECTS OF THIS MEDICINE

Side effects that should be reported to your doctor

RARE—Bloody or cloudy urine; continuing ulcers or sores in mouth; difficult, burning, or painful urination; frequent urge to urinate; sore throat and fever; unusual bleeding or bruising; unusual tiredness or weakness

Side effects that usually do not require medical attention

These possible side effects may go away during treatment; however, if they continue or are bothersome, check with your doctor, nurse, or pharmacist.

MORE COMMON—Abdominal or stomach pain

LESS COMMON—Chest pain; constipation; diarrhea or loose stools; dizziness; gas; headache; heartburn; muscle pain; nausea and vomiting; skin rash or itching; unusual drowsiness; unusual tiredness

Other side effects not listed above may also occur in some patients. If you notice any other effects, check with your doctor, nurse, or pharmacist.

$\mathcal{O}$NDANSETRON (INJECTION)

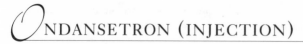

ABOUT YOUR MEDICINE

Ondansetron (on-DAN-se-tron) is used to prevent the nausea and vomiting that may occur after treatment with anticancer medicines (chemotherapy) or radiation, or after surgery.

If any of the information in this profile causes you special concern or if you want additional information about your medicine and its use, check with your doctor, nurse, or pharmacist. **Remember, keep this and all other medicines out of the reach of children and never share your medicines with others.**

BEFORE USING THIS MEDICINE

Tell your doctor, nurse, and pharmacist if you . . .
- are allergic to any medicine, either prescription or nonprescription (OTC);
- are pregnant or intend to become pregnant while using this medicine;

- are breast-feeding;
- are taking any other prescription or nonprescription (OTC) medicine;
- have any other medical problems.

PREPARATION FOR THIS TREATMENT

Your doctor may have special instructions for you in preparation for your treatment. If you have not received such instructions or if you do not understand them, check with your doctor in advance.

POSSIBLE SIDE EFFECTS OF THIS MEDICINE

Side effects that should be reported to your doctor immediately
> RARE—Chest pain; shortness of breath; skin rash, hives or itching; tightness in chest; troubled breathing; wheezing

Side effects that usually do not require medical attention
> These possible side effects may go away during treatment; however, if they continue or are bothersome, check with your doctor, nurse, or pharmacist.

> MORE COMMON—Constipation; diarrhea; fever; headache
> LESS COMMON—Abdominal pain or stomach cramps; dizziness or lightheadedness; drowsiness; dryness of mouth; unusual tiredness or weakness

> Other side effects not listed above may also occur in some patients. If you notice any other effects, check with your doctor, nurse, or pharmacist.

$\mathcal{O}$NDANSETRON (ORAL)

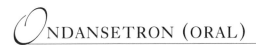

ABOUT YOUR MEDICINE

Ondansetron (on-DAN-se-tron) is used to prevent the nausea and vomiting that may occur after treatment with anticancer medicines (chemotherapy) or radiation, or after surgery.

If any of the information in this profile causes you special concern or if you want additional information about your medicine and its use, check with your doctor, nurse, or pharmacist. **Remember, keep this and all other medicines out of the reach of children and never share your medicines with others.**

BEFORE USING THIS MEDICINE

Tell your doctor, nurse, and pharmacist if you . . .
- are allergic to any medicine, either prescription or nonprescription (OTC);
- are pregnant or intend to become pregnant while using this medicine;

- are breast-feeding;
- are taking any other prescription or nonprescription (OTC) medicine;
- have any other medical problems.

PROPER USE OF THIS MEDICINE

If you vomit within 30 minutes after taking this medicine, take the same amount of medicine again. If vomiting continues, check with your doctor.

If you miss a dose of this medicine and you do not feel nauseous, skip the missed dose and go back to your regular dosing schedule. If you miss a dose of this medicine and you feel nauseous or you vomit, take the missed dose as soon as possible.

POSSIBLE SIDE EFFECTS OF THIS MEDICINE

Side effects that should be reported to your doctor immediately

> RARE—Chest pain, shortness of breath; skin rash, hives or itching; tightness in chest; troubled breathing; wheezing

Side effects that usually do not require medical attention

> These possible side effects may go away during treatment; however, if they continue or are bothersome, check with your doctor, nurse, or pharmacist.
>
> MORE COMMON—Constipation; diarrhea; fever; headache; unusual tiredness or weakness
>
> LESS COMMON—Abdominal pain or stomach cramps; dizziness or lightheadedness; drowsiness; dryness of mouth; unusual tiredness or weakness
>
> Other side effects not listed above may also occur in some patients. If you notice any other effects, check with your doctor, nurse, or pharmacist.

$\mathcal{O}$XYTOCIN (NASAL)

ABOUT YOUR MEDICINE

Oxytocin (ox-i-TOE-sin) is a hormone used to help milk secretion in breast-feeding.

Oxytocin may also be used for other conditions as determined by your doctor.

If any of the information in this profile causes you special concern or if you want additional information about your medicine and its use, check with your doctor, nurse, or pharmacist. **Remember, keep this and all other medicines out of the reach of children and never share your medicines with others.**

BEFORE USING THIS MEDICINE

Tell your doctor, nurse, and pharmacist if you . . .
- are allergic to any medicine, either prescription or nonprescription (OTC);
- are pregnant or intend to become pregnant while using this medicine;
- are breast-feeding;
- are taking any other prescription or nonprescription (OTC) medicine;
- have any other medical problems.

PROPER USE OF THIS MEDICINE

This medicine usually comes with directions for use. Read them carefully before using.

PRECAUTIONS WHILE USING THIS MEDICINE

Oxytocin nasal spray may not help milk secretion in some breast-feeding women. Call your doctor if this medicine is not working.

POSSIBLE SIDE EFFECTS OF THIS MEDICINE

Side effects that should be reported to your doctor
> RARE—Convulsions (seizures); mental disturbances; unexpected bleeding or contractions of the uterus

Side effects that usually do not require medical attention
> These possible side effects may go away during treatment; however, if they continue or are bothersome, check with your doctor, nurse, or pharmacist.

> RARE—Nasal irritation; runny nose; tearing of the eyes

> Other side effects not listed above may also occur in some patients. If you notice any other effects, check with your doctor, nurse, or pharmacist.

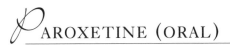

PAROXETINE (ORAL)

ABOUT YOUR MEDICINE

Paroxetine (pa-ROX-uh-teen) is used to treat mental depression.

If any of the information in this profile causes you special concern or if you want additional information about your medicine and its use, check with your doctor, nurse, or pharmacist. **Remember, keep this and all other medicines out of the reach of children and never share your medicines with others.**

BEFORE USING THIS MEDICINE

Tell your doctor, nurse, and pharmacist if you . . .
- are allergic to any medicine, either prescription or nonprescription (OTC);
- are pregnant or intend to become pregnant while using this medicine;
- are breast-feeding;
- are taking any other prescription or nonprescription (OTC) medicine, especially MAO inhibitors, tryptophan, or warfarin (a blood thinner);
- have any other medical problems.

PROPER USE OF THIS MEDICINE

Take this medicine only as directed by your doctor, to benefit your condition as much as possible. Do not take more of it, do not take it more often, and do not take it for a longer time than your doctor ordered.

You may have to take paroxetine for up to 4 weeks or longer before you begin to feel better.

Paroxetine may be taken with or without food. Take it as directed.

If you miss a dose of this medicine, take it as soon as possible. However, if it is almost time for your next dose, skip the missed dose and go back to your regular dosing schedule. Do not double doses.

PRECAUTIONS WHILE USING THIS MEDICINE

It is important that your doctor check your progress at regular visits, to allow for changes in your dose and to help lessen any side effects.

Do not stop taking this medicine without first checking with your doctor. Your doctor may want you to gradually reduce the amount you are taking before stopping completely. This is to decrease the chance of side effects.

This medicine may add to the effects of alcohol and other CNS depressants (medicines that slow down the nervous system). **Check with your doctor before taking any such depressants while you are using this medicine.**

This medicine may cause some people to become drowsy or have blurred vision. **Make sure you know how you react to paroxetine before you drive, use machines, or do other jobs that could be dangerous if you are not alert or able to see clearly.**

Dizziness, lightheadedness, or fainting may occur, especially when you get up from a lying or sitting position. Getting up slowly may help. If this problem continues or gets worse, check with your doctor.

This medicine may cause dryness of the mouth. For temporary relief, use sugarless gum or candy, melt bits of ice in your mouth, or use a saliva substitute. However, if your mouth continues to feel dry for more than 2 weeks, check with your physician or dentist. Continuing dryness of the mouth may increase the chance of dental disease, including tooth decay, gum disease, and fungus infections.

POSSIBLE SIDE EFFECTS OF THIS MEDICINE

Side effects that should be reported to your doctor

LESS COMMON—Agitation; lightheadedness or fainting; muscle pain or
weakness; rash

RARE—Diarrhea; difficulty in speaking; drowsiness; dryness of mouth; fever;
inability to move eyes; increased sweating; increased thirst; lack of energy;
loss of or decrease in body movements; mood or behavior changes;
overactive reflexes; racing heartbeat; restlessness; shivering or shaking;
sudden or unusual body or face movements; talking, feeling, and acting
with excitement and activity you cannot control

Side effects that usually do not require medical attention

These possible side effects may go away during treatment; however, if they
continue or are bothersome, check with your doctor, nurse, or pharmacist.

MORE COMMON—Constipation; decreased sexual ability; dizziness; headache;
nausea; problems in urinating; tremor; trouble in sleeping; unusual tiredness
or weakness; vomiting

LESS COMMON—Anxiety or nervousness; blurred vision; change in your sense
of taste; decreased or increased appetite; decreased sexual desire; fast or
irregular heartbeat; tingling, burning, or prickly sensations; weight loss or
gain

Other side effects not listed above may also occur in some patients. If you
notice any other effects, check with your doctor, nurse, or pharmacist.

After you stop using this medicine, your body may need time to adjust. During this
time, check with your doctor if you notice any unusual effects.

PENICILLINS (ORAL)

Including Amoxicillin; Ampicillin;
Bacampicillin; Carbenicillin; Cloxacillin;
Dicloxacillin; Nafcillin; Oxacillin; Penicillin G; Penicillin V

ABOUT YOUR MEDICINE

Penicillins (pen-i-SILL-ins) are used to treat infections caused by bacteria. They
will not work for colds, flu, or other virus infections. Some penicillins are also used to
prevent "strep" infections in patients with a history of rheumatic heart disease.

If any of the information in this profile causes you special concern or if you want
additional information about your medicine and its use, check with your doctor,

nurse, or pharmacist. **Remember, keep this and all other medicines out of the reach of children and never share your medicines with others.**

BEFORE USING THIS MEDICINE

Tell your doctor, nurse, and pharmacist if you . . .
- are allergic to any medicine, either prescription or nonprescription (OTC);
- are pregnant or intend to become pregnant while using this medicine;
- are breast-feeding;
- are taking any other prescription or nonprescription (OTC) medicine, especially birth control pills containing estrogen, cholestyramine, colestipol, methotrexate, or probenecid;
- have any other medical problems, especially kidney disease, mononucleosis ("mono"), or history of bleeding disorders or stomach or intestinal disease (such as colitis, including colitis caused by antibiotics).

PROPER USE OF THIS MEDICINE

Most penicillins are best taken with a full glass (8 ounces) of water on an empty stomach; however, some are best taken with a snack or meal. Follow your doctor's or pharmacist's directions on how to take your medicine.

If you are taking penicillin G, do not take acidic fruit juices (for example, orange or grapefruit juice) or other acidic beverages within 1 hour of the time you take penicillin G. To do so may keep the medicine from working properly.

Keep taking this medicine for the full time of treatment even if you begin to feel better after a few days; **do not miss any doses. This is especially important if you have a "strep" infection since serious heart problems could develop later** if your infection is not cleared up completely.

If you do miss a dose of this medicine, take it as soon as possible. However, if it is almost time for your next dose, skip the missed dose and go back to your regular dosing schedule. Do not double doses.

PRECAUTIONS WHILE USING THIS MEDICINE

If your symptoms do not improve within a few days, or if they become worse, check with your doctor.

In some patients, penicillins may cause diarrhea. Severe diarrhea may be a sign of a serious side effect. **Do not take any diarrhea medicine without first checking with your doctor.**

Oral contraceptives (birth control pills) containing estrogen may not work properly if you take them while you are taking ampicillin, bacampicillin, or penicillin V. Unplanned pregnancies may occur. Use a different or additional means of birth control while taking any of these penicillins.

Diabetics—Some penicillins may cause false test results with some urine sugar tests. Check with your doctor before changing your diet or the dosage of your diabetes medicine.

This medicine must not be given to other people or used for other infections unless you are otherwise directed by your doctor.

POSSIBLE SIDE EFFECTS OF THIS MEDICINE

Side effects that should be reported to your doctor immediately
Stop taking this medicine and get emergency help immediately if you notice:

LESS COMMON—Fast or irregular breathing; fever; joint pain; lightheadedness or fainting (sudden); puffiness or swelling around the face; red, scaly skin; shortness of breath; skin rash, hives, or itching

Other side effects that should be reported to your doctor immediately
RARE—Abdominal or stomach cramps and pain; abdominal tenderness; convulsions (seizures); decreased amount of urine; diarrhea (watery and severe) which may also be bloody; nausea or vomiting; sore throat and fever; unusual bleeding or bruising; yellow eyes or skin

Some of the above side effects may occur up to several weeks after you stop taking this medicine.

Side effects that usually do not require medical attention
These possible side effects may go away during treatment; however, if they continue or are bothersome, check with your doctor, nurse, or pharmacist.

MORE COMMON—Diarrhea (mild); headache; sore mouth or tongue; vaginal itching and discharge; white patches in the mouth and/or on the tongue

Other side effects not listed above may also occur in some patients. If you notice any other effects, check with your doctor, nurse, or pharmacist.

PHENOBARBITAL (FOR EPILEPSY—ORAL)

ABOUT YOUR MEDICINE

Phenobarbital (fee-noe-BAR-bi-tal) belongs to the group of medicines called central nervous system (CNS) depressants. It is used to help control seizures in certain disorders or diseases, such as epilepsy. Phenobarbital may also be used for other conditions as determined by your doctor.

If any of the information in this profile causes you special concern or if you want additional information about your medicine and its use, check with your doctor, nurse, or pharmacist. **Remember, keep this and all other medicines out of the reach of children and never share your medicines with others.**

BEFORE USING THIS MEDICINE

Tell your doctor, nurse, and pharmacist if you . . .
- are allergic to any medicine, either prescription or nonprescription (OTC);
- are pregnant or intend to become pregnant while using this medicine;
- are breast-feeding;
- compete in athletics;
- are taking **any** other prescription or nonprescription (OTC) medicine;
- have **any** other medical problems.

PROPER USE OF THIS MEDICINE

Use this medicine only as directed. If too much is used, it may become habit-forming. Even if you think this medicine is not working, **do not increase the dose.** Instead, check with your doctor.

Phenobarbital must be taken every day in regularly spaced doses in order for it to control your seizures.

If you are taking this medicine regularly and you miss a dose, take it as soon as possible. However, if it is almost time for your next dose, skip the missed dose and go back to your regular dosing schedule. Do not double doses.

PRECAUTIONS WHILE USING THIS MEDICINE

If you will be taking this medicine regularly for a long time, do not stop taking it without first checking with your doctor.

Phenobarbital will add to the effects of alcohol and other CNS depressants. **Check with your doctor before taking any such depressants while taking this medicine.**

Before you have any medical tests, tell the doctor in charge that you are taking this medicine. The results of some tests may be affected by this medicine.

This medicine may cause some people to become dizzy, lightheaded, drowsy, or less alert than they are normally. Even if taken at bedtime, it may cause these effects on arising. **Make sure you know how you react before you drive, use machines, or do other jobs that require you to be alert.**

If you think you or someone else may have taken an overdose, get emergency help at once. Taking an overdose of phenobarbital or taking alcohol or other CNS depressants with it may lead to death. Some signs of an overdose are decrease in or loss of reflexes, severe drowsiness, severe confusion, severe weakness, shortness of breath or slow or troubled breathing, slurred speech, staggering, and slow heartbeat.

POSSIBLE SIDE EFFECTS OF THIS MEDICINE

Side effects that should be reported to your doctor immediately
> RARE—Bleeding sores on lips; chest pain; muscle or joint pain; red, thickened, or scaly skin; skin rash or hives; sores or white spots in mouth (painful); sore throat; fever; swelling of eyelids, face, or lips; wheezing or tightness in chest

Other side effects that should be reported to your doctor
> LESS COMMON—Confusion; mental depression; unusual excitement
> RARE—Hallucinations; unusual bleeding, bruising, tiredness, or weakness
> WITH LONG-TERM OR CHRONIC USE—Bone pain or aching; loss of appetite; muscle weakness; weight loss (unusual); yellow eyes or skin

Side effects that usually do not require medical attention
> These possible side effects may go away during treatment; however, if they continue or are bothersome, check with your doctor, nurse, or pharmacist.

> MORE COMMON—Clumsiness or unsteadiness, dizziness or lightheadedness, drowsiness, "hangover" effect

> Other side effects not listed above may also occur in some patients. If you notice any other effects, check with your doctor, nurse, or pharmacist.

After you stop using this medicine, your body may need time to adjust. If you took this medicine in high doses or for a long time, this may take up to about 15 days. Check with your doctor if you experience anxiety; convulsions (seizures); dizziness or lightheadedness; faint feeling; hallucinations; muscle twitching; nausea or vomiting; trembling of hands; trouble in sleeping, increased dreaming, or nightmares; vision problems; or weakness.

$\mathscr{P}$HENOTHIAZINES (INJECTION)

Including Chlorpromazine; Fluphenazine;
Mesoridazine; Methotrimeprazine; Perphenazine; Pipotiazine;
Prochlorperazine; Promazine; Trifluoperazine; Triflupromazine

ABOUT YOUR MEDICINE

Phenothiazines (FEE-noe-THYE-a-zeens) are used to treat nervous, mental, and emotional disorders. Some are used also to control anxiety or agitation in certain patients, severe nausea and vomiting, severe hiccups, and moderate to severe pain. Chlorpromazine is also used in the treatment of certain types of porphyria, and with other medicines in the treatment of tetanus. Phenothiazines may also be used for other conditions as determined by your doctor.

If any of the information in this profile causes you special concern or if you want additional information about your medicine and its use, check with your doctor, nurse, or pharmacist. **Remember, keep this and all other medicines out of the reach of children and never share your medicines with others.**

BEFORE USING THIS MEDICINE

Discuss with your doctor possible side effects of this medicine. Some may be serious and/or permanent. For example, tardive dyskinesia (a movement disorder) may occur and may not go away after you stop using the medicine.

Tell your doctor, nurse, and pharmacist if you . . .
- are allergic to any medicine, either prescription or nonprescription (OTC);
- are pregnant or intend to become pregnant while using this medicine;
- are breast-feeding;
- are taking **any** other prescription or nonprescription (OTC) medicine;
- have **any** other medical problems.

PROPER USE OF THIS MEDICINE

If you miss a dose of this medicine, use it as soon as possible. However, if it is almost time for your next dose, skip the missed dose. Do not double doses.

PRECAUTIONS WHILE USING THIS MEDICINE

Do not stop using this medicine without first checking with your doctor. Your doctor may want you to reduce gradually the amount you are using.

This medicine will add to the effects of alcohol and other CNS depressants (medicines that may make you drowsy or less alert). **Check with your doctor before taking any such depressants while you are using this medicine.**

This medicine may cause changes in vision or cause some people to become drowsy or less alert than they are normally. **Make sure you know how you react before you drive or do jobs that require you to be alert and to see well.**

Dizziness, lightheadedness, or fainting may occur, especially when getting up from a lying or sitting position. Getting up slowly may help.

This medicine may make you sweat less, causing your body temperature to rise. **Do not become overheated during exercise or hot weather, since overheating may result in heat stroke.**

Before having any kind of surgery or dental or emergency treatment, tell the physician or dentist in charge that you are using this medicine.

Some people who use this medicine may become more sensitive to sunlight. Stay out of direct sunlight and protect yourself from getting too much sun.

The effects of the long-acting injection form of this medicine may last for up to 12 weeks. **The precautions and side effects information for this medicine applies during this time.**

POSSIBLE SIDE EFFECTS OF THIS MEDICINE

Side effects that should be reported to your doctor immediately

Stop using this medicine and check with your doctor or get emergency help immediately if any of the following side effects occur:

RARE—Convulsions (seizures); fast or irregular heartbeat; high fever; high or low blood pressure; increased sweating; loss of bladder control; muscle stiffness (severe); troubled breathing; unusually pale skin; unusual tiredness

Other side effects that should be reported to your doctor

MORE COMMON—Blurred vision or difficulty in seeing at night; difficulty in talking or swallowing; fainting; inability to move eyes; lip smacking or puckering; loss of balance control; mask-like face; muscle spasms of face, neck, or back; puffing of cheeks; restlessness; shuffling walk or stiff arms and legs; tic-like, twitching, or twisting movements; trembling of hands; uncontrolled chewing or tongue movements; uncontrolled movements or weakness of arms or legs

LESS COMMON—Difficulty in urinating; skin rash; sunburn (severe)

RARE—Abdominal or stomach pains; aching muscles and joints; confusion; fever and chills; hot, dry skin or lack of sweating; muscle weakness; nausea, vomiting, or diarrhea; painful, inappropriate penile erection (continuing); skin itching (severe) or discoloration (tan or blue-gray); sore throat and fever; unusual bleeding or bruising; yellow eyes or skin

Side effects that usually do not require medical attention

These possible side effects may go away during treatment; however, if they continue or are bothersome, check with your doctor, nurse, or pharmacist.

MORE COMMON—Constipation; decreased sweating; drowsiness; dryness of mouth; lightheadedness or dizziness; stuffy nose

Other side effects not listed above may also occur in some patients. If you notice any other effects, check with your doctor, nurse, or pharmacist.

After you stop using this medicine, your body may need time to adjust. Check with your doctor if you notice any of the above side effects.

PHENOTHIAZINES (ORAL)

Including Acetophenazine; Chlorpromazine;
Fluphenazine; Mesoridazine; Methotrimeprazine;
Pericyazine; Perphenazine; Prochlorperazine; Promazine;
Thiopropazate; Thioproperazine; Thioridazine; Trifluoperazin

ABOUT YOUR MEDICINE

Phenothiazines (fee-noe-THYE-a-zeens) are used to treat nervous, mental, and emotional disorders. Some are used also to control anxiety or agitation in certain patients, severe nausea and vomiting, severe hiccups, and moderate to severe pain. Chlorpromazine is also used in the treatment of certain types of porphyria, and with other medicines in the treatment of tetanus. Phenothiazines may also be used for other conditions as determined by your doctor.

If any of the information in this profile causes you special concern or if you want additional information about your medicine and its use, check with your doctor, nurse, or pharmacist. **Remember, keep this and all other medicines out of the reach of children and never share your medicines with others.**

BEFORE USING THIS MEDICINE

Discuss with your doctor possible side effects of this medicine. Some may be serious and/or permanent. For example, tardive dyskinesia (a movement disorder) may occur and may not go away after you stop using the medicine.

Tell your doctor, nurse, and pharmacist if you . . .
- are allergic to any medicine, either prescription or nonprescription (OTC);
- are pregnant or intend to become pregnant while using this medicine;
- are breast-feeding;
- are taking **any** other prescription or nonprescription (OTC) medicine;
- have **any** other medical problems.

PROPER USE OF THIS MEDICINE

Phenothiazines may be taken with food or a full glass (8 ounces) of water or milk to reduce stomach irritation.

If you miss a dose of this medicine, take it as soon as possible. However, if it is almost time for your next dose, skip the missed dose. Do not double doses.

PRECAUTIONS WHILE USING THIS MEDICINE

Do not stop taking this medicine without first checking with your doctor. Your doctor may want you to reduce gradually the amount you are taking.

This medicine will add to the effects of alcohol and other CNS depressants (medicines that may make you drowsy or less alert). **Check with your doctor before taking any such depressants while you are taking this medicine.**

This medicine may cause changes in vision or cause some people to become drowsy or less alert than they are normally. **Make sure you know how you react before you drive or do jobs that require you to be alert and to see well.**

Dizziness, lightheadedness, or fainting may occur, especially when getting up from a lying or sitting position. Getting up slowly may help.

This medicine may make you sweat less, causing your body temperature to rise. **Do not become overheated during exercise or hot weather, since overheating may result in heat stroke.**

Before having any kind of surgery or dental or emergency treatment, tell the physician or dentist in charge that you are using this medicine.

Some people who take this medicine may become more sensitive to sunlight. Stay out of direct sunlight and protect yourself from getting too much sun.

POSSIBLE SIDE EFFECTS OF THIS MEDICINE

Side effects that should be reported to your doctor immediately
Stop taking this medicine and check with your doctor or get emergency help immediately if any of the following side effects occur:

RARE—Convulsions (seizures); fast or irregular heartbeat; high fever; high or low blood pressure; increased sweating; loss of bladder control; muscle stiffness (severe); troubled breathing; unusually pale skin; unusual tiredness

Other side effects that should be reported to your doctor
MORE COMMON—Blurred vision or difficulty in seeing at night; difficulty in talking or swallowing; fainting; inability to move eyes; lip smacking or puckering; loss of balance control; mask-like face; muscle spasms of face, neck, or back; puffing of cheeks; restlessness; shuffling walk or stiff arms and legs; tic-like, twitching, or twisting movements; trembling of hands; uncontrolled chewing or tongue movements; uncontrolled movements or weakness of arms or legs
LESS COMMON—Difficulty in urinating; skin rash; sunburn (severe)
RARE—Abdominal or stomach pains; aching muscles and joints; confusion; fever and chills; hot, dry skin or lack of sweating; muscle weakness; nausea, vomiting, or diarrhea; painful, inappropriate penile erection (continuing); skin itching (severe) or discoloration (tan or blue-gray); sore throat and fever; unusual bleeding or bruising; yellow eyes or skin

Side effects that usually do not require medical attention
These possible side effects may go away during treatment; however, if they continue or are bothersome, check with your doctor, nurse, or pharmacist.

MORE COMMON—Constipation; decreased sweating; drowsiness; dryness of mouth; lightheadedness or dizziness; stuffy nose

Other side effects not listed above may also occur in some patients. If you notice any other effects, check with your doctor, nurse, or pharmacist.

After you stop using this medicine, your body may need time to adjust. Check with your doctor if you notice any of the above side effects.

PHENOTHIAZINES (FOR NAUSEA AND VOMITING—ORAL)

Including Chlorpromazine; Perphenazine; Prochlorperazine

ABOUT YOUR MEDICINE

Phenothiazines (FEE-noe-THYE-a-zeens) are used to treat severe nausea and vomiting. Phenothiazines may also be used for other conditions as determined by your doctor.

If any of the information in this profile causes you special concern or if you want additional information about your medicine and its use, check with your doctor, nurse, or pharmacist. **Remember, keep this and all other medicines out of the reach of children and never share your medicines with others.**

BEFORE USING THIS MEDICINE

Discuss with your doctor possible side effects of this medicine. Some may be serious and/or permanent. For example, tardive dyskinesia (a movement disorder) may occur and may not go away after you stop using the medicine.

Tell your doctor, nurse, and pharmacist if you . . .
- are allergic to any medicine, either prescription or nonprescription (OTC);
- are pregnant or intend to become pregnant while using this medicine;
- are breast-feeding;
- are taking **any** other prescription or nonprescription (OTC) medicine;
- have **any** other medical problems.

PROPER USE OF THIS MEDICINE

Phenothiazines may be taken with food or a full glass (8 ounces) of water or milk to reduce stomach irritation.

If you miss a dose of this medicine, take it as soon as possible. However, if it is almost time for your next dose, skip the missed dose. Do not double doses.

PRECAUTIONS WHILE USING THIS MEDICINE

Do not stop taking this medicine without first checking with your doctor. Your doctor may want you to reduce gradually the amount you are taking.

This medicine will add to the effects of alcohol and other CNS depressants (medicines that may make you drowsy or less alert). **Check with your doctor before taking any such depressants while you are taking this medicine.**

This medicine may cause changes in vision or cause some people to become drowsy or less alert than they are normally. **Make sure you know how you react before you drive or do jobs that require you to be alert and to see well.**

Dizziness, lightheadedness, or fainting may occur, especially when getting up from a lying or sitting position. Getting up slowly may help.

This medicine may make you sweat less, causing your body temperature to rise. **Do not become overheated during exercise or hot weather, since overheating may result in heat stroke.**

Before having any kind of surgery or dental or emergency treatment, tell the physician or dentist in charge that you are using this medicine.

Some people who take this medicine may become more sensitive to sunlight. Stay out of direct sunlight and protect yourself from getting too much sun.

POSSIBLE SIDE EFFECTS OF THIS MEDICINE

Side effects that should be reported to your doctor immediately
> **Stop taking this medicine and check with your doctor or get emergency help immediately** if any of the following side effects occur:
>
> RARE—Convulsions (seizures); fast or irregular heartbeat; high fever; high or low blood pressure; increased sweating; loss of bladder control; muscle stiffness (severe); troubled breathing; unusually pale skin; unusual tiredness

Other side effects that should be reported to your doctor
> MORE COMMON—Blurred vision or difficulty in seeing at night; difficulty in talking or swallowing; fainting; inability to move eyes; lip smacking or puckering; loss of balance control; mask-like face; muscle spasms of face, neck, or back; puffing of cheeks; restlessness; shuffling walk or stiff arms and legs; tic-like, twitching, or twisting movements; trembling of hands; uncontrolled chewing or tongue movements; uncontrolled movements or weakness of arms or legs
>
> LESS COMMON—Difficulty in urinating; skin rash; sunburn (severe)
>
> RARE—Abdominal or stomach pains; aching muscles and joints; confusion; fever and chills; hot, dry skin or lack of sweating; muscle weakness; nausea, vomiting, or diarrhea; painful, inappropriate penile erection (continuing); skin itching (severe) or discoloration (tan or blue-gray); sore throat and fever; unusual bleeding or bruising; yellow eyes or skin

Side effects that usually do not require medical attention

These possible side effects may go away during treatment; however, if they continue or are bothersome, check with your doctor, nurse, or pharmacist.

MORE COMMON—Constipation; decreased sweating; drowsiness; dryness of mouth; lightheadedness or dizziness; stuffy nose

Other side effects not listed above may also occur in some patients. If you notice any other effects, check with your doctor, nurse, or pharmacist.

After you stop using this medicine, your body may need time to adjust. Check with your doctor if you notice any of the above side effects.

PHENYLPROPANOLAMINE (ORAL)

ABOUT YOUR MEDICINE

Phenylpropanolamine (fen-ill-proe-pa-NOLE-a-meen), commonly known as PPA, is used as a nasal decongestant or as an appetite suppressant.

If any of the information in this profile causes you special concern or if you want additional information about your medicine and its use, check with your doctor, nurse, or pharmacist. **Remember, keep this and all other medicines out of the reach of children and never share your medicines with others.**

BEFORE USING THIS MEDICINE

If you are taking this medicine without a prescription, carefully read and follow any precautions on the label. You should be especially careful if you . . .
* are allergic to any medicine, either prescription or nonprescription (OTC);
* are pregnant, intend to become pregnant, or are breast-feeding;
* compete in athletics;
* are taking **any** other prescription or nonprescription (OTC) medicine;
* have any other medical problems, especially heart or blood vessel disease (including a history of heart attack or stroke), or high blood pressure.

If you have any questions, check with your doctor, nurse, or pharmacist.

PROPER USE OF THIS MEDICINE

For patients taking an extended-release form of this medicine:
* Swallow the capsule or tablet whole. Do not crush, break, or chew before swallowing.
* Take with a full glass (at least 8 ounces) of water.

- If taking only one dose of this medicine a day, take it in the morning around 10 a.m.

Take phenylpropanolamine (PPA) only as directed. Do not take more of it, do not take it more often, and do not take it for a longer time than directed. To do so may increase the chance of side effects.

For patients taking this medicine as an appetite suppressant:
- Do not take this medicine for longer than a few weeks without your doctor's permission.

If PPA causes trouble in sleeping, take the last dose for each day a few hours before bedtime. If you are taking an extended-release form of this medicine, take your daily dose at least 12 hours before bedtime.

Phenylpropanolamine should not be used for weight control in children under the age of 12 years. Children 12 to 18 years old should not take phenylpropanolamine for weight control unless its use is ordered and supervised by their doctor.

For patients taking phenylpropanolamine for nasal congestion:
- **If you miss a dose,** take it as soon as possible. However, if it is within 2 hours (or 12 hours for extended-release forms) of your next dose, skip the missed dose and go back to your regular dosing schedule. Do not double doses.

PRECAUTIONS WHILE USING THIS MEDICINE

This medicine may cause some people to become dizzy. **Make sure you know how you react to this medicine before you drive or use machines or do anything else that could be dangerous if you are dizzy or not alert.**

If you are taking this medicine for nasal congestion and cold symptoms do not improve within 7 days or if you also have a high fever, check with your doctor. These signs may mean that you have other medical problems.

POSSIBLE SIDE EFFECTS OF THIS MEDICINE

Side effects that should be reported to your doctor
> RARE—Headache (severe); increased blood pressure; painful or difficult urination; tightness in chest
>
> EARLY SIGNS OF OVERDOSE—Abdominal or stomach pain; fast, pounding, or irregular heartbeat; headache (severe); increased sweating not caused by exercise; nausea and vomiting (severe); nervousness or restlessness (severe)

Side effects that usually do not require medical attention
> These possible side effects may go away during treatment; however, if they continue or are bothersome, check with your doctor, nurse, or pharmacist.
>
> LESS COMMON (MORE COMMON WITH HIGH DOSES)—Dizziness; dryness of nose or mouth; headache (mild); nausea (mild); nervousness or restlessness (mild); trouble in sleeping; unusual feeling of well-being

Other side effects not listed above may also occur in some patients. If you notice any other effects, check with your doctor, nurse, or pharmacist.

PLATELET AGGREGATION INHIBITORS (ORAL)

Including Aspirin; Aspirin and Caffeine;
Aspirin, Sodium Bicarbonate, and Citric
Acid; Buffered Aspirin; Dipyridamole; Ticlopidine

ABOUT YOUR MEDICINE

Platelet aggregation inhibitors (PLAYT-let a-gre-GAY-shun in-HIB-i-ters) help to prevent dangerous blood clots that may cause problems such as a heart attack or stroke. These medicines are only used when there is a larger-than-usual chance that these problems may occur. **Do not take aspirin to prevent blood clots unless it has been ordered by your doctor.**

If any of the information in this profile causes you special concern or if you want additional information about your medicine and its use, check with your doctor, nurse, or pharmacist. **Remember, keep this and all other medicines out of the reach of children and never share your medicines with others.**

BEFORE USING THIS MEDICINE

Do not give aspirin to a child or a teenager with symptoms of flu or chickenpox without first discussing this with your child's doctor.
If you are taking this medicine without a prescription, carefully read and follow any precautions on the label. You should be especially careful if you . . .

- are allergic to any medicine, either prescription or nonprescription (OTC);
- are pregnant, intend to become pregnant, or are breast-feeding;
- are taking **any** other prescription or nonprescription (OTC) medicine;
- have **any** other medical problems, or are on a low-sodium diet.

If you have any questions, check with your doctor, nurse, or pharmacist.

PROPER USE OF THIS MEDICINE

Take this medicine only as directed. It will not work properly if you take less than directed. Taking more than directed may increase the chance of bleeding or other serious side effects without increasing the helpful effects.

Take aspirin with food (except for enteric-coated capsules or tablets) and a full glass (8 ounces) of water to lessen stomach irritation.

Aspirin, sodium bicarbonate, and citric acid combination tablets are used to prepare a liquid. **Do not swallow the tablets or any pieces of the tablets.** To make the liquid, add each tablet to 1/2 glass (4 ounces) of water.

Ticlopidine should be taken with food. This helps more of the medicine to be absorbed into the body. It may also lessen the chance of stomach upset.

Dipyridamole works best when taken with a full glass (8 ounces) of water at least 1 hour before or 2 hours after meals. However, to lessen stomach upset, your doctor may want you to take it with food or milk.

If you miss a dose of your medicine, take it as soon as possible. However, if it is almost time for your next dose, skip the missed dose and go back to your regular dosing schedule. Do not double doses.

PRECAUTIONS WHILE USING THIS MEDICINE

Tell all medical doctors, dentists, nurses, and pharmacists you go to that you are taking this medicine. This medicine may increase the risk of serious bleeding. If you need an operation or some kinds of dental work, treatment may have to be stopped about 10 days to 2 weeks ahead of time.

If you are taking ticlopidine, it is very important that blood tests be done every 2 weeks, for at least the first 3 months of treatment. Be sure that you do not miss any of these tests. They are needed to detect certain side effects.

Taking aspirin or certain other medicines for arthritis, pain, or fever while taking this medicine (including aspirin) may increase the chance of unwanted effects. Ask your doctor what to take for these conditions.

Platelet aggregation inhibitor treatment may cause serious bleeding after an injury. Ask your doctor if you should avoid certain activities, and **check with your doctor immediately if you are injured.**

Do not stop taking this medicine for any reason without first checking with the doctor who directed you to take it.

After you stop taking aspirin or ticlopidine, the chance of bleeding may continue for 1 or 2 weeks. Continue to follow the same precautions that you followed while you were taking the medicine.

POSSIBLE SIDE EFFECTS OF THIS MEDICINE

Side effects that should be reported to your doctor immediately

Any sign of bleeding, such as blood in eyes, bloody urine, bloody or black, tarry stools, bruising or purple areas on skin, coughing up blood, decreased alertness, dizziness, headache (severe), joint pain or swelling, nosebleeds, paralysis or problems with coordination, stammering or other difficulty in speaking, heavy bleeding or oozing from cuts or wounds, unusually heavy or unexpected menstrual bleeding, vomiting of blood or material that looks like coffee grounds; any sign of infection, such as fever, chills, or sore throat (ticlopidine only); difficulty in swallowing, shortness of breath, troubled breathing, or wheezing (aspirin only); pinpoint red spots on skin or sores, ulcers, or white spots in the mouth (ticlopidine only); tightness in chest (aspirin or dipyridamole only)

Other side effects that should be reported to your doctor

Abdominal or stomach pain, cramping, or burning (severe); back or chest pain; flushing; ringing or buzzing in ears; skin rash, hives, or itching; fever without other signs of infection (aspirin only); yellow eyes or skin

Other side effects not listed above may also occur in some patients. If you notice any other effects, check with your doctor, nurse, or pharmacist.

POTASSIUM-SPARING DIURETICS (ORAL)

Including Amiloride; Spironolactone; Triamterene

ABOUT YOUR MEDICINE

Potassium-sparing diuretics are commonly used to help reduce the amount of water in the body by increasing the flow of urine. Amiloride and spironolactone are also used to treat high blood pressure (hypertension). Unlike some other diuretics, these medicines do not cause your body to lose potassium. Spironolactone may also be used to help increase the amount of potassium in the body when it is getting too low. These medicines may also be used for other conditions as determined by your doctor.

If any of the information in this profile causes you special concern or if you want additional information about your medicine and its use, check with your doctor, nurse, or pharmacist. **Remember, keep this and all other medicines out of the reach of children and never share your medicines with others.**

BEFORE USING THIS MEDICINE

Tell your doctor, nurse, and pharmacist if you . . .
- are allergic to any medicine, either prescription or nonprescription (OTC);
- are pregnant or intend to become pregnant while using this medicine;
- are breast-feeding;
- compete in athletics;
- are taking any other prescription or nonprescription (OTC) medicine, especially angiotensin-converting enzyme (ACE) inhibitors; cyclosporine; digitalis; lithium; medicines for appetite control, asthma, colds, cough, hay fever, or sinus; potassium-containing medicines or supplements; or other potassium-sparing diuretics;
- have any other medical problems, especially kidney disease or liver disease.

PROPER USE OF THIS MEDICINE

This medicine may cause an unusual feeling of tiredness when you begin to take it. You may also notice an increase in urine or in frequency of urination. In order to keep this from affecting sleep:
- if you are to take a single dose a day, take it in the morning after breakfast.
- if you are to take more than one dose, take the last one no later than 6 p.m.

If this medicine upsets your stomach, it may be taken with meals or milk. If stomach upset continues, check with your doctor.

For patients taking this medicine for high blood pressure:
- This medicine will not cure your high blood pressure but it does help control it. You must continue to take it—even if you feel well—if you expect to keep your blood pressure down. **You may have to take high blood pressure medicine for the rest of your life.**

If you miss a dose of this medicine, take it as soon as possible. However, if it is almost time for your next dose, skip the missed dose and go back to your regular dosing schedule. Do not double doses.

PRECAUTIONS WHILE USING THIS MEDICINE

This medicine does not cause a loss of potassium from your body as some other diuretics (water pills) do. Therefore, it is not necessary for you to get extra potassium in your diet and too much potassium could even be harmful. Since salt substitutes and low-sodium milk may contain potassium, do not use them unless told to do so by your doctor.

POSSIBLE SIDE EFFECTS OF THIS MEDICINE

Side effects that should be reported to your doctor

> RARE—Skin rash or itching
>
> FOR SPIRONOLACTONE AND TRIAMTERENE ONLY (IN ADDITION TO EFFECTS LISTED ABOVE)—Cough or hoarseness; fever or chills; lower back or side pain; painful or difficult urination
>
> FOR TRIAMTERENE ONLY (IN ADDITION TO EFFECTS LISTED ABOVE)—Black, tarry stools; blood in urine or stools; bright red tongue; burning, inflamed feeling in tongue; cracked corners of mouth; pinpoint red spots on skin; unusual bleeding or bruising; weakness
>
> SIGNS OF TOO MUCH POTASSIUM—Confusion; irregular heartbeat; nervousness; numbness or tingling in hands, feet, or lips; shortness of breath or difficult breathing; unusual tiredness or weakness; weakness or heaviness of legs

Side effects that usually do not require medical attention

> These possible side effects may go away during treatment; however, if they continue or are bothersome, check with your doctor, nurse, or pharmacist.
>
> Diarrhea; dizziness; nausea; signs of too little sodium (drowsiness, dryness of mouth, increased thirst, lack of energy); stomach cramps; vomiting

In addition to the effects listed above:

FOR AMILORIDE—Constipation; decreased sexual ability; muscle cramps
FOR SPIRONOLACTONE—
IN WOMEN—Breast tenderness; deepening of voice; increased hair growth; irregular menstrual periods
IN MEN—Enlargement of breasts; inability to have or keep an erection
FOR TRIAMTERENE—Increased sensitivity of skin to sunlight

Other side effects not listed above may also occur in some patients. If you notice any other effects, check with your doctor, nurse, or pharmacist.

POTASSIUM SUPPLEMENTS (ORAL)

Including Potassium Acetate; Potassium Bicarbonate; Potassium Bicarbonate and Potassium Chloride; Potassium Bicarbonate and Potassium Citrate; Potassium Chloride; Potassium Chloride, Potassium Bicarbonate, and Potassium Citrate; Potassium Gluconate; Potassium Gluconate and Potassium Chloride; Potassium Gluconate and Potassium Citrate; Potassium Gluconate, Potassium Citrate, and Ammonium Chloride; Trikates

ABOUT YOUR MEDICINE

Potassium (poe-TASS-ee-um) is needed to maintain good health. A balanced diet usually supplies all the potassium a person needs. However, potassium supplements may be needed by patients who do not have enough potassium in their regular diet. Potassium supplements are also used in patients who have lost too much potassium because of illness or treatment with certain medicines.

If any of the information in this profile causes you special concern or if you want additional information about your medicine and its use, check with your doctor, nurse, or pharmacist. **Remember, keep this and all other medicines out of the reach of children and never share your medicines with others.**

BEFORE USING THIS MEDICINE

If you are taking this medicine without a prescription, carefully read and follow any precautions on the label. You should be especially careful if you . . .
- are allergic to any medicine, either prescription or nonprescription (OTC);
- are pregnant, intend to become pregnant, or are breast-feeding;
- are taking any other prescription or nonprescription (OTC) medicine,

especially captopril, cortisone-like medicine, digitalis glycosides (heart medicine), enalapril, heparin, medicine for inflammation or pain, medicine for stomach pain or cramps, other medicine containing potassium, potassium-sparing diuretics (amiloride, spironolactone, triamterene), or thiazide diuretics;

- have any other medical problems, especially Addison's disease, diarrhea (continuing or severe), heart disease, intestinal blockage, kidney disease, difficulty in urination, or stomach ulcer.

If you have any questions, check with your doctor, nurse, or pharmacist.

PROPER USE OF THIS MEDICINE

Take this medicine only as directed. Do not take more of it, do not take it more often, and do not take it for a longer time than your doctor ordered. **This is especially important if you are also taking diuretics (water pills) and digitalis medicines for your heart.**

Take this medicine immediately after meals or with food to lessen possible stomach upset or laxative action. Follow each dose, whether liquid, tablet, or capsule, with a glass of water.

If you miss a dose of this medicine and remember within 2 hours, take it as soon as possible. However, if you do not remember until later, skip the missed dose and go back to your regular dosing schedule. Do not double doses.

PRECAUTIONS WHILE USING THIS MEDICINE

Your doctor should check your progress at regular visits to make sure the medicine is working properly and that possible side effects are avoided. Laboratory tests may be necessary.

Since salt substitutes, low-sodium foods (especially some breads and canned foods), and low-sodium milk may contain potassium, do not use them unless told to do so by your doctor. It is important to read the labels carefully on all low-sodium food products.

Check with your doctor at once if you notice blackish stools or other signs of stomach or intestinal bleeding. This medicine, especially when taken in tablet form, may cause such a condition to become worse.

POSSIBLE SIDE EFFECTS OF THIS MEDICINE

Side effects that should be reported to your doctor immediately

Stop taking this medicine and check with your doctor immediately if any of the following side effects occur:

RARE—Confusion; irregular or slow heartbeat; numbness or tingling in hands, feet, or lips; shortness of breath or difficult breathing; unexplained anxiety; unusual tiredness or weakness; weakness or heaviness of legs

Other side effects that should be reported to your doctor

RARE—Abdominal or stomach pain, cramping, or soreness (continuing); chest or throat pain, especially when swallowing; stools with signs of blood (red or black color)

Side effects that usually do not require medical attention

These possible side effects may go away during treatment; however, if they continue or are bothersome, check with your doctor, nurse, or pharmacist.

MORE COMMON—Diarrhea; nausea; stomach pain, discomfort, or gas (mild); vomiting

Other side effects not listed above may also occur in some patients. If you notice any other effects, check with your doctor, nurse, or pharmacist.

PREDNISONE (ORAL)

ABOUT YOUR MEDICINE

Prednisone (PRED-ni-sone) is a cortisone-like substance. Cortisone is produced naturally by the body and is necessary to maintain good health. If your body does not make enough, your doctor may have prescribed this medicine to help make up the difference. Cortisone-like medicines are used also to provide relief for inflamed areas of the body. They are often used as part of treatment for a number of different diseases such as severe allergies or skin problems, asthma, or arthritis. Prednisone may also be used for other conditions as determined by your doctor.

If any of the information in this profile causes you special concern or if you want additional information about your medicine and its use, check with your doctor, nurse, or pharmacist. **Remember, keep this and all other medicines out of the reach of children and never share your medicines with others.**

BEFORE USING THIS MEDICINE

Tell your doctor, nurse, and pharmacist if you . . .

- are allergic to any medicine, either prescription or nonprescription (OTC);
- are pregnant or intend to become pregnant while using this medicine;
- are breast-feeding;
- are taking any other prescription or nonprescription (OTC) medicine, especially antacids; barbiturates; digitalis glycosides (heart medicine); diuretics (water pills); immunizations (vaccinations); medicine for arthritis, diabetes, or seizures; potassium supplements; rifampin; sodium-containing medicines or foods; somatrem; or somatropin;

- have any other medical problems, especially AIDS, diabetes, fungal infection, heart disease, herpes simplex of the eye, myasthenia gravis, stomach ulcer or other stomach problems, or tuberculosis (active, nonactive, or history of).

PROPER USE OF THIS MEDICINE

Use this medicine only as directed. Do not use more or less, more often, or for a longer time than ordered. To do so may cause unwanted effects.

Prednisone may slow or stop growth in children and teenagers (with long-term use). Discuss with the doctor the best way to lessen this effect and carefully follow the doctor's directions.

If you miss a dose of this medicine, and your dosing schedule is:
- One dose every other day—Take as soon as possible if you remember it the same morning, then go back to your regular schedule. If you do not remember until that afternoon, wait and take it the following morning. Then skip a day.
- One dose a day—Take as soon as possible, then go back to your regular schedule. If you do not remember until the next day, skip the missed dose.
- Several doses a day—Take as soon as possible, then go back to your regular schedule. If you do not remember until your next dose, double it.

PRECAUTIONS WHILE USING THIS MEDICINE

Do not stop using this medicine without first checking with your doctor. You may have to gradually reduce your dose before stopping completely.

Tell the doctor in charge that you are using this medicine:
- before having any immunizations, especially with live polio vaccine, or skin tests.
- before having any kind of surgery or emergency treatment.
- if you get a serious infection or injury.

Avoid close contact with anyone who has chickenpox or measles. This is especially important for children. **Tell the doctor right away if you think you have been exposed to chickenpox or measles.**

POSSIBLE SIDE EFFECTS OF THIS MEDICINE

Side effects that should be reported to your doctor

LESS COMMON—Decreased or blurred vision; frequent urination; increased thirst

RARE—Confusion; excitement; false sense of well-being; hallucinations; mental depression; mistaken feelings of self-importance or being mistreated; mood changes; restlessness

WITH LONG-TERM USE—Acne; back or rib pain; bloody or black, tarry stools; continuing stomach pain or burning; filling out of face; irregular heartbeats; menstrual problems; muscle cramps, pain, or weakness; reddish purple lines on skin; swelling of feet; thin, shiny skin; unusual tiredness; weight gain (rapid)

Side effects that usually do not require medical attention

These possible side effects may go away during treatment; however, if they continue or are bothersome, check with your doctor, nurse, or pharmacist.

MORE COMMON—Increase in appetite; indigestion; nervousness; restlessness; trouble in sleeping

LESS COMMON OR RARE—Headache; increased sweating; increase in hair growth

Other side effects not listed above may also occur in some patients. If you notice any other effects, check with your doctor, nurse, or pharmacist.

PROBUCOL (ORAL)

ABOUT YOUR MEDICINE

Probucol (proe-BYOO-kole) is used to lower levels of cholesterol (a fat-like substance) in the blood. This may help prevent medical problems caused by cholesterol clogging the blood vessels.

If any of the information in this profile causes you special concern or if you want additional information about your medicine and its use, check with your doctor, nurse, or pharmacist. **Remember, keep this and all other medicines out of the reach of children and never share your medicines with others.**

BEFORE USING THIS MEDICINE

Importance of diet—Before prescribing medicine for your condition, your doctor will probably try to control your condition by prescribing a personal diet for you. Such a diet may be low in fats, sugars, and/or cholesterol. Many people are able to control their condition by carefully following their doctor's orders for proper diet and exercise. Medicine is prescribed only when additional help is needed and is effective only when a schedule of diet and exercise is properly followed. **Follow carefully the special diet your doctor gave you.**

Also, this medicine is less effective if you are greatly overweight. It may be very important for you to go on a reducing diet. However, check with your doctor before going on any diet.

Tell your doctor, nurse, and pharmacist if you . . .

- are allergic to any medicine, either prescription or nonprescription (OTC);
- are pregnant or intend to become pregnant while using this medicine;

- are breast-feeding;
- are taking any other prescription or nonprescription (OTC) medicine;
- have any other medical problems, especially heart, liver, or gallbladder disease.

PROPER USE OF THIS MEDICINE

Many patients who have high cholesterol levels will not notice any signs of the problem. In fact, many may feel normal. **Take this medicine exactly as directed by your doctor, even though you may feel well.** Try not to miss any doses and do not take more medicine than your doctor ordered.

Remember that this medicine will not cure your condition but it does help control it. Therefore, you must continue to take this medicine as directed if you expect to keep your cholesterol levels down.

This medicine works better when taken with meals.

If you miss a dose of this medicine, take it as soon as possible. However, if it is almost time for your next dose, skip the missed dose and go back to your regular dosing schedule. Do not double doses.

PRECAUTIONS WHILE USING THIS MEDICINE

It is very important that your doctor check your progress at regular visits. This will allow your doctor to see if the medicine is working properly to lower your cholesterol levels and if you should continue to take it.

Do not stop taking this medicine without first checking with your doctor. When you stop taking this medicine, your blood fat levels may increase again. Your doctor may want you to follow a special diet to help prevent this.

POSSIBLE SIDE EFFECTS OF THIS MEDICINE

Side effects that should be reported to your doctor
>
> MORE COMMON—Dizziness or fainting; fast or irregular heartbeat
> RARE—Swellings on face, hands, or feet, or in mouth; unusual bleeding or bruising; unusual tiredness or weakness

Side effects that usually do not require medical attention
>
> These possible side effects may go away during treatment; however, if they continue or are bothersome, check with your doctor, nurse, or pharmacist.
>
> MORE COMMON—Bloating; diarrhea; nausea and vomiting; stomach pain
> LESS COMMON—Headache; numbness or tingling of fingers, toes, or face
>
> Other side effects not listed above may also occur in some patients. If you notice any other effects, check with your doctor, nurse, or pharmacist.

PROGESTINS (FOR CONTRACEPTIVE USE— ORAL)

Including Norethindrone; Norgestrel

ABOUT YOUR MEDICINE

Progestins (proe-JESS-tins) are used to prevent pregnancy. They may also be used for other conditions as determined by your doctor.

If any of the information in this profile causes you special concern or if you want additional information about your medicine and its use, check with your doctor, nurse, or pharmacist. **Remember, keep this and all other medicines out of the reach of children and never share your medicines with others.**

BEFORE USING THIS MEDICINE

Tell your doctor, nurse, and pharmacist if you . . .
- are allergic to any medicine, either prescription or nonprescription (OTC);
- are taking **any** other prescription or nonprescription (OTC) medicine;
- have any other medical problems, especially breast disease, such as breast lumps or cysts (history of), heart or circulation problems, or liver disease.

PROPER USE OF THIS MEDICINE

Progestins for contraception usually come with patient directions. Read them carefully before taking this medicine.

Progestins will not protect a woman from sexually transmitted diseases (STDs), including human immunodeficiency virus (HIV), or acquired immunodeficiency syndrome (AIDS). The use of latex (rubber) condoms or abstinence is recommended for protection from these diseases.

Take a tablet every 24 hours each day of the year. Taking your tablet 3 hours late is almost the same as missing a dose. The chance of getting pregnant is greater with each pill that is missed.

If you miss 1 dose of this medicine (or are more than 3 hours late taking your dose):
- Take the missed dose immediately and go back to your regular dosing schedule. Use another method of birth control for 2 days.

If you miss 2 doses of this medicine:
- Take 1 dose immediately, then go back to your regular dosing schedule. Use another method of birth control for 7 days.

If your doctor has other directions, follow that advice. **Any time you miss a menstrual period within 45 days of a missed or delayed dose, you will need to be tested for a possible pregnancy.**

PRECAUTIONS WHILE USING THIS MEDICINE

It is very important that your doctor check your progress at regular visits. Usually these visits will be made every 12 months.

Vaginal bleeding (called spotting when bleeding is slight and breakthrough bleeding when it is heavier) may occur between your regular periods during the first 3 months of use. Having vaginal bleeding or a delayed or missed period can be normal. Do not stop taking your medicine. **Check with your doctor** if bleeding continues for an unusually long time or if your period has not started within 45 days of your last period. **If you think you may be pregnant, call your doctor immediately.**

If you are scheduled for any laboratory tests, tell your doctor or nurse that you are taking a progestin. Progestins can change certain test results.

Use a second method of birth control:
- **for 3 weeks after you begin taking progestins. It takes time to have full protection from pregnancy.**
- during and for 4 weeks (a full cycle) after stopping medicines that reduce the contraceptive effects of progestins. These medicines include aminoglutethimide, carbamazepine, phenobarbital, phenytoin, rifabutin, and rifampin. Your doctor may ask that you use one or more of these medicines with your progestin but will give you special directions to make sure your birth control pill works properly.

POSSIBLE SIDE EFFECTS OF THIS MEDICINE

Side effects that should be reported to your doctor

MORE COMMON—Changes in uterine bleeding (increased amounts of menstrual bleeding at regular monthly periods; lighter or heavier bleeding between periods; stopping of menstrual periods)

LESS COMMON OR RARE—Mental depression; skin rash; unexpected or increased flow of breast milk

Side effects that usually do not require medical attention

These possible side effects may go away during treatment; however, if they continue or are bothersome, check with your doctor, nurse, or pharmacist.

MORE COMMON—Abdominal pain or cramping; delayed return to fertility; headache (mild); swelling of face, ankles, or feet; mood changes; nervousness; unusual tiredness or weakness; weight gain

LESS COMMON—Acne; breast pain or tenderness; brown spots on exposed skin, possibly long-lasting; hot flashes; loss or gain of body, facial, or scalp hair; loss of sexual desire; nausea; trouble in sleeping

Other side effects not listed above may also occur in some patients. If you notice any other effects, check with your doctor, nurse, or pharmacist.

PROGESTINS (INJECTION)

Including Hydroxyprogesterone; Medroxyprogesterone; Progesterone

ABOUT YOUR MEDICINE

Progestins (proe-JESS-tins) are produced by the body and are necessary during the childbearing years for the development of the milk-producing glands, and for the proper regulation of the menstrual cycle. They are also prescribed:

- to help treat selected cases of cancer of the breast, kidney, or uterus.
- to prevent pregnancy.
- for testing the body's production of certain hormones.

Progestins may also be used for other conditions as determined by your doctor.

If any of the information in this profile causes you special concern or if you want additional information about your medicine and its use, check with your doctor, nurse, or pharmacist.

BEFORE USING THIS MEDICINE

Tell your doctor, nurse, and pharmacist if you . . .

- are allergic to any medicine, either prescription or nonprescription (OTC);
- are pregnant or intend to become pregnant while using this medicine;
- are breast-feeding;
- are taking any other prescription or nonprescription (OTC) medicine, especially one that contains bromocriptine;
- have any other medical problems, especially blood clots, stroke, or cancer (or history of); changes in vaginal bleeding; or liver or gallbladder disease.

PROPER USE OF THIS MEDICINE

Most patients should receive with this medicine an information sheet regarding the benefits and risks specific to the product dispensed. **Be sure you have read and understand that information.** This profile does not replace that information sheet.

PRECAUTIONS WHILE USING THIS MEDICINE

It is very important that your doctor check your progress at regular visits. These visits will usually be every 3 to 12 months, but may be more often.

Check with your doctor right away:

- if vaginal bleeding continues for an unusually long time.
- if your menstrual period has not started within 45 days of your last period.
- **if you suspect that you may have become pregnant. You should stop using this medicine immediately.**

Possible Side Effects of This Medicine

Side effects that should be reported to your doctor immediately

Along with their needed effects, **progestins sometimes cause some unwanted effects,** such as blood clots, heart attack and stroke, and problems of the liver and eyes. Although these effects are rare, they can be very serious and may cause death. **Get emergency help immediately** if you have sudden or severe headache, loss of coordination, loss of or change in vision, shortness of breath, or slurred speech; pains in chest, groin, or leg (especially in calf of leg); or weakness, numbness, or pain in arm or leg.

Other side effects that should be reported to your doctor

MORE COMMON—Changes in vaginal bleeding

LESS COMMON OR RARE—Bulging eyes; discharge from breasts; double vision; loss of vision (gradual, partial, or complete); mental depression; pains in stomach, side, or abdomen; skin rash or itching; yellow eyes or skin

Side effects that usually do not require medical attention

These possible side effects may go away during treatment; however, if they continue or are bothersome, check with your doctor, nurse, or pharmacist.

MORE COMMON—Changes in appetite; changes in weight; pain or irritation at place of injection (with progesterone); swelling of ankles and feet; unusual tiredness or weakness

Other side effects not listed above may also occur in some patients. If you notice any other effects, check with your doctor, nurse, or pharmacist.

PROGESTINS (ORAL)

Including Medroxyprogesterone;
Megestrol; Norethindrone; Norgestrel

About Your Medicine

Progestins (proe-JESS-tins) are produced by the body and are necessary during the childbearing years for the development of the milk-producing glands, and for the proper regulation of the menstrual cycle. They are also prescribed:

- to treat a certain type of disorder of the uterus known as endometriosis.
- to prevent pregnancy, when used in birth-control pills.
- to help treat selected cases of cancer of the breast, kidney, or uterus.
- for testing the body's production of certain hormones.

Progestins may also be used for other conditions as determined by your doctor.

If any of the information in this profile causes you special concern or if you want additional information about your medicine and its use, check with your doctor, nurse, or pharmacist. **Remember, keep this and all other medicines out of the reach of children and never share your medicines with others.**

BEFORE USING THIS MEDICINE

Tell your doctor, nurse, and pharmacist if you . . .
- are allergic to any medicine, either prescription or nonprescription (OTC);
- are pregnant or intend to become pregnant while using this medicine;
- are breast-feeding;
- are taking any other prescription or nonprescription (OTC) medicine, especially one that contains bromocriptine;
- have any other medical problems, especially blood clots, stroke, or cancer (or history of); changes in vaginal bleeding; or liver or gallbladder disease.

PROPER USE OF THIS MEDICINE

Most patients should receive with this medicine an information sheet regarding the benefits and risks specific to the product dispensed. **Be sure you have read and understand that information.** This profile does not replace that information sheet.

Take this medicine only as directed. Do not take more of it and do not take it for a longer time than ordered. To do so may increase the chance of side effects. When used for birth control, this medicine should be taken every day of the year, with doses taken 24 hours apart.

If you miss a dose of this medicine and you are:
- *not* **taking it for birth control,** take the missed dose as soon as possible. However, if it is almost time for your next dose, skip the missed dose. Do not double doses.
- **taking it for birth control,** the safest thing to do is to stop taking the medicine immediately and use another method of birth control until your period begins or until your doctor determines that you are not pregnant.

PRECAUTIONS WHILE USING THIS MEDICINE

It is very important that your doctor check your progress at regular visits. These visits will usually be every 6 to 12 months, but may be more often.

Check with your doctor right away:
- if vaginal bleeding continues for an unusually long time.
- if your menstrual period has not started within 45 days of your last period.
- **if you suspect that you may have become pregnant. You should stop taking this medicine immediately.**

If you are taking this medicine for birth control:
- **When you begin to use birth control tablets** your body will need time to adjust before pregnancy will be prevented. **Use a second method of birth control for at least the first 3 weeks to ensure full protection.**

Possible Side Effects of This Medicine

Side effects that should be reported to your doctor immediately

Along with their needed effects, **progestins sometimes cause some unwanted effects,** such as blood clots, heart attack and stroke, and problems of the liver and eyes. Although these effects are rare, they can be very serious and may cause death. **Get emergency help immediately** if you have sudden or severe headache, loss of coordination, loss of or change in vision, shortness of breath, or slurred speech; pains in chest, groin, or leg (especially in calf of leg); or weakness, numbness, or pain in arm or leg.

Other side effects that should be reported to your doctor

MORE COMMON—Changes in vaginal bleeding

LESS COMMON OR RARE—Bulging eyes; discharge from breasts; double vision; loss of vision (gradual, partial, or complete); mental depression; pains in stomach, side, or abdomen; skin rash or itching; yellow eyes or skin

Side effects that usually do not require medical attention

These possible side effects may go away during treatment; however, if they continue or are bothersome, check with your doctor, nurse, or pharmacist.

MORE COMMON—Changes in appetite; changes in weight; swelling of ankles and feet; unusual tiredness or weakness

Other side effects not listed above may also occur in some patients. If you notice any other effects, check with your doctor, nurse, or pharmacist.

PROPRANOLOL (ORAL)

About Your Medicine

Propranolol (proh-PRAN-oh-lol) is used to treat high blood pressure. Propranolol is also used in the relief of angina (chest pain) and in heart attack patients to help prevent additional heart attacks. Propranolol is also used to correct irregular heartbeats, prevent migraine headaches, and treat tremors. It may also be used for other conditions as determined by your doctor.

If any of the information in this profile causes you special concern or if you want additional information about your medicine and its use, check with your doctor, nurse, or pharmacist. **Remember, keep this and all other medicines out of the reach of children and never share your medicines with others.**

BEFORE USING THIS MEDICINE

Tell your doctor, nurse, and pharmacist if you . . .
- are allergic to any medicine, either prescription or nonprescription (OTC);
- are pregnant or intend to become pregnant while using this medicine;
- are breast-feeding;
- are taking any other prescription or nonprescription (OTC) medicine, especially allergy shots or allergy skin testing; aminophylline; caffeine; calcium channel blockers; clonidine; diabetes medicine; dyphylline; guanabenz; insulin; MAO inhibitors; oxtriphylline; theophylline; or medicines for appetite control, asthma, colds, cough, hay fever, or sinus;
- have any other medical problems, especially allergy, asthma or other lung disease, diabetes, heart or blood vessel disease, mental depression, or overactive thyroid;
- use cocaine.

PROPER USE OF THIS MEDICINE

Even if you feel well, **take this medicine exactly as directed.**

Ask your doctor about your pulse rate before and after taking this medicine. Then, while you are taking this medicine, check your pulse regularly. If it is much slower than your usual rate (or less than 50 beats per minute), check with your doctor. A pulse rate that is too slow may cause circulation problems.

If you are taking this medicine for high blood pressure, remember that it will not cure your high blood pressure, but it does help control it. You must continue to take it—even if you feel well—if you expect to keep your blood pressure down. **You may have to take medicine for the rest of your life.**

Do not miss any doses, especially if you are taking only one dose a day. Some conditions may become worse when this medicine is not taken regularly.

If you do miss a dose of this medicine, take it as soon as possible. However, if it is within 4 hours of your next dose (8 hours when taking extended-release propranolol), skip the missed dose and go back to your regular dosing schedule. Do not double doses.

PRECAUTIONS WHILE USING THIS MEDICINE

Do not stop taking this medicine without first checking with your doctor.

For diabetic patients:
- **This medicine may cause your blood sugar levels to fall. Also, this medicine may cover up signs of hypoglycemia (low blood sugar).**

This medicine may cause some people to become dizzy, drowsy, or lightheaded. **Make sure you know how you react before you drive, use machines, or do other jobs that require you to be alert.**

Chest pain resulting from exercise or physical exertion is usually reduced or prevented by this medicine. This may tempt a patient to be overly active. **Make sure you discuss with your doctor a safe amount of exercise for you.**

POSSIBLE SIDE EFFECTS OF THIS MEDICINE

Side effects that should be reported to your doctor

LESS COMMON—Breathing difficulty; cold hands and feet; mental depression; shortness of breath; slow heartbeat (especially less than 50 beats per minute); swelling of ankles, feet, and/or lower legs

RARE—Back pain or joint pain; chest pain; confusion (especially in elderly); dizziness or lightheadedness when getting up from a lying or sitting position; fever and sore throat; hallucinations; irregular heartbeat; red, scaling, or crusted skin; skin rash; unusual bleeding and bruising

Side effects that usually do not require medical attention

These possible side effects may go away during treatment; however, if they continue or are bothersome, check with your doctor, nurse, or pharmacist.

MORE COMMON—Decreased sexual ability; dizziness or lightheadedness; drowsiness (slight); trouble in sleeping; unusual tiredness or weakness

After you have been taking this medicine for a while, it may cause unpleasant or even harmful effects if you stop taking it too suddenly. Check with your doctor right away if you notice chest pain, fast or irregular heartbeat, general feeling of body discomfort or weakness, shortness of breath (sudden), sweating, or trembling.

Other side effects not listed above may also occur in some patients. If you notice any other effects, check with your doctor, nurse, or pharmacist.

$\mathcal{P}$SEUDOEPHEDRINE (ORAL)

ABOUT YOUR MEDICINE

Pseudoephedrine (soo-doe-e-FED-rin) is used to relieve nasal or sinus congestion caused by the common cold, sinusitis, and hay fever and other respiratory allergies. It is also used to relieve ear congestion caused by ear inflammation or infection.

If any of the information in this profile causes you special concern or if you want additional information about your medicine and its use, check with your doctor, nurse, or pharmacist. **Remember, keep this and all other medicines out of the reach of children and never share your medicines with others.**

BEFORE USING THIS MEDICINE

If you are taking this medicine without a prescription, carefully read and follow any precautions on the label. You should be especially careful if you . . .
- are allergic to any medicine, either prescription or nonprescription (OTC);
- are pregnant, intend to become pregnant, or are breast-feeding;
- are taking **any** other prescription or nonprescription (OTC) medicine;
- have **any** other medical problems;
- are now using or have used cocaine.

If you have any questions, check with your doctor, nurse, or pharmacist.

PROPER USE OF THIS MEDICINE

Take this medicine only as directed. Do not take more of it, do not take it more often, and do not take it for a longer time than recommended on the label (usually 7 days), unless otherwise directed by your doctor. To do so may increase the chance of side effects.

To help prevent trouble in sleeping, **take the last dose of pseudoephedrine for each day a few hours before bedtime.** If you have any questions about this, check with your doctor.

For patients taking the extended-release capsule form of this medicine:
- Swallow the capsule whole. However, if the capsule is too large to swallow, you may mix the contents of the capsule with jam or jelly and swallow without chewing.
- Do not crush or chew before swallowing.

For patients taking the extended-release tablet form of this medicine:
- Swallow the tablet whole.
- Do not break, crush, or chew before swallowing.

If you miss a dose of this medicine and you remember within an hour or so of the missed dose, take it right away. However, if you do not remember until later, skip the missed dose and go back to your regular dosing schedule. Do not double doses.

PRECAUTIONS WHILE USING THIS MEDICINE

If symptoms do not improve within 7 days or if you also have a high fever, check with your doctor since these signs may mean that you have other medical problems.

POSSIBLE SIDE EFFECTS OF THIS MEDICINE

Side effects that should be reported to your doctor
> RARE (MORE COMMON WITH HIGH DOSES)—Convulsions (seizures); hallucinations; irregular heartbeat; slow heartbeat; shortness of breath; troubled breathing

Side effects that usually do not require medical attention

These possible side effects may go away during treatment; however, if they continue or are bothersome, check with your doctor, nurse, or pharmacist.

MORE COMMON—Nervousness; restlessness; trouble in sleeping

Other side effects not listed above may also occur in some patients. If you notice any other effects, check with your doctor, nurse, or pharmacist.

$\mathcal{R}$ADIOPHARMACEUTICALS (DIAGNOSTIC)

ABOUT THIS DIAGNOSTIC AGENT

Radiopharmaceuticals (ray-dee-oh-far-ma-SOO-ti-kals) are agents used to diagnose certain medical problems or treat certain diseases. They may be given to the patient in several different ways. For example, they may be given by mouth, given by injection, or placed into the eye or into the bladder.

Radiopharmaceuticals are radioactive agents. However, when small amounts are used, the radiation your body receives is very low and is considered safe. When larger amounts of these agents are given to treat disease, there may be different effects on the body.

If any of the information in this profile causes you special concern or if you want additional information about your medicine and its use, check with your doctor, nurse, or pharmacist.

BEFORE HAVING THIS TEST

Tell your doctor, nurse, and pharmacist if you . . .
- are allergic to any medicine, either prescription or nonprescription (OTC);
- are pregnant;
- are breast-feeding;
- are taking any other prescription or nonprescription (OTC) medicine;
- have any other medical problems.

PREPARATION FOR THIS TEST

The nuclear medicine doctor may have special instructions for you in preparation for your test. For example, before some tests you must fast for several hours, or the results of the test may be affected. For other tests you should drink plenty of liquids. If you do not understand the instructions you receive or if you have not received any instructions, check with the nuclear medicine doctor in advance.

For patients receiving radioactive iodine (sodium iodide I 123, sodium iodide I 131) or sodium pertechnetate Tc 99m for a thyroid test, since your test results may be affected, it is important that you tell your doctor if you:

- are taking iodine-containing medicines, including certain multivitamins and cough syrups.
- eat large amounts of iodine-containing foods, such as iodized salt, seafood, cabbage, kale, rape (turnip-like vegetable), or turnips.
- have had an x-ray test recently for which you were given a special dye that contained iodine.

PRECAUTIONS AFTER HAVING THIS TEST

There are usually no special precautions to take for radiopharmaceuticals when they are used in small amounts for diagnosis.

Some radiopharmaceuticals may collect in your bladder. Therefore, to increase the flow of urine and lessen the amount of radiation to your bladder, your doctor may tell you to drink plenty of liquids and urinate often after certain tests.

For patients receiving radioactive iodine (iodohippurate sodium I 123, iodohippurate sodium I 131, iofetamine I 123, iothalamate I 125, radioiodinated albumin, or radioiodinated iobenguane):

- Make sure your doctor knows if you are planning to have any future thyroid tests. Even after several weeks, the results of the thyroid test may be affected by the iodine solution that may be given before the radiopharmaceutical.

POSSIBLE SIDE EFFECTS OF THIS DIAGNOSTIC AGENT

Side effects that should be reported to your doctor immediately

RARE—Chills; difficulty breathing; drowsiness (severe); fainting; fast heartbeat; fever; flushing or redness of skin; headache (severe); nausea or vomiting; skin rash, hives, or itching; stomach pain; swelling of throat, hands, or feet

Other side effects not listed above may also occur in some patients. If you notice any other effects, check with your doctor, nurse, or pharmacist.

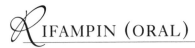IFAMPIN (ORAL)

ABOUT YOUR MEDICINE

Rifampin (rif-AM-pin) is used with other medicines to treat tuberculosis (TB). Rifampin is also taken alone by patients who may carry meningitis bacteria in their nose and throat (without feeling sick) and may spread these bacteria to others. This medicine may also be used for other problems as determined by your doctor. However, rifampin will not work for colds, flu, or other virus infections.

To help clear up your tuberculosis (TB) completely, you must keep taking this medicine for the full time of treatment, even if you begin to feel better. This is very important. It is also important that you do not miss any doses.

If any of the information in this profile causes you special concern or if you want additional information about your medicine and its use, check with your doctor, nurse, or pharmacist. **Remember, keep this and all other medicines out of the reach of children and never share your medicines with others.**

BEFORE USING THIS MEDICINE

Tell your doctor, nurse, and pharmacist if you . . .
- are allergic to any medicine, either prescription or nonprescription (OTC);
- are pregnant or intend to become pregnant while using this medicine;
- are breast-feeding;
- are taking **any** other prescription or nonprescription (OTC) medicine;
- have any other medical problems, especially alcohol abuse (or history of) or liver disease.

PROPER USE OF THIS MEDICINE

Rifampin is best taken with a full glass (8 ounces) of water on an empty stomach (either 1 hour before or 2 hours after a meal). However, if this medicine upsets your stomach, your doctor may want you to take it with food.

To help clear up your tuberculosis (TB) completely, **it is very important that you keep taking this medicine for the full time of treatment.** You may have to take it every day for 1 to 2 years or more. **Do not miss any doses.**

If you do miss a dose of this medicine, take it as soon as possible. However, if it is almost time for your next dose, skip the missed dose and go back to your regular schedule. Do not double doses. **If rifampin is taken on an irregular schedule, side effects may occur more often and may be more serious than usual.**

PRECAUTIONS WHILE USING THIS MEDICINE

Rifampin will cause the urine, stool, saliva, sputum, sweat, and tears to turn reddish orange to reddish brown. This is to be expected and does not usually need medical attention. This effect may cause soft contact lenses (but not hard contact lenses) to become permanently discolored. **Therefore, it is best not to wear soft contact lenses while taking rifampin.**

Oral contraceptives (birth control pills) containing estrogen may not work properly if you take them while you are taking rifampin. Unplanned pregnancies may occur. Use a different means of birth control while taking rifampin.

If your symptoms do not improve within 2 or 3 weeks, or if they become worse, check with your doctor.

If rifampin causes you to feel very tired or weak or causes a loss of appetite, nausea, or vomiting, stop taking it and check with your doctor immediately.

The regular use of alcohol may keep rifampin from working as well. Also, liver problems may be more likely to occur. Therefore, **you should not drink alcoholic beverages while you are taking this medicine.**

Rifampin can lower the number of white blood cells in your blood temporarily, increasing the chance of getting an infection. It can also lower the number of platelets, which are necessary for proper blood clotting. These problems may result in a greater chance of getting certain infections, slow healing, and bleeding of the gums. Be careful when using a regular toothbrush, dental floss, or a toothpick. Dental work should be delayed until your blood counts have returned to normal. Check with your physician or dentist if you have any questions.

This medicine must not be given to other people or used for other infections unless you are otherwise directed by your doctor.

POSSIBLE SIDE EFFECTS OF THIS MEDICINE

Side effects that should be reported to your doctor immediately
> LESS COMMON—Chills; difficult breathing; dizziness; fever; headache; itching; muscle and bone pain; shivering; skin rash and redness
> RARE—Bloody or cloudy urine; greatly decreased frequency of urination or amount of urine; loss of appetite; nausea or vomiting; sore throat; unusual bruising or bleeding; unusual tiredness or weakness; yellow eyes or skin

Side effects that usually do not require medical attention
> These possible side effects may go away during treatment; however, if they continue or are bothersome, check with your doctor, nurse, or pharmacist.

> MORE COMMON—Diarrhea; stomach cramps

> Other side effects not listed above may also occur in some patients. If you notice any other effects, check with your doctor, nurse, or pharmacist.

$\mathcal{R}$IFAMPIN AND ISONIAZID (ORAL)

ABOUT YOUR MEDICINE

Rifampin (rif-AM-pin) and **isoniazid** (eye-soe-NYE-a-zid) is a combination antibiotic medicine. It is used to treat tuberculosis (TB). It may be taken alone or with one or more other medicines for TB.

To help clear up your tuberculosis (TB) completely, you must keep taking this medicine for the full time of treatment, even if you begin to feel better. This is very important. It is also important that you do not miss any doses.

If any of the information in this profile causes you special concern or if you want additional information about your medicine and its use, check with your doctor, nurse, or pharmacist. **Remember, keep this and all other medicines out of the reach of children and never share your medicines with others.**

BEFORE USING THIS MEDICINE

Tell your doctor, nurse, and pharmacist if you . . .
- are allergic to any medicine, either prescription or nonprescription (OTC);
- are pregnant or intend to become pregnant while using this medicine;
- are breast-feeding;
- are taking **any** other prescription or nonprescription (OTC) medicine;
- have any other medical problems, especially alcohol abuse (or history of) or liver disease.

PROPER USE OF THIS MEDICINE

If this medicine upsets your stomach, take it with food. Antacids may also help. However, do not take aluminum-containing antacids within 1 hour of the time you take rifampin and isoniazid combination.

To help clear up your tuberculosis (TB) completely, **it is very important that you keep taking this medicine for the full time of treatment** even if you begin to feel better after a few weeks.

Your doctor may also want you to take pyridoxine (vitamin B$_6$) every day to help prevent or lessen some of the side effects of isoniazid. If it is needed, **it is very important to take pyridoxine every day along with this medicine. Do not miss any doses.**

If you miss a dose of either of these medicines, take it as soon as possible. However, if it is almost time for your next dose, skip the missed dose and go back to your regular dosing schedule. Do not double doses. **If rifampin and isoniazid combination is taken on an irregular schedule, side effects may occur more often and may be more serious than usual.**

PRECAUTIONS WHILE USING THIS MEDICINE

This medicine will cause the urine, stool, saliva, sputum, sweat, and tears to turn reddish orange to reddish brown. This is to be expected and does not usually require medical attention. This effect may cause soft contact lenses to become permanently discolored. **Therefore, it is best not to wear soft contact lenses while taking this medicine.** Hard contact lenses are not discolored by this medicine.

Oral contraceptives (birth control pills) containing estrogen may not work properly if you take them while you are taking rifampin and isoniazid combination. Unplanned pregnancies may occur. You should use a different means of birth control while you are taking this medicine.

If your symptoms do not improve within 2 to 3 weeks, or if they become worse, check with your doctor.

It is very important that your doctor check your progress at regular visits. In addition, you should **check with your doctor immediately if blurred vision or loss of vision, with or without eye pain, occurs during treatment.**

Liver problems may be more likely to occur if you drink alcoholic beverages regularly while you are taking this medicine. Also, the regular use of alcohol may keep this medicine from working properly. Therefore, **you should strictly limit the amount of alcoholic beverages you drink while you are taking this medicine.**

This medicine must not be given to other people or used for other infections unless you are otherwise directed by your doctor.

POSSIBLE SIDE EFFECTS OF THIS MEDICINE

Side effects that should be reported to your doctor immediately

MORE COMMON—Clumsiness or unsteadiness; dark urine; loss of appetite; nausea or vomiting; numbness, tingling, burning, or pain in hands and feet; unusual tiredness or weakness; yellow eyes or skin

LESS COMMON—Chills; difficult breathing; dizziness; fever; headache; itching; muscle and bone pain; shivering; skin rash and redness

RARE—Bloody or cloudy urine; blurred vision or loss of vision, with or without eye pain; convulsions (seizures); depression; greatly decreased frequency of urination or amount of urine; joint pain; mood or mental changes; sore throat; unusual bruising or bleeding

Side effects that usually do not require medical attention

These possible side effects may go away during treatment; however, if they continue or are bothersome, check with your doctor, nurse, or pharmacist.

MORE COMMON—Diarrhea; stomach cramps or upset

Dark urine and yellowing of the eyes or skin (signs of liver problems) are more likely to occur in patients over 50 years of age.

Other side effects not listed above may also occur in some patients. If you notice any other effects, check with your doctor, nurse, or pharmacist.

$\mathcal{S}$ALICYLATES (ORAL)

Including Aspirin; Aspirin and Caffeine; Buffered Aspirin; Buffered Aspirin and Caffeine; Choline Salicylate; Choline and Magnesium Salicylates; Magnesium Salicylate; Salsalate; Sodium Salicylate

ABOUT YOUR MEDICINE

Salicylates relieve pain and reduce fever. Most also relieve arthritis symptoms, such as swelling, stiffness, and joint pain. However, they do not cure arthritis and will help you only as long as you take them. Aspirin is also used to lessen the chance of stroke, heart attack, or other problems caused by blood clots. **However, do not take aspirin to prevent blood clots or a heart attack unless it has been ordered by your doctor.** Salicylates may also be used for other conditions as determined by your doctor.

If any of the information in this profile causes you special concern or if you want additional information about your medicine and its use, check with your doctor, nurse, or pharmacist. **Remember, keep this and all other medicines out of the reach of children and never share your medicines with others.**

BEFORE USING THIS MEDICINE

Do not give a medicine containing aspirin or other salicylates to a child or a teenager with symptoms of flu or chickenpox without first discussing this with your child's doctor.

If you are taking this medicine without a prescription, carefully read and follow any precautions on the label. You should be especially careful if you . . .
- are allergic to any medicine, either prescription or nonprescription (OTC);
- are pregnant, intend to become pregnant, or are breast-feeding;
- are taking any other prescription or nonprescription (OTC) medicine;
- have any other medical problems, especially asthma, hemophilia or other bleeding problems, or stomach ulcer or other stomach problems.

If you have any questions, check with your doctor, nurse, or pharmacist.

PROPER USE OF THIS MEDICINE

Take this medicine with food (except for enteric-coated capsules or tablets) and a full glass (8 ounces) of water to lessen stomach irritation.

Do not use any product that contains aspirin if it has a strong vinegar-like odor. This odor means the medicine is breaking down.

When used for arthritis, this medicine must be taken regularly as ordered. Several weeks may pass before you feel the full effects of this medicine.

If you are taking this medicine regularly and you miss a dose, take it as soon as possible. However, if it is almost time for your next dose, skip the missed dose and go back to your regular dosing schedule. Do not double doses.

PRECAUTIONS WHILE USING THIS MEDICINE

Check the labels of all over-the-counter (OTC), nonprescription, and prescription medicines you now take. If any contain aspirin or other salicylates, check with your doctor or pharmacist. Using other salicylate-containing products with this medicine may lead to overdose.

For patients taking **aspirin to lessen the chance of a heart attack, stroke, or other problems caused by blood clots:**
- Take only the amount of aspirin ordered by your doctor.
- Do not stop taking aspirin without first checking with your doctor.

Do not regularly take acetaminophen or ibuprofen or other anti-inflammatory analgesics while you are taking a salicylate unless your doctor directs you to do so.

It is best not to drink alcoholic beverages while taking this medicine because stomach problems may occur.

If you think that you or someone in your home may have taken an overdose, get emergency help at once. Taking an overdose may cause unconsciousness or death. Signs of overdose include changes in behavior; convulsions (seizures); hearing loss; confusion; ringing or buzzing in the ears; severe drowsiness, tiredness, excitement, or nervousness; and unusually fast or deep breathing.

POSSIBLE SIDE EFFECTS OF THIS MEDICINE

Side effects that should be reported to your doctor immediately
> Bloody urine; diarrhea (severe or continuing); difficulty in swallowing; dizziness, lightheadedness, or feeling faint (severe); hallucinations; increased thirst; nausea or vomiting (severe or continuing); shortness of breath, troubled breathing, tightness in chest, or wheezing; stomach pain (severe or continuing); swelling of eyelids, face, or lips; uncontrollable flapping movements of hands; unexplained fever; vision problems

Other side effects that should be reported to your doctor
> LESS COMMON OR RARE—Abdominal or stomach pain, cramping, or burning (severe); bloody or black, tarry stools; headache (severe or continuing); skin rash, hives, or itching; unusual tiredness or weakness; vomiting of blood or material that looks like coffee grounds

Side effects that usually do not require medical attention

> MORE COMMON—Abdominal or stomach cramps, pain, or discomfort (mild to
> moderate); heartburn or indigestion; nausea or vomiting

> Serious stomach problems are more likely to occur with aspirin products that do
> not have an enteric coating than with enteric-coated aspirin or with other
> salicylates.

> Other side effects not listed above may also occur in some patients. If you
> notice any other effects, check with your doctor, nurse, or pharmacist.

$\mathcal{S}$COPOLAMINE (TRANSDERMAL)

ABOUT YOUR MEDICINE

Transdermal scopolamine (scoe-POL-a-meen) is used to prevent nausea,
vomiting, and motion sickness. Scopolamine may also be used for other conditions as
determined by your doctor.

If any of the information in this profile causes you special concern or if you want
additional information about your medicine and its use, check with your doctor,
nurse, or pharmacist. **Remember, keep this and all other medicines out of the
reach of children and never share your medicines with others.**

BEFORE USING THIS MEDICINE

Tell your doctor, nurse, and pharmacist if you . . .
- are allergic to any medicine, either prescription or nonprescription (OTC);
- are pregnant or intend to become pregnant while using this medicine;
- are breast-feeding;
- are taking **any** other prescription or nonprescription (OTC) medicine;
- have **any** other medical problems.

PROPER USE OF THIS MEDICINE

Use this medicine only as directed. Do not use more of it, do not use it more
often, and do not use it for a longer period of time than ordered.

If you miss a dose of this medicine, use it as soon as possible. However, if it is
almost time for your next dose, skip the missed dose and go back to your regular
dosing schedule. Do not double doses.

To use the transdermal disk:
- This medicine usually comes with patient directions. Read them carefully
  before using this medicine.

- Wash and dry your hands thoroughly before and after handling.
- Put the disk on the hairless area of skin behind the ear. Do not put it on cuts, scars, or irritations.
- After taking off the used disk, discard it carefully out of the reach of children.

PRECAUTIONS WHILE USING THIS MEDICINE

High doses of this medicine may lead to overdose. An overdose of this medicine or its use with alcohol or other CNS depressants may lead to unconsciousness and possibly death. **Get emergency help at once if any of these signs of overdose occur:** clumsiness or unsteadiness; confusion; dizziness; fever; hallucinations (seeing, hearing, or feeling things that are not there); severe drowsiness; shortness of breath or troubled breathing; slurred speech; unusual excitement, nervousness, restlessness, or irritability; unusually fast heartbeat; or unusual warmth, dryness, and flushing of skin.

Scopolamine may make you sweat less, causing your body temperature to rise. **Use care not to become overheated during exercise or hot weather** since overheating may result in heat stroke. Also, hot baths or saunas may make you dizzy or faint while you are taking this medicine.

Scopolamine may cause some people to have blurred vision. **Make sure your vision is clear before you drive or do other jobs that require you to see well.** This medicine may also cause your eyes to become more sensitive to light. Wearing sunglasses may help lessen the discomfort from bright light.

Scopolamine, especially in high doses, may cause some people to become dizzy or drowsy. **Make sure you know how you react to this medicine before you drive, use machines, or do other jobs that require you to be alert.**

Scopolamine may cause dryness of the mouth, nose, and throat. For temporary relief of mouth dryness, use sugarless candy or gum, melt bits of ice in your mouth, or use a saliva substitute. However, if dry mouth continues for more than 2 weeks, check with your physician or dentist. Continuing dryness of the mouth may increase the chance of dental disease.

This medicine will add to the effects of alcohol and other CNS depressants (medicines that may make you drowsy or less alert). **Check with your doctor before taking any such depressants while you are taking this medicine.**

POSSIBLE SIDE EFFECTS OF THIS MEDICINE

Side effects that should be reported to your doctor
> RARE—Confusion (especially in the elderly); dizziness, lightheadedness (continuing), or fainting; eye pain; skin rash or hives

Side effects that usually do not require medical attention
> These possible side effects may go away during treatment; however, if they continue or are bothersome, check with your doctor, nurse, or pharmacist.

MORE COMMON—Constipation; decrease in sweating; dryness of mouth, nose, throat, or skin

Other side effects not listed above may also occur in some patients. If you notice any other effects, check with your doctor, nurse, or pharmacist.

After you stop using scopolamine, your body may need time to adjust. The length of time this takes depends on the amount of scopolamine you were using and how long you used it. During this time check with your doctor if you notice anxiety, irritability, nightmares, or trouble in sleeping.

SERTRALINE (ORAL)

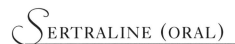

ABOUT YOUR MEDICINE

Sertraline (SER-tra-leen) is used to treat mental depression.

If any of the information in this profile causes you special concern or if you want additional information about your medicine and its use, check with your doctor, nurse, or pharmacist. **Remember, keep this and all other medicines out of the reach of children and never share your medicines with others.**

BEFORE USING THIS MEDICINE

Tell your doctor, nurse, and pharmacist if you . . .
- are allergic to any medicine, either prescription or nonprescription (OTC);
- are pregnant or intend to become pregnant while using this medicine;
- are breast-feeding;
- are taking any other prescription or nonprescription (OTC) medicine, especially digitoxin, MAO inhibitors, or warfarin;
- have any other medical problems.

PROPER USE OF THIS MEDICINE

Take this medicine only as directed by your doctor, to benefit your condition as much as possible. Do not take more of it, do not take it more often, and do not take it for a longer time than your doctor ordered.

You may have to take sertraline for up to 4 weeks or longer before you begin to feel better. Your doctor should check your progress at regular visits during this time.

Always take this medicine at the same time in relation to meals and snacks. You may take it on a full or empty stomach, but always take it the same way. This is to make sure that your body absorbs the medicine the same way.

Because sertraline is taken by different patients at different times of the day, you and your doctor should discuss what to do about any missed doses.

PRECAUTIONS WHILE USING THIS MEDICINE

It is important that your doctor check your progress at regular visits, to allow for changes in your dose and help reduce any side effects.

This medicine may add to the effects of alcohol and other CNS depressants (medicines that slow down the nervous system). **Check with your doctor before taking any such depressants while you are using this medicine.**

This medicine may cause some people to become drowsy. **Make sure you know how you react to this medicine before you drive, use machines, or do other jobs that require you to be alert.**

This medicine may cause dryness of the mouth. **For temporary relief, use sugarless gum or candy, melt bits of ice in your mouth, or use a saliva substitute.** However, if your mouth feels dry for more than 2 weeks, check with your physician or dentist. Continuing dryness of the mouth may increase the chance of dental disease, including tooth decay, gum disease, and fungus infections.

POSSIBLE SIDE EFFECTS OF THIS MEDICINE

Side effects that should be reported to your doctor

LESS COMMON OR RARE—Fast talking and excited feelings or actions that are out of control; fever; skin rash, hives, or itching

Side effects that usually do not require medical attention

These possible side effects may go away during treatment; however, if they continue or are bothersome, check with your doctor, nurse, or pharmacist.

MORE COMMON—Decreased appetite or weight loss; decreased sexual drive or ability; diarrhea; drowsiness; dryness of mouth; headache; nausea; stomach cramps, gas, or pain; tiredness or weakness; tremor; trouble in sleeping

Other side effects not listed above may also occur in some patients. If you notice any other effects, check with your doctor, nurse, or pharmacist.

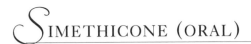 SIMETHICONE (ORAL)

ABOUT YOUR MEDICINE

Simethicone (si-METH-i-kone) is used to relieve the painful symptoms of too much gas in the stomach and intestines. Simethicone may also be used for other conditions as determined by your doctor.

If any of the information in this profile causes you special concern or if you want additional information about your medicine and its use, check with your doctor, nurse, or pharmacist. **Remember, keep this and all other medicines out of the reach of children and never share your medicines with others.**

BEFORE USING THIS MEDICINE

Importance of proper diet and exercise to prevent gas problem—Avoid foods that seem to increase gas. Chew food thoroughly and slowly. Reduce air swallowing by avoiding fizzy, carbonated drinks. Do not smoke before meals. Develop regular bowel habits and exercise regularly.

If you are taking this medicine without a prescription, carefully read and follow any precautions on the label. You should be especially careful if you . . .
- are allergic to any medicine, either prescription or nonprescription (OTC);
- are pregnant or intend to become pregnant while using this medicine;
- are breast-feeding;
- are taking any other prescription or nonprescription (OTC) medicine;
- have any other medical problems.

If you have any questions, check with your doctor, nurse, or pharmacist.

PROPER USE OF THIS MEDICINE

Take this medicine after meals and at bedtime for best results.

For patients taking the chewable tablet form of this medicine:
- It is important that you chew the tablets thoroughly before swallowing. This is to allow the medicine to work faster and more completely.

For patients taking the oral liquid form of this medicine:
- This medicine is to be taken by mouth even if it comes in a dropper bottle. The amount you should take is to be measured with the specially marked dropper or measuring spoon.

If you must take this medicine regularly and you miss a dose, take it as soon as possible. However, if it is almost time for your next dose, skip the missed dose and go back to your regular dosing schedule. Do not double doses.

POSSIBLE SIDE EFFECTS OF THIS MEDICINE

There have not been any common or important side effects reported with this medicine. However, if you notice any side effects, check with your doctor, nurse, or pharmacist.

SPERMICIDES (VAGINAL)

Including Benzalkonium Chloride; Nonoxynol 9; Octoxynol 9

ABOUT YOUR MEDICINE

Vaginal spermicides are a type of contraceptive (birth control). They are inserted into the vagina **before** any genital contact or sexual intercourse begins.

Vaginal spermicides when used alone are much less effective in preventing pregnancy than birth control pills (the Pill) or intrauterine devices (IUDs) or spermicides used with another form of birth control such as the condom, cervical cap, or diaphragm. The number of pregnancies is reduced when spermicides are used with another method, especially the condom.

Although it has **not** been proven in **human** studies, some scientists **believe** that if spermicides are put into the vagina or on the inside and outside of a latex (rubber) condom, they **may** kill germs that cause gonorrhea, chlamydia, syphilis, trichomoniasis, herpes, HIV infection, and other sexually transmitted diseases (venereal disease, VD, STDs), before they are able to come in contact with the vagina or rectum (lower bowel).

The sure way to protect against STDs is by not having sex or by having only one partner, who is not already infected and is not going to get an STD. Otherwise, using latex condoms with a spermicide is the best way to protect yourself.

The use of a spermicide and condoms is recommended even when you are using the Pill or IUDs, since they do not offer any protection from STDs.

If any of the information in this profile causes you special concern or if you want additional information about your medicine and its use, check with your doctor, nurse, or pharmacist. **Remember, keep this and all other medicines out of the reach of children and never share your medicines with others.**

BEFORE USING THIS MEDICINE

Tell your doctor, nurse, and pharmacist if you . . .
- are allergic to any medicine, either prescription or nonprescription (OTC);
- are pregnant or intend to become pregnant while using this medicine;

- are breast-feeding;
- are taking any other prescription or nonprescription (OTC) medicine, especially vaginal medicines, douches, or rinses;
- have any other medical problems, especially allergies, irritations, infections or sores of the genitals; or toxic shock syndrome;
- are menstruating.

PROPER USE OF THIS MEDICINE

It is very important that the spermicide be placed properly in the vagina. Make sure you carefully read and follow the instructions that come with each product.

For spermicides to prevent pregnancy, they must stay in contact with the sperm in the vagina for at least 6 or 8 hours (depending upon which brand of spermicide you use) after sexual intercourse. Washing or rinsing the vaginal or rectal area may also make the spermicide ineffective in preventing STDs.

If you are using spermicide with another birth control method (latex diaphragm, cervical cap, or condom), make sure the spermicide you choose is labeled as being safe for use with these devices. Otherwise, it may cause the diaphragm, cervical cap, or condom to weaken and leak or even break during intercourse. If there is a leak or break during intercourse, it may be a good idea to immediately place more spermicide in the vagina or rectum.

To be most effective at preventing pregnancy, the cervical cap or diaphragm must always be used with a spermicide and every time you have sexual intercourse. Condoms do not have to be used with spermicides, but the spermicide may provide a back-up in case the condom breaks or leaks.

PRECAUTIONS WHILE USING THIS MEDICINE

Spermicides may cause either partner to notice burning, stinging, warmth, itching, or other irritation of the skin, sex organs, anus, or rectum. Using a weaker strength of vaginal spermicide or one with different ingredients may be necessary. If you are using benzalkonium chloride suppositories, it may help to wet them before they are inserted into the vagina. Check with your doctor if these effects continue after you have changed products. You may have an allergy or infection.

POSSIBLE SIDE EFFECTS OF THIS MEDICINE

Side effects that should be reported to your doctor immediately
For the cervical cap or diaphragm only

RARE (SIGNS OF **TOXIC-SHOCK SYNDROME** SUCH AS)—Chills; confusion; dizziness; fever; lightheadedness; muscle aches; sunburn-like rash that is followed by peeling of the skin; unusual redness of the inside of the nose, mouth, throat, vagina, or insides of the eyelids

Other side effects that should be reported to your doctor

For females and males

RARE—Skin rash, redness, irritation, or itching that does not go away

For females only

RARE (SIGNS OF URINARY TRACT INFECTION OR VAGINAL ALLERGY OR
INFECTION)—Cloudy or bloody urine; increased frequency of urination;
pain in the bladder or lower abdomen; pain on urination; thick, white, or
curd-like vaginal discharge (with use of the cervical cap or diaphragm only);
vaginal irritation, redness, rash, dryness, or whitish discharge

Other side effects not listed above may also occur in some patients. If you
notice any other effects, check with your doctor, nurse, or pharmacist.

STATIN CHOLESTEROL-LOWERING MEDICINES (ORAL)

Including Fluvastatin; Lovastatin; Pravastatin; Simvastatin

ABOUT YOUR MEDICINE

Statin cholesterol-lowering medicines are used to lower levels of cholesterol and
other fats in the blood. This may help prevent medical problems caused by
cholesterol clogging the blood vessels.

If any of the information in this profile causes you special concern or if you want
additional information about your medicine and its use, check with your doctor,
nurse, or pharmacist. **Remember, keep this and all other medicines out of the
reach of children and never share your medicines with others.**

BEFORE USING THIS MEDICINE

Importance of diet—Before prescribing medicine to lower your cholesterol, your
doctor will probably try to control your condition by prescribing a personal diet for
you. Such a diet may be low in fats, sugars, and/or cholesterol. Many people are able
to control their condition by carefully following their doctor's orders for proper diet
and exercise. **Medicine is prescribed only when additional help is needed** and is
effective only when a schedule of diet and exercise is properly followed.

Also, this medicine is less effective if you are greatly overweight. It may be very
important for you to go on a reducing diet. However, check with your doctor before
going on any diet.

Tell your doctor, nurse, and pharmacist if you . . .
- are allergic to any medicine, either prescription or nonprescription (OTC);
- **are pregnant or intend to become pregnant while using this medicine;**
- are breast-feeding;
- are taking any other prescription or nonprescription (OTC) medicine, especially cyclosporine, gemfibrozil, or niacin;
- have had major surgery, especially a heart transplant;
- have any other medical problems, especially convulsions (seizures) or liver disease.

PROPER USE OF THIS MEDICINE

Use this medicine only as directed by your doctor. Do not use more or less of it, and do not use it more often or for a longer time than ordered.

Remember that this medicine will not cure your condition but it does help control it. Therefore, you must continue to take it as directed if you expect to keep your cholesterol levels down.

For patients taking lovastatin:
- This medicine works better when it is taken with food. If you are taking this medicine once a day, take it with the evening meal. If you are taking more than one dose a day, take with meals or snacks.

If you miss a dose of this medicine, take it as soon as possible. However, if it is almost time for your next dose, skip the missed dose and go back to your regular dosing schedule. Do not double doses.

PRECAUTIONS WHILE USING THIS MEDICINE

It is very important that your doctor check your progress at regular visits. This will allow your doctor to see if the medicine is working properly to lower your cholesterol levels and that it does not cause unwanted effects.

Check with your doctor immediately if you think that you may be pregnant. This medicine may cause birth defects or other problems in the baby if taken during pregnancy.

Do not stop taking this medicine without first checking with your doctor. When you stop taking this medicine, your blood cholesterol levels may increase again. Your doctor may want you to follow a special diet to help prevent this from happening.

Before having any kind of surgery or dental or emergency treatment, tell the physician or dentist in charge that you are taking this medicine.

POSSIBLE SIDE EFFECTS OF THIS MEDICINE

Side effects that should be reported to your doctor
LESS COMMON OR RARE—Fever; muscle aches or cramps; stomach pain (severe); unusual tiredness or weakness

Side effects that usually do not require medical attention

These possible side effects may go away during treatment; however, if they continue or are bothersome, check with your doctor, nurse, or pharmacist.

MORE COMMON—Constipation; diarrhea; dizziness; headache; heartburn; nausea; skin rash; stomach pain

RARE—Decreased sexual ability; trouble in sleeping

Other side effects not listed above may also occur in some patients. If you notice any other effects, check with your doctor, nurse, or pharmacist.

$\mathcal{S}$UCRALFATE (ORAL)

ABOUT YOUR MEDICINE

Sucralfate (soo-KRAL-fate) is used to treat and prevent duodenal ulcer. It may also be used for other conditions as determined by your doctor.

Sucralfate contains an aluminum salt.

If any of the information in this profile causes you special concern or if you want additional information about your medicine and its use, check with your doctor, nurse, or pharmacist. **Remember, keep this and all other medicines out of the reach of children and never share your medicines with others.**

BEFORE USING THIS MEDICINE

Tell your doctor, nurse, and pharmacist if you . . .

- are allergic to any medicine, either prescription or nonprescription (OTC);
- are pregnant or intend to become pregnant while using this medicine;
- are breast-feeding;
- are taking any other prescription or nonprescription (OTC) medicine, especially ciprofloxacin, digoxin, norfloxacin, ofloxacin, phenytoin, or theophylline;
- have any other medical problems.

PROPER USE OF THIS MEDICINE

Sucralfate is best taken with water on an empty stomach 1 hour before meals and at bedtime, unless otherwise directed by your doctor.

Take this medicine for the full time of treatment, even if you begin to feel better. Also, it is important that you keep your doctor's appointments for check-ups so that your doctor will be better able to tell you when to stop taking this medicine.

If you miss a dose of this medicine, take it as soon as possible. However, if it is almost time for your next dose, skip the missed dose and go back to your regular dosing schedule. Do not double doses.

PRECAUTIONS WHILE USING THIS MEDICINE

Antacids may be taken with sucralfate to help relieve any stomach pain, unless your doctor has told you not to use them. **However, antacids should not be taken within 30 minutes before or after sucralfate.** Taking these medicines too close together may keep sucralfate from working properly.

POSSIBLE SIDE EFFECTS OF THIS MEDICINE

Side effects that should be reported to your doctor immediately
> SIGNS OF TOO MUCH ALUMINUM IN THE BODY—Drowsiness; seizures

Side effects that usually do not require medical attention
> These possible side effects may go away during treatment; however, if they continue or are bothersome, check with your doctor, nurse, or pharmacist.
>
> MORE COMMON—Constipation
> LESS COMMON OR RARE—Backache; diarrhea; dizziness or lightheadedness; dryness of mouth; indigestion; nausea; skin rash, hives, or itching; stomach cramps or pain
>
> Other side effects not listed above may also occur in some patients. If you notice any other effects, check with your doctor, nurse, or pharmacist.

SULFAMETHOXAZOLE AND TRIMETHOPRIM (ORAL)

ABOUT YOUR MEDICINE

Sulfamethoxazole and trimethoprim (sul-fa-meth-OX-a-zole and trye-METH-oh-prim) combination is used to treat infections such as bronchitis, middle ear infection, urinary tract infection and traveler's diarrhea. It is also used for the prevention and treatment of *Pneumocystis carinii* (noo-moe-siss-tis ka-RIN-ee-eye) pneumonia (PCP). However, it will not work for colds, flu, or other virus infections. Sulfamethoxazole and trimethoprim may also be used for other conditions as determined by your doctor.

If any of the information in this profile causes you special concern or if you want additional information about your medicine and its use, check with your doctor, nurse, or pharmacist. **Remember, keep this and all other medicines out of the reach of children and never share your medicines with others.**

Before Using This Medicine

Tell your doctor, nurse, and pharmacist if you . . .
- are allergic to any medicine, either prescription or nonprescription (OTC);
- are pregnant or intend to become pregnant while using this medicine;
- are breast-feeding;
- are taking **any** other prescription or nonprescription (OTC) medicine;
- have any other medical problems, especially anemia or other blood problems, glucose-6-phosphate dehydrogenase (G6PD) deficiency, kidney disease, liver disease, or porphyria.

Proper Use of This Medicine

Sulfamethoxazole and trimethoprim is best taken with a full glass (8 ounces) of water. Several additional glasses of water should be taken every day, unless otherwise directed by your doctor. Drinking extra water will help to prevent some unwanted effects of sulfamethoxazole and trimethoprim.

To help clear up your infection completely, **keep taking this medicine for the full time of treatment** even if you feel better after a few days; **do not miss any doses.**

If you do miss a dose of this medicine, take it as soon as possible. However, if it is almost time for your next dose, skip the missed dose and go back to your regular dosing schedule. Do not double doses.

Precautions While Using This Medicine

It is very important that your doctor check your progress at regular visits. This medicine may cause blood problems, especially if it is taken for a long time.

If your symptoms do not improve within a few days, or if they become worse, check with your doctor.

Some people who take this medicine may become more sensitive to sunlight than they are normally. **When you begin taking this medicine, avoid too much sun and do not use a sunlamp until you see how you react to the sun,** especially if you tend to burn easily. This sensitivity may last for many months after you stop taking this medicine. **If you have a severe reaction, check with your doctor.**

This medicine may also cause some people to become dizzy. **Make sure you know how you react to this medicine before you drive, use machines, or do other jobs that require you to be alert.** If this reaction is especially bothersome, check with your doctor.

This medicine must not be given to other people or used for other infections unless you are otherwise directed by your doctor.

POSSIBLE SIDE EFFECTS OF THIS MEDICINE

Side effects that should be reported to your doctor immediately

MORE COMMON—Itching or skin rash

LESS COMMON—Aching of joints and muscles; difficulty in swallowing; pale skin; redness, blistering, peeling, or loosening of skin; sore throat and fever; unusual bleeding or bruising; unusual tiredness or weakness; yellow eyes or skin

RARE—Blood in urine; bluish fingernails, lips, or skin; difficult breathing; greatly increased or decreased frequency of urination or amount of urine; increased thirst; lower back pain; pain or burning while urinating; swelling of front part of neck

Other side effects that should be reported to your doctor

MORE COMMON—Increased sensitivity of skin to sunlight

Side effects that usually do not require medical attention

These possible side effects may go away during treatment; however, if they continue or are bothersome, check with your doctor, nurse, or pharmacist.

MORE COMMON—Diarrhea; dizziness; headache; loss of appetite; nausea or vomiting

Other side effects not listed above may also occur in some patients. If you notice any other effects, check with your doctor, nurse, or pharmacist.

$\int$ ULFASALAZINE (ORAL)
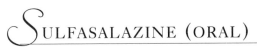

ABOUT YOUR MEDICINE

Sulfasalazine (sul-fa-SAL-a-zeen), a sulfa medicine, is used to prevent and treat inflammatory bowel disease, such as ulcerative colitis. Sulfasalazine is sometimes given with other medicines to treat inflammatory bowel disease. Sulfasalazine may also be used for other conditions as determined by your doctor.

If any of the information in this profile causes you special concern or if you want additional information about your medicine and its use, check with your doctor, nurse, or pharmacist. **Remember, keep this and all other medicines out of the reach of children and never share your medicines with others.**

BEFORE USING THIS MEDICINE

Tell your doctor, nurse, and pharmacist if you . . .

- are allergic to any medicine, either prescription or nonprescription (OTC);
- are pregnant or intend to become pregnant while using this medicine;

- are breast-feeding;
- are taking **any** other prescription or nonprescription (OTC) medicine;
- have any other medical problems, especially blood problems; glucose-6-phosphate dehydrogenase (G6PD) deficiency; kidney disease; liver disease; or porphyria.

PROPER USE OF THIS MEDICINE

Do not give sulfasalazine to infants and children up to 2 years of age unless otherwise directed by your doctor. It may cause brain problems.

Sulfasalazine is best taken right after meals or with food to lessen stomach upset. If stomach upset continues or is bothersome, check with your doctor.

Each dose of sulfasalazine should also be taken with a full glass (8 ounces) of water. Several additional glasses of water should be taken every day, unless otherwise directed by your doctor. Drinking extra water will help to prevent some unwanted effects of the sulfa medicine.

For patients taking the oral suspension form of this medicine:
- Use a specially marked measuring spoon or other device to measure each dose accurately. The average household teaspoon may not hold the right amount of liquid.

If you are taking the enteric-coated tablet form of this medicine, swallow the tablets whole. Do not break or crush them.

Keep taking this medicine for the full time of treatment even if you begin to feel better after a few days; **do not miss any doses.**

If you do miss a dose of this medicine, take it as soon as possible. However, if it is almost time for your next dose, skip the missed dose and go back to your regular dosing schedule. Do not double doses.

PRECAUTIONS WHILE USING THIS MEDICINE

If your symptoms (including diarrhea) do not improve within 1 or 2 months, or if they become worse, check with your doctor.

It is very important that your doctor check your progress at regular visits. This medicine may cause blood problems, especially if it is taken for a long time. These problems may result in a greater chance of certain infections, slow healing, and bleeding of the gums. Be careful when using regular toothbrushes, dental floss, and toothpicks. Dental work should be delayed until your blood counts have returned to normal. Check with your medical doctor or dentist if you have any questions.

Sulfasalazine may cause your skin to be more sensitive to sunlight than it is normally. Do not use a sunlamp or go out in the sun without clothing or sunblock to protect you until you see how you react. You may still be more sensitive to sunlight or sunlamps for many months after you stop taking this medicine. **If you have a severe reaction, check with your doctor.**

This medicine may also cause some people to become dizzy. **Make sure you know how you react to this medicine before you drive, use machines, or do other jobs that require you to be alert.** If this reaction is especially bothersome, check with your doctor.

POSSIBLE SIDE EFFECTS OF THIS MEDICINE

Side effects that should be reported to your doctor immediately
> MORE COMMON—Aching of joints; headache (continuing); itching; skin rash
> LESS COMMON OR RARE—Aching of joints and muscles; back, leg, or stomach pains; bloody diarrhea; bluish fingernails, lips, or skin; chest pain; cough; difficult breathing; difficulty in swallowing; fever and sore throat; general feeling of discomfort or illness; loss of appetite; pale skin; redness, blistering, peeling, or loosening of skin; unusual bleeding or bruising; unusual tiredness or weakness; yellow eyes or skin

Other side effects that should be reported to your doctor
> MORE COMMON—Increased sensitivity of skin to sunlight

Side effects that usually do not require medical attention
> These possible side effects may go away during treatment; however, if they continue or are bothersome, check with your doctor, nurse, or pharmacist.
>
> MORE COMMON—Abdominal or stomach pain or upset; diarrhea; nausea or vomiting
>
> In some patients, this medicine may also cause the urine or skin to become orange-yellow. This side effect does not need medical attention.
>
> Other side effects not listed above may also occur in some patients. If you notice any other effects, check with your doctor, nurse, or pharmacist.

SUMATRIPTAN (INJECTION)

ABOUT YOUR MEDICINE

Sumatriptan (soo-ma-TRIP-tan) is used to treat severe migraine headaches. It will not relieve any kind of pain other than headaches. However, sumatriptan often relieves other symptoms that occur together with a migraine headache, such as nausea, vomiting, sensitivity to light, and sensitivity to sound.

If any of the information in this profile causes you special concern or if you want additional information about your medicine and its use, check with your doctor, nurse, or pharmacist. **Remember, keep this and all other medicines out of the reach of children and never share your medicines with others.**

BEFORE USING THIS MEDICINE

Tell your doctor, nurse, and pharmacist if you . . .

- are allergic to any medicine, either prescription or nonprescription (OTC);
- are pregnant or intend to become pregnant while using this medicine;
- are breast-feeding;
- are taking any other prescription or nonprescription (OTC) medicine;
- have any other medical problems, especially heart or blood vessel disease.

PROPER USE OF THIS MEDICINE

To relieve your migraine as soon as possible, use sumatriptan at the first sign that the headache is coming. If you get warning signals of a coming migraine (an aura), you may use the medicine before the headache pain actually starts. However, even if you do not use sumatriptan until your migraine has been present for several hours, the medicine will still work.

Lying down in a quiet, dark room for a while after you use this medicine may help relieve your migraine.

If you do not feel much better in 1 to 2 hours after an injection of sumatriptan, **do not use any more of this medicine for the same migraine.** A migraine that is not relieved by the first dose of sumatriptan will probably not be relieved by a second dose, either. Ask your doctor ahead of time about other medicine to be used if sumatriptan does not work. However, even if sumatriptan does not relieve one migraine, it may still relieve the next one.

If you feel much better after a dose of sumatriptan, but your headache comes back or gets worse after a while, you may use more sumatriptan. However, **use this medicine only as directed by your doctor. Do not use more of it, and do not use it more often than directed.** Using too much sumatriptan may increase the chance of side effects.

Your doctor may direct you to use another medicine to help prevent headaches. **It is important that you follow your doctor's directions, even if your headaches continue to occur.**

This medicine comes with patient directions. **Read them carefully before using the medicine,** and check with your doctor or pharmacist if you have any questions.

Your doctor or nurse will teach you how to inject yourself with the medicine. **Be sure to follow the directions carefully. Check with your doctor or nurse if you have any problems using the medicine.**

Be sure to follow the patient directions about safely discarding the empty cartridge and the needle. Keep the autoinjector unit, because refills are available.

PRECAUTIONS WHILE USING THIS MEDICINE

Check with your doctor if you have used sumatriptan for 3 headaches, and have not had good relief. Also, check with your doctor if your migraine headaches are worse, or if they occur more often, than before you started using sumatriptan.

Drinking alcoholic beverages can cause headaches or make them worse. People who suffer from severe headaches should probably avoid alcoholic beverages, especially during a headache.

Some people feel drowsy or dizzy during or after a migraine, or after using sumatriptan. As long as you are feeling drowsy or dizzy, **do not drive, use machines, or do other jobs that require you to be alert and clearheaded.**

POSSIBLE SIDE EFFECTS OF THIS MEDICINE

Side effects that should be reported to your doctor immediately
> **Stop using this medicine and check with your doctor immediately** if any of the following side effects occur:

> RARE—Chest pain (severe); swelling of eyelids, face, or lips; wheezing

> **Check with your doctor right away if any of the following side effects continue for more than 1 hour.** Even if they go away in less than 1 hour, **check with your doctor before using any more sumatriptan if the following side effects occur:**

> LESS COMMON—Chest pain (mild); heaviness, tightness, or pressure in chest or neck

Side effects that should be reported to your doctor
> LESS COMMON—Difficulty in swallowing; pounding heartbeat; skin rash or bumps on skin

Side effects that usually do not require medical attention
> These possible side effects may go away during treatment; however, if they continue or are bothersome, check with your doctor, nurse, or pharmacist.

> MORE COMMON—Burning, pain, or redness at place of injection; discomfort in jaw, mouth, tongue, throat, nose, or sinuses; dizziness; drowsiness; feeling cold, "strange," or weak; feeling of burning, warmth, heat, numbness, tightness, or tingling; flushing; lightheadedness; muscle aches, cramps, or stiffness; nausea or vomiting

> Other side effects not listed above may also occur in some patients. If you notice any other effects, check with your doctor, nurse, or pharmacist.

Sumatriptan (oral)

About Your Medicine

Sumatriptan (soo-ma-TRIP-tan) is used to treat severe migraine headaches. It will not relieve any kind of pain other than headaches. However, sumatriptan often relieves other symptoms that occur together with a migraine headache, such as nausea, vomiting, sensitivity to light, and sensitivity to sound.

If any of the information in this profile causes you special concern or if you want additional information about your medicine and its use, check with your doctor, nurse, or pharmacist. **Remember, keep this and all other medicines out of the reach of children and never share your medicines with others.**

Before Using This Medicine

Tell your doctor, nurse, and pharmacist if you . . .
- are allergic to any medicine, either prescription or nonprescription (OTC);
- are pregnant or intend to become pregnant while using this medicine;
- are breast-feeding;
- are taking any other prescription or nonprescription (OTC) medicine;
- have any other medical problems, especially heart or blood vessel disease.

Proper Use of This Medicine

To relieve your migraine as soon as possible, take sumatriptan at the first sign that the headache is coming. If you get warning signals of a coming migraine (an aura), you may take the medicine before the headache pain actually starts. However, even if you do not take sumatriptan until your migraine has been present for several hours, the medicine will still work.

Lying down in a quiet, dark room for a while after you take this medicine may help relieve your migraine.

If you do not feel much better in 2 to 4 hours after a tablet is taken, **do not take any more of this medicine for the same migraine.** A migraine that is not relieved by the first dose of sumatriptan will probably not be relieved by a second dose, either. Ask your doctor ahead of time about other medicine to be taken if sumatriptan does not work. However, even if sumatriptan does not relieve one migraine, it may still relieve the next one.

If you feel much better after a dose of sumatriptan, but your headache comes back or gets worse after a while, you may take more sumatriptan. However, **take this medicine only as directed by your doctor. Do not take more of it, and do not take it more often than directed.** Using too much sumatriptan may increase the chance of side effects.

Your doctor may direct you to take another medicine to help prevent headaches. **It is important that you follow your doctor's directions, even if your headaches continue to occur.**

Sumatriptan tablets are to be swallowed whole. **Do not break, crush, or chew the tablets before swallowing them.**

Precautions While Using This Medicine

Check with your doctor if you have taken sumatriptan for 3 headaches, and have not had good relief. Also, check with your doctor if your migraine headaches are worse, or if they occur more often, than before you started taking sumatriptan.

Drinking alcoholic beverages can cause headaches or make them worse. People who suffer from severe headaches should probably avoid alcoholic beverages, especially during a headache.

Some people feel drowsy or dizzy during or after a migraine, or after taking sumatriptan. As long as you are feeling drowsy or dizzy, **do not drive, use machines, or do other jobs that require you to be alert and clearheaded.**

Possible Side Effects of This Medicine

Side effects that should be reported to your doctor immediately
> **Stop taking this medicine and check with your doctor immediately** if any of the following side effects occur:

> RARE—Chest pain (severe); swelling of eyelids, face, or lips; wheezing

> **Check with your doctor right away if any of the following side effects continue for more than 1 hour.** Even if they go away in less than 1 hour, **check with your doctor before using any more sumatriptan if the following side effects occur:**

> LESS COMMON—Chest pain (mild); heaviness, tightness, or pressure in chest or neck

Side effects that should be reported to your doctor
> LESS COMMON—Difficulty in swallowing; pounding heartbeat; skin rash or bumps on skin

Side effects that usually do not require medical attention
> These possible side effects may go away during treatment; however, if they continue or are bothersome, check with your doctor, nurse, or pharmacist.

> MORE COMMON—Discomfort in jaw, mouth, tongue, throat, nose, or sinuses; dizziness; drowsiness; feeling cold, "strange," or weak; feeling of burning, warmth, heat, numbness, tightness, or tingling; flushing; lightheadedness; muscle aches, cramps, or stiffness; nausea or vomiting

> Other side effects not listed above may also occur in some patients. If you notice any other effects, check with your doctor, nurse, or pharmacist.

$\mathcal{T}$AMOXIFEN (ORAL)

ABOUT YOUR MEDICINE

Tamoxifen (ta-MOX-i-fen) is a medicine that blocks the effects of the hormone estrogen in the body. It is used to treat some cases of breast cancer in women or men.

If any of the information in this profile causes you special concern or if you want additional information about your medicine and its use, check with your doctor, nurse, or pharmacist. **Remember, keep this and all other medicines out of the reach of children and never share your medicines with others.**

BEFORE USING THIS MEDICINE

Discuss with your doctor the possible side effects that may be caused by this medicine. Some of them may be serious and/or long-term.

Tell your doctor, nurse, and pharmacist if you . . .
- are allergic to any medicine, either prescription or nonprescription (OTC);
- are pregnant or intend to become pregnant while using this medicine;
- are breast-feeding;
- are taking **any** other prescription or nonprescription (OTC) medicine;
- have any other medical problems.

PROPER USE OF THIS MEDICINE

Use this medicine only as directed by your doctor. Do not use more or less of it, and do not use it more often than your doctor ordered.

Tamoxifen sometimes causes mild nausea and vomiting. However, it is very important that you continue to use the medicine, even if you begin to feel ill. Ask your doctor, nurse, or pharmacist for ways to lessen these effects.

If you vomit shortly after taking a dose of tamoxifen, check with your doctor.

If you miss a dose of this medicine, do not take the missed dose at all and do not double the next one. Instead, go back to your regular dosing schedule and check with your doctor.

PRECAUTIONS WHILE USING THIS MEDICINE

It is very important that your doctor check your progress at regular visits to make sure this medicine is working properly and to check for unwanted effects.

For women: Tamoxifen may make you more fertile. It is best to use some type of birth control while you are taking it. However, do not use oral contraceptives (the "Pill") since they may change the effects of tamoxifen. Tell your doctor right away if you think you have become pregnant while taking this medicine.

POSSIBLE SIDE EFFECTS OF THIS MEDICINE

Tamoxifen has been reported to increase the chance of cancer of the uterus (womb) in some women taking it. Discuss this possible effect with your doctor.

Side effects that should be reported to your doctor

FOR FEMALES AND MALES—LESS COMMON OR RARE—Blurred vision; confusion; pain or swelling in legs; shortness of breath; weakness or sleepiness; yellow eyes or skin

FOR FEMALES ONLY—LESS COMMON OR RARE—Change in vaginal discharge; pain or feeling of pressure in pelvis; vaginal bleeding

Side effects that usually do not require medical attention

These possible side effects may go away during treatment; however, if they continue or are bothersome, check with your doctor, nurse, or pharmacist.

FOR FEMALES AND MALES—LESS COMMON—Bone pain; headache; nausea and/or vomiting (mild); skin rash or dryness

FOR FEMALES ONLY—MORE COMMON—Hot flashes; weight gain

FOR FEMALES ONLY—LESS COMMON—Changes in menstrual period; itching in genital area; vaginal discharge

FOR MALES ONLY—LESS COMMON—Impotence or decreased sexual interest

Other side effects not listed above may also occur in some patients. If you notice any other effects, check with your doctor, nurse, or pharmacist.

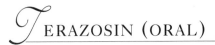 ERAZOSIN (ORAL)

ABOUT YOUR MEDICINE

Terazosin (ter-AY-zoe-sin) is used to treat high blood pressure (hypertension) or benign enlargement of the prostate (benign prostatic hyperplasia [BPH]).

If any of the information in this profile causes you special concern or if you want additional information about your medicine and its use, check with your doctor, nurse, or pharmacist. **Remember, keep this and all other medicines out of the reach of children and never share your medicines with others.**

BEFORE USING THIS MEDICINE

Tell your doctor, nurse, and pharmacist if you . . .
- are allergic to any medicine, either prescription or nonprescription (OTC);
- are pregnant or intend to become pregnant while using this medicine;
- are breast-feeding;

- are taking any other prescription or nonprescription (OTC) medicine;
- have any other medical problems.

PROPER USE OF THIS MEDICINE

For patients taking this medicine for high blood pressure:
- This medicine will not cure your high blood pressure but it does help control it. You must continue to take it—even if you feel well—if you expect to keep your blood pressure down. **You may have to take high blood pressure medicine for the rest of your life.**

For patients taking this medicine for benign enlargement of the prostate:
- Remember that terazosin will not shrink the size of your prostate, but it does help to relieve the symptoms.
- It may take up to 6 weeks before your symptoms get better.

To help you remember to take your medicine, try to get into the habit of taking it at the same time each day.

If you miss a dose of this medicine, take it as soon as possible the same day. However, if you do not remember the missed dose until the next day, skip the missed dose and go back to your regular dosing schedule. Do not double doses.

PRECAUTIONS WHILE USING THIS MEDICINE

It is important that your doctor check your progress at regular visits to make sure that this medicine is working properly.

For patients taking this medicine for high blood pressure:
- **Do not take other medicines unless they have been discussed with your doctor.** This especially includes over-the-counter (nonprescription) medicines for appetite control, asthma, colds, cough, hay fever, or sinus problems, since they may tend to increase your blood pressure.

Dizziness, lightheadedness, or sudden fainting may occur after you take this medicine, especially when you get up from a sitting or lying position. These effects are more likely to occur when you take the first dose of this medicine. Taking the first dose at bedtime may prevent problems. However, **be especially careful if you need to get up during the night.** These effects may also occur with any doses you take after the first dose. Getting up slowly may help lessen this problem. **If you feel dizzy, lie down so that you do not faint.** Then sit for a few minutes before standing to prevent the dizziness from returning.

The dizziness, lightheadedness, or fainting is more likely to occur if you drink alcohol, stand for long periods of time, exercise, or if the weather is hot. **While you are taking this medicine, be careful to limit the amount of alcohol you drink. Also, use extra care during exercise or hot weather or if you must stand for long periods of time.**

This medicine may cause some people to become drowsy or less alert than they are normally. **Make sure you know how you react to this medicine before you** drive, use machines, or do other jobs that could be dangerous if you are dizzy, drowsy, or are not alert. After you have taken several doses of this medicine, these effects should lessen.

POSSIBLE SIDE EFFECTS OF THIS MEDICINE

Side effects that should be reported to your doctor

MORE COMMON—Dizziness

LESS COMMON—Chest pain; dizziness or lightheadedness when standing up; fainting (sudden); fast or irregular heartbeat; pounding heartbeat; shortness of breath; swelling of feet or lower legs

RARE—Weight gain

Side effects that usually do not require medical attention

These possible side effects may go away during treatment; however, if they continue or are bothersome, check with your doctor, nurse, or pharmacist.

MORE COMMON—Headache; unusual tiredness or weakness

LESS COMMON—Back or joint pain; blurred vision; drowsiness; nausea and vomiting; stuffy nose

Other side effects not listed above may also occur in some patients. If you notice any other effects, check with your doctor, nurse, or pharmacist.

TERFENADINE (ORAL)

ABOUT YOUR MEDICINE

Terfenadine (ter-FEN-a-deen) is used to relieve or prevent the symptoms of hay fever and other types of allergy. Terfenadine may also be used for other conditions as determined by your doctor.

If any of the information in this profile causes you special concern or if you want additional information about your medicine and its use, check with your doctor, nurse, or pharmacist. Remember, keep this and all other medicines out of the reach of children and never share your medicines with others.

BEFORE USING THIS MEDICINE

Tell your doctor, nurse, or pharmacist if you . . .
- are allergic to any medicine, either prescription or nonprescription (OTC);
- are pregnant or intend to become pregnant;
- are breast-feeding;
- are taking any other prescription or nonprescription (OTC) medicine, especially bepridil, clarithromycin, disopyramide, erythromycin,

itraconazole, ketoconazole, maprotiline, phenothiazines, pimozide, procainamide, quinidine, tricyclic antidepressants, or troleandomycin;
- have any other medical problems, especially difficult urination, enlarged prostate, glaucoma, heart rhythm problems (history of), liver disease, low potassium blood levels, or urinary tract blockage.

PROPER USE OF THIS MEDICINE

Terfenadine is used to relieve or prevent the symptoms of your medical problem. Take it only as directed. Do not take more of it and do not take it more often than your doctor ordered. To do so may increase the chance of side effects.

Terfenadine can be taken with food or a glass of water or milk to lessen stomach irritation if necessary.

If you must take this medicine regularly and you miss a dose, take it as soon as possible. However, if it is almost time for your next dose, skip the missed dose and go back to your regular dosing schedule. Do not double doses.

POSSIBLE SIDE EFFECTS OF THIS MEDICINE

Side effects that should be reported to your doctor immediately
> LESS COMMON OR RARE (WITH HIGH DOSES)—Fast or irregular heartbeat

Other side effects that should be reported to your doctor
> LESS COMMON OR RARE—Sore throat and fever; unusual bleeding or bruising; unusual tiredness or weakness

Side effects that usually do not require medical attention
> These possible side effects may go away during treatment; however, if they continue or are bothersome, check with your doctor, nurse, or pharmacist.
>
> RARE—Drowsiness; thickening of mucus
>
> Other side effects not listed above may also occur in some patients. If you notice any other effects, check with your doctor, nurse, or pharmacist.

$\mathcal{T}$ETRACYCLINES (ORAL)

Including Demeclocycline; Doxycycline;
Minocycline; Oxytetracycline; Tetracycline

ABOUT YOUR MEDICINE

Tetracyclines (te-tra-SYE-kleens) are used to treat certain infections and also to help control acne. Demeclocycline and doxycycline may also be used for other problems as determined by your doctor. Tetracyclines will not work for colds, flu, or other virus infections.

If any of the information in this profile causes you special concern or if you want additional information about your medicine and its use, check with your doctor, nurse, or pharmacist. **Remember, keep this and all other medicines out of the reach of children and never share your medicines with others.**

BEFORE USING THIS MEDICINE

Tell your doctor, nurse, and pharmacist if you . . .
- are allergic to any medicine, either prescription or nonprescription (OTC);
- are pregnant or intend to become pregnant while using this medicine; tetracyclines should not be used during the last half of pregnancy;
- are breast-feeding;
- are taking any other prescription or nonprescription (OTC) medicine, especially antacids, calcium or iron supplements, cholestyramine, colestipol, magnesium-containing laxatives, oral contraceptives (birth control pills) containing estrogen, or other medicines containing calcium, iron, or magnesium;
- have any other medical problems, especially diabetes insipidus (water diabetes—demeclocycline only), or kidney disease.

PROPER USE OF THIS MEDICINE

Tetracyclines should be taken with a full glass (8 ounces) of water to prevent irritation of the esophagus or stomach. In addition, most tetracyclines are best taken on an empty stomach (either 1 hour before or 2 hours after meals). However, if this medicine upsets your stomach, your doctor may want you to take it with food; **but do not take milk or other dairy products within 1 or 2 hours of the time you take tetracyclines** (except doxycycline or minocycline).

Do not give tetracyclines to infants or children under 8 years of age unless directed by your doctor. Tetracyclines may cause permanently discolored teeth and other problems in this age group.

To help clear up your infection completely, **keep taking this medicine for the full time of treatment** even if you begin to feel better; **do not miss any doses.**

If you do miss a dose of this medicine, take it as soon as possible. However, if it is almost time for your next dose, skip the missed dose and go back to your regular dosing schedule. Do not double doses.

PRECAUTIONS WHILE USING THIS MEDICINE

If your symptoms do not improve within a few days (or a few weeks or months for acne patients), or if they become worse, check with your doctor.

Oral contraceptives (birth control pills) containing estrogen may not work properly if you take them while you are taking tetracyclines. Unplanned pregnancies may occur. You should use a different or additional means of birth control while you are taking tetracyclines. If you have any questions about this, check with your doctor or pharmacist.

Tetracyclines may cause your skin to be more sensitive to sunlight than it is normally. When you begin taking this medicine, avoid too much sun and do not use a sunlamp until you see how you react. This sensitivity may last for 2 weeks to several months or more after you stop taking this medicine. **If you have a severe reaction, check with your doctor.**

This medicine must not be given to other people or used for other infections unless you are otherwise directed by your doctor.

POSSIBLE SIDE EFFECTS OF THIS MEDICINE

Side effects that should be reported to your doctor

FOR ALL TETRACYCLINES—MORE COMMON—Increased sensitivity of skin to sunlight (rare with minocycline)

RARE—Abdominal pain; bulging fontanel (soft spot on head) of infants; discolored teeth (in infants and children); headache; loss of appetite; nausea and vomiting; yellow skin; visual changes

FOR DEMECLOCYCLINE (IN ADDITION TO THE ABOVE)—Greatly increased frequency of urination or amount of urine; increased thirst; unusual tiredness or weakness

FOR MINOCYCLINE (IN ADDITION TO THE ABOVE)—Discoloration of skin and mucous membranes

Side effects that usually do not require medical attention

These possible side effects may go away during treatment; however, if they continue or are bothersome, check with your doctor, nurse, or pharmacist.

MORE COMMON—Cramps or burning of the stomach; diarrhea; dizziness, lightheadedness, or unsteadiness (minocycline only); nausea or vomiting

LESS COMMON—Itching of the rectal or genital (sex organ) areas; sore mouth or tongue

In some patients tetracyclines may cause the tongue to become darkened or discolored. This will go away when you stop taking this medicine.

Other side effects not listed above may also occur in some patients. If you notice any other effects, check with your doctor, nurse, or pharmacist.

ᴛETRACYCLINES (TOPICAL)

Including Chlortetracycline; Meclocycline; Tetracycline

ABOUT YOUR MEDICINE

Tetracyclines (te-tra-SYE-kleens) belong to the family of medicines called antibiotics. The topical ointment forms are used to treat infections of the skin. Meclocycline (me-kloe-SYE-kleen) cream and the topical liquid form of tetracycline are used to help control acne. They may be used alone or with one or more other medicines that are applied to the skin or taken by mouth for acne.

If any of the information in this profile causes you special concern or if you want additional information about your medicine and its use, check with your doctor, nurse, or pharmacist. **Remember, keep this and all other medicines out of the reach of children and never share your medicines with others.**

BEFORE USING THIS MEDICINE

Tell your doctor, nurse, and pharmacist if you . . .
- are allergic to any medicine, either prescription or nonprescription (OTC);
- are pregnant or intend to become pregnant while using this medicine;
- are breast-feeding;
- are taking any other prescription or nonprescription (OTC) medicine;
- have any other medical problems.

PROPER USE OF THIS MEDICINE

To help clear up your infection or acne completely, **keep using this medicine for the full time of treatment,** even if your symptoms begin to clear up after a few days. If you stop using this medicine too soon, your symptoms may return.

You should apply the medicine to the whole area usually affected by acne, not just the pimples themselves.

Do not get this medicine on your clothing since it may stain.

The liquid form of this medicine contains alcohol and is flammable. **Do not use near heat, near open flame, or while smoking.**

If you are using this medicine without a prescription, do not use it to treat deep wounds, puncture wounds, or serious burns without first checking with your doctor or pharmacist.

Since this medicine contains alcohol, it will sting or burn. Therefore, **do not get this medicine in the eyes, nose, mouth, or on other mucous membranes.**

If you miss a dose of this medicine, apply it as soon as possible. However, if it is almost time for your next dose, skip the missed dose and go back to your regular dosing schedule.

PRECAUTIONS WHILE USING THIS MEDICINE

For patients using either the cream form or the topical liquid form of this medicine for acne:

- Some people may notice improvement in their acne within 4 to 6 weeks. However, if there is no improvement in your acne after you have used this medicine for 6 to 8 weeks or if it becomes worse, check with your doctor or pharmacist. The treatment of acne may take up to 8 to 12 weeks before full improvement is seen.

For patients using the topical ointment form of this medicine:

- If there is no improvement in your skin infection after you have used this medicine for 2 weeks, or if it becomes worse, check with your doctor or pharmacist.

POSSIBLE SIDE EFFECTS OF THIS MEDICINE

Side effects that should be reported to your doctor

LESS COMMON—Pain, redness, swelling, or other sign of irritation not present before use of this medicine

Side effects that usually do not require medical attention

These possible side effects may go away during treatment; however, if they continue or are bothersome, check with your doctor, nurse, or pharmacist.

MORE COMMON (FOR TOPICAL LIQUID FORM ONLY)—Dry or scaly skin; stinging or burning feeling

MORE COMMON (FOR CREAM AND TOPICAL LIQUID FORMS ONLY)—Faint yellowing of the skin, especially around hair roots

Other side effects not listed above may also occur in some patients. If you notice any other effects, check with your doctor, nurse, or pharmacist.

$\mathcal{T}$HIAZIDE DIURETICS (ORAL)

Including Bendroflumethiazide; Benzthiazide;
Chlorothiazide; Chlorthalidone; Cyclothiazide;
Hydrochlorothiazide; Hydroflumethiazide; Methyclothiazide;
Metolazone; Polythiazide; Quinethazone; Trichlormethiazide

ABOUT YOUR MEDICINE

Thiazide diuretics are commonly used to treat high blood pressure (hypertension). They are used also to help reduce the amount of water in the body by increasing the flow of urine. Thiazide diuretics may also be used for other conditions as determined by your doctor.

If any of the information in this profile causes you special concern or if you want additional information about your medicine and its use, check with your doctor, nurse, or pharmacist. **Remember, keep this and all other medicines out of the reach of children and never share your medicines with others.**

BEFORE USING THIS MEDICINE

Tell your doctor, nurse, and pharmacist if you . . .
- are allergic to any medicine, either prescription or nonprescription (OTC);
- are pregnant or intend to become pregnant while using this medicine;
- are breast-feeding;
- compete in athletics;
- are taking any other prescription or nonprescription (OTC) medicine, especially cholestyramine, colestipol, digitalis glycosides (heart medicine), or lithium;
- have any other medical problems, especially severe kidney disease.

PROPER USE OF THIS MEDICINE

Thiazide diuretics may cause an unusual feeling of tiredness when you begin to take them. You may also notice an increase in urine or in frequency of urination. To keep this from affecting sleep:
- if you are to take a single dose a day, take it in the morning after breakfast.
- if you are to take more than one dose, take the last one no later than 6 p.m.

For patients taking this medicine for high blood pressure:
- This medicine will not cure your high blood pressure but it does help control it. You must continue to take it—even if you feel well—if you expect to keep your blood pressure down. **You may have to take high blood pressure medicine for the rest of your life.**

If you miss a dose of this medicine, take it as soon as possible. However, if it is almost time for your next dose, skip the missed dose and go back to your regular dosing schedule. Do not double doses.

PRECAUTIONS WHILE USING THIS MEDICINE

This medicine may cause a loss of potassium from your body. To help prevent this, your doctor **may** want you to eat or drink foods that have a high potassium content, take a potassium supplement, or take another medicine to help prevent loss of the potassium in the first place. It is very important to follow these directions. Also, it is important not to change your diet on your own and to check with your doctor if you become sick and have severe or continuing vomiting or diarrhea.

POSSIBLE SIDE EFFECTS OF THIS MEDICINE

Side effects that should be reported to your doctor

RARE—Black, tarry stools; blood in urine or stools; cough or hoarseness; fever or chills; joint pain; lower back or side pain; painful or difficult urination; pinpoint red spots on skin; skin rash or hives; stomach pain (severe) with nausea and vomiting; unusual bleeding or bruising; yellow eyes or skin

SIGNS OF TOO MUCH POTASSIUM LOSS—Dryness of mouth; increased thirst; mood changes; muscle cramps or pain; nausea or vomiting; unusual tiredness or weakness; weak or irregular heartbeat

SIGNS OF TOO MUCH SODIUM LOSS—Confusion; convulsions; decreased mental activity; irritability; muscle cramps; unusual tiredness or weakness

Side effects that usually do not require medical attention

These possible side effects may go away during treatment; however, if they continue or are bothersome, check with your doctor, nurse, or pharmacist.

LESS COMMON—Decreased sexual ability; diarrhea; dizziness or lightheadedness when standing up; increased sensitivity of skin to sunlight; loss of appetite; upset stomach

Other side effects not listed above may also occur in some patients. If you notice any other effects, check with your doctor, nurse, or pharmacist.

---

*T*ICLOPIDINE (ORAL)

ABOUT YOUR MEDICINE

Ticlopidine (tye-KLOE-pi-deen) is used to lower the chance of having a stroke. It is given to people who have already had a stroke and to people with certain medical problems that may lead to a stroke. Because ticlopidine can cause serious side effects, especially during the first three months of treatment, it is used mostly for people who cannot take aspirin to prevent strokes.

If any of the information in this profile causes you special concern or if you want additional information about your medicine and its use, check with your doctor, nurse, or pharmacist. **Remember, keep this and all other medicines out of the reach of children and never share your medicines with others.**

BEFORE USING THIS MEDICINE

Tell your doctor, nurse, and pharmacist if you . . .
- are allergic to any medicine, either prescription or nonprescription (OTC);
- are pregnant or intend to become pregnant while using this medicine;
- are breast-feeding;
- are taking any other prescription or nonprescription (OTC) medicine, especially anticoagulants (blood thinners), aspirin, or heparin;
- have any other medical problems, especially blood clotting problems, such as hemophilia; blood disease; kidney disease (severe); or stomach ulcers.

PROPER USE OF THIS MEDICINE

Ticlopidine should be taken with food. This helps more of the medicine to be absorbed into the body. It may also lessen the chance of stomach upset.

Take this medicine only as directed. It will not work properly if you take less of it than directed. Taking more than directed may increase the chance of bleeding or other serious side effects without increasing the helpful effects.

If you miss a dose of this medicine, take it as soon as possible. However, if it is almost time for your next dose, skip the missed dose and go back to your regular dosing schedule. Do not double doses.

PRECAUTIONS WHILE USING THIS MEDICINE

It is very important that blood tests be done every 2 weeks for at least the first 3 months of treatment. The tests are needed to find out whether certain side effects are occurring. Finding these side effects early helps to prevent them from becoming serious. Your doctor will arrange for the blood tests to be done. **Be sure that you do not miss any of these tests.**

Tell all medical doctors, dentists, nurses, and pharmacists you go to that you are taking this medicine. Ticlopidine may increase the risk of serious bleeding during an operation or some kinds of dental work. Therefore, treatment may have to be stopped about 10 days to 2 weeks ahead of time.

Ticlopidine may cause serious bleeding, especially after an injury. Sometimes, bleeding inside the body can occur without your knowing about it. Ask your doctor whether there are certain activities you should avoid while taking this medicine, and **check with your doctor immediately if you are injured while being treated with ticlopidine.**

Check with your doctor immediately if you notice bleeding or bruising, especially bleeding that is hard to stop; any sign of infection, such as fever, chills, or sore throat; or sores, ulcers, or white spots in the mouth.

After you stop taking ticlopidine, the chance of bleeding may continue for 1 or 2 weeks. During this time, continue to follow the same precautions that you followed while you were taking the medicine.

POSSIBLE SIDE EFFECTS OF THIS MEDICINE

Side effects that should be reported to your doctor immediately
LESS COMMON OR RARE—Abdominal or stomach pain (severe) or swelling; back pain; blood in eyes; blood in urine; bloody or black, tarry stools; bruising or purple areas on skin; coughing up blood; decreased alertness; dizziness; fever, chills, or sore throat; headache (severe); joint pain or swelling; nosebleeds; paralysis or problems with coordination; pinpoint red spots on skin; sores, ulcers, or white spots in mouth; stammering or other difficulty in speaking; unusually heavy bleeding or oozing from cuts or wounds; unusually heavy or unexpected menstrual bleeding; vomiting of blood or material that looks like coffee grounds

Other side effects that should be reported to your doctor
MORE COMMON—Skin rash

LESS COMMON OR RARE—Hives or itching of skin; ringing or buzzing in ears; yellow eyes or skin

Side effects that usually do not require medical attention
These possible side effects may go away during treatment; however, if they continue or are bothersome, check with your doctor, nurse, or pharmacist.

MORE COMMON—Abdominal or stomach pain (mild); bloating or gas; diarrhea; nausea

Other side effects not listed above may also occur in some patients. If you notice any other effects, check with your doctor, nurse, or pharmacist.

$\mathcal{T}$RICYCLIC ANTIDEPRESSANTS (ORAL)

Including Amitriptyline; Amoxapine; Clomipramine; Desipramine; Doxepin; Imipramine; Nortriptyline; Protriptyline; Trimipramine.

ABOUT YOUR MEDICINE

Tricyclic antidepressants are used to relieve mental depression and depression that sometimes occurs with anxiety. One form of this medicine (imipramine) may also be used to treat enuresis (bedwetting). Another form (clomipramine) is used to treat obsessive-compulsive disorders. Tricyclic antidepressants may also be used for other conditions as determined by your doctor.

If any of the information in this profile causes you special concern or if you want additional information about your medicine and its use, check with your doctor, nurse, or pharmacist. **Remember, keep this and all other medicines out of the reach of children and never share your medicines with others.**

BEFORE USING THIS MEDICINE

Tell your doctor, nurse, and pharmacist if you . . .
- are allergic to any medicine, either prescription or nonprescription (OTC);
- are pregnant or intend to become pregnant while using this medicine;
- are breast-feeding;
- are taking **any** other prescription or nonprescription (OTC) medicine;
- have **any** other medical problems.

PROPER USE OF THIS MEDICINE

Take this medicine only as directed by your doctor. Sometimes tricyclic antidepressants must be taken for several weeks before you feel better.

If you miss a dose of this medicine, take it as soon as possible. However, if it is almost time for your next dose, skip the missed dose. Do not double doses. If a once-a-day bedtime dose is missed, do not take that dose in the morning since it may cause disturbing side effects during waking hours.

PRECAUTIONS WHILE USING THIS MEDICINE

Do not stop taking this medicine without first checking with your doctor.

This medicine will add to the effects of alcohol and other CNS depressants (medicines that make you drowsy or less alert). **Check with your doctor before taking any such depressants while you are taking this medicine.**

This medicine may cause some people to become drowsy or less alert than they are normally. **Make sure you know how you react before you drive, use machines, or do other jobs that require you to be alert.**

Dizziness, lightheadedness, or fainting may occur, especially when getting up from a lying or sitting position. Getting up slowly may help.

Before having any kind of surgery or dental or emergency treatment, tell the physician or dentist in charge that you are taking this medicine.

The effects of this medicine may last for 3 to 7 days after you stop taking it. Make sure you continue to follow the precautions during this time.

POSSIBLE SIDE EFFECTS OF THIS MEDICINE

Side effects that should be reported to your doctor

LESS COMMON—Blurred vision; confusion or delirium; constipation (especially in the elderly); decreased sexual ability (more common with amoxapine and clomipramine); difficulty in swallowing or speaking; eye pain; fainting; fast or irregular heartbeat; hallucinations; loss of balance control; mask-like face; nervousness or restlessness; problems in urinating; shakiness or trembling; shuffling walk; slowed movements; stiff arms and legs

RARE—Breast enlargement; hair loss; inappropriate secretion of milk (in females); increased sensitivity to sunlight; irritability; muscle twitching; red or brownish spots on skin; ringing, buzzing, or other unexplained noises in the ears; seizures (more common with clomipramine); skin rash and itching; sore throat and fever; swelling of face and tongue; swelling of testicles (more common with amoxapine); trouble with teeth or gums (more common with clomipramine); unusual bleeding or bruising; yellow eyes or skin

FOR AMOXAPINE ONLY (IN ADDITION TO THE ABOVE)—**Stop taking this medicine and get emergency help immediately** if any of the following side effects occur: Convulsions (seizures); fever with increased sweating; high or low blood pressure; loss of bladder control; muscle stiffness (severe); tiredness or weakness; troubled breathing; unusually pale skin. Other side effects of amoxapine that need medical attention include: Lip smacking or puckering; puffing of cheeks; rapid or worm-like movements of the tongue; uncontrolled chewing movements; uncontrolled movements of hands, arms, or legs

Side effects that usually do not require medical attention

These possible side effects may go away during treatment; however, if they continue or are bothersome, check with your doctor, nurse, or pharmacist.

MORE COMMON—Dizziness or lightheadedness; drowsiness (mild); dryness of mouth; headache; increased appetite (may include craving for sweets); nausea; unpleasant taste; weight gain

Other side effects not listed above may also occur in some patients. If you notice any other effects, check with your doctor, nurse, or pharmacist.

After you stop taking this medicine, your body may need time to adjust. Check with your doctor if you notice headache; irritability; nausea, vomiting, or diarrhea; restlessness; trouble in sleeping, with vivid dreams; uncontrolled movements of mouth, tongue, jaw, arms, or legs; or unusual excitement.

Xanthine Bronchodilators (Oral)

Including Aminophylline; Dyphylline; Oxtriphylline; Theophylline

About Your Medicine

Xanthine bronchodilators are used to treat and/or prevent the symptoms of bronchial asthma, chronic bronchitis, and emphysema. These medicines relieve cough, wheezing, shortness of breath, and troubled breathing. Aminophylline and theophylline may also be used for other conditions as determined by your doctor.

If any of the information in this profile causes you special concern or if you want additional information about your medicine and its use, check with your doctor, nurse, or pharmacist. **Remember, keep this and all other medicines out of the reach of children and never share your medicines with others.**

Before Using This Medicine

Tell your doctor, nurse, and pharmacist if you . . .
- are allergic to any medicine, either prescription or nonprescription (OTC);
- are pregnant or intend to become pregnant while using this medicine;
- are breast-feeding;
- are taking any other prescription or nonprescription (OTC) medicine, especially beta-blockers, cimetidine, ciprofloxacin, corticosteroids (cortisone-like medicine), erythromycin, nicotine chewing gum, norfloxacin, phenytoin, ranitidine, or troleandomycin;
- smoke or have smoked (tobacco or marijuana) within the last 2 years;
- have any other medical problems, especially stomach ulcer (or history of) or other stomach problems.

Proper Use of This Medicine

For patients taking the capsule, tablet, liquid, or extended-release (not including the once-a-day capsule or tablet) form of this medicine:
- **This medicine works best when taken with a glass of water on an empty stomach** (either 30 minutes to 1 hour before or 2 hours after meals) since that way it will get into the blood sooner. However, in some cases your doctor may want you to take this medicine with or right after meals to lessen stomach upset.

For patients taking the once-a-day capsule or tablet form of this medicine:
- **Some products are to be taken each morning after fasting overnight and at least 1 hour before eating. However, other products are to be taken in the morning or evening with or without food. Be sure you understand exactly how to take the medicine prescribed for you.** Try to take the medicine at about the same time each day.

Use this medicine only as directed by your doctor. Do not use more of it, do not use it more often, and do not use it for a longer time than your doctor ordered. To do so may increase the chance of serious side effects.

In order for this medicine to help your medical problem, it must be taken every day in regularly spaced doses.

If you miss a dose of this medicine, take it as soon as possible. However, if it is almost time for your next dose, skip the missed dose and go back to your regular dosing schedule. Do not double doses.

PRECAUTIONS WHILE USING THIS MEDICINE

Your doctor should check your progress at regular visits, especially for the first few weeks after you begin using this medicine.

Do not change brands or dosage forms of this medicine without first checking with your doctor. Different products may not work the same way.

This medicine may add to the central nervous system (CNS) stimulant effects of caffeine-containing foods or beverages such as chocolate, cocoa, tea, coffee, and cola drinks. **Avoid eating or drinking large amounts of these foods or beverages while using this medicine.**

Check with your doctor at once if you develop symptoms of influenza (flu) or a fever since either of these may increase the chance of side effects with this medicine. Also, **check with your doctor if diarrhea occurs** because the dose of this medicine may need to be changed.

POSSIBLE SIDE EFFECTS OF THIS MEDICINE

Side effects that should be reported to your doctor

LESS COMMON—Heartburn and/or vomiting

RARE—Skin rash or hives

SIGNS OF OVERDOSE—Bloody or black tarry stools; confusion or change in behavior; convulsions (seizures); diarrhea; dizziness or lightheadedness; fast breathing; fast, pounding, or irregular heartbeat; flushing or redness of face; headache; increased urination; irritability; loss of appetite; muscle twitching; stomach cramps or pain; trembling; trouble in sleeping; unusual tiredness or weakness; vomiting of blood or material that looks like coffee grounds

Side effects that usually do not require medical attention

These possible side effects may go away during treatment; however, if they continue or are bothersome, check with your doctor, nurse, or pharmacist.

MORE COMMON—Nausea; nervousness or restlessness

Other side effects not listed above may also occur in some patients. If you notice any other effects, check with your doctor, nurse, or pharmacist.

DRUG
IDENTIFICATION
GUIDE INDEX

DRUG INDEX

THIS INDEX CONTAINS generic and brand-name drugs that are covered by the profiles. There are many brand names on the market. The index includes the most common names for ease of reference only. The inclusion of a brand name is not an endorsement of that product, nor is the omission of a brand name a rejection of its quality.

A brand name that appears on your bottle or label will probably not appear in the profile itself.

A general index to the book follows this index. There, you will find listings of other topics that are related to your health questions. For example, if you are looking up Estrogens and Progestins (Oral Contraceptives), you will also be interested in the information in the first part of the book about the pill and other contraceptive methods.

NOTE: An asterisk (*) following the drug name indicates that it is not available in the United States.

A

*Abenol**—See Acetaminophen (Oral), 329–30

Accupril (Quinapril)—See ACE Inhibitors (Oral), 325–27

Accutane—See Isotretinoin (Oral), 514–16

*Accutane Roche**—See Isotretinoin (Oral), 514–16

ACE Inhibitors (Oral), 325–26

ACE Inhibitors and Hydrochlorothiazide (Oral), 327–28

Acebutolol—See Beta-blockers (Oral), 397–99

Aceta with Codeine (Acetaminophen and Codeine)—See Narcotic Analgesics and Acetaminophen (Oral), 574–76

Aceta Elixir—See Acetaminophen (Oral), 329–30

Aceta Tablets—See Acetaminophen (Oral), 329–30

Acetaco (Acetaminophen and Codeine)—See Narcotic Analgesics and Acetaminophen (Oral), 574–76

Acetaminophen (Oral), 329–30

Acetaminophen and Caffeine—See Acetaminophen (Oral), 329–30

Acetaminophen and Codeine—See Narcotic Analgesics and Acetaminophen (Oral), 574–76

Acetaminophen, Codeine, and Caffeine—See Narcotic Analgesics and Acetaminophen (Oral), 574–76

Acetohexamide—See Antidiabetics (Oral), 364–66

Acetophenazine—See Phenothiazines (Oral), 602–4

Achromycin (Tetracycline)—See Tetracyclines (Topical), 661–62

Achromycin V (Tetracycline)—See Tetracyclines (Oral), 659–61

Aclophen (Chlorpheniramine, Phenylephrine, and Acetaminophen)—See Antihistamines, Decongestants, and Analgesics (Oral), 372–74

Aclovate (Alclometasone)—See Corticosteroids (Topical—Low Potency), 447–48

Acrivastine and Pseudoephedrine—See Antihistamines and Decongestants (Oral), 370–72

Actagen (Triprolidine and Pseudoephedrine)—See Antihistamines and Decongestants (Oral), 370–72

Actagen-C Cough—See Cough/Cold Combinations (Oral), 451–52

Actamin—See Acetaminophen (Oral), 329–30

Actamin Extra—See Acetaminophen (Oral), 329–30

Actamin Super (Acetaminophen and Caffeine)—See Acetaminophen (Oral), 329–30

Acticort 100 (Hydrocortisone)—See Corticosteroids (Topical—Low Potency), 447–48

Actifed (Triprolidine and Pseudoephedrine)—See Antihistamines and Decongestants (Oral), 370–72

Actifed Allergy Nighttime Caplets (Diphenhydramine and Pseudoephedrine)—See Antihistamines and Decongestants (Oral), 370–72

Actifed with Codeine Cough—See Cough/Cold Combinations (Oral), 451–52

*Actifed DM**—See Cough/Cold Combinations (Oral), 451–52

Actifed Head Cold and Allergy Medicine (Triprolidine and Pseudoephedrine)—See Antihistamines and Decongestants (Oral), 370–72

Actifed Plus (Triprolidine, Pseudoephedrine, and Acetaminophen)—See Antihistamines, Decongestants, and Analgesics (Oral), 372–74

Actifed Plus Caplets (Triprolidine, Pseudoephedrine, and Acetaminophen)—See Antihistamines, Decongestants, and Analgesics (Oral), 372–74

Actifed Sinus Daytime (Pseudoephedrine and Acetaminophen)—See Decongestants and Analgesics (Oral), 456–58

Apo-Biscodyl* (Biscodyl)—See Laxatives, Stimulant (Rectal), 524–26

Apo-Cal* (Calcium Carbonate)—See Calcium Supplements (Oral), 415–17

Apo-Carbamazepine*—See Carbamazepine (Oral), 419–21

Apo-Cephalex* (Cephalexin)—See Cephalosporins (Oral), 421–23

Apo-Chlordiazepoxide* (Chlordiazepoxide)—See Benzodiazepines (Oral), 389–91; Benzodiazepines (For Anxiety—Oral), 391–93; Benzodiazepines (For Insomnia—Oral), 395–96

Apo-Chlorpropamide* (Chlorpropamide)—See Antidiabetics (Oral), 364–66

Apo-Chlorthalidone* (Chlorthalidone)—See Thiazide Diuretics (Oral), 663–64

Apo-Cimetidine* (Cimetidine)—See H$_2$–blockers (Oral), 493–94

Apo-Clorazepate* (Clorazepate)—See Benzodiazepines (Oral), 389–91; Benzodiazepines (For Anxiety—Oral), 391–93; Benzodiazepines (For Epilepsy—Oral), 393–95; Benzodiazepines (For Insomnia—Oral), 395–96

Apo-Cloxi* (Cloxacillin)—See Penicillins (Oral), 595–97

Apo-Diazepam* (Diazepam)—See Benzodiazepines (Oral), 389–91; Benzodiazepines (For Anxiety—Oral), 391–93; Benzodiazepines (For Epilepsy—Oral), 393–95; Benzodiazepines (For Insomnia—Oral), 395–96

Apo-Diflunisal* (Diflunisal)—See Anti-inflammatory Drugs (NSAIDs) (Oral), 374–76

Apo-Diltiaz* (Diltiazem)—See Calcium Channel Blockers (Oral), 413–15

Apo-Dimenhydrinate* (Dimenhydrinate)—See Antihistamines (Oral), 368–70

Apo-Dipyridamole (Dipyridamole)—See Platelet Aggregation Inhibitors (Oral), 608–10

Apo-Doxy* (Doxycycline)—See Tetracyclines (Oral), 659–61

Apo-Erythro* (Erythromycin)—See Erythromycins (Oral), 467–68

Apo-Erythro-EC* (Erythromycin)—See Erythromycins (Oral), 467–68

Apo-Erythro-ES* (Erythromycin Ethylsuccinate)—See Erythromycins (Oral), 467–68

Apo-Erythro-S* (Erythromycin Stearate)—See Erythromycins (Oral), 467–68

Apo-Ferrous Gluconate* (Ferrous Gluconate)—See Iron Supplements (Oral), 510–12

Apo-Ferrous Sulfate* (Ferrous Sulfate)—See Iron Supplements (Oral), 510–12

Apo-Fluphenazine* (Fluphenazine)—See Phenothiazines (Oral), 602–4

Apo-Flurazepam* (Flurazepam)—See Benzodiazepines (Oral), 389–91; Benzodiazepines (For Insomnia—Oral), 395–96

Apo-Flurbiprofen* (Flurbiprofen)—See Anti-inflammatory Drugs (NSAIDs) (Oral), 374–76

Apo-Folic*—See Folic Acid (Vitamin B$_9$) (Oral), 490–91

Apo-Furosemide* (Furosemide)—See Loop Diuretics (Oral), 539–40

Apo-Glyburide* (Glyburide)—See Antidiabetics (Oral), 364–66

Apo-Haloperidol*—See Haloperidol (Oral), 497–99

Apo-Hydro* (Hydrochlorothiazide)—See Thiazide Diuretics (Oral), 663–64

Apo-Hydroxyzine* (Hydroxyzine)—See Antihistamines (Oral), 368–70; Hydroxyzine (Oral/Injection), 505–6

Apo-Ibuprofen* (Ibuprofen)—See Anti-inflammatory Drugs (NSAIDs) (Oral), 374–76

Apo-Imipramine* (Imipramine)—See Tricyclic Antidepressants (Oral), 667–68

Apo-Indomethacin* (Indomethacin)—See Anti-inflammatory Drugs (NSAIDs) (Oral), 374–76

Apo-Ipravent*—See Ipratropium (Inhalation), 508–10

Apo-ISDN* (Isosorbide Dinitrate)—See Nitrates (Oral), 582–84; Nitrates (Sublingual), 584–86

Apo-K* (Potassium Chloride)—See Potassium Supplements (Oral), 612–14

Apo-Keto* (Ketoprofen)—See Anti-inflammatory Drugs (NSAIDs) (Oral), 374–76

Apo-Keto-E* (Ketoprofen)—See Anti-inflammatory Drugs (NSAIDs) (Oral), 374–76

Apo-Lorazepam* (Lorazepam)—See Benzodiazepines (Oral), 389–91; Benzodiazepines (For Anxiety—Oral), 391–93; Benzodiazepines (For Insomnia—Oral), 395–96

Apo-Methyldopa*—See Methyldopa (Oral), 556–57

Apo-Metoclop*—See Metoclopramide (Oral), 557–59

Apo-Metoprolol* (Metoprolol)—See Beta-blockers (Oral), 397–99

Apo-Metoprolol (Type L)* (Metoprolol)—See Beta-blockers (Oral), 397–99

Apo-Metronidazole*—See Metronidazole (Oral), 559–61

Apo-Napro-Na* (Naproxen)—See Anti-inflammatory Drugs (NSAIDs) (Oral), 374–76

Apo-Naproxen* (Naproxen)—See Anti-inflammatory Drugs (NSAIDs) (Oral), 374–76

Apo-Nifed* (Nifedipine)—See Calcium Channel Blockers (Oral), 413–15

Apo-Oxazepam* (Oxazepam)—See Benzodiazepines (Oral), 389–91; Benzodiazepines (For Anxiety—Oral), 391–93; Benzodiazepines (For Insomnia—Oral), 395–96

Apo-Oxtriphylline* (Oxtriphylline)—See Xanthine Bronchodilators (Oral), 669–70

Apo-Pen VK* (Penicillin V)—See Penicillins (Oral), 595–97

Apo-Perphenazine* (Perphenazine)—See Phenothiazines (Oral), 602–4; Phenothiazines (For Nausea and Vomiting—Oral), 604–6

Apo-Phenylbutazone* (Phenylbutazone)—See Anti-inflammatory Drugs (NSAIDs) (Oral), 374–76

Apo-Piroxicam* (Piroxicam)—See Anti-inflammatory Drugs (NSAIDs) (Oral), 374–76

Apo-Prednisone* (Prednisone)—See Corticosteroids (Oral), 445; Prednisone (Oral), 614–16

Apo-Propranolol* (Propranolol)—See Beta-blockers (Oral), 397–99; Propranolol (Oral), 623–25

H

M

N

Pediacof Cough—See Cough/Cold Combinations (Oral), 451–52

Pediapred (Prednisolone)—See Corticosteroids (Oral), 445–47

Pedituss Cough—See Cough/Cold Combinations (Oral), 451–52

Peganone (Ethotoin)—See Hydantoin Anticonvulsants (Oral), 501–2

Pelamine (Tripelennamine)—See Antihistamines (Oral), 368–70

*Pen Vee** (Penicillin V)—See Penicillins (Oral), 595–97

Pen Vee K (Penicillin V)—See Penicillins (Oral), 595–97

*Penbritin** (Ampicillin)—See Penicillins (Oral), 595–97

Penbutolol—See Beta-blockers (Oral), 397–99

Penecort (Hydrocortisone)—See Corticosteroids (Topical—Low Potency), 447–48

Penetrex (Enoxacin)—See Fluoroquinolones (Oral), 484–86

*Penglobe** (Bacampicillin)—See Penicillins (Oral), 595–97

Penicillin G—See Penicillins (Oral), 595–97

Penicillin V—See Penicillins (Oral), 595–97

Penicillins (Oral), 595–97

Pentacort (Hydrocortisone)—See Corticosteroids (Topical—Low Potency), 447–48

Pentaerythritol Tetranitrate—See Nitrates (Oral), 582–84

Pentasa—See Mesalamine (Oral), 548–50

Pentazine VC w/Codeine—See Cough/Cold Combinations (Oral), 451–52

Pentazocine—See Narcotic Analgesics (Injection), 570–72; Narcotic Analgesics (Oral), 572–74

Pentazocine and Acetaminophen—See Narcotic Analgesics and Acetaminophen (Oral), 574–76

Pentazocine and Aspirin—See Narcotic Analgesics and Aspirin (Oral), 576–78

Pentazocine and Naloxone—See Narcotic Analgesics (Oral), 572–74

Pentids (Penicillin G)—See Penicillins (Oral), 595–97

Pentobarbital—See Barbiturates (Oral), 387–89

Pentylan (Pentaerythritol Tetranitrate)—See Nitrates (Oral), 582–84

Pepcid (Famotidine)—See H_2–blockers (Oral), 493–94

*Peptol** (Cimetidine)—See H_2–blockers (Oral), 493–94

Percocet (Oxycodone and Acetaminophen)—See Narcotic Analgesics and Acetaminophen (Oral), 574–76

*Percocet-Demi** (Oxycodone and Acetaminophen)—See Narcotic Analgesics and Acetaminophen (Oral), 574–76

Percodan (Oxycodone and Aspirin)—See Narcotic Analgesics and Aspirin (Oral), 576–78

Percodan-Demi (Oxycodone and Aspirin)—See Narcotic Analgesics and Aspirin (Oral), 576–78

Perdiem (Psyllium and Senna)—See Laxatives, Bulk-forming and Stimulant Combination (Oral), 527–28

Perdiem Fiber (Psyllium)—See Laxatives, Bulk-forming (Oral), 518–20

Pergonal—See Menotropins (Injection), 547–48

Periactin (Cyproheptadine)—See Antihistamines (Oral), 368–70

Peri-Colace (Casanthranol and Docusate)—See Laxatives, Stimulant and Stool Softener Combination (Oral), 527–28

Pericyazine—See Phenothiazines (Oral), 602–4

*Peridol**—See Haloperidol (Oral), 497–99

Peritrate (Pentaerythritol Tetranitrate)—See Nitrates (Oral), 582–84

*Peritrate Forte** (Pentaerythritol Tetranitrate)—See Nitrates (Oral), 582–84

Peritrate SA (Pentaerythritol Tetranitrate)—See Nitrates (Oral), 582–84

Permitil (Fluphenazine)—See Phenothiazines (Oral), 602–4

Permitil Concentrate (Fluphenazine)—See Phenothiazines (Oral), 602–4

Perphenazine—See Phenothiazines (Injection), 599–601; Phenothiazines (Oral), 602–4; Phenothiazines (For Nausea and Vomiting—Oral), 604–6

Persantine (Dipyridamole)—See Platelet Aggregation Inhibitors (Oral), 608–10

*Pertofrane** (Desipramine)—See Tricyclic Antidepressants (Oral), 667–68

Pertussin All Night CS—See Cough/Cold Combinations (Oral), 451–52

Pertussin All Night PM—See Cough/Cold Combinations (Oral), 451–52

Pfeiffer's Allergy (Chlorpheniramine)—See Antihistamines (Oral), 368–70

Phanadex—See Cough/Cold Combinations (Oral), 451–52

Phanatuss—See Cough/Cold Combinations (Oral), 451–52

Pharma-Cort (Hydrocortisone Acetate)—See Corticosteroids (Topical—Low Potency), 447–48

Pharmagesic (Butalbital, Acetaminophen, and Caffeine)—See Butalbital and Acetaminophen (Oral), 404–6

*Pharmatex** (Benzalkonium Chloride)—See Spermicides (Vaginal), 640–42

Phazyme—See Simethicone (Oral), 639–40

*Phazyme Drops**—See Simethicone (Oral), 639–40

Phazyme-95—See Simethicone (Oral), 639–40

*Phazyme-125**—See Simethicone (Oral), 639–40

Phenameth DM—See Cough/Cold Combinations (Oral), 451–52

Phenameth VC with Codeine—See Cough/Cold Combinations (Oral), 451–52

PhenAPAP No. 2 (Phenylpropanolamine and Acetaminophen)—See Decongestants and Analgesics (Oral), 456–58

Phenapap Sinus Headache & Congestion (Chlorpheniramine, Pseudoephedrine, and Acetaminophen)—See Antihistamines, Decongestants, and Analgesics (Oral), 372–74

Phenaphen Caplets—See Acetaminophen (Oral), 329–30

Phenaphen with Codeine No.2 (Acetaminophen and Codeine)—See Narcotic Analgesics and Acetaminophen (Oral), 574–76

Procaterol*—See Adrenergic Bronchodilators (Inhalation), 335–36

Prochlorperazine—See Phenothiazines (Injection), 599–601; Phenothiazines (Oral), 602–4; Phenothiazines (For Nausea and Vomiting—Oral), 604–6

*Procyclid** (Procyclidine)—See Antidyskinetics (Oral), 366–68

Procyclidine—See Antidyskinetics (Oral), 366–68

Pro-Depo (Hydroxyprogesterone)—See Progestins (Injection), 620–21

*Prodiem Plain** (Psyllium Hydrophilic Mucilloid)—See Laxatives, Bulk-forming (Oral), 518–20

*Prodiem Plus** (Psyllium Hydrophilic Mucilloid and Senna)—See Laxatives, Bulk-forming and Stimulant Combination (Oral), 520–22

Prodrox (Hydroxyprogesterone)—See Progestins (Injection), 620–21

Profasi—See Chorionic Gonadotropin (Injection), 425–27

Progesterone—See Progestins (Injection), 620–21

Progestins (For Contraceptive Use—Oral), 618–19

Progestins (Injection), 620–21

Progestins (Oral), 621–23

Prolamine—See Phenylpropanolamine (Oral), 606–8

Pro-Lax (Psyllium Hydrophilic Mucilloid)—See Laxatives, Bulk-forming (Oral), 518–20

Prolixin (Fluphenazine)—See Phenothiazines (Injection), 599–601; Phenothiazines (Oral), 602–4

Prolixin Concentrate (Fluphenazine)—See Phenothiazines (Oral), 602–4

Prolixin Decanoate (Fluphenazine)—See Phenothiazines (Injection), 599–601

Prolixin Enanthate (Fluphenazine)—See Phenothiazines (Injection), 599–601

Promazine—See Phenothiazines (Injection), 599–601; Phenothiazines (Oral), 602–4

Prometh VC with Codeine—See Cough/Cold Combinations (Oral), 451–52

Prometh VC Plain (Promethazine and Phenylephrine)—See Antihistamines and Decongestants (Oral), 370–72

Prometh w/Dextromethorphan—See Cough/Cold Combinations (Oral), 451–52

Promethazine DM—See Cough/Cold Combinations (Oral), 451–52

Promethazine and Phenylephrine—See Antihistamines and Decongestants (Oral), 370–72

Promethazine VC (Promethazine and Phenylephrine)—See Antihistamines and Decongestants (Oral), 370–72

Promethazine VC w/Codeine—See Cough/Cold Combinations (Oral), 451–52

Promethist w/Codeine—See Cough/Cold Combinations (Oral), 451–52

Promine (Procainamide)—See Antiarrhythmics, Type I (Oral), 358–60

Prominic Expectorant—See Cough/Cold Combinations (Oral), 451–52; Decongestants/Expectorants (Oral), 458–60

Prominicol Cough—See Cough/Cold Combinations (Oral), 451–52

Promist HD Liquid—See Cough/Cold Combinations (Oral), 451–52

Prompt (Psyllium Hydrophilic Mucilloid and Sennosides)—See Laxatives, Bulk-forming and Stimulant Combination (Oral), 520–22

Prompt Insulin Zinc*—See Insulin (Injection), 506–8

Pronestyl (Procainamide)—See Antiarrhythmics, Type I (Oral), 358–60

Pronestyl-SR (Procainamide)—See Antiarrhythmics, Type I (Oral), 358–60

Propacet 100 (Propoxyphene and Acetaminophen)—See Narcotic Analgesics and Acetaminophen (Oral), 574–76

*Propaderm** (Beclomethasone)—See Corticosteroids (Topical—Medium to Very High Potency), 449–50

Propafenone—See Antiarrhythmics, Type I (Oral), 358–60

Propagest—See Phenylpropanolamine (Oral), 606–8

Propain-HC (Hydrocodone and Acetaminophen)—See Narcotic Analgesics and Acetaminophen (Oral), 574–76

*Propanthel** (Propantheline)—See Anticholinergics/Antispasmodics (Oral), 360–62

Propantheline—See Anticholinergics/Antispasmodics (Oral), 360–62

Propoxycaine and Procaine—See Anesthetics, Local (Injection), 348–49

Propoxyphene—See Narcotic Analgesics (Oral), 572–74

Propoxyphene and Acetaminophen—See Narcotic Analgesics and Acetaminophen (Oral), 574–76

Propoxyphene and Aspirin*—See Narcotic Analgesics and Aspirin (Oral), 576–78

Propoxyphene, Aspirin, and Caffeine—See Narcotic Analgesics and Aspirin (Oral), 576–78

Propoxyphene Compound-65 (Propoxyphene, Aspirin, and Caffeine)—See Narcotic Analgesics and Aspirin (Oral), 576–78

Propranolol—See Beta-blockers (Oral), 397–99; Propranolol (Oral), 623–25

Propulsid—See Cisapride (Oral), 427–28

Propylthiouracil—See Antithyroid Agents (Oral), 376–78

*Propyl-Thyracil** (Propylthiouracil)—See Antithyroid Agents (Oral), 376–78

*Prorazin** (Prochlorperazine)—See Phenothiazines (Oral), 602–4; Phenothiazines (For Nausea and Vomiting—Oral), 604–6

Pro-Sof (Docusate)—See Laxatives, Stool Softener (Oral), 529–30

Pro-Sof Plus (Casanthranol and Docusate)—See Laxatives, Stimulant and Stool Softener Combination (Oral), 527–28

ProSom (Estazolam)—See Benzodiazepines (Oral), 389–91; Benzodiazepines (For Insomnia—Oral), 395–96

Pro-Span (Hydroxyprogesterone)—See Progestins (Injection), 620–21

Prostaphlin (Oxacillin)—See Penicillins (Oral), 595–97

Rhinatate (Chlorpheniramine, Pyrilamine, and Phenylephrine)—See Antihistamines and Decongestants (Oral), 370–72

Rhinocaps (Phenylpropanolamine, Acetaminophen, and Aspirin)—See Decongestants and Analgesics (Oral), 456–58

*Rhinocort Aqua** (Budesonide)—See Corticosteroids (Nasal), 443–45

*Rhinocort Turbuhaler** (Budesonide)—See Corticosteroids (Nasal), 443–45

Rhinogesic (Chlorpheniramine, Phenylephrine, Acetaminophen, and Salicylamide)—See Antihistamines, Decongestants, and Analgesics (Oral), 372–74

Rhinolar-EX (Chlorpheniramine and Phenylpropanolamine)—See Antihistamines and Decongestants (Oral), 370–72

Rhinolar-EX 12 (Chlorpheniramine and Phenylpropanolamine)—See Antihistamines and Decongestants (Oral), 370–72

Rhinosyn (Chlorpheniramine and Pseudoephedrine)—See Antihistamines and Decongestants (Oral), 370–72

Rhinosyn-DM—See Cough/Cold Combinations (Oral), 451–52

Rhinosyn-DMX Expectorant—See Cough/Cold Combinations (Oral), 451–52

Rhinosyn-PD (Chlorpheniramine and Pseudoephedrine)—See Antihistamines and Decongestants (Oral), 370–72

Rhinosyn-X—See Cough/Cold Combinations (Oral), 451–52

*Rhodis** (Ketoprofen)—See Anti-inflammatory Drugs (NSAIDs) (Oral), 374–76

*Rhodis-E** (Ketoprofen)—See Anti-inflammatory Drugs (NSAIDs) (Oral), 374–76

*Rhodis-EC** (Ketoprofen)—See Anti-inflammatory Drugs (NSAIDs) (Oral), 374–76

*Rhotrimine** (Trimipramine)—See Tricyclic Antidepressants (Oral), 667–68

Rhulicort (Hydrocortisone Acetate)—See Corticosteroids (Topical—Low Potency), 447–48

Rifadin—See Rifampin (Oral), 629–30

Rifamate—See Rifampin and Isoniazid (Oral), 631–33

Rifampin (Oral), 629–30

Rifampin and Isoniazid (Oral), 631–33

Rimactane—See Rifampin (Oral), 629–30

Rinade B.I.D. (Chlorpheniramine and Pseudoephedrine)—See Antihistamines and Decongestants (Oral), 370–72

*Riphen** (Aspirin)—See Salicylates (Oral), 633–35

*Rivotril** (Clonazepam)—See Benzodiazepines (Oral), 389–91; Benzodiazepines (For Epilepsy—Oral), 393–95

Robafen AC Cough—See Cough/Cold Combinations (Oral), 451–52

Robafen CF—See Cough/Cold Combinations (Oral), 451–52

Robafen DAC—See Cough/Cold Combinations (Oral), 451–52

Robafen DM—See Cough/Cold Combinations (Oral), 451–52

*Robidone** (Hydrocodone)—See Narcotic Analgesics (Oral), 572–74

*Robidrine**—See Pseudoephedrine (Oral), 625–27

*Robigesic**—See Acetaminophen (Oral), 329–30

Robinul (Glycopyrrolate)—See Anticholinergics/Antispasmodics (Oral), 360–62

Robinul Forte (Glycopyrrolate)—See Anticholinergics/Antispasmodics (Oral), 360–62

Robitet (Tetracycline)—See Tetracyclines (Oral), 659–61

Robitussin A-C—See Cough/Cold Combinations (Oral), 451–52

*Robitussin with Codeine**—See Cough/Cold Combinations (Oral), 451–52

Robitussin Cold and Cough Liqui-Gels—See Cough/Cold Combinations (Oral), 451–52

Robitussin Maximum Strength Cough and Cold—See Cough/Cold Combinations (Oral), 451–52

Robitussin Night Relief—See Cough/Cold Combinations (Oral), 451–52

Robitussin Severe Congestion Liqui-Gels—See Cough/Cold Combinations (Oral), 451–52; Decongestants/Expectorants (Oral), 458–60

Robitussin-CF—See Cough/Cold Combinations (Oral), 451–52

Robitussin-DAC—See Cough/Cold Combinations (Oral), 451–52

Robitussin-DM—See Cough/Cold Combinations (Oral), 451–52

Robitussin-PE—See Cough/Cold Combinations (Oral), 451–52; Decongestants/Expectorants (Oral), 458–60

*Rofact**—See Rifampin (Oral), 629–30

Rogesic No. 3 (Hydrocodone and Acetaminophen)—See Narcotic Analgesics and Acetaminophen (Oral), 574–76

Rolaids Calcium Rich (Calcium Carbonate)—See Antacids, Calcium Carbonate–containing (Oral), 356–57; Calcium Supplements (Oral), 415–17

Rolatuss Expectorant—See Cough/Cold Combinations (Oral), 451–52

Rolatuss Plain (Chlorpheniramine and Phenylephrine)—See Antihistamines and Decongestants (Oral), 370–72

Rolatuss w/Hydrocodone—See Cough/Cold Combinations (Oral), 451–52

Rondamine-DM Drops—See Cough/Cold Combinations (Oral), 451–52

Rondec (Carbinoxamine and Pseudoephedrine)—See Antihistamines and Decongestants (Oral), 370–72

Rondec Drops (Carbinoxamine and Pseudoephedrine)—See Antihistamines and Decongestants (Oral), 370–72

Rondec-DM—See Cough/Cold Combinations (Oral), 451–52

Rondec-TR (Carbinoxamine and Pseudoephedrine)—See Antihistamines and Decongestants (Oral), 370–72

Roubac*—See Sulfamethoxazole and Trimethoprim (Oral), 645–47

Rounox*—See Acetaminophen (Oral), 329–30

Rounox and Codeine 15* (Acetaminophen and Codeine)—See Narcotic Analgesics and Acetaminophen (Oral), 574–76

Rounox and Codeine 30* (Acetaminophen and Codeine)—See Narcotic Analgesics and Acetaminophen (Oral), 574–76

Rounox and Codeine 60* (Acetaminophen and Codeine)—See Narcotic Analgesics and Acetaminophen (Oral), 574–76

Rowasa—See Mesalamine (Rectal), 550–52

Roxanol (Morphine)—See Narcotic Analgesics (Oral), 572–74

Roxanol UD (Morphine)—See Narcotic Analgesics (Oral), 572–74

Roxanol 100 (Morphine)—See Narcotic Analgesics (Oral), 572–74

Roxicet (Oxycodone and Acetaminophen)—See Narcotic Analgesics and Acetaminophen (Oral), 574–76

Roxicet 5/500 (Oxycodone and Acetaminophen)—See Narcotic Analgesics and Acetaminophen (Oral), 574–76

Roxicodone (Oxycodone)—See Narcotic Analgesics (Oral), 572–74

Roxicodone Intensol (Oxycodone)—See Narcotic Analgesics (Oral), 572–74

Roxiprin (Oxycodone and Aspirin)—See Narcotic Analgesics and Aspirin (Oral), 576–78

Roychlor-10%* (Potassium Chloride)—See Potassium Supplements (Oral), 612–14

Roychlor-20%* (Potassium Chloride)—See Potassium Supplements (Oral), 612–14

Royonate* (Potassium Gluconate)—See Potassium Supplements (Oral), 612–14

R-Tannamine (Chlorpheniramine, Pyrilamine, and Phenylephrine)—See Antihistamines and Decongestants (Oral), 370–72

R-Tannate (Chlorpheniramine, Pyrilamine, and Phenylephrine)—See Antihistamines and Decongestants (Oral), 370–72

Rubidium Rb 82—See Radiopharmaceuticals (Diagnostic), 627–28

Rufen (Ibuprofen)—See Anti-inflammatory Drugs (NSAIDs) (Oral), 374–76

Rulox (Alumina and Magnesia)—See Antacids, Aluminum- and Magnesium-containing (Oral), 354–55

Rulox No. 1 (Alumina and Magnesia)—See Antacids, Aluminum- and Magnesium-containing (Oral), 354–55

Rulox No. 2 (Alumina and Magnesia)—See Antacids, Aluminum- and Magnesium-containing (Oral), 354–55

Rum-K (Potassium Chloride)—See Potassium Supplements (Oral), 612–14

Ru-Tuss (Chlorpheniramine and Phenylephrine)—See Antihistamines and Decongestants (Oral), 370–72

Ru-Tuss DE—See Cough/Cold Combinations (Oral), 451–52; Decongestants/Expectorants (Oral), 458–60

Ru-Tuss Expectorant—See Cough/Cold Combinations (Oral), 451–52

Ru-Tuss with Hydrocodone Liquid—See Cough/Cold Combinations (Oral), 451–52

Rymed—See Cough/Cold Combinations (Oral), 451–52; Decongestants/Expectorants (Oral), 458–60

Rymed Liquid—See Cough/Cold Combinations (Oral), 451–52; Decongestants/Expectorants (Oral), 458–60

Rymed-TR Caplets—See Cough/Cold Combinations (Oral), 451–52; Decongestants/Expectorants (Oral), 458–60

Ryna (Chlorpheniramine and Pseudoephedrine)—See Antihistamines and Decongestants (Oral), 370–72

Ryna-C Liquid—See Cough/Cold Combinations (Oral), 451–52

Ryna-CX Liquid—See Cough/Cold Combinations (Oral), 451–52

Rynatan (Chlorpheniramine, Pyrilamine, and Phenylephrine)—See Antihistamines and Decongestants (Oral), 370–72

Rynatuss—See Cough/Cold Combinations (Oral), 451–52

Rythmodan* (Disopyramide)—See Antiarrhythmics, Type I (Oral), 358–60

Rythmodan-LA* (Disopyramide)—See Antiarrhythmics, Type I (Oral), 358–60

Rythmol (Propafenone)—See Antiarrhythmics, Type I (Oral), 358–60

S

Safe Tussin 30—See Cough/Cold Combinations (Oral), 451–52

Salazopyrin*—See Sulfasalazine (Oral), 647–49

Salazopyrin EN-Tabs*—See Sulfasalazine (Oral), 647–49

Salcylic Acid (Salsalate)—See Salicylates (Oral), 633–35

Saleto D (Phenylpropanolamine, Acetaminophen, Salicylamide, and Caffeine)—See Decongestants and Analgesics (Oral), 456–58

Saleto-CF—See Cough/Cold Combinations (Oral), 451–52

Salflex (Salsalate)—See Salicylates (Oral), 633–35

Salgesic (Salsalate)—See Salicylates (Oral), 633–35

Salicylates (Oral), 633–35

Salofalk*—See Mesalamine (Rectal), 550–52

Salphenyl (Chlorpheniramine, Phenylephrine, Acetaminophen, and Salicylamide)—See Antihistamines, Decongestants, and Analgesics (Oral), 372–74

Salsalate—See Salicylates (Oral), 633–35

Salsitab (Salsalate)—See Salicylates (Oral), 633–35

Saluron (Hydroflumethiazide)—See Thiazide Diuretics (Oral), 663–64

Sanorex (Mazindol)—See Appetite Suppressants (Oral), 378–80

Sarisol No. 2 (Butabarbital)—See Barbiturates (Oral), 387–89

Sarna HC 1.0% (Hydrocortisone)—See Corticosteroids (Topical—Low Potency), 447–48

S.A.S. Enteric-500*—See Sulfasalazine (Oral), 647–49

S.A.S.-500*—See Sulfasalazine (Oral), 647–49

Scopolamine—See Anticholinergics/Antispasmodics (Oral), 360–62; Scopolamine (Transdermal), 635–37

Scott-tussin Original 5–Action Cold Medicine (Pheniramine, Phenylephrine, Sodium Salicylate, and Caffeine)—See Antihistamines, Decongestants, and Analgesics (Oral), 372–74

Scot-Tussin DM—See Cough/Cold Combinations (Oral), 451–52

Scot-tussin Original 5–Action Cold Formula (Pheniramine, Phenylephrine, Sodium Salicylate, and Caffeine)—See Antihistamines, Decongestants, and Analgesics (Oral), 372–74

Secobarbital—See Barbiturates (Oral), 387–89

Secobarbital and Amobarbital—See Barbiturates (Oral), 387–89

Seconal (Secobarbital)—See Barbiturates (Oral), 387–89

Sectral (Acebutolol)—See Beta-blockers (Oral), 397–99

Sedapap—See Butalbital and Acetaminophen (Oral), 404–6

Seldane (Terfenadine)—See Antihistamines (Oral), 368–70; Terfenadine (Oral), 657–58

Seldane Caplets* (Terfenadine)—See Antihistamines (Oral), 368–70; Terfenadine (Oral), 657–58

Seldane-D (Terfenadine and Pseudoephedrine)—See Antihistamines and Decongestants (Oral), 370–72

Selexid* (Pivmecillinam)—See Penicillins (Oral), 595–97

Semicid (Nonoxynol 9)—See Spermicides (Vaginal), 640–42

Semilente Insulin* (Prompt Insulin Zinc)—See Insulin (Injection), 506–8

Semprex-D (Acrivastine and Pseudoephedrine)—See Antihistamines and Decongestants (Oral), 370–72

Senefen III (Hydrocodone and Acetaminophen)—See Narcotic Analgesics and Acetaminophen (Oral), 574–76

Senexon (Senna)—See Laxatives, Stimulant (Oral), 522–24

Senna—See Laxatives, Stimulant (Oral), 522–24; Laxatives, Stimulant (Rectal), 524–26

Senna and Docusate—See Laxatives, Stimulant and Stool Softener Combination (Oral), 527–28

Sennosides—See Laxatives, Stimulant (Oral), 522–24

Senokot* (Senna and Docusate)—See Laxatives, Stimulant and Stool Softener Combination (Oral), 527–28

Senokot (Senna)—See Laxatives, Stimulant (Oral), 522–24; Laxatives, Stimulant (Rectal), 524–26

Senokot XTRA (Senna)—See Laxatives, Stimulant (Oral), 522–24

Senokot-S (Senna and Docusate)—See Laxatives, Stimulant and Stool Softener Combination (Oral), 527–28

Senolax (Senna)—See Laxatives, Stimulant (Oral), 522–24

Sensorcaine (Bupivacaine)—See Anesthetics, Local (Injection), 348–49

Sensorcaine-MPF (Bupivacaine)—See Anesthetics, Local (Injection), 348–49

Sensorcaine-MPF Spinal (Bupivacaine)—See Anesthetics, Local (Injection), 348–49

Septra—See Sulfamethoxazole and Trimethoprim (Oral), 645–47

Septra DS—See Sulfamethoxazole and Trimethoprim (Oral), 645–47

Serax (Oxazepam)—See Benzodiazepines (Oral), 389–91; Benzodiazepines (For Anxiety—Oral), 391–93; Benzodiazepines (For Insomnia—Oral), 395–96

Serentil (Mesoridazine)—See Phenothiazines (Injection), 599–601; Phenothiazines (Oral), 602–4

Serentil Concentrate (Mesoridazine)—See Phenothiazines (Oral), 602–4

Serophene—See Clomiphene (Oral), 431–33

Sertraline (Oral), 637–38

Serutan (Psyllium Hydrophilic Mucilloid)—See Laxatives, Bulk-forming (Oral), 518–20

Serutan Toasted Granules (Psyllium Hydrophilic Mucilloid and Carboxymethylcellulose)—See Laxatives, Bulk-forming (Oral), 518–20

Shields Bernasept Spray (Benzocaine)—See Anesthetics (Topical), 346–48

Shur-Seal (Nonoxynol 9)—See Spermicides (Vaginal), 640–42

Sibelium* (Flunarizine)—See Calcium Channel Blockers (Oral), 413–15

Siladryl (Diphenhydramine)—See Antihistamines (Oral), 368–70

Silexin Cough—See Cough/Cold Combinations (Oral), 451–52

Silphen Cough Syrup (Diphenhydramine)—See Antihistamines (Oral), 368–70

Simaal Gel (Alumina, Magnesia, and Simethicone)—See Antacids, Aluminum- and Magnesium-containing (Oral), 354–55

Simaal 2 Gel (Alumina, Magnesia, and Simethicone)—See Antacids, Aluminum- and Magnesium-containing (Oral), 354–55

Simethicone (Oral), 639–40

Simethicone, Alumina, Calcium Carbonate, and Magnesia—See Antacids, Aluminum-, Calcium-, and Magnesium-containing (Oral), 352–53

Simethicone, Alumina, Magnesium Carbonate, and Magnesia—See Antacids, Aluminum- and Magnesium-containing (Oral), 354–55

Simplet (Chlorpheniramine, Pseudoephedrine, and Acetaminophen)—See Antihistamines, Decongestants, and Analgesics (Oral), 372–74

Simron (Ferrous Gluconate)—See Iron Supplements (Oral), 510–12

Simvastatin—See Statin Cholesterol-lowering Medicines (Oral), 642–44

Sinapils (Chlorpheniramine, Phenylpropanolamine, Acetaminophen, and Caffeine)—See Antihistamines, Decongestants, and Analgesics (Oral), 372–74

Sinarest (Chlorpheniramine, Pseudoephedrine, and

Slow-Trasicor* (Oxprenolol)—See Beta-blockers (Oral), 397–99

Snaplets-D (Chlorpheniramine and Phenylpropanolamine)—See Antihistamines and Decongestants (Oral), 370–72

Snaplets-DM—See Cough/Cold Combinations (Oral), 451–52

Snaplets-EX—See Cough/Cold Combinations (Oral), 451–52; Decongestants/Expectorants (Oral), 458–60

Snaplets-FR—See Acetaminophen (Oral), 329–30

Snaplets-Multi—See Cough/Cold Combinations (Oral), 451–52

Sodium Chromate Cr 51—See Radiopharmaceuticals (Diagnostic), 627–28

Sodium Iodide I 123—See Radiopharmaceuticals (Diagnostic), 627–28

Sodium Iodide I 131—See Radiopharmaceuticals (Diagnostic), 627–28

Sodium Pertechnetate Tc 99m—See Radiopharmaceuticals (Diagnostic), 627–28

Sodium Salicylate—See Salicylates (Oral), 633–35

Sofarin (Warfarin)—See Anticoagulants (Oral), 362–64

Solazine* (Trifluoperazine)—See Phenothiazines (Oral), 602–4

Solfoton (Phenobarbital)—See Barbiturates (Oral), 387–89; Phenobarbital (For Epilepsy—Oral), 597–99

Solium* (Chlordiazepoxide)—See Benzodiazepines (Oral), 389–91; Benzodiazepines (For Anxiety—Oral), 391–93; Benzodiazepines (For Insomnia—Oral), 395–96

Solu-Phyllin (Theophylline)—See Xanthine Bronchodilators (Oral), 669–70

Sominex Formula 2 (Diphenhydramine)—See Antihistamines (Oral), 368–70

Somnol* (Flurazepam)—See Benzodiazepines (Oral), 389–91; Benzodiazepines (For Insomnia—Oral), 395–96

Somophyllin-12* (Theophylline)—See Xanthine Bronchodilators (Oral), 669–70

Sorbitrate (Isosorbide Dinitrate)—See Nitrates (Oral), 582–84; Nitrates (Sublingual), 584–86

Sorbitrate SA (Isosorbide Dinitrate)—See Nitrates (Oral), 582–84

Sotacor* (Sotalol)—See Beta-blockers (Oral), 397–99

Sotalol—See Beta-blockers (Oral), 397–99

Span-FF (Ferrous Fumarate)—See Iron Supplements (Oral), 510–12

Sparine (Promazine)—See Phenothiazines (Injection), 599–601; Phenothiazines (Oral), 602–4

Spasmoban* (Dicyclomine)—See Anticholinergics/Antispasmodics (Oral), 360–62

Spectrobid (Bacampicillin)—See Penicillins (Oral), 595–97

Spermicides (Vaginal), 640–42

Spironolactone—See Potassium-sparing Diuretics (Oral), 610–12

Sporanox (Itraconazole)—See Azole Antifungals (Oral), 383–84

SRC Expectorant—See Cough/Cold Combinations (Oral), 451–52

S-T Cort (Hydrocortisone)—See Corticosteroids (Topical—Low Potency), 447–48

S-T Forte—See Cough/Cold Combinations (Oral), 451–52

S-T Forte 2—See Cough/Cold Combinations (Oral), 451–52

St. Joseph Adult Chewable Aspirin (Aspirin)—See Platelet Aggregation Inhibitors (Oral), 608–10; Salicylates (Oral), 633–35

Stadol (Butorphanol)—See Narcotic Analgesics (Injection), 570–72

Stamoist E—See Cough/Cold Combinations (Oral), 451–52; Decongestants/Expectorants (Oral), 458–60

Stamoist LA—See Cough/Cold Combinations (Oral), 451–52; Decongestants/Expectorants (Oral), 458–60

Statex* (Morphine)—See Narcotic Analgesics (Oral), 572–74

Statex Drops* (Morphine)—See Narcotic Analgesics (Oral), 572–74

Statin Cholesterol-lowering Medicines (Oral), 642–44

Statuss Expectorant—See Cough/Cold Combinations (Oral), 451–52

Statuss Green—See Cough/Cold Combinations (Oral), 451–52

Stelazine (Trifluoperazine)—See Phenothiazines (Injection), 599–601; Phenothiazines (Oral), 602–4

Stelazine Concentrate (Trifluoperazine)—See Phenothiazines (Oral), 602–4

Stemetil* (Prochlorperazine)—See Phenothiazines (Injection), 599–601; Phenothiazines (Oral), 602–4; Phenothiazines (For Nausea and Vomiting—Oral), 604–6

Stemetil Liquid* (Prochlorperazine)—See Phenothiazines (Oral), 602–4; Phenothiazines (For Nausea and Vomiting—Oral), 604–6

Sterapred (Prednisone)—See Corticosteroids (Oral), 445–47; Prednisone (Oral), 614–16

Sterapred DS (Prednisone)—See Corticosteroids (Oral), 445–47; Prednisone (Oral), 614–16

Stilphostrol (Diethylstilbestrol)—See Estrogens (Injection), 470–72; Estrogens (Oral), 472–74

Stresstabs—See Multivitamins (Oral), 567–68

Stress-600—See Multivitamins (Oral), 567–68

Stulex (Docusate)—See Laxatives, Stool Softener (Oral), 529–30

Sucralfate (Oral), 644–46

Sudafed—See Pseudoephedrine (Oral), 625–27

Sudafed Cold and Cough Extra Strength Non-Drowsy*—See Cough/Cold Combinations (Oral), 451–52

Sudafed Cold & Cough Liquid Caps—See Cough/Cold Combinations (Oral), 451–52

Sudafed Cough—See Cough/Cold Combinations (Oral), 451–52

Sudafed DM*—See Cough/Cold Combinations (Oral), 451–52

Sudafed Plus (Chlorpheniramine and Pseudoephedrine)—See Antihistamines and Decongestants (Oral), 370–72

Sudafed Severe Cold Formula Caplets—See Cough/Cold Combinations (Oral), 451–52

U

V

𝒲

𝒳-𝒴

𝒵

INDEX

C